Pediatric Radiology

SERIES EDITOR **James H. Thrall, MD**
Radiologist-in-Chief
Massachusetts General Hospital
Juan M. Taveras Professor of Radiology
Harvard Medical School
Boston, Massachusetts

OTHER VOLUMES IN
THE REQUISITES IN RADIOLOGY SERIES

Breast Imaging
Cardiac Imaging
Genitourinary Radiology
Musculoskeletal Imaging
Neuroradiology
Nuclear Medicine
Ultrasound
Thoracic Radiology
Vascular & Interventional Radiology

THE REQUISITES

Pediatric Radiology

Third Edition

Johan G. Blickman, MD, PhD
Professor and Chairman
Department of Radiology
Radboud University Medical Center
Nijmegen, The Netherlands

Bruce R. Parker, MD
Professor
Departments of Radiology and Pediatrics
Baylor College of Medicine
Chairman Emeritus
Department of Diagnostic Imaging
Texas Children's Hospital
Houston, Texas
Professor (Emeritus) of Radiology and Pediatrics
Department of Radiology
Stanford University School of Medicine
Stanford, California

Patrick D. Barnes, MD
Professor
Department of Radiology
Stanford University School of Medicine
Stanford, California
Chief, Section of Pediatric Neuroradiology
Director, Pediatric MRI and CT Center
Department of Radiology
Lucile Packard Children's Hospital
Palo Alto, California

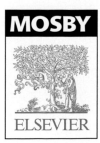

MOSBY

ELSEVIER

1600 John F. Kennedy Blvd.
Ste 1800
Philadelphia, PA 19103-2899

PEDIATRIC RADIOLOGY: THE REQUISITES   ISBN: 978-0-323-03125-7

Notice

Knowledge and best practice in this field are constantly changing. As new research and experience broaden our knowledge, changes in practice, treatment, and drug therapy may become necessary or appropriate. Readers are advised to check the most current information provided (i) on procedures featured or (ii) by the manufacturer of each product to be administered, to verify the recommended dose or formula, the method and duration of administration, and contraindications. It is the responsibility of the practitioner, relying on his or her own experience and knowledge of the patient, to make diagnoses, to determine dosages and the best treatment for each individual patient, and to take all appropriate safety precautions. To the fullest extent of the law, neither the publisher nor the editors assume any liability for any injury and/or damage to persons or property arising out of or related to any use of the material contained in this book.

The Publisher

Library of Congress Cataloging-in-Publication Data
Blickman, Johan G.
  Pediatric radiology : the requisites / Johan G. Blickman, Bruce R. Parker, Patrick D. Barnes. -- 3rd ed.
    p. ; cm. -- (Requisites series)
  Includes bibliographical references and index.
  ISBN 978-0-323-03125-7
  1. Pediatric radiology. I. Parker, Bruce R. II. Barnes, Patrick D. III. Title. IV. Series:
Requisites series.
  [DNLM: 1. Diagnostic Imaging. 2. Child. 3. Infant. WN 240 B648p 2009]
  RJ51.R3B55 2009
  618.92'00757--dc22   2009007873

Acquisitions Editor: Rebecca Gaertner
Developmental Editor: Martha Limbach
Publishing Services Manager: Tina Rebane
Project Manager: Norm Stellander
Design Direction: Lou Forgione

Printed in The United States of America

Last digit is the print number: 9 8 7 6 5 4 3 2 1

To All My Children

JOHAN. G. (HANS) BLICKMAN

Contributors

Patrick D. Barnes, MD
Professor
Department of Radiology
Stanford University School of Medicine
Stanford, California
Chief, Section of Pediatric Neuroradiology
Director, Pediatric MRI and CT Center
Department of Radiology
Lucile Packard Children's Hospital
Palo Alto, California

Johan G. (Hans) Blickman, MD, PhD
Professor and Chairman
Department of Radiology
Radboud University Medical Center
Nijmegen, The Netherlands

Carla Boetes, MD, PhD
Professor of Radiology
Director of Mammography
Department of Radiology
Maastricht University Medical Center
Maastricht, The Netherlands

Lya Van Die, MD
Assistant Professor of Radiology
Radboud University Medical Center
Nijmegen, The Netherlands

Rajesh Krishnamurthy, MD
Clinical Professor of Radiology
Baylor College of Medicine
Staff Radiologist
Texas Children's Hospital
Houston, Texas

Bruce R. Parker, MD
Professor
Departments of Radiology and Pediatrics
Baylor College of Medicine
Chairman Emeritus
Department of Diagnostic Imaging
Texas Children's Hospital
Houston, Texas
Professor (Emeritus) of Radiology and Pediatrics
Department of Radiology
Stanford University School of Medicine
Stanford, California

Geert Vanderschueren, MD, PhD
Staff Radiologist
Department of Musculoskeletal Radiology
Leuven University Hospital
Leuven, Belgium

Foreword

THE REQUISITES is a series of textbooks encompassing the fundamental building blocks of radiology practice. This series is approaching its third decade and continues to flourish due to the diligence and success of the authors in producing such high quality work. *Pediatric Imaging: THE REQUISITES,* authored by Dr. Hans Blickman and colleagues, again exemplifies this high standard.

Pediatric imaging has evolved in many extremely important ways since the publication of the first and second editions of *Pediatric Imaging: THE REQUISITES.* Among other trends, CT and MRI have taken on progressively important roles in the imaging of children, 3D imaging is playing a role, and ultrasound has continued to progress technologically. The increase in utilization of CT in children is the subject of public concern, and the need to keep radiation exposure as low as reasonably achievable (ALARA) is highlighted by Dr. Blickman in his opening remarks.

Dr. Blickman has assembled a terrific team for the current edition, including Drs. Lya Van Die, Rajesh Krishnamurthy, Bruce Parker, Carla Boetas, Geert Vandershueren, and Patrick Barnes. The addition of new authors reflects the expansion of knowledge and the rising importance of subspecialization in pediatric imaging. In keeping with the philosophy of THE REQUISITES series, Dr. Blickman and his team are to be congratulated for capturing the most important aspects of pediatric imaging and putting the knowledge and information into an accessible and useful form.

Some aspects of pediatric imaging are enduring. Certainly knowledge of imaging anatomy and disease pathophysiology will never go out of style. However, the particular imaging methods of choice and the development of new protocols are very dynamic, making it challenging to stay current. Dr. Blickman and his team have done a great job capturing these changes.

Dr. Blickman has maintained the design of his book based on an organ system approach, with each chapter introduced by a discussion of methods of importance to the respective organ system. This approach brings the discussion of technology and applications together in a very efficient way for the reader. The illustrations have been widely updated, especially for cross-sectional imaging.

One of the features of THE REQUISITES series most noted and appreciated in reader feedback is the use of tables and boxes to restate and summarize essential information in concise form. This reinforces the narrative discussion, and the liberal use of this approach again highlights *Pediatric Imaging: THE REQUISITES.*

THE REQUISITES have now become old friends to two or three generations of medical imagers. We have tried to remain true to the original intent of the series, which was to provide the resident, fellow, or practicing physician with a text that might reasonably be read within several days. In practice, we see residents and fellows doing exactly that at the beginning of each subspecialty rotation. The concise presentation and reasonable length of THE REQUISITES books allows them to be read and reread several times during subsequent rotations and during preparation for board examinations.

THE REQUISITES are not intended to be exhaustive but rather to provide basic conceptional, factual, and interpretative material required for clinical practice. Each book is written by nationally recognized authorities in the respective subspecialty areas. Each author is challenged to present material in the context of today's practice of radiology rather than grafting information about new imaging methods onto old out-of-date material.

Dr. Blickman and his coauthors have done an outstanding job in sustaining the philosophy of THE REQUISITES in this radiology series. They have produced another truly contemporary text for pediatric imaging. I believe that *Pediatric Imaging: THE REQUISITES* will serve radiologists, pediatricians, and pediatric surgeons as a concise and useful introduction to the subject and will also serve as a very manageable text for review by fellows and practicing radiologists and cardiologists.

James H. Thrall, MD
Radiologist-in-Chief
Massachusetts General Hospital
Juan M. Taveras Professor of Radiology
Harvard Medical School
Boston, Massachusetts

Contents

COLOR PLATES

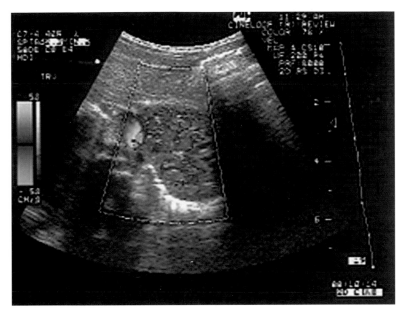

PLATE 1. Transverse color-flow Doppler image of a sequestration. See discussion in Chapter 2 of Fig. 2-34, D (plate 1 reproduced in black-and-white).

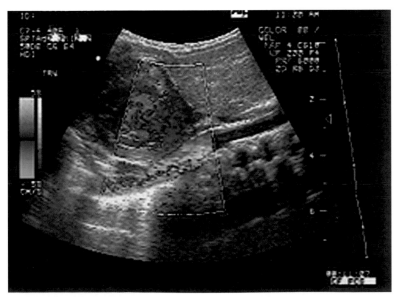

PLATE 2. Sagittal color-flow Doppler image of a sequestration. See discussion in Chapter 2 of Fig. 2-34, E (plate 2 reproduced in black-and-white).

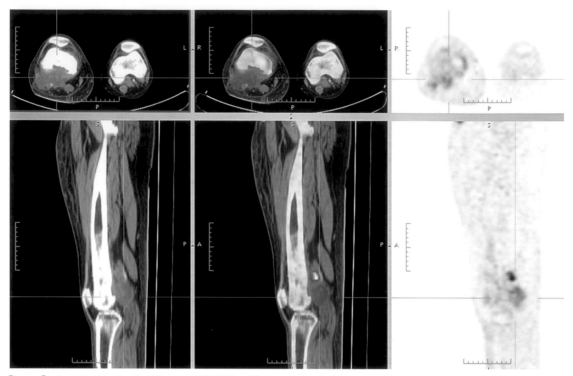

PLATE 3. Lytic lesion in distal femur. PET/CT of knee shows uptake. See discussion in Chapter 2 of Fig. 2-61, B (plate 3 reproduced in black-and-white). (Courtesy Rick van Rijn, MD, PhD, Academic Medical Centre Amsterdam, The Netherlands).

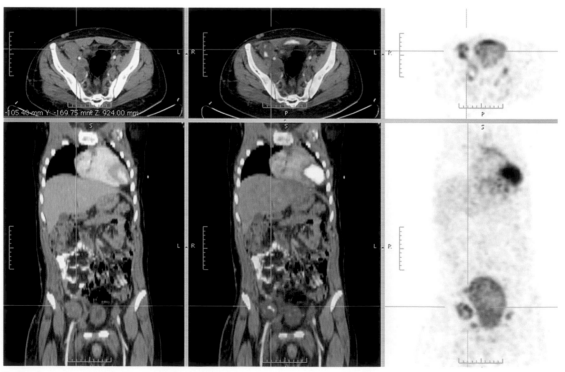

PLATE 4. Abdominal PET/CT reveals metastatic lesions in the pelvic and right inguinal regions. The lungs are clear. See discussion in Chapter 2 of Fig. 2-61, C (plate 4 reproduced in black-and-white). (Courtesy Rick van Rijn, MD, PhD, Academic Medical Centre Amsterdam, The Netherlands).

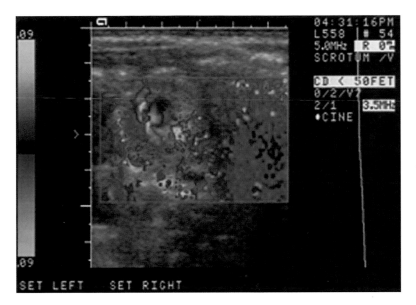

PLATE 5. Transverse color-flow Doppler image illustrates the "whirlpool" sign. See discussion in Chapter 4 of Fig. 4-9, C (plate 5 reproduced in black-and-white).

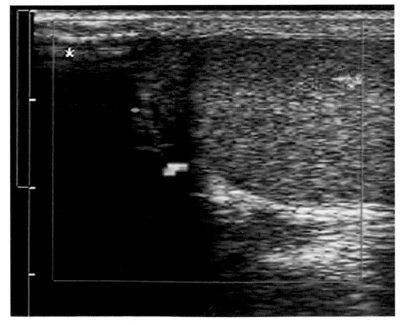

PLATE 6. Normal testicular echogenicity and flow. See discussion in Chapter 6 of Fig. 6-49 (plate 6 reproduced in black-and-white).

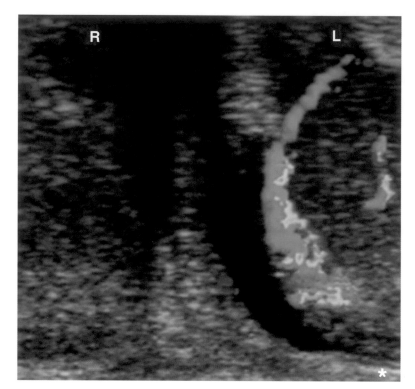

PLATE 7. Color-flow Doppler US demonstrates increased flow in the epididymis consistent with epididymitis. See discussion in Chapter 6 of Fig. 6-50.

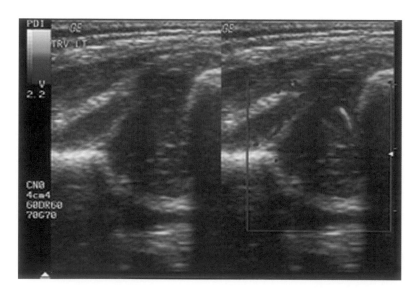

PLATE 8. Coronal left hip color-flow Doppler US showing normal alignment and normal vascular supply. See discussion in Chapter 7 of Fig. 7-73, D (Plate 8 reproduced in black-and-white).

CHAPTER 1

Pediatric Imaging

Johan G. (Hans) Blickman

On the one hand, the imaging of children is in many ways a microcosm of diagnostic imaging in general. Put another way, pediatric radiologists are the last of the general radiologists, those who are capable of using all modalities expertly. Although conventional radiography and fluoroscopy are still the cornerstones of their practice, maybe even more so than in adult practice, the cross-sectional imaging modalities such as ultrasonography (US), computed tomography (CT), and magnetic resonance imaging (MRI) do have their rightful place in the imaging armamentarium that is available today to imagers and clinicians who are caring for sick children.

US clearly remains the favorite screening modality in children's imaging, more so in Europe than in the United States. This is probably a reflection of the many years that CT (and MRI) was heavily regulated by European governmental agencies so that more energy and resultant experience were given to US. It probably also reflects the greater reliance on contrast-enhanced and post-processing US in renal and cardiac imaging in Europe, not in the least because there is no European agency comparable to the U.S. Food and Drug Administration to temporize the introduction of newer contrast agents.

Because reimbursement schemes in countries other than the United States are more favorable to "experimenting" with MRI, this "non-ionizing" modality is also used more intensively and routinely in urinary tract and cardiac imaging in those countries, as reflected in the origin of the relevant literature.

With regard to CT, there is a real catch-up (or Americanization) going on in Europe, led by the emergence of trauma centers as well as the ever-growing demand for what we radiologists call "non-focused imaging." Everywhere there is a shortage of time and physicians, thus leading to an unfortunate increase in the use of CT as a "stethoscope."

This is—of course, to older-generation imagers, regrettably—a natural evolution. On the positive side, this movement is also fueled by the move toward imaging time and resolution to near-pixel level, leading eventually to molecular and functional imaging.

None of these issues is unique to pediatric imaging. Especially in children, however, the radiation exposure aspect of imaging tends to be attention grabbing. Although the practice of using an ALARA (as low as reasonably achievable) radiation dose is widely accepted and followed, concern about radiation deaths is an issue everywhere. Vigilance about indications, proper (low mAs) protocols, and the actual presence of pediatric imagers are required to guarantee optimal imaging of children. Fortunately, the rapidly expanding digitalization of our practice makes this process easier.

The proper indication, use, and order of the different imaging modalities are the legal responsibility of a properly trained and practicing radiologist. American College of Radiology guidelines and cost reimbursement patterns are changing the way imaging is being performed today, and we imagers must thus practice what we preach.

A powerful influence is the ever-present legal challenge in the United States, which is sadly making slight inroads in other parts of the world as well. Protocols therefore must be as evidence-based as possible, and the indications must be well managed if order management systems in electronic patient records of all-digital medical centers are to be optimally implemented.

As far as the radiologist's being present: it is unavoidable, and rightly so. If we demand to be fully responsible medical specialist doctors, we must be on the playing field with our colleagues "24/7." The digital age has afforded us at the very least the possibility to render our interpretations at any time of day or night, making the decision to be physically present ours.

In the past 35 years, pediatric radiology has evolved so that it fully merits its status as a subspecialty, pediatric imaging. Radiologists in training are tested in pediatric imaging at the end of their 4 (or, in Europe, 5) years of training. Also, pediatric radiology is one of the four subspecialties in 2005 for which the first group of reexaminations were conducted for a time-limited certificate of additional qualification (CAQ). The Society of Pediatric Radiology is the oldest specialty organization within radiology; a global pediatric imaging meeting is held every 5 years alternatively in Europe and the United States, with full participation of the Australasian Society of Pediatric Imaging.

Teaching pediatric radiology presents some unique challenges. It is not enough to rely on statements such as "A child is a small adult" and "If it were your child, you would do every imaging modality as well." But it is difficult to quantify what must be known by a general radiologist about pediatric imaging. In addition, retaining that knowledge is often a problem because children usually are only a small part of a general radiology practice. Also, many general radiologists and technologists are not comfortable dealing with infants or young children.

In addition to their knowledge of general radiology, those who image children must be fully conversant with anatomy, embryology, and basic pediatrics. General radiologists should be familiar with these pediatric issues as well, although to a somewhat lesser degree. Meticulous attention to indications for diagnostic studies, standards of practice, and sensitivity to radiation dosage are just as much a part of pediatric imaging as they are in other radiologic subspecialties. However, the pediatric radiologist is often more conscious of these issues. Indeed, the practice of imaging children demands special attention, knowledge, and understanding.

This book, designed with the neophyte radiology resident in mind, attempts to answer the question what one could reasonably read and retain during the usual 12- to 16-week rotation through pediatric radiology. The radiology resident must go from little or no knowledge of pediatric radiology to a more or less working knowledge in a short training interval. The radiologist in training must also understand pediatric disease processes and their diagnosis, therapy, and follow-up. Finally, this knowledge must be retained in some form throughout one's radiology career.

Consequently, the manner in which the clinical phases, from initial diagnosis through therapy and follow-up, can be assessed most efficiently by the different imaging modalities is the ultimate challenge of pediatric imaging and is the major focus of this book. Therefore, it is hoped that this book will serve as a quick reference for the more common vignettes that may have temporarily slipped the mind of a general radiologist who is interpreting imaging findings in a child.

Although pediatric radiology is a problem-oriented specialty, an organ system approach is used in this book as a tool for presenting these essentials and as a method for systematic review. The remainder of this book is divided into nine main chapters according to organ system. Within each chapter, the imaging techniques as they pertain to pediatric patients are briefly reviewed. Emphasis is then placed on the anatomic and embryologic aspects of each region, because congenital lesions are an essential part of the differential diagnostic possibilities. Understanding these, even in rudimentary form, is of significant value.

Each organ system is discussed in a logical anatomic sequence. Within this framework, the most common imaging approaches and clinical highlights are presented. When applicable, pathology rounds out the discussion. Practical differential diagnostic possibilities, which often help guide the process of interpretation, are offered. Suggestions for further reading are made at the end of each chapter. General pediatric imaging reference texts are listed first, with pertinent page numbers. Then, selected review and seminal articles are listed that should enhance the reader's understanding of selected common and specific pediatric imaging topics.

For general radiologists, some observations may be useful to assist in the efficient and practical performance of basic pediatric imaging. Neonates must be kept warm. The help of the nursing staff should be enlisted in the care of neonates, and parents can also be asked to help with infants and children. The patient's history and the indications for the study must be reviewed. When it comes to interpreting pediatric images, taking the age of the child into account is paramount in determining the appropriate list of differential diagnostic possibilities: A toddler cannot climb stairs with alternate feet, and hypertrophy of the pylorus muscle seldom occurs at day 1 of life!

One must be organized and meticulous and must remember that teamwork (technologists are the radiologist's best ally) works wonders for imaging children. Following are other specific observations, adhering to the organ system outline of the ensuing chapters, that have been culled from many different experiences over the past decades of practice.

Regarding the pediatric chest, newer imaging is not necessarily better. Expensive cross-sectional imaging such as CT and MRI may necessitate sedating the child and should be contemplated only if a real, diagnostic AND therapeutic question needs to be (and possibly can be) answered by the procedure.

A conventional radiographic or fluoroscopic examination may be sufficient, without the added risk and exposure of a CT scan or the potential for claustrophobia with MRI. A plain film, and there is some discussion of whether a lateral film is always necessary in infants and young children, should be the initial step in all instances.

Imaging findings in the pediatric chest are influenced by the immature lung physiology, which differs significantly from lung physiology in adults with respect to histology, immunology, and anatomy. The presence of the thymus also affects the overall appearance of the cardiomediastinal silhouette.

Most important, particularly in the chest, an acceptable, technically adequate radiograph must be obtained to arrive at a proper interpretation. To achieve this objective, proper immobilization of the child is important because it decreases the duration and retake rate of the study. Techniques and devices in use include the Pigg-O-Stat Pediatric Immobilizer and Positioner (Modern Way Immobilizers, Inc., Clifton, Tenn), a clear plastic device that envelops an infant, and the Universal Octopaque (Octostop, Laval, Quebec, Canada), a wooden board with an octagon at each end. The main drawback of the Pigg-O-Stat is that it causes anxiety in both the infant and the parents; it also creates artifacts (artificial lines, and so on) that may cause anxiety in the interpreter. The Tame-EM Immobilizer (Cone Instruments, LLC, Solon, Ohio) uses hook-and-loop tape bands applied around the child's arms and legs, a method that is easier on everyone involved. The Pigg-O-Stat allows for upright imaging; sandbags and the Tame-EM Immobilizer necessitate supine positioning. The Universal Octopaque's main use is to facilitate fluoroscopic positioning, particularly in infants. In most instances, however, sandbags, adhesive tape, foam rubber wedges, or towels accomplish the immobilization cheaply and effectively, with the help of technical staff and even parents or caretakers.

Furthermore, one must keep in mind that fluoroscopy of the chest is quicker and easier to interpret than inspiratory-expiratory or oblique radiographs. Fluoroscopy is especially useful if conventional chest radiographs do not answer clinical questions about the presence or absence of a check-valve airway obstruction (foreign body) or retropharyngeal pathology, or for the elucidation of the mediastinal contour. In the pediatric chest, horizontal beam (decubitus) radiographs are seldom necessary to answer any more serious diagnostic dilemmas than the layering of a pleural effusion.

For imaging of the gastrointestinal tract or the genitourinary tract of a child, it is even more imperative than in an adult that the radiologist review prior examinations and pertinent clinical information. More important yet is to prepare the patient and parents before they enter the imaging suite. During the introduction to the child and parents, one must again verify the indication for the study, check for contraindications and allergies, and establish rapport to ensure a cooperative patient for an efficient and complete study. This process also helps assess whether parents will be a help or a hindrance if they accompany the child during the examination. The overwhelming majority of children benefit from the presence of a parent in the room, to help with both positioning and reassuring of the child. In the final analysis, however, allowing parents to be present is a personal choice for the radiologist.

During fluoroscopy, immobilization can be achieved by having the technologist at the head of the fluoroscopy table while the imager holds the child at the knees with one hand. As mentioned, some prefer using the Octopaque cradle device. "Papoosing" the child with towels or elastic bandages also works well. No matter which technique is used, during fluoroscopy, the right hand of the radiologist should not let go of the patient being examined. "One hand for the fluoroscopy unit (machine), one for the patient" should be the motto.

All upper gastrointestinal tract studies should include fluoroscopic observation of the respiratory motion of the diaphragm. The contour and motion of the mediastinum should also be assessed. With the administration of contrast material, assessment of the swallowing mechanism in the lateral position and an evaluation of the anatomic integrity from the oral cavity to the ligament of Treitz should be standard. A small-bowel follow-through study generally is not necessary for children younger than 9 years except in a workup for malabsorption.

In cases necessitating a contrast agent enema, bowel preparation depends on the clinical scenario. Children with potential Hirschsprung disease, for instance, should not undergo bowel preparation because the cleansing process could obscure a possible transition zone. Prohibiting the child from taking anything by mouth for 2 to 3 hours beforehand is often sufficient for most upper gastrointestinal studies.

In skeletal radiology, comparison views are recommended only if the observer is confused by the appearance of an epiphysis or other ossification center on a certain projection; comparison views should never be obtained on a routine basis.

Radiographs of a hip should always include an evaluation of the entire pelvis. If the pelvis is to be imaged in both a frog-leg lateral and a neutral (anteroposterior [AP]) projection, one of the exposures should be accompanied by proper gonadal shielding; in practice this is often the frog-leg lateral view. Screening for developmental dysplasia of the hip (DDH) should be done with US, with ionizing radiation reserved for follow-up if screening results are positive.

Regarding the cervical spine, odontoid views may be difficult to obtain in young children. Fluoroscopy of the area is preferred over repeated attempts or CT. In a trauma setting, if cranial CT is going to be performed, the odontoid can be assessed by extending this examination through C3, obviating repeated attempts to see the C1 to C2 region.

In general, for children younger than 12 years, coned-down views of the skeleton are not recommended, particularly in the L5 to S1 region. Oblique views of the spine are also not routinely obtained in children. More importantly, in the lumbosacral region, these views represent the single highest gonadal dose and thus should be avoided whenever possible.

A skeletal series to determine child abuse should comprise at the minimum AP and lateral views of the skull and entire spine and an AP view of the chest, abdomen, and extremities, including the hands and feet. Skeletal maturation is assessed on a single AP view of either hand and wrist in children older than 1 year. In those younger than 1 year, a single view of the knee may be useful. MRI and CT are the modalities of choice in cases in which the standard AP and lateral radiographs do not supply adequate information.

All cross-sectional imaging deserves special attention in the pediatric age group. Patients seldom require sedation for US examinations, but particularly active children may need to be immobilized. In general, children 4 months to 4 years of age should be sedated for MRI. This rule used to apply to CT as well, but spiral acquisition of data by CT has drastically reduced the need for sedation, by about 90%. The slice thickness and slice interval must be adjusted from case to case, which is why there is no such thing as a routine cross-sectional imaging study in the pediatric age group. All studies should be monitored by a radiologist. The use of oral contrast agents is almost always preferable for CT studies of the abdomen and pelvis, but the use of intravenous contrast agents should be considered routine, especially in cases of abdominal trauma.

Tailored, problem-oriented imaging is stressed throughout this book. To achieve it, the imaging team should be familiar with the indications for, and the limitations and possible results of, the various imaging procedures.

Providing optimal imaging care to children of all ages requires a team effort.

CHAPTER 2

Chest

Johan G. (Hans) Blickman and Lya Van Die

▬ IMAGING TECHNIQUES

About 40% of all pediatric imaging consists of chest radiographs. Conventional radiographs of the chest are frequently done with a portable machine and with the patient younger than 2 years placed supine. Upright films can be obtained after age 2. Frontal views are often the only ones necessary, but lateral views can be obtained depending on local custom. Proper immobilization and positioning are mandatory. There is no appreciable difference in magnification between the anteroposterior (AP) supine and the erect AP or posteroanterior (PA) view of the chest in the child younger than 4 years, assuming equal tube-to-film distance.

The conventional examination may be expanded by expiratory, decubitus, or high–kV technique films. Common clinical questions that prompt request for these special views are (foreign body) aspiration, the detection of pleural fluid, and determination of the presence and size of a pneumothorax. However, to evaluate for normal respiratory motion, especially to assess airway patency, fluoroscopy is often invaluable in the pediatric patient because it allows for more accurate localization of some lesions as well as for dynamic observation of the entire airway, hemidiaphragms, mediastinum, and bony thorax (Fig. 2-1).

The gonadal dose for AP and lateral views of the chest with proper coning and gonadal shielding is approximately 1 mR.

Computed Tomography

Modern-day, spiral computed tomography (CT) scanning provides excellent image quality, particularly in the less-than-cooperative patient, and has virtually eliminated the need for sedation (used in <2% of patients younger than 4 years). The airway, metastatic disease, and mediastinal pathology are optimally assessed, as are subpleural lesions. In congenital cardiac anomalies, CT angiography (CTA) has an established role (see Chapter 3). High-resolution CT (HRCT) demonstrates the morphologic characteristics of normal and abnormal lung parenchyma and the interstitium better—in evaluations for cystic fibrosis (CF), bronchiectasis, or fever in the immunocompromised patient—and can image the lung with excellent spatial resolution. CT of the mediastinum is done after intravenous administration of a non-ionic contrast agent (2 mL/kg).

Magnetic Resonance Imaging

Extremely useful in the determination of the extent of mediastinal masses, especially in the posterior mediastinum by itself, gated magnetic resonance imaging (MRI) and magnetic resonance angiography (MRA) are becoming more widely used in the evaluation of mediastinal vasculature, rings, and slings as well as of congenital cardiac lesions and anomalies of the great vessels. Both modalities are also useful for characterization and assessment of the vascular supply of bronchopulmonary foregut malformations and of vascular lesions of the lung. The cardiac and vascular lesions are discussed in Chapter 3.

Radionuclide Imaging

Radionuclide imaging may be used to evaluate for pulmonary embolism (in sickle cell disease), although CTA has made inroads in this area. Radionuclide imaging can also assess cardiac structure

and function and neoplastic/inflammatory lesions. These issues are covered extensively in another volume of this series, *Nuclear Medicine: The Requisites*.

Ultrasound

Conventional ultrasonography (US) has been used in the chest to determine the cystic or solid nature of neck masses as well as lesions in the superior mediastinum. Doppler US allows for the evaluation of intravascular access lines, patency of vessels, and/or clot formation. Cardiac structure and function can also be exquisitely assessed easily by US without ionizing radiation or (catheter) contrast administration. The US evaluation of cardiac structure and function, however, is now performed primarily by the pediatric cardiology team rather than the radiologist.

Further noncardiac evaluation by US is useful in the assessment of diaphragmatic motion, for determining the presence or absence of pleural fluid, and occasionally for mediastinal (thymic) diagnostic dilemmas. Furthermore, US evaluation has the benefit of being portable and therefore able to be performed at the bedside.

▬ DEVELOPMENT OF AIRWAY AND LUNGS

Structural Development

In the 4th week of gestation, the trachea first appears as a ventral diverticulum arising from the foregut. At 5 weeks' gestation, the lobar bronchi appear, and at 6 weeks', all subsegmental bronchi are present. By the 16th week, all airway branches are present and contain air sacs, but no alveoli are present yet. The sacs proliferate during the remainder of gestation. The right upper lobe bronchus arises from the trachea ("pig" bronchus) in 0.1% of all newborns.

With the first few breaths of life, complete aeration of the normal newborn chest is accomplished. This breathing effort has been practiced by the fetus. Intrauterine fetal respiratory activity has been well documented on prenatal US, and it occurs at a variable rate and low tidal volume during the last half of gestation.

After birth the alveoli develop from the air sacs, increasing in number until age 8 years. Alveolar size then increases until growth of the chest wall is complete. Concomitantly, the preacinar vessels (pulmonary arteries and veins) follow the development of the airway; the intra-acinar bronchial vessels follow that of the alveoli.

The first differentiation of tracheal cartilage occurs during the fourth week of gestation, and distinct rings of cartilage are present along the trachea and main bronchi by 11 weeks' gestation. The development of cartilage lags behind the branching of the airways; this is why cartilage does not extend to the periphery of the airway. Any derangements of this orderly sequence may result in a predictable set of developmental aberrations, often referred to as *bronchopulmonary foregut malformations* (Box 2-1). The submucosal glands are even slower to appear than cartilage. Insults (e.g., viruses) to the lungs in young children affect primarily the terminal and respiratory bronchioles, whereas in adults, such insults primarily affect the interstitium or the airspace.

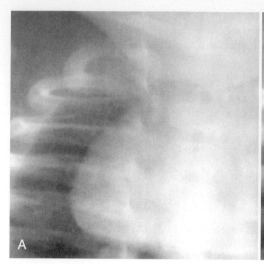
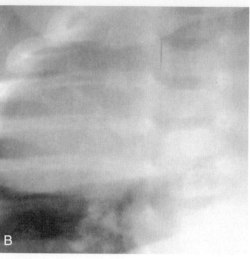

FIGURE 2-1. Inspiratory (**A**) and expiratory (**B**) views of the thymus confirm its change in shape with respiration.

Box 2-1. **Spectrum of Pulmonary Developmental Anomalies in Relation to the Pulmonary Vasculature**

Aplastic or hypo-plastic lung Arteriovenous malformation Scimitar syndrome }→	Intralobar or extralobar sequestration (Cystic) adenomatoid malformation }→	Bronchogenic cyst Congenital lobar emphysema/ obstruction
↓	↓	↓
Normal lung **Abnormal** vasculature	**Abnormal** lung **Abnormal** vasculature	**Abnormal** lung **Normal** vasculature

---

Functional Development

As noted previously, the pediatric tracheobronchial tree is not a miniature version of the adult tracheobronchial tree. During development its structure and function are still maturing. The laryngeal tissues are softer and more flaccid, and the aryepiglottic and arytenoid folds are larger and more loosely attached to the underlying cartilage. Anatomically, the overall size of the peripheral airways is smaller. Physiologically, there is more production of mucus per square millimeter in the pediatric airway, and the mucus is of a different composition from that in an adult. The pediatric immune system is not as well developed as an adult's. Likewise, the collateral air circulation through the pores of Kohn and channels of Lambert is not fully operational until at least 1 year of age. All of these differences result in greater susceptibility of the airway to irritants of all kinds and often such consequences as edema and swelling of the interstitium and increased mucus production. This combination of events may in turn lead the terminal bronchioles to collapse because of their increased weight, to be obstructed by the copious mucus, or both, resulting in "disordered aeration": areas of hyperinflation (air trapping) and atelectasis (hypoaeration).

Physiologically, therefore, the respiratory cycles of a healthy infant are markedly different from those of an infant suffering from peripheral airway disease. In children with diffuse peripheral airway disease (bronchiolitis), the tidal volume is smaller and the residual volume is significantly higher than normal, resulting in air trapping. In severe cases the air trapping may approach total lung capacity. On radiographs this condition is manifested by hyperinflation associated with thickened (visible) bronchial walls and areas of atelectasis. This peribronchial "cuffing" is best seen on the lateral radiograph. Other (concomitant) radiographic signs are flattened diaphragms, anterior bowing of the sternum, and more "horizontal" ribs (Fig. 2-2). These findings on radiographs reflect the physiologic changes and may vary over time. Before age 2 years, *bronchiolitis, diffuse airway disease,* and *viral pneumonitis* are the terms used; after age 2 years, the term *reactive airway disease*—previously known as "asthma"—is currently recommended.

UPPER AIRWAY

Pharynx

Normal and Variants
The pharynx is divided into the nasopharynx, oropharynx, and hypopharynx. Important nonosseous structures are the components of the Waldeyer ring: the adenoids superiorly, the palatine tonsils laterally, and the lingual tonsils inferiorly, all of which are evident when one inspects the oral cavity. The retropharyngeal soft tissues extend from the adenoids, which are visible by 3 to 6 months of age, to the origin of the esophagus at the level of C4 to C5. Prominent adenoids become pathologic when they encroach on the nasopharyngeal airway (Fig. 2-3). The palatine tonsils are outlined by air only with marked dilatation of the hypopharynx. The lingual tonsils are occasionally visible radiographically at the base of the tongue. Measurements of these structures are neither reliable nor useful. A useful ratio, however, is that of the retropharyngeal soft tissue to (C2) vertebral body width. The ratio varies in inspiration from almost 1.00 before 1 year of age to 0.5 by 6 years of age: To be prudent, the soft tissue width should not exceed 50% of the accompanying vertebral body to C4.

Congenital Anomalies
The most common anomaly of the upper airway, choanal atresia, occurs in 1 in 5000 live births. It is usually present bilaterally and consists of a bony obstruction to airflow in 90% of cases, with membranous obstruction accounting for the other 10%. It is commonly associated with craniofacial anomalies, tracheoesophageal fistula, and congenital heart disease (CHD). Because neonates are obligate nose breathers, newborns with choanal atresia present clinically with respiratory distress immediately after birth. This respiratory distress is severe if bilateral atresia is present. CT should reveal enlargement of the vomer and fusion of the bony aspects of the pterygoid process and palatine bone (see Fig. 10-6).

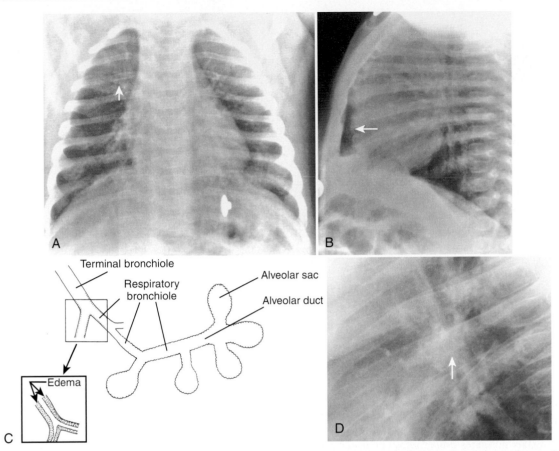

FIGURE 2-2. PA (**A**) and lateral (**B**) chest radiographs demonstrate flattening of diaphragms and anterior bowing of sternum consistent with hyperinflation; lung is seen "anterior" to the heart *(long arrow)*. Increased interstitial markings and evidence of disordered aeration are exemplified by mild hyperinflation of the right lower lobe and decreased aeration in the right upper lobe *(short arrow)*. **C**, Diagram illustrating the difference between pediatric and adult airways. Peribronchial thickening caused by edema narrows the effective diameter of the airway, necessitating increased effort at breathing. **D**, "Donuts" or peribronchial "cuffing" *(arrow)*.

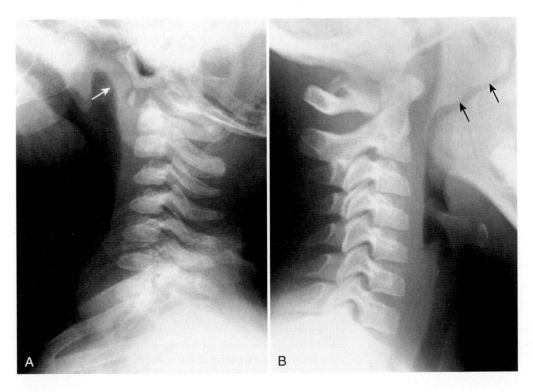

FIGURE 2-3. **A**, Normal lateral neck radiograph with the normal adenoidal "pad" *(arrow)*. **B**, Adenoidal tissue encroaching on the nasopharyngeal airway *(arrows)*.

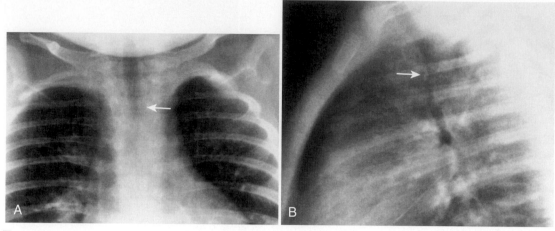

FIGURE 2-4. Tracheal stenosis. Note narrowing *(arrow)* in a prematurely born infant requiring 3 months of endotracheal intubation. **A,** AP view. **B,** Lateral view.

Tracheal stenosis may be due to a continuous cartilage ring or to underdevelopment of a short segment of the airway. It may also be caused by prolonged intubation (Fig. 2-4).

Tracheobronchomegaly (Mounier-Kuhn syndrome) is of unknown etiology and is rare in children, but a similar disorder has been noted in premature infants, possibly secondary to long-term respirator therapy. The disorder consists of a floppy, bulging trachea that variably extends into the (mainstem) bronchi and collapses on inspiration. Children with the disorder often have recurrent pulmonary infiltrates and/or fibrosis or emphysema.

Inflammatory Lesions

A retropharyngeal abscess is usually seen in children younger than 1 year, and the most common causative organisms are group B streptococci or staphylococci from the oropharynx. Clinical presentation consists of fever, stiff neck, and dysphagia. Cervical adenopathy is common. Because prevertebral lymph nodes and channels drain the posterior nasal structures and form a communication in the retropharyngeal space between lateral soft tissues of the neck, infection or obstruction to lymph flow predisposes the area to abscess formation. On conventional radiographs the presence of air in the retropharyngeal space strongly suggests a retropharyngeal abscess. Dissection of air cephalad from the pleura or mediastinum due to air block phenomenon (CF, asthma) or trauma may mimic this finding. Retropharyngeal soft tissue fullness may be either inflammatory in origin or the normal soft tissue prominence seen especially well in expiration. Fluoroscopy will distinguish fixed soft tissue swelling from the normal respiratory soft tissue variation. As previously discussed, in inspiration the width of the retropharyngeal soft tissues between C1 and C4 to C5 should not exceed one half the width of the accompanying vertebral body (Fig. 2-5). If the retropharyngeal space is pathologically widened, this finding may be accompanied by straightening or reversal of the normal lordotic cervical spine (Fig. 2-5A and B). Straightening or reversal of the normal lordotic curve in turn often results in pseudosubluxation of C2 on C3 (C3 on C4, C4 on C5 less common). This finding is also seen in trauma situations when the reversal of the lordotic curve is either caused by muscle spasm or secondary to the soft-collar immobilization device that is often used in these situations. Reversal of the lordotic curve is thus frequently associated with pseudosubluxation; any subluxation in a normally aligned (lordotic) cervical spine is pathologic until proven otherwise (Fig. 2-6A).

Inflammatory lesions are best imaged by MRI or CT, both of which are better for evaluation of the extent of a lesion and may assist in treatment planning (Fig. 2-6B).

After age 3 years, the common pathway of prevertebral (retropharyngeal) lymph nodes, which drains the posterior nasal structures and the nasopharynx as well as lymphatic tissue in the neck, disappears. Therefore, after the patient's age has been determined, the differential diagnosis of a retropharyngeal soft tissue mass should include—in addition to hemorrhage and inflammatory lesion—trauma (from intubation) or infection, lymphadenopathy caused by leukemia/lymphoma, and (rarely) neuroblastoma or a retropharyngeal goiter. If the mass is associated with enlarged palatine tonsils or adenoids, and (occasionally) preauricular nodes, infectious mononucleosis may also be considered.

Larynx

Normal and Variants

The larynx extends from the base of the tongue to the trachea and is composed of three major cartilaginous structures: the epiglottis, the thyroid cartilage, and the cricoid cartilage. There are, in addition, three small paired cartilaginous structures: the arytenoid, cuneiform, and corniculate cartilages. A practical anatomic division of the larynx consists of three regions: (1) a supraglottic region, which contains the epiglottis, aryepiglottic folds, and false vocal cords; (2) a glottic portion, which contains the laryngeal ventricle and the true vocal cords; and (3) a subglottic region, which is immediately distal to the true vocal cords and extends to the lower cricoid cartilage. Calcification in respiratory cartilage, although very rare in children, is pathologic; such rare conditions include chondrodysplasia punctata and relapsing polychondritis.

Other anatomic hallmarks are the hyoid bone, body, and horns, which may be ossified at birth. The horns are oriented in such a way that they "point" to the epiglottis on a conventional lateral radiograph of the neck (Fig. 2-7).

Supraglottic Region
Developmental Lesions
Developmental lesions are often midline or off-midline structures that manifest as a mass. Sixty-five percent are below the level of the hyoid bone, often embedded in the strap muscles. Centrally located masses carry a differential diagnosis that includes dermoid, lingual thyroid, thyroglossal duct cyst (Figs. 2-8 and 10.24), lingual tonsil, and remula (epithelial retention cyst). The differential diagnosis of laterally located masses consists of branchial cleft cyst, hemangiomas, and lymphangiomas (or cystic hygromas) as well as inflamed (matted) lymph nodes. All may manifest as upper airway obstruction, most often with inspiratory

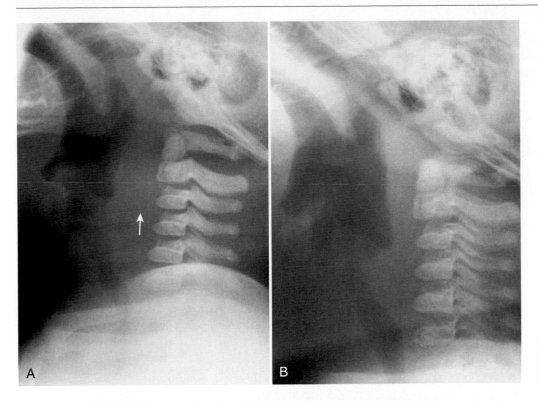

FIGURE 2-5. **A**, *Arrow* demonstrates the prevertebral soft tissue widening on expiration that disappears on inspiration (**B**).

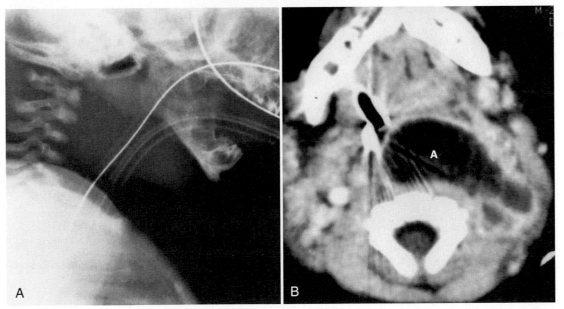

FIGURE 2-6. **A**, Lateral radiograph of the neck demonstrates a soft tissue mass encroaching on the airway and esophagus. Note also "straightening" of the cervical spine (reverse lordosis). **B**, CT demonstrates the abscess cavity (A) displacing the nasogastric and endotracheal tube laterally.

stridor. Two thirds of lymphangiomas manifest in the posterior cervical triangle, often at birth. Extension of such a lesion into the mediastinum occurs in 10% of cases (Fig. 2-9). Branchial cleft cysts occur in the anterior cervical triangle, most commonly at the angle of the jaw (Fig. 2-10, see also Figs. 10-21 and 10-22). They are often infected at presentation.

Conventional imaging may delineate air, fat, or calcium in these structures. US is the screening modality used to differentiate cystic from solid masses. CT delineates the extent of these masses and bone destruction, whereas MRI has better tissue plane resolution. The most common appearance of these masses

is cystic with a rim of enhancing tissue. The presence of functioning thyroid tissue can be determined by scintigraphy.

Laryngomalacia (Supraglottic Hypermobility Syndrome)

Laryngomalacia is a common cause of inspiratory stridor in the first year of life. It is self-limiting and is caused by infolding of the aryepiglottic folds, with inspiration leading to collapse and obstruction of the airway (hypermobility). As the arytenoid tissues strengthen and become more firmly attached to the underlying cartilage by 1 to 2 years of age, the hypermobility and resultant stridor resolve spontaneously. This is one of the very

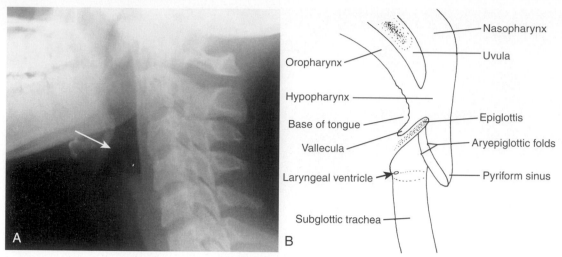

FIGURE 2-7. A, Lateral radiograph of the normal neck. Horns of the hyoid "point" to the epiglottis *(arrowhead).* **B,** Normal anatomy of the upper airway.

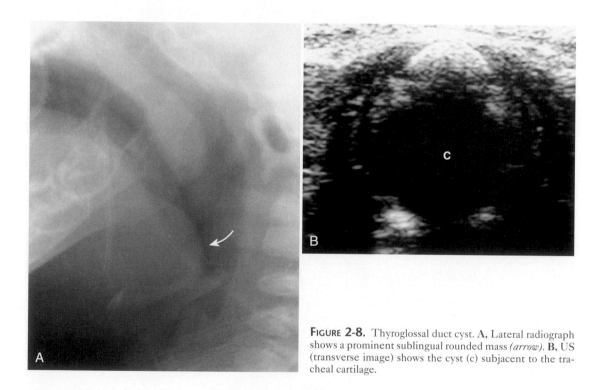

FIGURE 2-8. Thyroglossal duct cyst. **A,** Lateral radiograph shows a prominent sublingual rounded mass *(arrow).* **B,** US (transverse image) shows the cyst (c) subjacent to the tracheal cartilage.

few conditions in which stridor improves with increasing activity of the child.

Hereditary Angioneurotic Edema

Hereditary angioneurotic edema is an autosomal dominant inherited disease that is characterized by a deficiency of a C1 esterase inhibitor, which results in vascular damage, increased vascular permeability, and edema. It affects the airway usually in the first decade of life and produces stridor in 50% of cases. The stridor can be life threatening. The radiographic findings may mimic those of epiglottitis. The gastrointestinal tract or extremities can also be involved with angioneurotic edema, generally manifesting as swelling of the affected tissues.

Acute Epiglottitis

Acute epiglottitis is most often caused by *Haemophilus influenzae* type B (HIB) and manifests as a high fever, dysphagia, and sore throat. The overall incidence is minimal because the HIB vaccine is routinely administered at 6 months of age. Classically, the child in severe respiratory distress assumes a bold upright position, with the head held forward and a protruding tongue (and panic-stricken eyes)—all the result of the rapidly progressive respiratory obstruction. Peak incidence is at 3 to 6 years of age. Immediate treatment consists of intubation, with verification of the diagnosis by endoscopy. Imaging should not be done with the child in a recumbent position nor without accompanying qualified personnel.

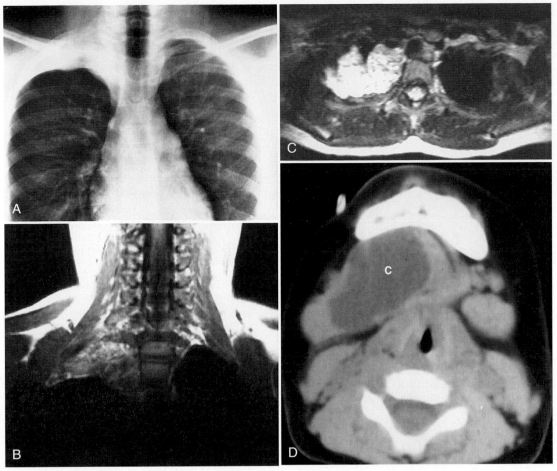

FIGURE 2-9. Cystic hygroma. **A,** Frontal chest radiograph reveals a right apical soft tissue mass without bony erosion, displacing the trachea to the left. Coronal T1-weighted (**B**) and axial T2-weighted (**C**) MR images delineate the cystic character and extent of this lesion. **D,** CT demonstrating a cystic hygroma (c) in a different patient.

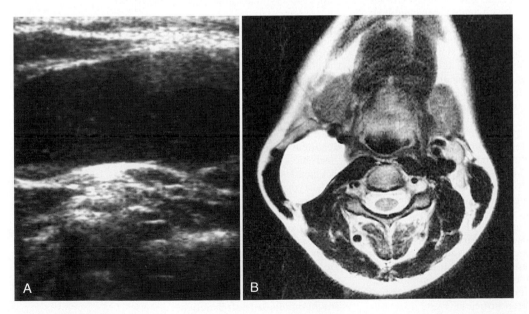

FIGURE 2-10. Branchial cleft cyst. **A,** Sagittal US scan demonstrates a clear cystic lesion. **B,** MRI shows its extent optimally.

A lateral soft tissue radiograph of the neck shows an enlarged, dilated hypopharynx that is the result of a reflex—the tongue goes up, the larynx goes down, and the retropharyngeal soft tissues flatten. There is swelling of the epiglottis and thickening of the aryepiglottic folds, with the latter finding being the real cause for the stridor and dysplasia. The vallecula is barely identifiable because of the soft tissue swelling of the epiglottis and aryepiglottic folds. This may result in the classic "thumb" sign (Fig. 2-11). Approximately one fourth of children also have accompanying subglottic edema that is indistinguishable from that seen in croup.

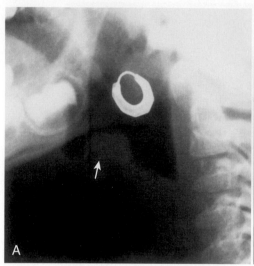
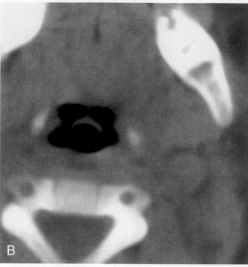

FIGURE 2-11. **A,** Lateral radiograph of a neck demonstrates the "thumb" sign of an acute epiglottitis *(arrow).* Note horns of hyoid bone pointing to the general area of the epiglottis. **B,** Appearance of a normal epiglottis in an axial plane (CT), illustrating the reason that the epiglottis appears "fuzzy" on a lateral view ("omega" shape).

The differential diagnosis includes angioneurotic edema, epiglottic cysts, and hematoma secondary to trauma or hemophilia.

Neoplasms

Neoplasms of the supraglottic region are very uncommon, and benign growths outnumber malignant ones.

Benign lesions include fibromatosis colli and juvenile angiofibroma.

Torticollis, or fibromatosis colli, which is not uncommon, is due to shortening of the sternocleidomastoid muscle. It typically manifests shortly after birth, most often in the second week. About a third of patients recover spontaneously within a few weeks to months. Facial asymmetry and head tilt may persist to varying degrees in the remaining children. The main contribution of radiography is the exclusion of underlying skeletal deformity or a vascular origin (calcification). On US a mixed echogenic, well-circumscribed mass is seen in an often enlarged sternocleidomastoid muscle (Fig. 2-12).

Juvenile angiofibroma is a vascular, locally invasive mass located posteriorly in the nasal cavity and occurring almost exclusively in adolescent boys. It often manifests initially as epistaxis (95%) or nasal obstruction (80%). Conventional radiographs of the sinus show anterior bowing of the posterior wall of the maxillary antrum, displacement of the nasal septum, and/or a large soft tissue mass in the nasopharynx that can be associated with bony erosion. CT and MRI accurately depict the anatomic extent of the mass and allow for staging. CT demonstrates bony involvement better, but MRI permits differentiation between sinus extension of the tumor and obstruction of the sinus by the tumor (i.e., different echo characterization; see Fig. 10-64). Preoperative embolization of this highly vascular structure is useful. The recurrence rate after resection is 25% to 30%.

The most common *malignant* supraglottic neoplasms are embryonal rhabdomyosarcomas. These lesions grow rapidly, infiltrate the surrounding tissues rapidly, and metastasize widely. Hodgkin lymphoma is the second most common malignant neoplasm, the retropharyngeal and lateral neck being the most common locations. MRI is the imaging modality of choice to delineate the extent of these lesions, but CT is often sufficient (Fig. 2-13).

Glottic Region
Congenital Lesions
Congenital lesions of the glottic region include laryngeal web and laryngocele, which most often manifest as stridor.

A membranous or cartilaginous laryngeal web (very rare) results from failure of recanalization of the larynx in fetal week 10.

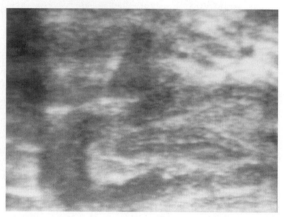

FIGURE 2-12. US representation of a "pseudotumor" in the sternocleidomastoid muscle, fibromatosis colli.

It most often involves the anterior portion of the vocal cords, and the child often has crouplike symptoms.

A laryngocele, also a rare occurrence, arises from the laryngeal ventricle, is air filled, and extends laterally into the soft tissues. The child usually presents with inspiratory stridor.

Infection
Recurrent respiratory papillomatosis (RRP) is a clinically aggressive (hoarseness, airway hemorrhage) but histologically benign lesion that manifests between the ages of 2 and 5 years. It is the most common laryngeal tumor. The lesions may prolapse into the subglottic region or, in less than 20%, metastasize to the lungs (Fig. 2-14).

A viral etiology has been suggested for RRP. The presence of genital papillomavirus does not lead to RRP in the infant necessarily, yet condylomata acuminata cultured from the maternal cervix or vagina have been reported in half of children with RRP. Treatment with laser therapy may be curative.

Subglottic Region
Tracheomalacia (Soft Trachea)
In the normal infant, there is respiratory "buckling" of the trachea, anteriorly and to the right (Figs. 2-5A and 2-15). Normally a slight deviation to the right of the trachea is noted in the frontal plane that is due to the aortic arch that normally passes on the left. The caliber of the trachea does not change when this "buckling" occurs; the angle of the "buckling" may reach 90 degrees and is exaggerated in inspiration and decreased in expiration. Any

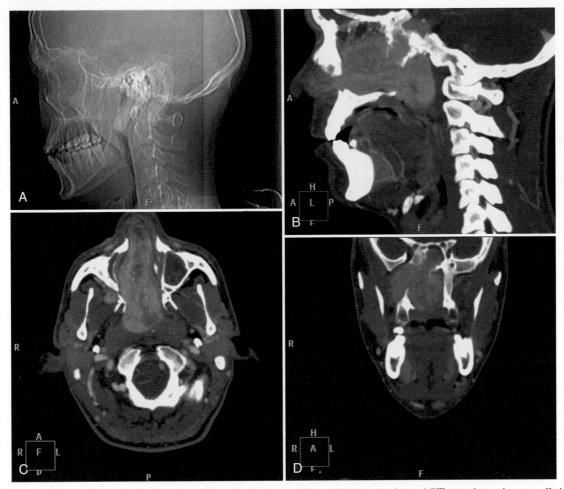

FIGURE 2-13. **A,** Lateral sinus film shows opacification of the maxillary antra. **B,** Coronal contrast-enhanced CT scan shows the same. **C,** Axial CT scan. **D,** Coronal scan. (Courtesy of Dr Ari Weinstein, Witwatersrand Group of Teaching Hospitals, Johannesburg, South Africa.)

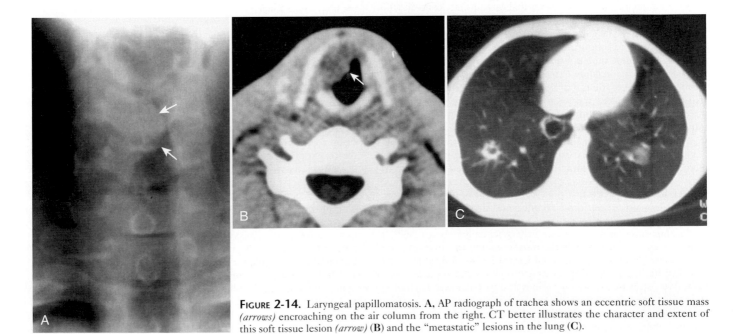

FIGURE 2-14. Laryngeal papillomatosis. **A,** AP radiograph of trachea shows an eccentric soft tissue mass *(arrows)* encroaching on the air column from the right. CT better illustrates the character and extent of this soft tissue lesion *(arrow)* (**B**) and the "metastatic" lesions in the lung (**C**).

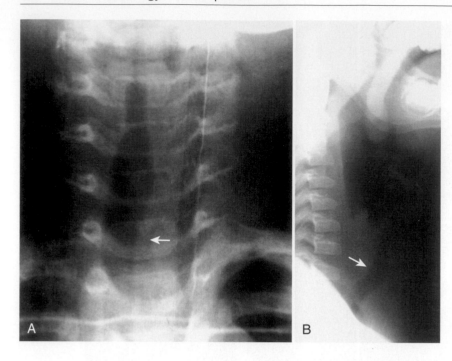

deviation of the trachea toward the midline or to the left should be explained; it may be caused by aberrant vessels, masses, or a unilateral disturbance of pulmonary aeration.

A soft trachea may have intrinsic or extrinsic causes. Intrinsic causes include weak supporting cartilage and/or muscles of the trachea, and the infant usually outgrows these problems. Extrinsic causes are more common. The severity of clinical features varies according to the cause. Expiratory or, at times, biphasic stridor is the clinical hallmark; it results from extrathoracic or intrathoracic tracheal stenosis or mass effect distal to the carina, respectively.

1. Primary tracheomalacia can be caused by chondromalacia, relapsing polychondritis, or prematurity, or it may be idiopathic.
2. Secondary tracheomalacia is usually due to a congenital anomaly such as a vascular ring or mediastinal mass.

Anterior tracheal narrowing, a normal variant that occurs in 30% of all infants younger than 2 years, was thought to be the result of compression of the trachea by an "aberrant" innominate vessel during its oblique ascent into the mediastinum and neck. The reasoning was that the superior mediastinum at the level of the thoracic inlet can become "crowded," and that the innominate artery originated to the left of the trachea. The former is probably still true, and the latter has been clearly shown to be the case in all people. Fluoroscopy, endoscopy, CT, and MRI can all aid in establishing the severity and extent of tracheal compromise. There may be an association with esophageal atresia and tracheoesophageal fistula, which may be an indication that segmental tracheomalacia (caused by inflammation or tracheal underdevelopment) may also be present. The decision for surgical intervention must be weighed against the fact that, as the infant grows older, more "room" develops in the thoracic inlet, and the indentation often disappears. Current thinking leans toward the latter (Fig. 2-16A).

Another vascular indentation of the trachea may be caused by a double aortic arch, which is the most common vascular ring and may be associated with congenital heart disease. A double aortic arch has its origin in the persistence of both the right and left primitive aortic arches, resulting in a true vascular ring encircling the trachea and esophagus. There are characteristic impressions on both the trachea and esophagus that are readily seen with use of fluoroscopy with contrast (barium) in the esophagus. The posterior indentation, because the right posterior arch is the larger of the two, is usually the most prominent (Fig. 2-16B).

Other conditions have been implicated as occasional causes of tracheomalacia. They include a right aortic arch and a pulmonary "sling" (occurring when the left pulmonary artery arises from the right pulmonary artery and crosses between the trachea and the esophagus) (Fig. 2-16C and D) as well as a high (cervical) aortic arch.

Primary Tracheal Stenosis

Primary tracheal stenosis is almost always a lethal condition caused by intact tracheal rings (i.e., the cartilaginous rings are not "open" posteriorly). The diagnosis is usually made on bronchoscopy, although conventional radiographs of the chest may show a narrow trachea in both dimensions. The stenosis is usually associated with vascular rings, pulmonary slings, and H-type tracheoesophageal fistulae.

Secondary Narrowing of the Trachea

Subglottic hemangioma is the most common soft tissue mass causing respiratory tract obstruction in the first 3 months of life. It is accompanied by dyspnea, a "croupy" cough, and inspiratory stridor. There is a 50% association with cutaneous hemangiomas. The lesion is usually asymmetric and eccentrically located in the trachea, and it deforms the subglottic portion of the trachea on conventional AP radiographs (Fig. 2-17A). Endoscopy is indicated to confirm the diagnosis, and laser excision is the current treatment of choice.

Acute laryngotracheobronchitis (croup) is the most common cause of upper airway obstruction in children. The peak age range at which it occurs is between 6 months and 3 years. (Pseudo)croup is viral in origin, with the most common offenders being parainfluenza and respiratory syncytial virus. The child has upper respiratory symptoms, a "barking" cough, and inspiratory stridor. Croup is usually a self-limited disease of 3 to 7 days' duration, and it is unusual for a child with croup to require intubation and hospitalization. There is a seasonal component in children younger than 2 years, who are afflicted more frequently in fall and winter.

Effective imaging includes a lateral soft tissue radiograph of the neck that demonstrates distention of the hypopharynx, a normal epiglottis, and (symmetric) subglottic narrowing. The normal trachea does not change in diameter from the false vocal cords

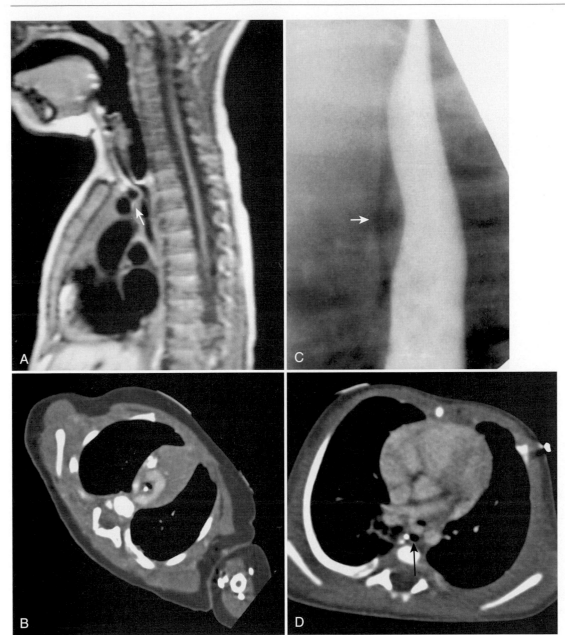

FIGURE 2-16. A, T$_1$-weighted sagittal MR image illustrating the innominate artery *(arrow)* that is causing an anterior impression of the trachea. **B,** Contrast-enhanced CT scan demonstrates a double aortic arch. A contrast-enhanced CT scan of the chest (**D**) and an esophagram (**C**) both demonstrate a lesion between trachea and esophagus: a pulmonary "sling *(arrow)*."

to the thoracic inlet, so the subglottic narrowing caused by the edema is easily appreciated. A lateral neck radiograph also allows for exclusion of foreign body and retropharyngeal abscess as a cause of the symptoms. On an AP radiograph, symmetric narrowing (the classic "steeple" sign) of the subglottic region may be seen with normal expiration but is classically noted in patients with croup (Fig. 2-17B-E). Often chest radiographs taken at the same time will show changes of bronchiolitis, most commonly hyperinflation.

Acute bacterial tracheitis (membranous croup) is more severe but has similar radiographic signs, and the characteristic membrane can be seen only endoscopically.

Foreign bodies that lodge in the airway can cause a croup-like clinical picture. If the foreign body is radiopaque, it can usually be identified on conventional radiographs. Fluoroscopy can evaluate better for nonopaque foreign bodies by demonstrating a check-valve mechanism: On expiration, the lung segment involved stays inflated, and the mediastinum may shift

away from the side of the foreign body, returning to normal on inspiration. Decubitus views and an expiration film may be difficult to interpret. The latter technique relies on the phenomenon that the affected lung, when dependent, should remain inflated. Endoscopic removal of the foreign body is the rule (Fig. 2-18A-D).

◼ THORACIC SKELETON

Developmental Aspects

At least five ossification centers of the sternum should be present at 6 months of life. Usually there is one main ossification center for the manubrium and the first sternal segment, whereas the other segments consist of variably paired centers. The first three of these centers are ossified at birth. Hypersegmentation is seen in Down syndrome 85% of the time. Early fusion is seen in 50% of children with cyanotic CHD but can be seen normally in 15%

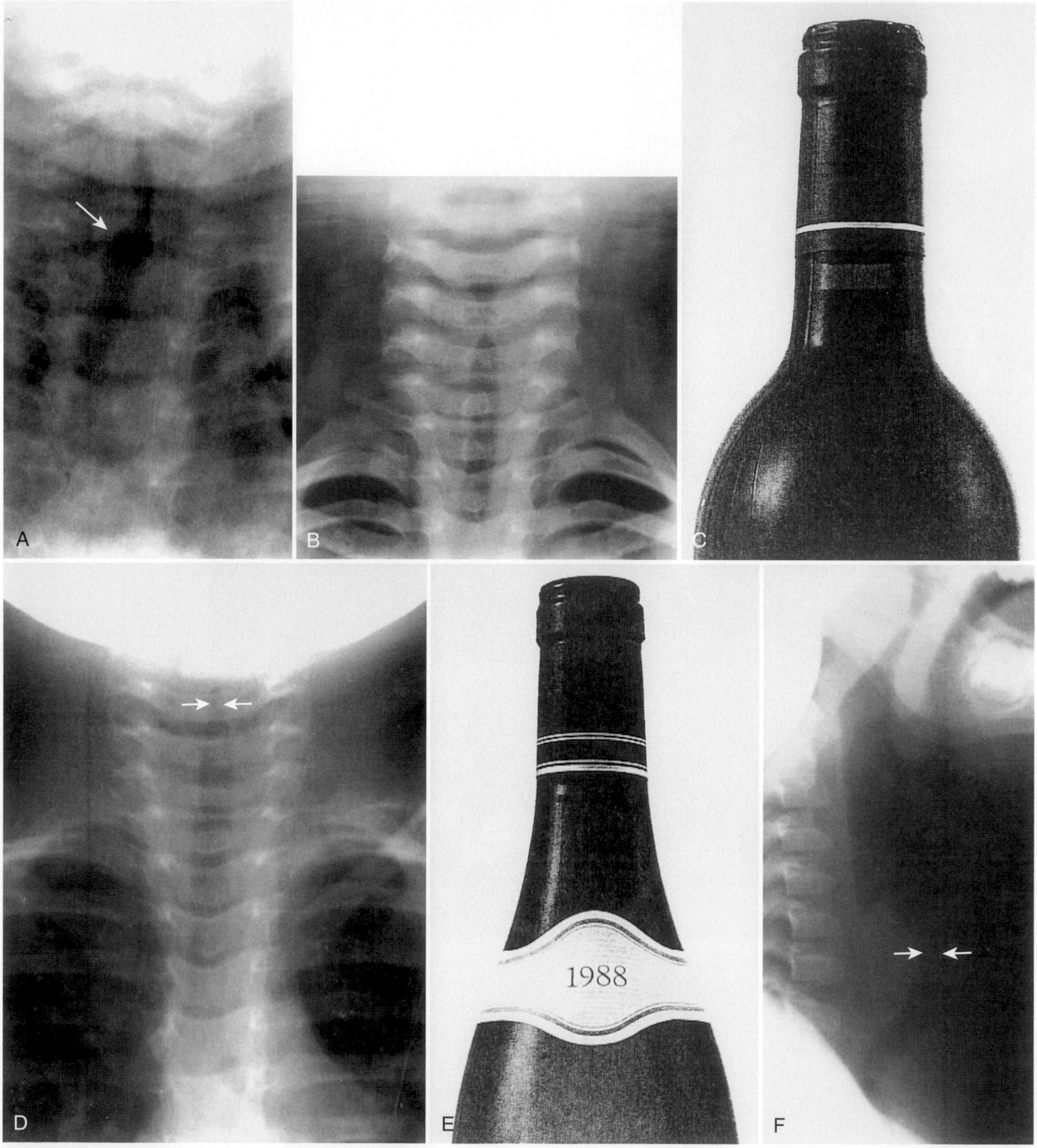

FIGURE 2-17. **A,** AP radiograph of the trachea demonstrating an eccentric, asymmetric soft tissue mass encroaching on the subglottic trachea: a hemangioma *(arrow)*. **B,** Normal "Bordeaux bottle" appearance of the subglottic region. **C,** Actual Bordeaux bottle. **D** through **F,** Croup: **D,** AP radiograph reveals symmetric subglottic narrowing *(arrows)*, often referred to as "steepling" in croup (or "white wine bottle" appearance). **E,** Actual white wine bottle. (The original concept for this book occurred in 1988!) **F,** Lateral view shows the subglottic narrowing *(arrows)* as well; the subglottic trachea on the lateral view should be of one diameter.

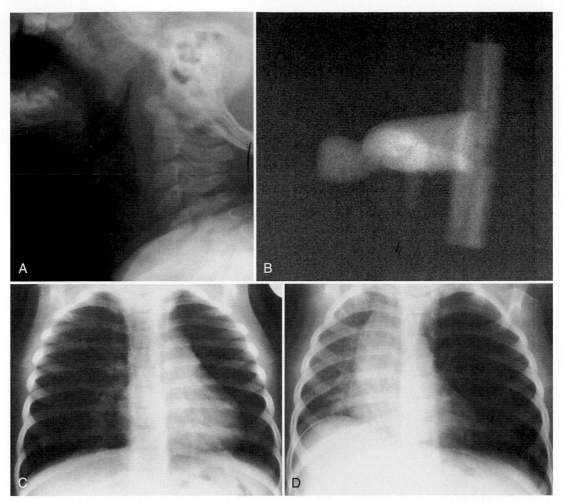

FIGURE 2-18. **A,** Pharyngeal foreign body on lateral radiograph: Note the "not-clear" hypopharynx. **B,** Specimen. Check-valve mechanism (see text for explanation). **C,** Virtually normal AP chest radiograph in a child who aspirated a peanut into the left mainstem bronchus. **D,** Expiratory film confirms the air trapping.

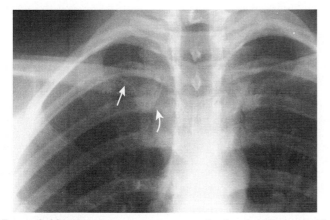

FIGURE 2-19. AP radiograph demonstrates the rhomboid fossa *(straight arrow)* and clavicular growth plate *(curved arrow)*.

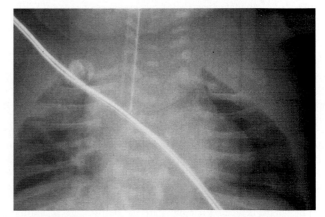

FIGURE 2-20. Cleidocranial dysostosis: absence of the clavicles.

of patients. Early fusion may result in pectus carinatum (pigeon breast). Pectus excavatum (funnel breast) occurs in about 1% of the general population and is more common in boys than in girls. Most of the affected children are asymptomatic.

The clavicle may contain a prominent rhomboid fossa in its inferior medial aspect, at the site where the sternoclavicular ligament attaches. In addition, its medial growth plate is the last

epiphysis to close; at about 20 years of age, all are closed (Fig. 2-19). On the inferior surface of the midclavicle, the midclavicular nerve canal is often identified. Absence of the clavicle is associated with cleidocranial dysostosis (Fig. 2-20).

Failure of descent of the scapula (Sprengel deformity) leads to persistence of a ligament, occasionally ossified (the omovertebral bone), extending from the spine to the scapula. Vertebral

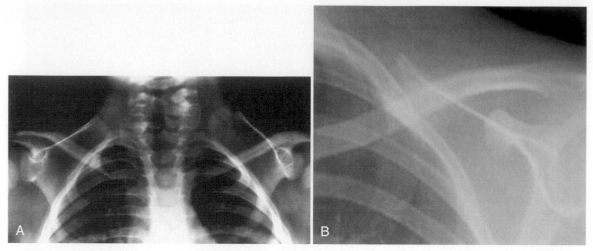

FIGURE 2-21. **A,** AP radiograph demonstrates segmentation anomalies of the cervicothoracic junction (Klippel-Feil syndrome) and failure of descent of both scapulae (Sprengel deformity). **B,** Normal appearance.

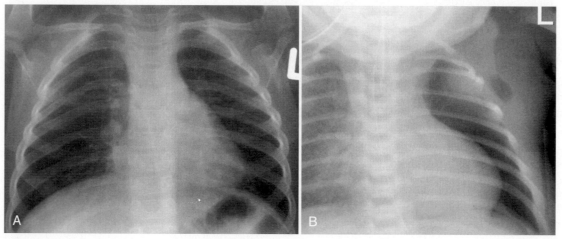

FIGURE 2-22. Frontal radiographs showing effects of surgery. **A,** Right lateral rib crowding after EA repair. **B,** Left lateral rib crowding after patent ductus arteriosus repair.

segmentation anomalies associated with Sprengel deformity of the scapulae are known as the Klippel-Feil syndrome (Fig. 2-21). This syndrome may be associated with congenital deafness and renal agenesis.

The ribs may show segmentation abnormalities and may be fused or bifid. Normally there are 12 paired ribs; the presence of 11 paired ribs is characteristic of Down syndrome. Rib fractures occur less often in children than in adults and are often lateral or anterior. Posterior (medial) rib fractures are virtually pathognomonic for child abuse.

The shape of the rib cage can be helpful. It is normally slightly bell-shaped after birth. An extreme bell shape may be seen in thanatophoric dwarfs, whereas postoperative rib changes can suggest what conditions have been treated—left lateral crowding after closure of patent ductus arteriosus, for example, and right-sided crowding in esophageal atresia repair (Fig. 2-22).

Systemic Involvement

Expansile lesions of the ribs are noted in Langerhans cell histiocytosis (LCH) and multiple hereditary osteochondromatosis.

Expansion of an entire rib may occur with secondary involvement of the ribs in systemic conditions such as hyperparathyroidism, thalassemia, and the mucopolysaccharidoses. Hyperostosis of the ribs may be seen in osteopetrosis (Fig 2-23A) and in Caffey disease, although less commonly in the latter than mandibular and scapular hyperostosis. Erosion of the undersurface of the ribs is seen in neurofibromatosis (ribbon ribs) and as a result of collateral circulation (left ribs 4 to 8 most commonly) in severe coarctation of the aorta (Fig. 2-23B-D).

Neoplasms

All tumors of the chest wall are rare. Soft tissue masses (lipomas, fibromas, sarcomas) do occur and arise from the cutaneous or subcutaneous tissues. Tumors originating from the skeletal system can be benign or malignant. The benign lesions include LCH and multiple hereditary exostoses. However, most skeletal tumors in children are of the *malignant variety*.

In the thorax the most common primary skeletal lesion is Ewing sarcoma. A variant of Ewing sarcoma is the primitive neuroectodermal tumor (PNET), which simulates the former clinically, histologically, and radiographically. Askin first described this

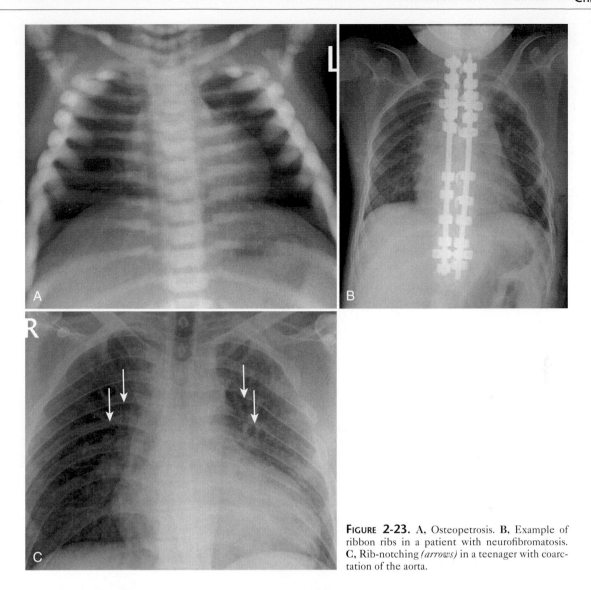

FIGURE 2-23. **A,** Osteopetrosis. **B,** Example of ribbon ribs in a patient with neurofibromatosis. **C,** Rib-notching *(arrows)* in a teenager with coarctation of the aorta.

lesion of the thoracic wall, which contains rhabdoid elements, in adolescent girls. Metastatic diseases of the rib cage include neuroblastoma, Ewing sarcoma, and leukemia/lymphoma. Imaging may reveal rib destruction, a pleura-based soft tissue mass, and/or a pleural effusion. CT is the modality of choice to best delineate the extent of the lesion (Fig. 2-24); US may help elucidate its character.

▬ LUNG

Developmental Anomalies

Primary Anomalies

Agenesis of the Lung

Pulmonary agenesis refers to complete absence of a lung or lobe and its bronchi. *Aplasia* refers to absence of lung tissue, in which rudimentary lobar bronchi are present. *Hypoplasia* refers to an underdeveloped lobe that contains both alveoli and bronchi.

Agenesis of the lung is a very uncommon lesion in which there is a single lung with alveolae equivalent in number and size to those of two lungs. The number of airways is that of a single lung (Fig. 2-25). The mediastinum and the heart are displaced toward the hemithorax of the agenetic site. The volume of the hemithorax containing the agenetic lung is shallow.

Approximately 1 in 15,000 children are born with congenital absence of one lung and the associated bronchus. Pulmonary agenesis occurs with equal frequency on the left and right sides. Right-sided agenesis, however, is associated with a much worse prognosis owing to a greater anatomic distortion of the airway and great vessels as well as recurrent infections, and tracheobronchomalacia.

Lobar Underdevelopment

Pulmonary hypoplasia is characterized by a decrease in volume, a decrease in the size of the pulmonary artery, and a shift of the mediastinal structures to the affected side (Fig. 2-26A). There is usually compensatory hyperinflation (overgrowth?) of the contralateral lung and loss of the heart border. In children with pulmonary hypoplasia, the lateral radiograph reveals a retrosternal "band," which is caused by the interface of the shifted mediastinum, possibly aided by extrapleural areolar tissue and the anterior border of the underdeveloped lung (Fig. 2-26B). This band has also been erroneously referred to as an "accessory" hemidiaphragm.

In most cases pulmonary hypoplasia is secondary to an underlying abnormality. The pathogenesis of pulmonary hypoplasia is not fully understood, but a normal thoracic cavity, fetal breathing movements, fetal lung liquid at positive pressure, and normal amniotic fluid volume are all required for normal lung growth in utero. Entities associated with pulmonary hypoplasia therefore include congenital diaphragmatic hernia, renal agenesis and dysgenesis, polycystic renal disease, and anterior wall defects.

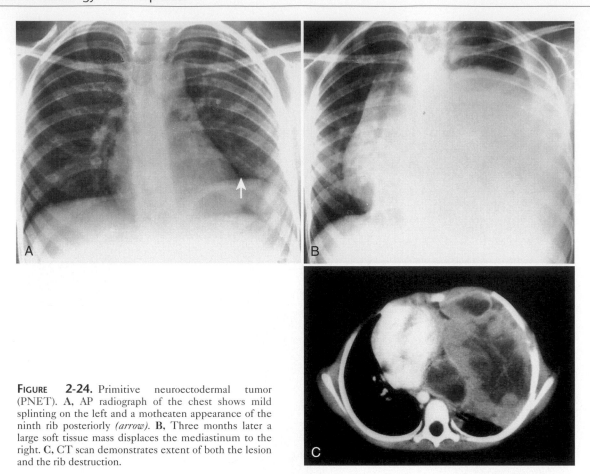

FIGURE 2-24. Primitive neuroectodermal tumor (PNET). **A,** AP radiograph of the chest shows mild splinting on the left and a motheaten appearance of the ninth rib posteriorly *(arrow)*. **B,** Three months later a large soft tissue mass displaces the mediastinum to the right. **C,** CT scan demonstrates extent of both the lesion and the rib destruction.

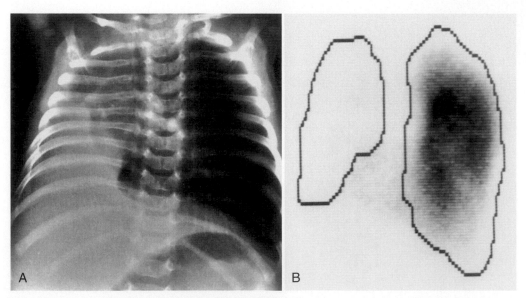

FIGURE 2-25. Agenesis of the lung. **A,** AP radiograph reveals a mediastinal shift to the right and an overexpanded left lung. **B,** Radionuclide pulmonary angiogram demonstrates normal left pulmonary perfusion and absence of perfusion on the right. There was no right pulmonary artery on PA gram (not shown). (A from Merten DF: Pediatric Learning File. Reston, Va, American College of Radiology Institute, 1987.)

Pulmonary hypoplasia is most often an incidental and insignificant anomaly except when it is part of the scimitar syndrome (Fig. 2-27), also called congenital pulmonary venolobar syndrome (CPVS). This syndrome consists of hypoplasia or aplasia of one or more lobes of the right lung, with partial anomalous pulmonary venous return below the diaphragm, absence or small size of the pulmonary artery, and occasional rib and vertebral body anomalies. It is slightly more common in girls (1.4:1) and may be inherited. Imaging findings on the conventional chest radiograph may consist of the anomalous vein draining medially and inferiorly into

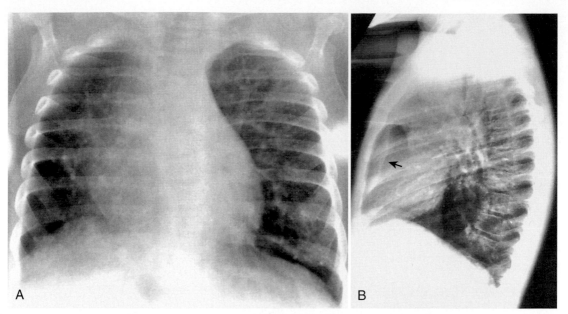

FIGURE 2-26. Hypoplasia of the lung. **A,** AP radiograph demonstrates shift of the mediastinum to the right because of decreased right lung volume, evidenced by longer interrib distance on the right than on the left. **B,** Retrosternal band *(arrow)* is the attempt by extrapleural areolar tissue to fill in the empty space.

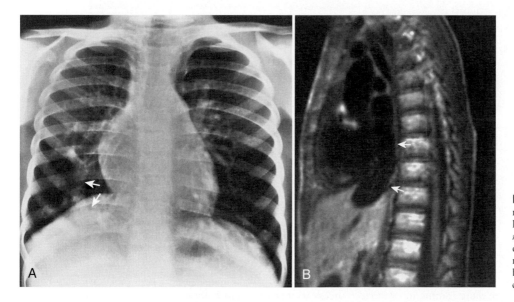

FIGURE 2-27. Scimitar syndrome. **A,** AP radiograph demonstrates decreased right lung volume and a tubular structure *(arrows)* coursing inferomedially below the diaphragm. **B,** Partial anomalous pulmonary venous return is confirmed on MRI by the flow void in the anomalous venous channel *(arrows).*

the inferior vena cava in proximity to the right hemidiaphragm. This venous structure often has the shape of a Turkish sword (scimitar). This syndrome may be associated with tetrad of Fallot or truncus arteriosus and hemivertebrae with resultant scoliosis. An atrial septal defect occurs in 25% of affected children. The differential diagnosis of pulmonary hypoplasia includes Swyer-James syndrome, effects of radiation therapy, and small lung volume as a result of scoliosis or after aspiration of toxic substances with pulmonary necrosis.

Secondary Anomalies
Congenital Diaphragmatic Hernia
Impaired development of the airways and resultant pulmonary hypoplasia is caused by the mass effect of the presence of bowel in the thorax. The herniated bowel passes through a defect in the diaphragm, the pleuroperitoneal canal. The closure of the pleuroperitoneal canal coincides with the return of the bowel to the

coelomic cavity. If the bowel is "early" or the diaphragm closure is "late," a hernia may occur. The hernia occurs in 1 in 2500 live births with a 2:1 male-to female ratio.

Prenatal US usually detects the hernia. There is hope that in utero palliation may improve the outcome of this condition. Postnatal conventional radiographs are also often diagnostic (Fig. 2-28 A and B), especially once swallowed or injected air has entered the loops of bowel.

Anomalies associated with congenital diaphragmatic hernia include neural tube defects (30% of infants), malrotation (95%), and cardiovascular anomalies (20%). The severity of the hypoplasia depends on the amount of bowel in the hemithorax as well as on the timing of the herniation.

The herniation occurs on the left side 90% of the time. Overall, a posterior *Bochdalek* hernia occurs in 85% (back of diaphragm, big babies), and a herniation through the foramen of *Morgagni* occurs in 3% to 5% (middle of diaphragm, mature,

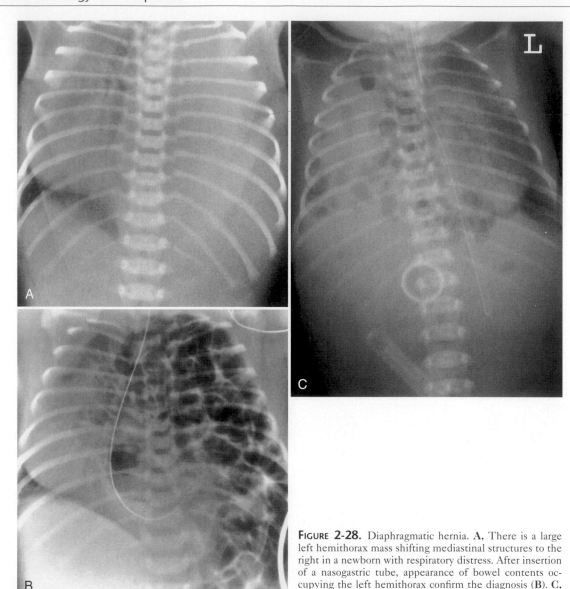

FIGURE 2-28. Diaphragmatic hernia. **A,** There is a large left hemithorax mass shifting mediastinal structures to the right in a newborn with respiratory distress. After insertion of a nasogastric tube, appearance of bowel contents occupying the left hemithorax confirm the diagnosis (**B**). **C,** Right-sided diaphragmatic hernia.

minuscule baby). These latter hernias are more commonly right-sided; the heart "protects" on the left (Fig. 2-28C). Contralateral hypoplasia of the lung is commonly present, probably caused to some degree by lung compression from the mediastinal shift. Treatment consists of repositioning the herniated bowel into the abdomen. To allow the lung to regenerate and heal, extracorporeal membrane oxygenation (ECMO) is often used, although it has improved the prognosis only marginally. Overall mortality of congenital diaphragmatic hernia remains at about 30% in most centers today.

Acquired hypoplasia can also be caused by bronchiolitis obliterans (the Swyer-James or Macleod syndrome). This condition is the sequela of a necrotizing viral lower respiratory tract infection leading to destruction and scarring of bronchi and bronchioles. This loss of volume eventually results in a small yet hyperlucent lung on a conventional chest radiograph (Fig. 2-29). Other causes of acquired pulmonary hypoplasia are rare yet include thromboembolism with infarction of the lung (Westermark sign), irradiation therapy, severe dehydration, and nephrotic syndrome.

Accessory Fissures and Lobes

A fissure caused by the azygos vein is a common entity and involves of part of the right upper lobe separated from itself by the azygos vein within four layers of pleura, the "azygos fissure" (Fig. 2-30).

In an inferior fissure, the medial part of the lower lobe may be separated from the lateral portion by a more or less vertical fissure, creating an inferior lobe, usually on the right side behind or adjacent to the right atrium.

A superior fissure may separate the apical segment from the rest of the left lower lobe at approximately the level of the minor fissure on the right.

Congenital (Cystic) Masses

Masses of congenital origin can be solid, cystic, or mixed lesions that usually manifest when they cause respiratory distress or become infected. This continuum of pulmonary developmental anomalies is based on the relationship between lung and vascular tissue, ranging from normal vasculature and abnormal lung (congenital lobar emphysema) to normal lung and

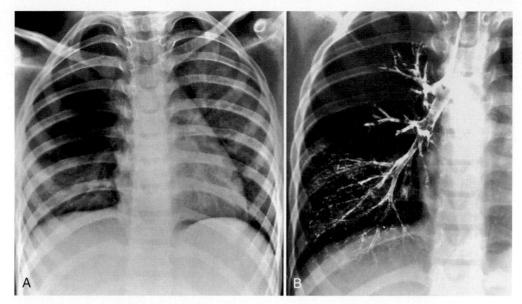

FIGURE 2-29. Swyer-James syndrome. A, Unilateral hyperlucent right upper lung with overall low right lung volume. B, Bronchography confirms obliterated lung tissue in right upper and middle lobes. (From Merten DF: Pediatric Learning File. Reston, Va, American College of Radiology Institute, 1987.)

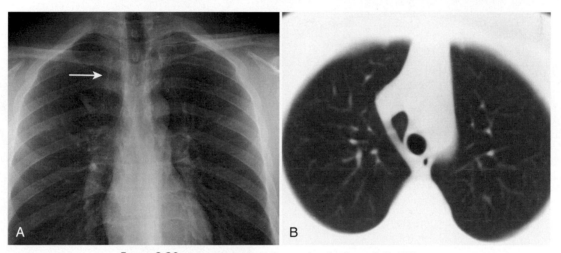

FIGURE 2-30. Azygos fissure. A, Conventional radiograph. B, CT scan.

abnormal vasculature (pulmonary arteriovenous malformation) (see Box 2-1).

Congenital Lobar Overinflation/Emphysema

The presumed cause of congenital lobar emphysema (overinflation) (CLO) is a progressive overdistention of a lobe secondary to bronchial cartilage deficiency, dysplasia, or immaturity, which in turn is caused by either an intrinsic cartilage anomaly or compression from an extrinsic vascular structure or mass (e.g., pulmonary vessel, lymph node, bronchogenic cyst). The affected pulmonary tissue may be emphysematous or may contain an increased number of alveoli. The lesion may encroach on the airway or may become infected. Destruction of alveolar walls may take place if infection occurs. Thus CLO manifests as respiratory distress and/or fever in the first 6 months of life; it occurs in boys three times more often than in girls. It involves the upper lobes in two thirds of patients, with the left upper lobe involved twice as often as the right upper lobe; the right middle lobe is involved in approximately 30% of patients (Fig. 2-31). Lower lobe involvement is rare (1%). There is an associated ventricular septal defect or patent ductus arteriosus in 15% of patients with CLO. The radiographic appearance again depends on the extent of resorption of the fetal lung fluid, the degree of emphysematous change, and the presence or absence of infection. The lesion may thus range from solid to reticular to hyperlucent with mass effect. Definitive treatment is surgical resection, especially in cases of acute respiratory distress.

Bronchogenic Cysts

Bronchogenic cysts are thought to be due to abnormal ectopic bronchial budding during lung development. Such a cyst, which does not usually communicate with the airway, consists of an oval or round lesion, frequently noted incidentally unless the child is in respiratory distress or the lesion becomes infected. Bronchogenic cysts are often found in either a pulmonary or a mediastinal (subcarinal) location, are twice as often located in the lower lobes, and are more common on the right. This variation in location depends on the timing of the abnormal budding: An "early" occurrence results in a mediastinal lesion; a "late" occurrence becomes an intraparenchymal lesion. There is an equal gender incidence. Bronchogenic cysts consist of serous or mucous material as well as cartilage rests.

Imaging reveals an oval or round mass, which is found to be cystic on CT and to have a characteristic high T2 signal on MRI

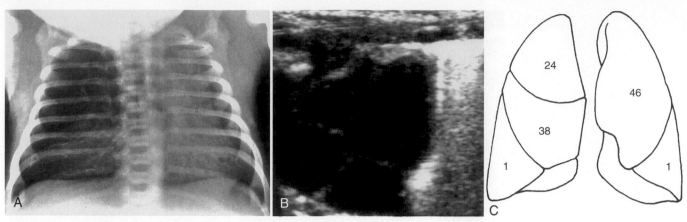

FIGURE 2-31. Congenital lobar emphysema (CLE) or overinfation (CLO). **A,** AP radiograph at 2 weeks of age demonstrates a hyperaerated right upper lobe with mass effect on the lower lung and mediastinum, causing it to shift to the left. **B,** US evaluation of this area at birth had shown a fluid-filled septated lesion. **C,** Relative lobar incidence of CLE/CLO. (After Hendren WH, McKee DN: Lobar emphysema of infancy. J Pediatr Surg 1966;1:24.)

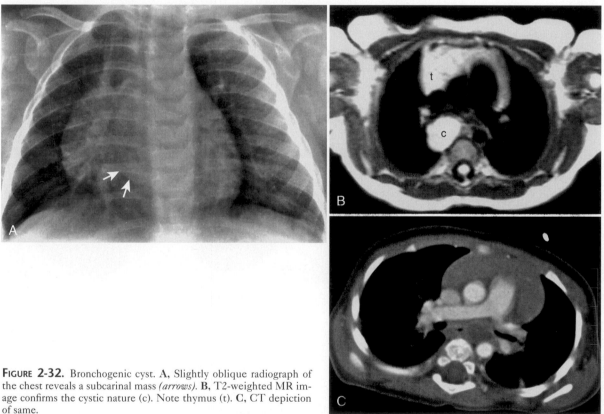

FIGURE 2-32. Bronchogenic cyst. **A,** Slightly oblique radiograph of the chest reveals a subcarinal mass *(arrows)*. **B,** T2-weighted MR image confirms the cystic nature (c). Note thymus (t). **C,** CT depiction of same.

(Fig. 2-32). These lesions may grow because of either recurrent infection or accumulating secretions. If growth and (therefore) symptoms occur, the lesions must be resected.

Neurenteric Cysts
Neurenteric cysts occur with failure of complete separation of the lung bud from the notochordal (primitive neural crest) structures during the third week of gestation. Occasionally there is communication with the enteric canal by a fibrous band or canal (neurenteric canal of Kovalevsky). Vertebral anomalies are almost always seen, including hemivertebrae, anterior spina bifida, and butterfly vertebrae. Thus a posterior mediastinal mass with dysraphic changes is pathognomonic of a neurenteric cyst. More than 50%

of children with neurenteric cyst have neurologic symptoms. Imaging is definitive, with MRI showing a cyst containing fluid that is consistent with a cerebrospinal fluid signal (see Chapter 9).

Congenital Cystic Adenomatoid Malformation
A congenital cystic adenomatoid malformation (CCAM) is characterized by anomalous fetal development of terminal respiratory structures, which results in a dysplastic, multicystic mass with a variable amount of proliferating bronchial structures. These cysts then interfere with alveolar development. A CCAM is now commonly diagnosed antenatally, often enlarges after birth, manifests in the first month of life (in 70% of cases) as a cause of respiratory distress, and has an equal gender distribution. It is most

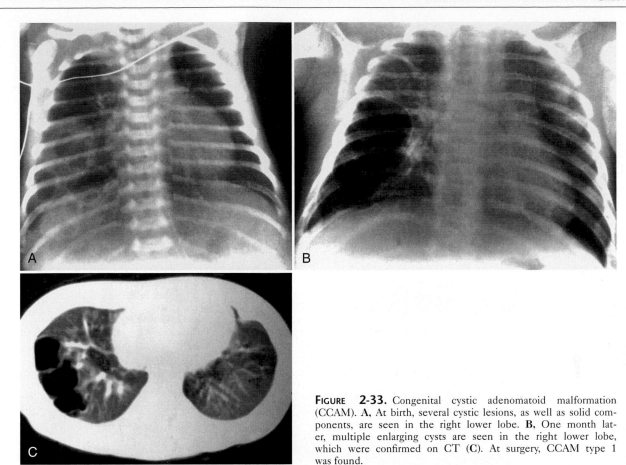

FIGURE 2-33. Congenital cystic adenomatoid malformation (CCAM). **A,** At birth, several cystic lesions, as well as solid components, are seen in the right lower lobe. **B,** One month later, multiple enlarging cysts are seen in the right lower lobe, which were confirmed on CT (**C**). At surgery, CCAM type 1 was found.

often unilobar, and 90% of infants are presented at less than age 1 year with increasing respiratory distress. CCAM can be divided into three types: (1) single or multiple air-filled cysts, often more than 2 cm in size (most common); (2) cysts smaller than 2 cm and mixed with solid tissue; and (3) solitary solid mass (rare). The imaging appearance on chest radiographs and CT depends on the amount of air replacing fluid in the cysts as they communicate with the airway. These imaging findings may mimic staphylococcal pneumonia or diaphragmatic hernia (Fig. 2-33). Treatment is controversial, with some advocating that a normal chest radiograph after prenatal detection of a CCAM warrants expectant therapy, whereas others point to the occurrence of malignancy in the cyst wall. Traditional thinking says that surgical lobectomy is curative in type 1; in types 2 and 3, however, the lesions are large at presentation and the prognosis parallels that of a diaphragmatic hernia with respect to morbidity and mortality (40%). Prenatal US detection has, on the other hand, improved morbidity and mortality because earlier measures can be taken to increase lung capacity.

Sequestration

Pulmonary sequestration, accessory lung, and *bronchopulmonary foregut malformation* probably all describe the same entity.

A *sequestration* is defined as a congenital mass of aberrant pulmonary tissue that has no normal connection with the bronchial tree or with the pulmonary arterial system. The lung parenchyma contained in this tissue mass may be normal or dysplastic. The most common vascular supply is through persistent fetal vessels with variable venous drainage. The intralobar and extralobar variants can most reliably be differentiated on the basis of this venous drainage. "Intralobar" drainage occurs primarily via the

left atrium or pulmonary veins; "extralobar" drainage is primarily via the systemic venous plexus, including the inferior vena cava or azygos system. Both intralobar and extralobar sequestrations have a vascular supply consisting of systemic arteries arising from the aorta or its branches, often from below the diaphragm. The majority of reported sequestrations are intralobar; relatively few are of the extralobar variety. Commonly, an intralobar sequestration is supplied by a large systemic vessel, is contained within the lung without a separate pleural covering, occurs on the left side (70% of the time), and manifests in teenagers. An extralobar sequestration is often supplied by a small systemic vessel, has its own pleural covering, occurs on the left side, and presents in boys (60% of the time). The extralobar variety often manifests in the first month of life.

Most sequestrations are located in the posterior basilar segments of the lower lobes and are only occasionally bilateral. Gastroenteric communication is not common. Conventional radiographs may have normal findings or may show a (recurrent) lower lobe consolidation or a relatively lucent, "cystic" lower lobe component. MRA often delineates the vascular supply; US may do so (Fig. 2-34). Complete surgical removal to treat recurrent infection is the therapy of choice; if the sequestration is an incidental finding, removal is not necessary. The intralobar variety may actually represent a CCAM with systemic vasculature or may be an acquired CCAM, usually diagnosed in later childhood.

The differential diagnostic possibilities of "cystic" thoracic (lung) lesions in the neonate or infant thus include the bronchopulmonary foregut malformations, such as CLO, CCAM, sequestration, and neurenteric or bronchogenic cysts, as well as a diaphragmatic hernia. Rarely are pulmonary vascular malformations present.

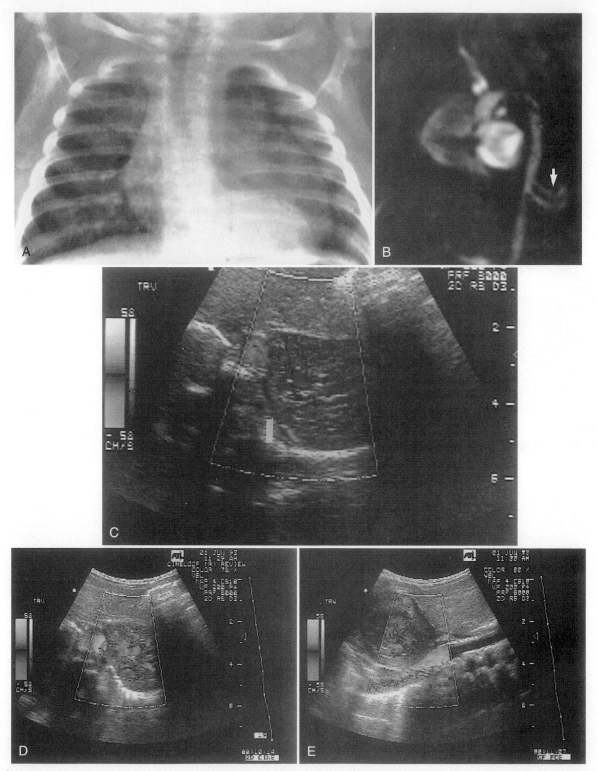

FIGURE 2-34. Sequestration. **A,** Frontal radiograph demonstrates a left lower lobe consolidation that persisted more than 4 weeks despite appropriate therapy. **B,** MRA shows the vascular supply of the sequestration *(arrow)* on lateral coronal projection. **C,** US scan shows the feeding vessel. **D** and **E,** Transverse and sagittal color-flow Doppler images. See Plates 1 and 2 for color reproductions.

Pulmonary Arteriovenous Malformation

A pulmonary arteriovenous malformation may be single or multiple in 40% of cases; the remaining 60% occur in patients with hereditary hemorrhagic telangiectasia (Osler-Weber-Rendu disease). Affected children may present with cyanosis, dyspnea or hemoptysis, and clubbing as well as polycythemia. The malformations are most often subpleural in location and are best treated with coiling (Fig 2-35).

Neonatal Chest

See Table 2-1.

Infant Respiratory Distress Syndrome

Also described as surfactant deficiency disease and hyaline membrane disease (HMD), infant respiratory distress syndrome (IRDS) is the most common cause of respiratory distress in the

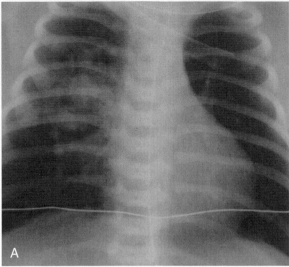

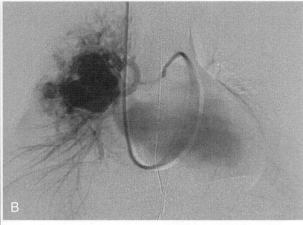

FIGURE 2-35. A, Abnormal density in the right upper lobe in a child with hemoptysis. **B,** S/P coiling of lung arteriovenous malformation.

TABLE 2-1. Neonatal Chest Vignettes

	Hyaline Membrane Disease	Transient Tachypnea of the Newborn	Meconium Aspiration	Neonatal Pneumonia
Typical patient	Premature	Term Cesarean section	Post-term Meconium-stained fluid below the vocal cords	Premature rupture of membranes
Time course	Within hours	24-48 hr	12-24 hr	Onset <6 hr
Lung volume	Decreased	Increased	Increased	Increased
Radiographic characteristics	Ground-glass, granular	Interstitial edema	Coarse, nodular, asymmetric	Perihilar "streaking"
Effusions	No	Yes	No	Maybe
Complications and possible therapy	Pulmonary interstitial emphysema or pneumothorax, respiratory distress syndrome, patent ductus arteriosus	None	Persistent fetal circulation, extracorporeal membrane oxygenation (ECMO)	Sepsis, ECMO

neonatal period. It almost always occurs in premature infants, although term infants of diabetic mothers and infants delivered by cesarean section are occasionally at risk. Underinflated lungs caused by generalized air sac atelectasis are the hallmark of this entity. In the premature infant, approximately 95% of the surface of the air sacs is covered by type I pneumocytes, where air exchange occurs, and 5% is covered by type II pneumocytes, which contain osmiophilic lamellar inclusion bodies that are responsible for the synthesis and storage of a lipoprotein: pulmonary surfactant. Pulmonary surfactant lowers the surface tension in the air sacs, increases pulmonary compliance, and thus decreases the work of breathing. The ability of air sacs to stay distended is part of the "driving force" preventing pulmonary edema (Starling forces). Surfactant synthesis begins at 24 to 28 weeks' gestation, and it gradually increases during gestation to reach normal levels at birth. It is the lack of surfactant and resulting poor compliance of the lungs that causes debris consisting of damaged or desquamated cells, exudative necrosis, and mucus (protein seepage) to line the alveolar sacs. This lining stains like hyaline cartilage under the microscope; hence the term *hyaline membrane disease.* A decreased lecithin-to-sphingomyelin ratio is present in the amniotic fluid of mothers who are carrying infants lacking surfactant; this indicator is useful prenatally to predict the development of IRDS in the infant. Clinically, infants with IRDS are identified

in the first few hours of life. Respiratory distress beginning *after* 8 hours of life is unlikely to be caused by surfactant deficiency.

Conventional radiographs show the low lung volumes, the typical "ground glass" (finely granular) appearance of the lungs, the poor definition of the pulmonary vessels, and an often more pronounced "bell-shaped" thorax. Air bronchograms are often evident and may extend to the periphery. Low lung volumes can also be seen in infants with neonatal pneumonia or pulmonary hemorrhage or edema, but hyperinflation in nonventilated infants virtually excludes IRDS. An effusion is seldom present, but a pneumothorax or pneumomediastinum at presentation is a bad predictor for survival (Fig. 2-36).

To prevent acidosis and hypoxemia in a child with IRDS, the diseased lungs must be ventilated and oxygenated to maintain open terminal air sacs and appropriate arterial blood gas levels. Positive-pressure ventilation (positive end-expiratory pressure [PEEP], continuous positive airway pressure [CPAP]) or oscillating jet ventilatory support is instituted after placement of an endotracheal tube. The "classic" surfactant-deficient lung with low volume often becomes relatively hyperinflated at this juncture.

In addition to supportive therapy with oxygen and diuretics, exogenous surfactant replacement has become a routine adjunct to increase pulmonary compliance and gas exchange; its use has been shown to reduce mortality. The effect on the chest

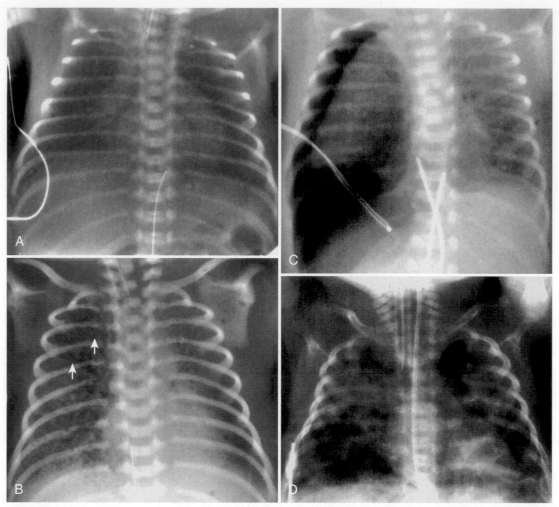

Figure 2-36. **A,** Typical "ground-glass" appearance in the lungs of a 27-week-gestation infant: hyaline membrane disease (HMD). **B,** Pulmonary interstitial emphysema *(arrows)* in the right hemithorax, and generalized atelectasis with air bronchograms almost to the periphery in the left. **C,** Right-sided pneumothorax. **D,** Dysplastic changes of pulmonary parenchyma bilaterally in a 28-week-gestation 1-month-old infant: bronchopulmonary dysplasia (BPD). Proper endotracheal tube tip position is about 1.5 vertebral bodies above the carina.

radiograph is variable. Clinical improvement even after one administered dose has been reported and may be evident as clearing of the lung fields on chest radiographs (Fig. 2-37). From this moment, the imaging findings of IRDS are the result of the *complications of therapy.*

Complications of ventilatory therapy include the following:

Overdistention of the air sacs in poorly compliant lungs may lead to rupture of the air sacs and a subsequent air leak into the pulmonary interstitium. This is referred to as *pulmonary interstitial emphysema* (PIE). PIE may develop as early as the first 24 hours of life, during which it carries a poor prognosis. Usually it occurs on day 2 or 3 of life and is characterized by peripheral streaks or bubbles of air in the interstitium. The air is presumably located in the lymphatics, and the condition can be unilateral or bilateral as well as asymptomatic. The air may migrate centrally, resulting in a pneumomediastinum, or it may migrate peripherally and rupture into the pleural space, resulting in a pneumothorax. Because infants are supine and because air rises to the highest point of the thorax, a pneumothorax is located paramediastinally and at the bases—resulting in the "sharp mediastinum" sign (Figs. 2-38A and 2-36C). The air may also dissect into the neck. One can distinguish this entity from a pneumopericardium by recalling that pericardial air (1) can rise only as high as the pericardial reflection at the level of the pulmonary arteries and (2) goes around the "bottom" of the heart. Extra-alveolar air collections may also be identified adjacent to the inferior pulmonary ligament (Fig. 2-38B).

In these premature infants, the ductus arteriosus may remain patent or may even become patent again because of persistent high intrapulmonary pressure. This most commonly becomes clinically evident at about 5 to 7 days of life. The increased interstitial markings caused by congestive failure secondary to this *persistent fetal circulation* (PFC) may complicate the radiographic findings and are often not recognized unless a series of radiographs are completed and evaluated over time.

After 28 days of ventilatory support and the resultant insults to the pulmonary parenchyma, interstitial pulmonary fibrosis may develop in about 10% of these premature infants. This fibrosis is often accompanied by exudative necrosis and a "honeycomb" appearance to the lungs on chest radiographs. This phase in the disease process is referred to as *bronchopulmonary dysplasia* (BPD).

Originally, BPD was defined as occurring when a premature newborn was treated with high oxygen concentration for more than 150 continuous hours under high pressure (CPAP, PEEP) on a respirator, resulting in injury to the lungs at the cellular level. Currently, BPD is defined as follows: After the initial destruction of the type I alveolar lining epithelium—in addition to mucosal necrosis, peribronchial edema, and hemorrhage—the result over time is a clinical and radiographic picture of interstitial fibrosis, cystlike emphysematous changes, and increased lung volume (see Fig. 2-36D). By 4 weeks (28 days) of age these changes are considered chronic and, in the presence of oxygen dependency and respiratory symptoms, constitute the syndrome of BPD.

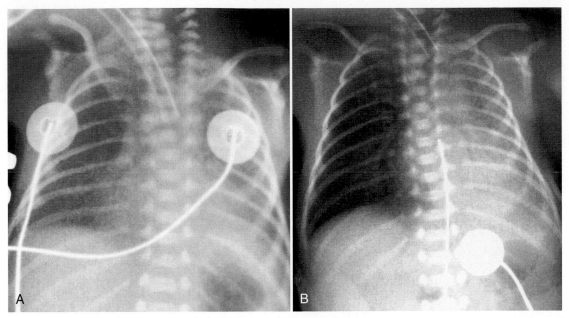

FIGURE 2-37. Hyaline membrane disease (HMD). Before (**A**) and 24 hours after (**B**) surfactant therapy. Radiographic appearances markedly improve on the right, probably after preferential infusion of surfactant mostly into the right mainstem bronchus.

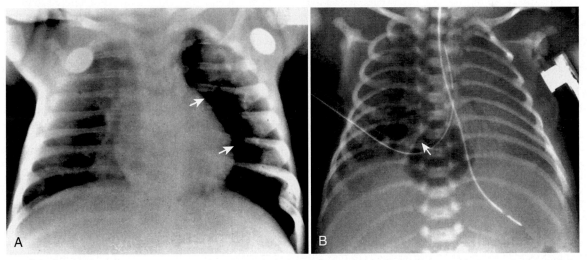

FIGURE 2-38. A, "Sharp mediastinum" sign caused by a medial pneumothorax *(arrows).* **B,** Extra-alveolar air collection outlines an inferior pulmonary ligament *(arrow).*

The radiographic appearance of BPD used to be classified into four stages, analogous to pathologic changes. This classification nicely reflected the course of the insults caused by the treatment of immature lungs. Today, the radiographic findings of HMD start at day 3, and by day 7, interstitial edema caused by leaking capillaries appears. Diuretics, pneumothoraces, and surfactant administration can all or individually clear these finding rapidly, and the "bubbly" stages III and IV are seldom seen today (see Fig. 2-37). The current use of this classification is thus not so much for staging per se, but rather as an easy way to remember the sequence of imaging findings for which one should be on the lookout. The stages are as follows:

- Stage I represents the classic granularity described as "ground glass" at birth.
- Stage II develops between 4 and 10 days of age, exhibiting a bilateral increased density caused by exudative necrosis.
- Stage III develops between 10 and 20 days of age and is characterized by the "honeycomb" appearance caused by

overdistention of alveoli and terminal air sacs within dysplastic interstitium.

- Stage IV develops after 1 month of age. There are fibrotic changes and scattered (cystic) emphysematous changes. This stage is associated with a mortality rate of between 40% and 50%.

If the infant survives (mortality 25% to 30%), there often is improvement in the appearance of the chest radiographs, progressing even to a normal chest radiograph at 3 to 5 years of age (in about 10% of BPD patients). Unfortunately, pulmonary function parameters remain abnormal, with restrictive changes evident as late as the teenage years, and there is an overall increased incidence of lower respiratory tract infections in these children.

Wilson-Mikity syndrome, a very rare condition seen in premature infants, is characterized by respiratory symptoms at 2 to 4 weeks of age. Some even doubt its existence, but others deem it a form of pre-HMD at 23 to 25 weeks that does not require early ventilatory support. Characteristically, chest radiographic findings are normal at birth yet reveal the typical changes indistinguishable

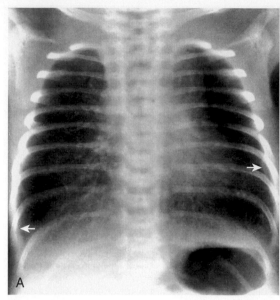

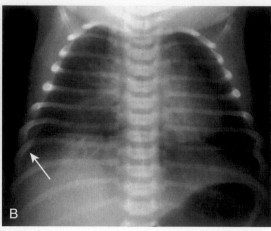

FIGURE 2-39. Transient tachypnea of a newborn. **A,** Hyperinflation, mild interstitial prominence. **B,** Occasional small effusions *(arrows)* may be noted. All findings had cleared by 24 to 48 hours after birth.

from BPD by 6 weeks. These changes are considered to be due to injury of the air sacs by room air as opposed to high oxygen concentration or toxicity. A virus has also been suggested as the cause of this condition. In most cases that have been described (50% to 70%), the infants survive.

In summary, a premature infant presents with an underinflated chest; all other (term) infants present with hyperinflation, which is discussed next.

Retained Fetal Lung Liquid (Transient Tachypnea of the Newborn)

The fetal lung is filled with fluid that, in turn, contributes to the amniotic fluid. During delivery, part of this fetal lung fluid is expressed from the airways (the birth canal "squeeze"), part is coughed or suctioned out, and part is resorbed by the lymphatics and the pulmonary veins. Impairment or delay of this process leads to difficulty in breathing, clinically evident as respiratory distress, in the newborn infant. This clearing process can be quantified as follows: lung fluid being cleared by the birth canal squeeze of the infant thorax during delivery, 30%, that being resorbed by lymphatics, 30%, and that being resorbed by the capillaries, 40%. Impairment or absence of any one of these mechanisms may exacerbate the "wet lung," or retained fetal lung liquid, and resultant tachypnea. Cesarean section, prolonged labor, and maternal anesthesia or diabetes, as well as a precipitous delivery, have all been shown to be contributing factors.

The typical infant with retained fetal lung fluid manifests tachypnea during the first 6 hours of life, displaying a peak of symptoms at 1 day of age and normalizing by 48 hours. Mild cyanosis, retraction, and grunting can occur. This condition affects about 5% of all term infants. There is an equal gender distribution. Conventional chest radiographs may show a mildly enlarged cardiothymic silhouette, interstitial edema, fluid within the fissures, and small pleural effusions (Fig. 2-39). The lungs are hyperinflated and start to clear at 12 hours, a process that should be complete (resulting in a normal chest radiograph) by 48 hours after birth. Differential diagnostic possibilities include cyanotic CHD with congestive heart failure, pneumonia or (meconium) aspiration, and hypervolemia or PFC.

Meconium Aspiration Syndrome

Approximately 10% of all term deliveries are accompanied by meconium staining of the amniotic fluid. Aspiration of this meconium-containing fluid in about half of these infants may result in presence of meconium below the level of the vocal cords; in about half of these cases, clinical symptoms occur. Meconium aspiration syndrome (MAS) is related to perinatal stress (hypoxia, prolonged labor), with a vagal response postulated as the triggering factor for intrauterine evacuation of meconium by the fetus. Concomitant fetal gasping caused by the intrauterine distress may facilitate the aspiration.

The aspirated meconium particles may produce bronchial obstruction and air trapping (check-valve mechanism), as well as a chemical pneumonitis. Secondary infection may occur, and the resultant hypoxia and vasospasm increases the risk of pulmonary hypertension and persistent fetal circulation. Conventional radiographs of the chest typically show bilateral asymmetric areas of atelectasis and hyperaeration caused by this check-valve mechanism of meconium aspiration as well as atelectasis caused by the irritative effect of meconium on the bronchial tree. The lungs are often hyperinflated, and there may be a concomitant pneumomediastinum or pneumothorax in about 25% of patients (Fig. 2-40).

Treatment is supportive and consists of antibiotics and oxygen. In severe cases, when oxygenation cannot be maintained by the infant, one option is ECMO. Another is high-frequency jet flow ventilation to allow for healing of the pneumonitis. Because the intrapulmonary pressure may remain high, meconium aspiration is often complicated by PFC as well.

Extracorporeal membrane oxygenation (ECMO) comes in two forms, venoarterial (classic) and the less common venovenous (Fig 2-40B and C). The latter is performed via a double-lumen catheter placed in the right atrium; this difference prevents the placement and injury of the carotid artery associated with the classic form of ECMO. The lungs become radiopaque, and fluid retention leads to anasarca and pleural effusions. In MAS, survival is 95% with ECMO; whereas in CDH, it has not significantly improved survival (45% mortality).

Neonatal Pneumonia

Neonatal pneumonia may be acquired in utero or perinatally. Prolonged labor, premature rupture of membranes, placental infection, and ascending infection from the perineum are predisposing factors. Respiratory distress with tachypnea and metabolic acidosis (occasionally progressing to shock) is the most common clinical scenario. The most common cause is group B hemolytic streptococcal infection, acquired in the birth canal. Other etiologic agents are *Pseudomonas, Enterobacter, Staphylococcus,* and *Klebsiella.* The incidence of neonatal pneumonia is

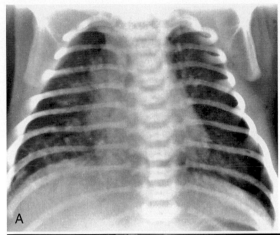

FIGURE 2-40. **A,** Meconium aspiration resulting in an asymmetric, somewhat nodular pattern in both lung fields, in addition to areas of mild hyperaeration (right apex). **B,** Venoarterial extracorporeal membrane oxygenation catheters in appropriate positions. **C,** Venovenous catheter in right atrium.

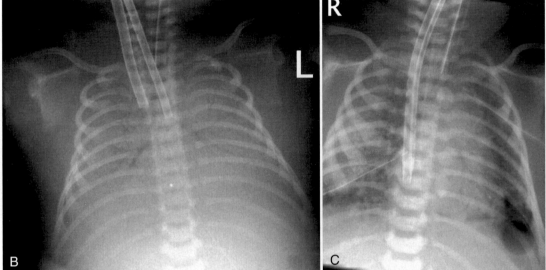

about 1 in 200 live births. Transplacentally acquired infections are rare.

The radiologic appearance of neonatal pneumonia is often identical to that of transient tachypnea of the newborn (TTN) or early HMD. A patchy, occasionally asymmetric, radiating, bilateral interstitial infiltrate is common (Fig. 2-41). A nodular pattern may predominate in hazy lungs, and an effusion is a common occurrence. Empyemas may develop and may suggest infection by *Staphylococcus* or *Klebsiella*. If neonatal pneumonia is untreated, mortality and morbidity rates are high; therefore early confirmation of the diagnosis and the institution of appropriate antibiotic therapy are critical.

Persistent Fetal Circulation

A physiologic event of right-to-left shunting persisting after birth, persistent fetal circulation has no clear cause. Normally, the ductus arteriosus functionally closes by 15 hours after birth, although anatomic closure may take days to weeks. In 1 in 1500 deliveries, fetal circulation persists. Increased sensitivity to intrauterine hypoxia, altered fetal pulmonary flow, and arterial muscle derangement have been implicated. It also may just be a transition phenomenon like TTN, in which time and maturation allow for an eventual return to normal as the high intrapulmonary pressure diminishes. Any of the neonatal pulmonary abnormalities discussed previously may be associated with PFC, likely secondary to increased pulmonary (interstitial) vascular resistance (pressure). There are no specific imaging findings.

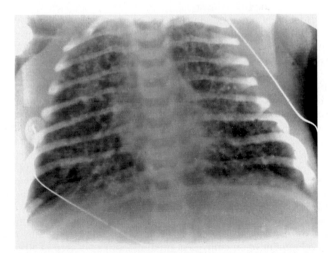

FIGURE 2-41. Neonatal pneumonia. Bilateral, coarse interstitial infiltrate, which may occasionally be nodular, is common.

Pulmonary Lymphangiectasia and Pulmonary Hemorrhage

Lymphangiectasia is defined as dilated lymph channels. In utero, embryologic lymph channels diminish in size to their expected neonatal caliber during weeks 6 to 20 of gestation. This process

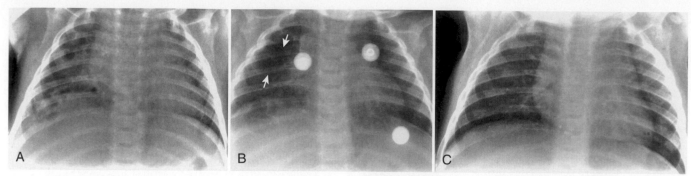

Figure 2-42. Staphylococcal pneumonia. AP radiographs of the chest show progressive clearing of the consolidation of pneumatocele formation *(arrows)* within 1 week (**A** and **B**), then clearing totally by 6 weeks (**C**).

may be interfered with by pulmonary venous obstruction or by the dilated lymph channels that may result from an anomalous development of the lymphatic system. About one third of cases occur in association with congenital cardiac defects that cause pulmonary venous obstruction (total anomalous pulmonary venous return, hypoplastic left heart syndrome). Conventional radiographs of pulmonary lymphangiectasia mimic the changes seen in TTN, or there may be a more nodular pattern. The condition is often fatal early in life.

Pulmonary hemorrhage, which is rare, is thought to be a form of pulmonary edema secondary to cardiac failure or to be related to the effects of exogenously administered surfactant. Its radiographic appearance is no different from that of edema fluid.

Inflammatory Lung Disease

There are four fairly distinct clinical syndromes in infection of the childhood lower respiratory (tracheobronchial tree and lung parenchyma) infection: croup, tracheobronchitis, bronchiolitis, and pneumonia. Croup was discussed earlier.

It is impossible to determine whether virus or bacterium causes the changes on a chest radiograph, and only an educated guess allows for identification an agent that causes a particular chest radiographic pattern.

In infancy and childhood, viruses cause most upper and lower respiratory tract infections, accounting for more than 90% of cases in children younger than 2 years, with respiratory syncytial virus (RSV) the causative agent in a third of these cases.

Bacterial Causes

Bacterial infection tends to cause alveolar exudates and lobar and segmental consolidations, as well as effusions. Most commonly caused by pneumococcus, HIB, and *Staphylococcus aureus*, clinically these infections have little to distinguish themselves from each other. Staphylococcal pneumonia occurs more commonly in early infancy, *H. influenzae* pneumonia most often between 6 and 12 months, and pneumococcal pneumonia more commonly between 1 and 3 years. Children with pneumonias due to these agents all have cough, chest pain, and (often) high fevers, which usually occur after an upper respiratory infection. Staphylococcal pneumonia and *H. influenzae* pneumonia can also be complicated by the development of an empyema. Pneumatoceles develop in 50% of patients with staphylococcal infection; they are thought to be a form of PIE and local emphysema caused by airway obstruction and subsequent check-valve mechanism. They are often multiple but resolve completely in about 6 weeks (Fig. 2-42). Pneumatoceles are less likely to occur with a streptococcal pneumonia.

Imaging is usually not helpful in determining the organism in pneumonia. Consolidation is usually lobar, may be accompanied by air bronchograms, and resolves in 2 to 3 weeks. In children younger than 8 years, a staphylococcal or pneumococcal

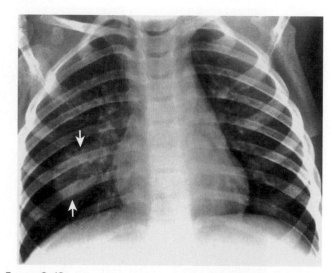

Figure 2-43. "Round pneumonia" in a 3-year-old child with pneumococcal pneumonia *(arrows)*. The lesion resolved in 2 weeks.

pneumonia can sometimes be sphere-shaped with unsharp edges. Such a rounded lesion may mimic a metastatic lesion and is often called a "round pneumonia" (Fig. 2-43). These pneumonias resolve completely after proper antimicrobial therapy. The round shape is probably a result of centrifugal spread of the multiplying organisms through the pores of Kohn and the channels of Lambert. CT may be able to demonstrate an enhancing rim around an empyema.

Pertussis Pneumonia

Pertussis pneumonia is a contagious disease most common in children younger than 5 years. Translated as "severe cough" from the Latin and as "100 days" from the Chinese, pertussis is caused by *Bordetella pertussis* and occurs more commonly in girls. Conventional radiographs reveal streaky perihilar infiltrates with (most often) unilateral hilar adenopathy, a pattern sometimes called the "shaggy heart" appearance (see Fig. 2-47).

Mycoplasma pneumoniae

Mycoplasma pneumoniae is a ubiquitous agent causing epidemics of respiratory infection, primarily in older school-age children and adolescents. It is the most common cause of pneumonia in children older than 5 years. Of those infected, 50% have tracheobronchitis, 30% pneumonia, and 10% each pharyngitis and otitis media. Clinically, symptoms are less severe but more common than in true bacterial pneumonias. Chest radiographs may reveal segmental, subsegmental, or reticulonodular interstitial infiltrates. Lobar involvement may be seen predominantly in the

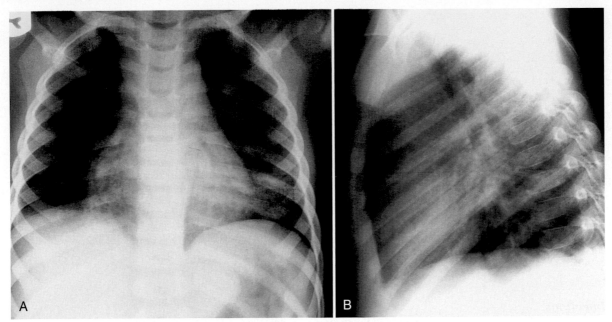

FIGURE 2-44. Chest radiographs illustrate pneumonia due to *Mycoplasma pneumoniae,* characterized by multiple areas of atelectasis in the lower lobes (**A**) and by hyperinflation (**B**).

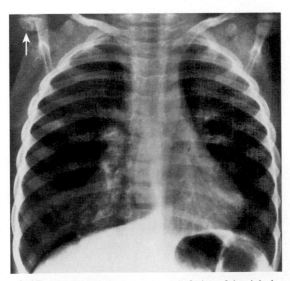

FIGURE 2-45. AP radiograph reveals hyperinflation of the right lung and right middle lobe atelectasis, and a well-circumscribed right humeral proximal epiphyseal lesion *(arrow)* in a patient with tuberculosis.

lower lobes. Effusions occur in about 20% of patients (Fig. 2-44). Treatment is supportive and recovery slow (1 week or more).

Mycobacterial Infection

Primary tuberculosis caused by *Mycobacterium tuberculosis* initially affects the lung but may spread throughout the body. Almost all cases in the infant and young child begin in the lung after exposure through inhalation. Initially there is an exudate that, over approximately 3 to 8 weeks as hypersensitivity develops, is followed by enlarging hilar and mediastinal nodes. Calcification and caseation, as well as parenchymal scarring, may ensue. Radiographically, this infiltrative process, with local lymphatic and node involvement and parenchymal scarring, is called the primary complex of Ranke (Fig. 2-45). With the development of resistance, postprimary tuberculosis occurs, manifesting as consolidation of

an entire segment or lobe and central lymph node enlargement, as well as pleural effusions and pulmonary cavitation. Seeding of organisms in the lungs through lymphatics and the venous system results in miliary (secondary) tuberculosis (2- to 3-mm nodules) within 6 months (Fig. 2-46).

The differential diagnosis of miliary nodular interstitial lesions in the lung is listed in Box 2-2

Chlamydia trachomatis *Pneumonia*

Pneumonia caused by *Chlamydia trachomatis* fits in neither the bacterial nor the viral group. *C. trachomatis* is probably an obligate intracellular parasite, and it usually causes a neonatal infection acquired after passage of the fetus through the cervix and vagina. The infant typically is presented at 3 to 6 weeks of age with respiratory symptoms and occasional associated pulmonary hemorrhage. The infant often (30% of the time) also has concomitant chlamydial conjunctivitis. Clinical and radiologic findings mimic those of bronchiolitis, with diffuse perihilar interstitial infiltrates in hyperexpanded chest radiographs (Fig. 2-47). Effusions may occur; consolidations are rare.

Viral Etiologies

As noted, airspace disease, segmental or lobar, is more likely to be bacterial in origin. Airway disease that manifests as peribronchial thickening, hyperinflation, and scattered atelectasis ("disordered aeration") is more likely to be viral in origin.

In children younger than 2 years, infection with respiratory syncytial virus—as well as parainfluenza types 1, 2, and 3, influenza, and adenovirus—leads to inflammatory edema, surface cell necrosis, and increased mucus production. Radiographs of the chest show peribronchial cuffing and hyperinflation. The terminal and respiratory bronchioles are most involved, but the alveoli are not. Often there are clear manifestations of disordered aeration— areas of atelectasis that, if sequential films were obtained, would be seen to clear within 24 to 48 hours and might reappear in other areas in the chest (see Fig. 2-2). The apices are spared; effusions and empyemas are rare. Resolution of these findings can take up to 2 weeks. In children older than 2 years, this appearance and course are characteristic of reactive airway disease (asthma). Cystic fibrosis should be considered if repeated episodes of bronchiolitis occur in the appropriate patient population.

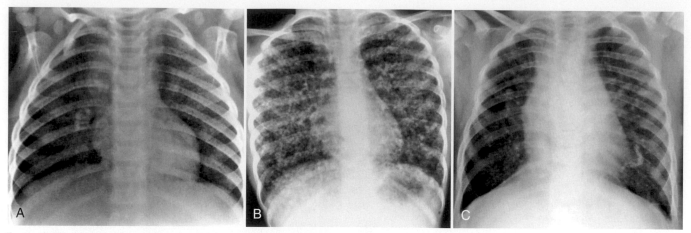

FIGURE 2-46. Nodular interstitial changes. **A,** AP chest radiograph reveals multiple miliary (millet seed) interstitial nodules as well as right hilar and paratracheal lymph node enlargement in miliary tuberculosis. **B,** Metastatic papillary carcinoma of the thyroid in an 11-year-old girl. Note deviation of the trachea to the right. **C,** Lymphoid interstitial pneumonitis (biopsy-proven).

Other Infections

Pulmonary mycotic infections are relatively rare in children except in endemic areas. Histoplasmosis is endemic in the mid-central United States, whereas coccidiomycosis is endemic in the southwestern United States. Radiographic findings are often lacking, but affected children may have clinical findings similar to those in primary tuberculosis, with characteristic hilar and mediastinal adenopathy and miliary granulomas in the pulmonary interstitium after 3 to 5 days.

In histoplasmosis, late calcification of the parenchymal lesions and nodes is common. Effusions are rare.

Opportunistic infections occur in the patient with an altered immune response state (acquired immunodeficiency syndrome [AIDS], after chemotherapy for leukemia/lymphoma, or after transplant surgery). *Pneumocystis carinii* pneumonia, varicella, and certain fungi are the more common entities that may cause infection in the lungs.

Infection with *P. carinii* (a protozoon) occurs in debilitated or otherwise immunocompromised children and is seen most often in those treated for leukemia or lymphoma. The child clinically presents with cough, tachypnea, and malaise, and the infection is often fatal. It is the most common opportunistic pulmonary infection in children with AIDS. Lung biopsy is necessary to confirm the diagnosis. Early chest radiographs may mimic those in children with a viral respiratory infection and then may progress from a reticulonodular interstitial process to a diffuse alveolar consolidation predominantly affecting the hila and bases. Lung volumes are normal to low. Pleural effusions may occur, but hilar adenopathy is uncommon (Fig. 2-48).

Chickenpox (varicella) is a highly contagious viral disease of childhood, with mortality highest in adults and immunocompromised hosts. Clinically, cough, fever, and a vesicular rash are generally accompanied by mild constitutional symptoms. Airspace disease (1% of all cases) associated with chickenpox in children occurs most often in the immunocompromised host. The younger the child, the less likely chickenpox complicated by airspace disease will develop. Radiographs of the chest initially show nodular infiltrates that may progress to large segmental areas of patchy consolidation, predominantly in the bases and perihilar regions. Total clearing is virtually guaranteed, although punctate calcifications may be evident within 2 years after the acute illness and may persist through life.

Aspergillosis is one of the more common sporadic infections that frequently affects children with underlying conditions such as asthma, cystic fibrosis, or chronic granulomatous disease of childhood and, as such, is regarded as a hypersensitivity reaction. It is almost always a complication in neutropenic

> **BOX 2-2. Differential Diagnosis of Miliary Nodular Interstitial Disease**
>
> Tuberculosis
> Histoplasmosis, blastomycosis, cryptococcosis, and coccidioidomycosis
> Varicella (airspace disease is rare)
> Lymphoid interstitial pneumonitis (human immunodeficiency virus–positive mother)
> Langerhans cell histiocytosis (Hand-Schüller-Christian disease)
> Metastatic (papillary) thyroid carcinoma (rare)
> Niemann-Pick disease or Gaucher disease (rare)

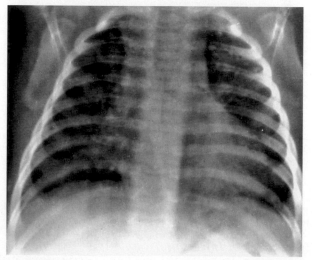

FIGURE 2-47. Perihilar, diffuse interstitial infiltrates resulting in the "shaggy heart" sometimes seen in pertussis and *C. trachomatis* infection.

immunocompromised patients, in whom it is considered invasive. A suprainfection in a preexisting cavitary lesion, called a "mycetoma," is rare in children.

The radiographs of the chest of the first variant, the angioinvasive *Aspergillus* infection, are characterized by a consolidation with a "halo" sign, a ground-glass zone surrounding the nodule.

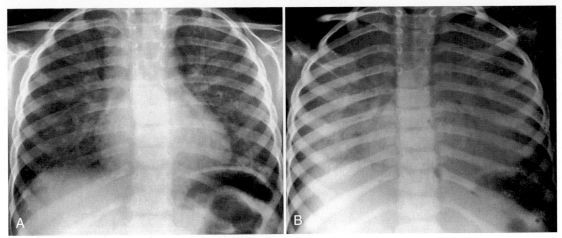

Figure 2-48. A, *P. carinii* pneumonia manifests as a diffuse reticular granular infiltrate bilaterally, progressing (**B**) to consolidation without hilar enlargement but with a right-sided effusion.

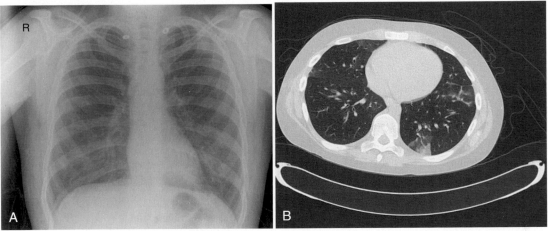

Figure 2-49. A, Chest radiograph in a teenager with acute lymphocytic leukemia reveals left upper lobe streaky densities. B, CT scan shows additional lesion in the left lower lobe as well as bronchiectasis in the right lower lobe.

In a later stage an "air crescent" sign can be seen, an air collection surrounding a necrotic mass in the area of consolidation.

Although rare in children, a mycetoma may subsequently form in a preexisting cavity. The mycetoma consists of *Aspergillus* spores.

Hypersensitivity or allergic aspergillosis mimics the imaging finding of bronchiolitis and can be characterized by mucus plugging, the "gloved finger" sign (Fig. 2-49).

Bronchiectasis is seen well on CT, allowing for early intervention with steroids to prevent damage to the airway.

Aspiration Pneumonia

Aspiration pneumonia often mimics ordinary pneumonia, may lead to superimposed infection, may be acute or chronic, and may have either fulminant pulmonary involvement or no effect at all. The degree of lung involvement depends to a large extent on what, how much, and how long (often) the child has aspirated. Aspiration is gravity dependent. If an infant (who preferably lies supine) aspirates, the right upper lobe and right lower lobe are common sites of involvement. The right mainstem bronchus is a "straight shot." If an older child (who spends more time in the vertical position) aspirates, the lower lobes are predominantly affected. Chest radiographic findings range from patchy airspace consolidation, with or without confluent areas, to atelectasis to a mixture of both. Perihilar peribronchial involvement is also common, mimicking bronchiolitis. Effusions are rare.

In the diagnostic evaluation of aspiration pneumonia, it is important to search for an anatomic anomaly—such as gastroesophageal reflux, an abnormal connection (tracheoesophageal fistula or cleft) between the trachea and esophagus, or swallowing dysfunction—that may predispose the child to aspiration. For the search for a tracheoesophageal connection, the child should be evaluated in the prone position, using a nasogastric tube that is withdrawn in small increments while contrast material is injected. Although occasionally helpful, this technique was originally designed to evaluate for a recurrent a tracheoesophageal fistula. Endoscopy may also be useful. An upper gastrointestinal examination evaluates for the other two possibilities.

Populations at risk for aspiration pneumonia include anesthetized children, near-drowning victims, and children suffering seizures (postictal).

Asthma (Reactive Airway Disease)

Asthma is a chronic and diffuse lung disease characterized by hypersensitivity (immunoglobulin E mediated) of the airways to irritants of all kinds (e.g., allergens, cigarette smoke, pollen), resulting in bronchospasm. This leads to recurrent bouts of wheezing, cough, and dyspnea and often results in recurrent

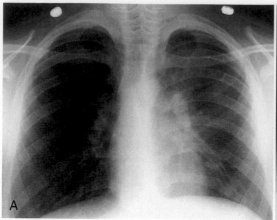

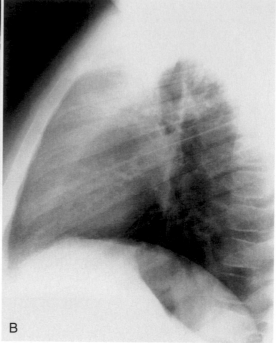

FIGURE 2-50. Teenager with asthma. **A,** AP chest radiograph demonstrates volume loss, increased overall density, and hilar prominence on the left. **B,** Lateral view confirms left upper lobe collapse. Subsequent reexpansion occurred after pulmonary physical therapy.

pulmonary infections. Approximately 50% of children suffering from reactive airway disease become symptomatic before 2 years of age, with 80% to 90% diagnosed by age 5 years. Chest imaging may show hyperaeration with peribronchial thickening and may demonstrate complications, including atelectasis, effusions, pneumothorax, and pneumomediastinum (Fig. 2-50). Most often, though, the chest radiograph in a child with an exacerbation of "asthma" is normal.

Cystic Lung Disease

Cystic Fibrosis

Cystic fibrosis is inherited as a single autosomal recessive trait caused by any one of more than 900 mutations in the CF transmembrane regulator gene (CFTG), and is the most common lethal genetic disease affecting Caucasians . It is a generalized dysfunction of the exocrine (mucous) glands, affecting approximately 1 in 2000 white individuals. It is very uncommon in African Americans (1 in 20,000) and Asians (even lower incidence at 1 in 90,000). Patients may have respiratory symptoms at all ages, although in a small proportion (approximately 5%) the earliest symptoms (related to the gastrointestinal tract: meconium ileus, malabsorption, and failure to thrive) can occur at birth or in infancy.

Pulmonary involvement—ranging from bronchiolitis in infants to chronic cough and recurrent respiratory infections in older children to chronic pulmonary disease in adolescents—eventually occurs in almost all patients. Fatigue and weight loss from malabsorption and recurrent pulmonary infections eventually develop. When respiratory insufficiency and progressive pulmonary arterial hypertension supervene, death usually occurs by the fourth decade, primarily because of pulmonary complications, including pulmonary hemorrhage.

Imaging findings on chest radiographs may range initially from completely normal to those indistinguishable from findings in bronchiolitis in infants and children. Often there is hyperinflation, and when progressive mucus plugging with superimposed infection injures the pulmonary parenchyma, the result is bronchial wall thickening, mucoid impaction, and bronchiectatic cavities located predominantly in the upper lobes (Fig. 2-51). Prominent hilar regions are often seen secondary to reactive nodal enlargement caused by recurrent bouts of infection. This constellation of findings (reactive nodal hyperplasia) is caused by the recurrent infections (*P. aeruginosa* and *S. aureus*) in the early stages of CF. Eventually, large pulmonary arteries that result from developing pulmonary arterial hypertension can also contribute to a prominent hilar region.

Complications of CF include pneumothorax, occasionally of the tension variety. Only in 65% of patients is such a pneumothorax evacuated by chest tube, because stiffening of the lung parenchyma caused by fibrosis prevents it. In addition, lobar atelectasis and pulmonary hypertension with cor pulmonale also frequently develop. Bronchial artery hemorrhage is a grave complication, and the finding of cardiac silhouette enlargement in a patient with CF is ominous for the development of congestive heart failure.

In the evaluation of chest radiographs, a number of scoring methods have been devised. Of these, the method of Brassfield (0 = normal, 4 = severe changes) is most often used. This scoring system correlates well with pulmonary function parameters, clinical criteria, and morbidity and has a high degree of interobserver reproducibility. It is most often used by pulmonary specialists and surgeons to help decide long-term therapy.

Kartagener Syndrome

Kartagener syndrome is an autosomal recessive disorder that is characterized by thoracic and abdominal situs inversus as well as the presence of immotile cilia that predispose to sinusitis, otitis media, and bronchiectasis. The ciliary immotility is due to a deficiency of the dynein arms of the cilia. These immotile cilia are also present in other areas in which cilia occur, namely in the inner ear and seminiferous tubules. Affected patients therefore suffer from deafness and infertility.

Imaging frequently suggests the diagnosis of Kartagener syndrome by demonstrating situs inversus along with two or more of the sinus, ear, or bronchiectatic components (Fig. 2-52). With a history of infertility or deafness, the diagnosis is confirmed.

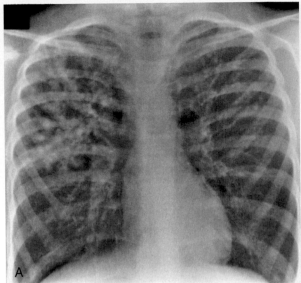

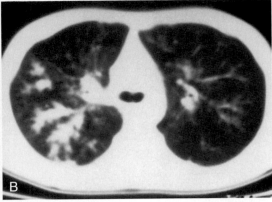

FIGURE 2-51. Cystic fibrosis. **A,** Chest radiograph with classic upper lobe bronchiectatic changes with a superimposed *P. aeruginosa* infection in the right upper lobe. **B,** CT examination confirms these changes.

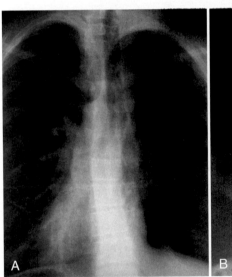

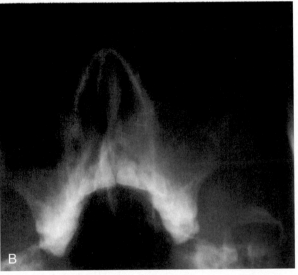

FIGURE 2-52. Kartagener's syndrome. **A,** Chest radiograph demonstrates situs inversus totalis. **B,** Waters view reveals opaque maxillary sinuses.

Bronchiectasis

Localized bronchiectasis is most often due to postinfectious causes, such as tuberculosis (TB), viral or bacterial pneumonias, and measles, or is secondary to infections superimposed on immune deficiency syndromes. Bronchiectatic change occurs less commonly than in the past because of improved medical therapy. Thin-section high-resolution CT can demonstrate the bronchiectasis. It can reliably differentiate between cylindric (tubular dilatation), varicose (resembling varicose veins), and cystic or saccular (balloon-like dilatation) types of bronchiectasis. An association of bronchiectasis with tracheal ectasia and defective elastic tissue has been described (Mounier-Kuhn syndrome).

Swyer-James Syndrome

Idiopathic unilateral hyperlucent lung (Swyer-James or Macleod syndrome) is characterized by unilateral hyperlucency of the lung associated with a decrease in the number and size of the airways and pulmonary vessels. It is thought to be due to a preceding viral pneumonitis that progresses to a necrotizing bronchiolitis. The resultant fibrosis produces a "bronchiolitis obliterans," manifested on chest radiographs as hyperlucency,

diminished lung markings, and a lung often decreased in size (see Fig. 2-29).

The differential diagnosis of a unilateral hyperlucent lung includes endobronchial foreign body, pneumothorax, congenital lobar emphysema, hypoplasia of the lung or pulmonary artery and compensatory hyperinflation, and post–radiation therapy shrinkage of the lungs.

Cysts
Solitary

The differential diagnostic possibilities of solitary cysts include pneumatocele (from *Staphylococcus*, tuberculosis, trauma), inflammation (from *Staphylococcus*, *Klebsiella*), pulmonary foregut malformation, and bronchogenic or neurenteric cysts. Necrotic tumor is a rare occurrence, as are echinococcal cysts (Fig. 2-53).

Multiple

Multiple cysts may be due to multiple occurrences of some of the aforementioned causes (e.g., pneumatocele or metastatic disease, such as papillomatosis, metastatic osteosarcoma, or Wilms tumor).

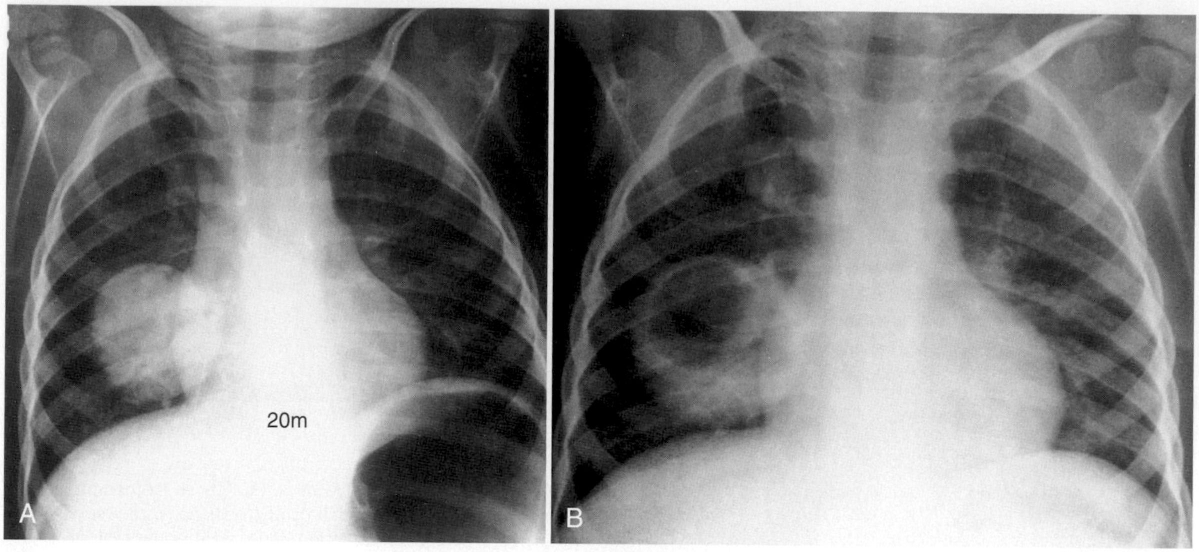

FIGURE 2-53. **A,** AP chest radiograph shows necrotic metastatic rhabdomyosarcoma in a 2-year-old child. **B,** Radiograph obtained 2 weeks later in same patient.

In addition, a diaphragmatic hernia in a neonate may manifest as multiple cysts once air replaces fluid after birth.

Less commonly, the cystic changes seen in surfactant deficiency disease (HMD) may manifest as multiple, occasionally bilateral, cysts. Bilateral cystic lesions may also be seen in CF, septic emboli, and posttraumatic cysts. Very rare causes are Wegener granulomatosis and hyperimmunoglobulinemia E (Buckley syndrome), the latter being additionally characterized by skin lesions and abdominal abscesses.

Lung Neoplasms

See Box 2-3.

Malignant

Metastatic disease to the lung is far more common than a primary lung tumor, with Wilms tumor being the most common primary lesion in infants and children. Osteosarcoma and Ewing sarcoma follow in incidence. Osteogenic sarcoma and rhabdomyosarcoma may be associated with pneumothorax or effusion.

Primary malignant lung tumors are extremely rare. The most common, previously known as bronchial adenomas, implying benign disease, are really lesions such as bronchial carcinoids arising from Kulchitsky (neuroendocrine) cell or APUD system cells and account for 75% of these; cylindromas and mucoepidermoid carcinomas account for the rest. Endobronchial in location, symptoms depend on size and location. Others are sarcomatous in origin.

Benign

Rare benign neoplastic lesions include pulmonary blastoma, bronchial adenoma, and postinflammatory pseudotumor. About half exhibit low-grade malignant characterization. The carcinoid type of bronchial adenoma is more common; the majority of these are located in the (right) mainstem bronchi and often manifest as foreign bodies with or without hemoptysis. Small nodules include hamartomas and granulomas (TB, histoplasmosis) (see Fig. 2-47); larger nodules include postinflammatory pseudotumors (plasma cell granulomas) (Fig. 2-54). Both arteriovenous malformations and hemangiomas are extremely rare in childhood. Bronchogenic cysts that are located in the parenchyma appear as lung masses that seldom contain calcium and may be solid or air-filled, depending on the extent of communication with the airways.

Box 2-3. Pulmonary Nodules

SOLITARY PULMONARY NODULES

Congenital
Bronchogenic cyst
Arteriovenous malformation or varix (lower lobes)
Sequestration

Inflammatory
Round pneumonia
Abscess
Granuloma (tuberculosis, fungus)
Plasma cell granuloma (pulmonary blastoma, inflammatory pseudotumor)

Neoplastic
Bronchial adenoma
Metastasis (e.g., Wilms tumor, osteosarcoma)
Hamartoma, pulmonary blastoma

MULTIPLE PULMONARY NODULES

Inflammatory
Viral (varicella)
Granuloma (tuberculosis, histoplasmosis, sarcoidosis)
Lymphocytic interstitial pneumonitis

Neoplastic
Metastatic (Wilms tumor, osteosarcoma, papillary thyroid cancer)
Laryngeal papillomatosis

Congenital
Multiple arteriovenous malformations (rare)
Lymphangiectasia

Miscellaneous Diffuse Interstitial Lung Diseases

Chronic Granulomatous Disease

Chronic granulomatous disease of childhood is an X-linked recessive disorder that usually manifests before the age of 3 years—because of increased susceptibility to infection by

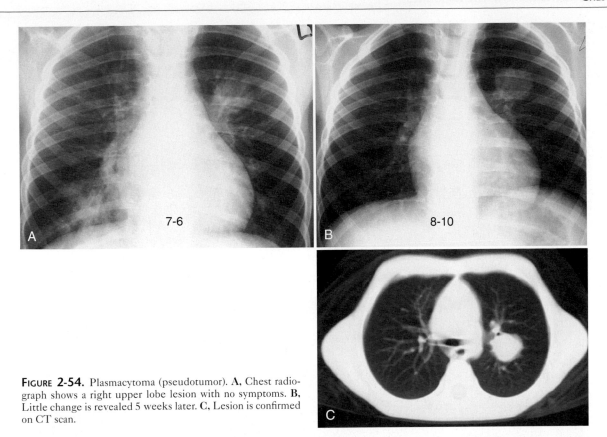

7-6

8-10

FIGURE 2-54. Plasmacytoma (pseudotumor). **A,** Chest radiograph shows a right upper lobe lesion with no symptoms. **B,** Little change is revealed 5 weeks later. **C,** Lesion is confirmed on CT scan.

usually nonpathogenic organisms—with lymphadenopathy, hepatosplenomegaly, and pneumonia. The pathophysiology rests in an enzymatic defect that prohibits the intracellular killing of bacteria and fungi. Granuloma formation in lung, liver, and lymph nodes as well as in the wall of the gastrointestinal tract may cause symptoms. Radiographs of the chest may show hilar enlargement; hepatomegaly and antral or esophageal narrowing (demonstrated after administration of oral contrast agents) are other abnormalities that can occur (see Chapter 4).

Sarcoidosis
Although relatively rare in children, sarcoidosis does occur between the ages of 5 and 15 years, predominantly in the African-American population and without gender predominance. It manifests as respiratory distress in 25% of cases. Pulmonary function testing reveals restrictive change that may be especially severe in the acute phase of disease. A rash, arthritis, and uveitis are much more frequent presenting symptoms in young infants.

In older children the imaging findings always include bilateral hilar lymphadenopathy, almost always in association with bilateral paratracheal lymphadenopathy (80%). Reticulonodular parenchymal involvement during childhood is seen in about two thirds of patients, about the same proportion as seen in adults (Fig. 2-55).

Acquired Immunodeficiency Syndrome
Approximately 2% of all AIDS cases occur in children, with about 80% diagnosed before 2 years of age. The major risk factors are maternal transmission and blood transfusions of the virus (human immunodeficiency virus), leading to infection of the infant that is clinically manifested as impaired helper T-cell function. The lung disease in pediatric patients consists of acute pulmonary infections caused predominantly by *P. carinii* and cytomegalovirus and eventually leading to chronic lymphocytic infiltration

or lymphatic interstitial pneumonia. Serious bacterial infections *(Streptococcus, H. influenzae)* may then supervene. The finding on radiographs of the chest in the early phases is predominantly a central, parahilar interstitial infiltrate (Fig. 2-47C), which may become more diffuse and nodular in appearance, mimicking miliary TB. Lung biopsy is the diagnostic test of choice.

Primary Pulmonary Histiocytosis X
Langerhans cell histiocytosis (LCH) may affect the lung parenchyma in about one half of patients with the disease. Males are affected more often than females. Clinical signs include cough and dyspnea. Conventional chest radiographs show overaeration, peribronchial thickening resulting in perihilar infiltrates, and occasional nodular appearance of the interstitium (Fig. 2-56). Imaging findings may (rarely) be confused with thoracic sarcoidosis in teenagers or with BPD in infants and children.

MEDIASTINUM
Mediastinal masses are the most common thoracic masses in children (Box 2-4). Eighty percent are made up by the lesions listed in boldface in Box 2-4. Approximately 30% develop before age 12 years, and about 30% occur in the anterior compartment, 30% in the middle compartment, and 40% in the posterior compartment.

Compartmentalization of the mediastinum represents an arbitrary classification. Classically the mediastinum has been divided into a superior portion and an inferior portion (a line drawn between the manubrial sternal junction and the T4 to T5 disc space); the inferior portion has been divided into anterior, middle, and posterior portions in slightly different ways by, among others, Felson and Hope. This division is slightly more difficult to apply to the mediastinum of infants and children, but for practical purposes the *anterior* mediastinum (A) consists of structures anterior to a line drawn along the anterior edge of the vascular

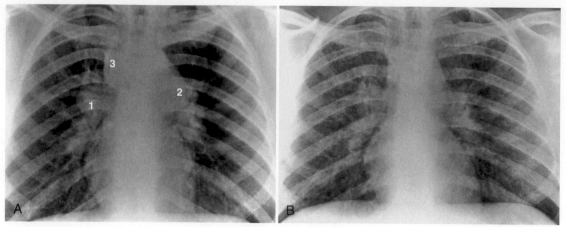

Figure 2-55. Sarcoidosis. **A,** Bilateral hilar (1, 2) and paratracheal (3) adenopathy. **B,** Reticulonodular parenchymal involvement.

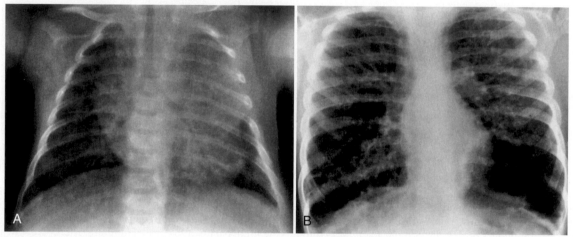

Figure 2-56. A, Nodular interstitial changes of Langerhans cell histiocytosis (LCH). **B,** Chronic interstitial changes of LCH resembling those of bronchopulmonary dysplasia.

pedicle, the prevascular space between the sternum and the pericardium, and the *posterior* mediastinum (P) consists of the structures posterior to a line drawn through the anterior edge of the vertebral bodies. The *middle* mediastinum (M) is the resultant compartment between these two, which contains the heart and great vessels, tracheobronchial tree, vagus and phrenic nerves, and lymph nodes. These compartments are easily superimposed on transverse imaging modalities such as CT and MRI (Fig. 2-57). After identification of a mediastinal lesion on conventional chest radiographs, CT and MRI are the preferred modalities for further evaluation of the middle and anterior mediastinum, but MRI is definitely the preferred modality for posterior mediastinal lesions.

Anterior Mediastinum

Thymus

The major occupant of the anterior mediastinum is the thymus, formed of two asymmetric lobes whose variability in size and shape is virtually limitless. The thymus shrinks quite dramatically under the stress of systemic illness or steroid therapy; it regenerates upon resolution of the stress or discontinuation of steroid therapy and may revert to the same shape or size.

A "rebound" thymus is larger than before the insult in 25% of children. Marked lobularity is never normal. The thymus also adapts to its surrounding structures yet normally does not displace structures such as vessels and the trachea. On conventional

---

Box 2-4. Mediastinal Masses

ANTERIOR
Thymus: normal, rebound hypertrophy, thymoma
Teratoma (three layers), dermoid (two layers)
Terrible lymphoma
Ectopic thyroid
Bronchogenic cyst

MIDDLE
Inflammatory lymph nodes or lymphoma
Foregut abnormalities (esophageal duplication, bronchogenic cysts)
Prominent pulmonary vessels, aortic dilatation or aneurysm
Pericardial abnormalities

POSTERIOR
Neurally based tumors: ganglioneuroma, ganglioneuroblastoma, neuroblastoma
Congenital pulmonary or pleural lesions: sequestration, bronchogenic or neurenteric cyst

SUPERIOR
Cystic hygroma
Bronchogenic cyst
Neurally based tumors
Rare vascular lesions

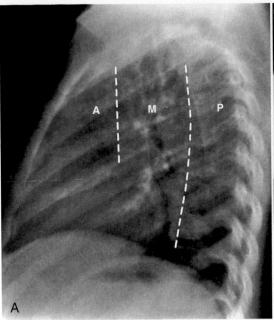
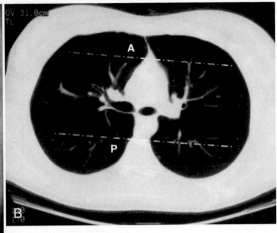

FIGURE 2-57. Mediastinal compartmentalization on lateral radiograph (**A**) and CT scan (**B**).

radiographs, because of its location, the thymus margins may be indented by the anterior ribs (thymic wave) (Fig. 2-58A). The thymus changes shape during respiration (by elongating and narrowing on inspiration), which can be visualized better at fluoroscopy (see Fig. 2-1). Occasionally a notch may be seen along the left cardiothymic border, delineating the junction of heart and thymus. The right lobe of the thymus can insinuate itself into the minor fissure (the "sail" sign) (Fig. 2-58B and C). On conventional radiographs of the chest, thymic tissue *is* visible in children up to 3 years of age and *may be* visible in children up to 8 or 9 years. On CT, thymic tissue may be distinct until the early teens (see Fig. 2-32C). Hyperthyroidism or Addison disease may cause the thymus to enlarge abnormally; infiltrative disorders such as lymphoma and leukemia and Langerhans cell histiocytosis may do so as well. On US, the thymus is homogeneous in density, although the follicular structure can be seen with the increasing resolving power of modern US equipment. On CT or MRI, the thymus is homogeneous throughout childhood, with an attenuation similar to or slightly greater than that of adjacent chest wall muscle on unenhanced studies. On MRI, the thymus is slightly hyperintense on T_1-weighted images and slightly less intense than fat on T_2-weighted images (see Fig. 2-32B).

A hypoplastic thymus is often present in premature infants because of stress. In aplasia of the thymus (DiGeorge syndrome), infants are born with little or no thymic tissue (or parathyroid glands) because of maldevelopment of the third and fourth pharyngeal pouches during the 6th to 12th weeks of gestational life. Congenital anomalies associated with DiGeorge syndrome include the tetralogy of Fallot, truncus arteriosus, transposition of the great vessels, ventricular septal defect, and absence of the pulmonary valve.

Neoplasms
About 30% of all mediastinal masses occur in the anterior mediastinum.

Lymphoma
After leukemia and central nervous system tumors, lymphoma is the third most common neoplasm of childhood. It is the most common anterior mediastinal mass, accounting for a quarter of all mediastinal masses. In about 30% of patients with lymphoma there is (bilateral) mediastinal lymphadenopathy. These findings

occur also in about 50% of children with acute lymphocytic leukemia (ALL), giving rise to the "leukemia/lymphoma" syndrome (Fig. 2-59). There are two major groups of lymphoma, as follows:

Non-Hodgkin lymphoma (NHL) usually manifests in an insidious fashion, with few specific symptoms. NHL makes up more than half (60%) of lymphomas in children, which represent 6% of all childhood cancers. There are marked clinical and laboratory similarities to ALL, which is the reason why leukemia and lymphoma are often referred to as a single entity in the pediatric age group. The peak age of presentation of NHL is around 9 years, and boys outnumber girls 3:1. More than 70% of patients have disseminated disease at the time of presentation.

There are four major types of NHL (Table 2-2). Type I usually occurs in a supradiaphragmatic location, types II and III are usually subdiaphragmatic in location, and type IV can occur anywhere but is rare in the mediastinum. Of note is that abdominal NHL is often of B-cell origin, whereas mediastinal NHL is often of T-cell origin. In addition, NHL manifests primarily in *extranodal* form, and overall, the most common primary site is the ileocecal region, followed by the mediastinum. NHL spreads hematogenously, and there is a mediastinal mass in about 50% of affected patients. A pleural effusion often occurs in this setting, and tracheobronchial compression occurs in 85%.

Hodgkin lymphoma occurs in the pediatric age group in about 10% of all cases. In children its incidence is slightly less than that of NHL (40%). There is no difference from the adult disease in mode of presentation, imaging appearance, histologic features, treatment, or prognosis, except for a male preponderance. The diagnosis is made on biopsy, with the Reed-Sternberg cell the classic marker. The nodular sclerotic type occurs in 60% and the mixed cellularity type in 25% of cases; the lymphocyte-prominent type (10%) and lymphocyte-depleted type (5%) account for the rest.

The site of origin is almost invariably nodal, and the disease spreads by direct continuity (Fig. 2-60). Most patients (85%) initially present with a mediastinal mass, 30% with hilar adenopathy. Hodgkin lymphoma most commonly manifests as cervical lymphadenopathy, almost always occurring concomitantly with mediastinal involvement (in 90%). Para-aortic and celiac nodes are much more commonly involved than mesenteric lymph nodes. In contradistinction to NHL, the initial clinical onset of Hodgkin

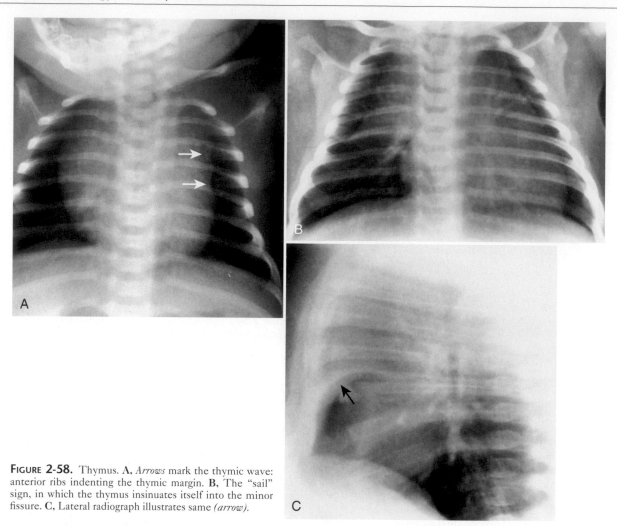

FIGURE 2-58. Thymus. **A,** *Arrows* mark the thymic wave: anterior ribs indenting the thymic margin. **B,** The "sail" sign, in which the thymus insinuates itself into the minor fissure. **C,** Lateral radiograph illustrates same *(arrow)*.

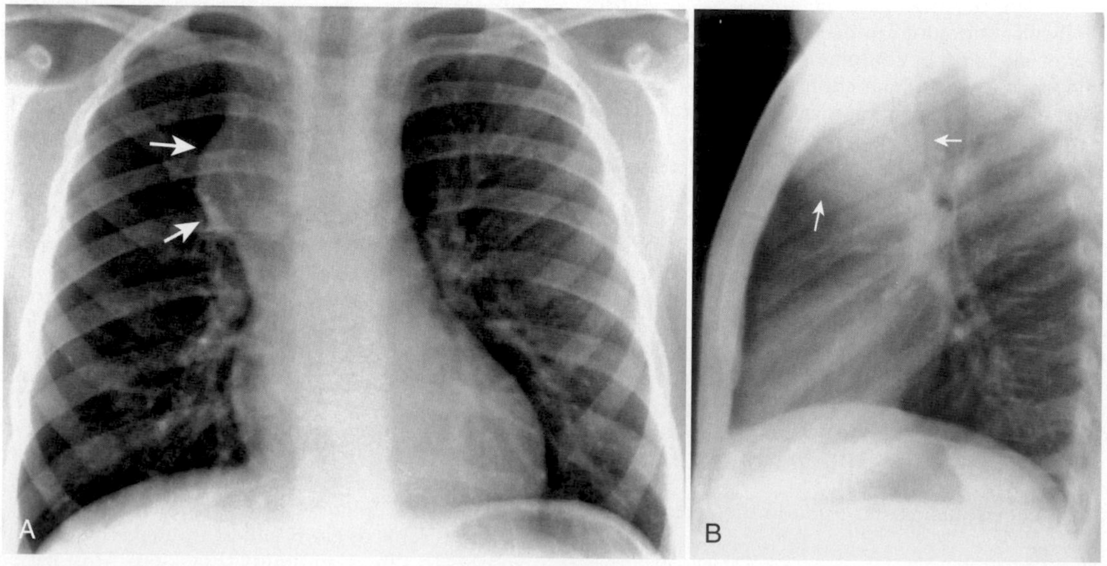

FIGURE 2-59. A, Frontal radiograph in a child with "leukemia/lymphoma" syndrome, demonstrating an anterior mediastinal mass *(arrows)*. **B,** Lateral film illustrates a posteriorly displaced and narrowed trachea *(arrows)*.

disease is anything but insidious. Fatigue, malaise, night sweats, and lymphadenopathy are frequent clinical symptoms.

Treatment revolves around chemotherapy, and the critical prognostic factor is bone marrow involvement: The less bone marrow involvement, the better the prognosis.

Staging, therefore, is extremely important in determining mode of therapy. CT and MRI are the modalities of choice. Contrast-enhanced CT, especially in the abdomen, is mandatory. If tracheobronchial compression occurs, in up to half of the patients at presentation with Hodgkin lymphoma, emergency radiation therapy may be needed. Scintigraphy (gallium Ga 67 citrate) but also positron emission tomography (PET) is useful for addressing response to therapy (Fig. 2-61).

Thymoma (Unilocular)

Thymic cysts, thymolipomas, and thymomas are rare in children. Approximately 15% of thymomas are malignant. Associated paraneoplastic syndromes include, most commonly, myasthenia gravis and red cell aplasia. Half of patients with thymoma have myasthenia gravis, and thymoma develops in 10% to 15% of all patients with myasthenia gravis. Calcification occurs in 25% of thymomas. MRI and CT complement conventional radiography for evaluation of the extent of the lesion.

Germ Cell Tumors

Germ cell tumors include teratoma, dermoid, and endodermal sinus (yolk sac) tumors, which can be distinguished from other masses on CT through identification of calcium and fat when present. A teratoma is the most common germ cell tumor. It is derived from multipotential cells in the third pharyngeal pouch that have descended into the mediastinum with the thymus. Most benign teratomas are cystic, containing a thick wall and fat. Calcification and local invasion occur often and are best demonstrated on CT. A malignant teratoma is much less common than its benign counterpart and occurs in (male) adolescents. It occurs more commonly in the sacrococcygeal region; only 10% occur in the mediastinum.

Middle Mediastinum

Lesions in the middle mediastinum also constitute about 30% of all mediastinal masses. The differential diagnosis of middle mediastinal lesions includes nodes, esophagus-related abnormalities such as duplication cysts, hiatal hernia, and bronchopulmonary foregut abnormalities, including bronchogenic cysts. In the assessment of lymphadenopathy, common considerations are neoplastic entities (such as in lymphoma/leukemia), infectious entities (primarily granulomatous, such as TB, histoplasmosis, and sarcoidosis), and immunocompromise-related entities (such as *P. carinii*). Classic vascular lesions include vascular rings and slings (see Fig 2-16) as well as aortic arch abnormalities, an aberrant left pulmonary artery, aortic dilatation, and enlarged pulmonary arteries (Fig. 2-62).

Foregut cysts are usually single and round. Depending on their communication with the gastrointestinal tract (enteric), the airways (bronchogenic), or the spinal canal (neurenteric), they may be solid, may contain an air-fluid level, or may be air-filled (see Fig. 2-32). All foregut-related cystic lesions are more common on the right than on the left and are often related to the carina.

CT and (increasingly) MRI are the imaging modalities of choice after initial demonstration of the mass on conventional (contrast) studies.

Tumors of the pericardium are rare in childhood. Lymphoma, lipomas, and cysts have been described.

Posterior Mediastinum

Posterior mediastinal masses account for about 40% of all pediatric mediastinal masses.

Neurogenic tumors constitute 90% of these mediastinal masses in the pediatric age group. Neuroblastoma, ganglioneuroblastoma, and ganglioneuroma represent a group of neurogenic

TABLE 2-2. Types of Non-Hodgkin Lymphoma

I	Lymphoblastic (30%)—supradiaphragmatic	T cell
II	Undifferentiated non-Burkitt type (30%)—abdomen	B cell
III	Undifferentiated Burkitt type (20%)—abdomen	B cell
IV	Large cell (histiocytic) (15%)—various locations	B, T cell

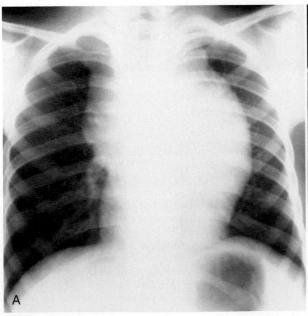

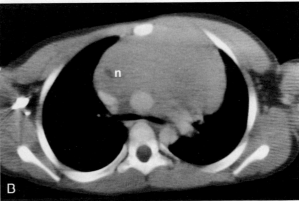

Figure 2-60. Hodgkin lymphoma. A, Chest radiograph demonstrating an anterior mediastinal mass with ipsilateral hilar adenopathy. B, Contrast-enhanced CT scan confirms the extent of the mediastinal lesion and the necrosis (n).

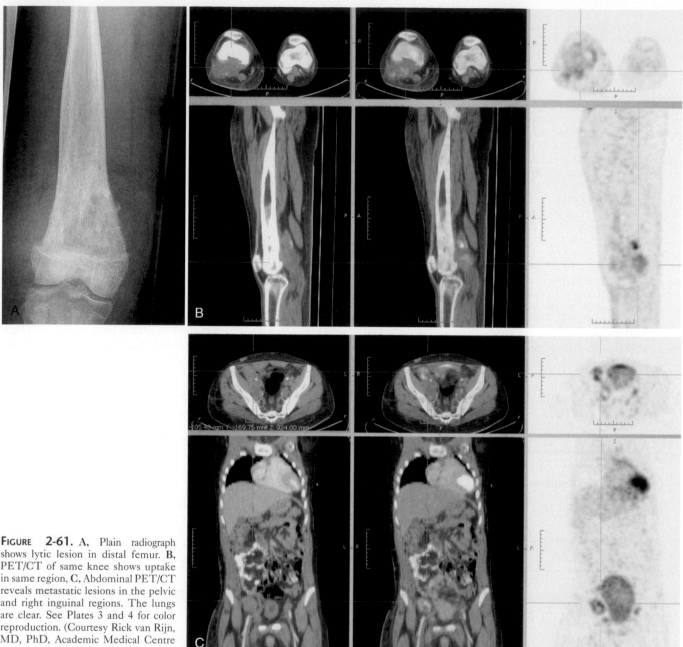

FIGURE 2-61. A, Plain radiograph shows lytic lesion in distal femur. B, PET/CT of same knee shows uptake in same region, C, Abdominal PET/CT reveals metastatic lesions in the pelvic and right inguinal regions. The lungs are clear. See Plates 3 and 4 for color reproduction. (Courtesy Rick van Rijn, MD, PhD, Academic Medical Centre Amsterdam, The Netherlands).

tumors with, in order shown, increasingly higher benign cell compositions. Neuroblastoma is by far the most common (15% of all neuroblastomas occur in the mediastinum), followed by ganglioneuroblastoma (more highly differentiated and with a better prognosis than neuroblastoma) and ganglioneuroma (a benign lesion occurring in older children, with an excellent prognosis). Schwannomas, neurofibromas (seldom solitary), and paragangliomas occur more rarely in children than in adults.

Mediastinal neuroblastoma is also associated with a more favorable prognosis when diagnosed in a child younger than 1 year. Usually a neuroblastoma occurs in the mediastinum before 2 years of age (Fig. 2-63).

Neurenteric cysts are histologically identical to broncho-genic or duplication (foregut) cysts, except for the association

with vertebral anomalies. These anomalies can vary from hemivertebrae and spina bifida to block vertebrae and clefts.

Extramedullary hematopoiesis is usually unilateral because the aorta "protects" on the left, can result from severe hereditary anemias (thalassemia, hereditary spherocytosis), and is usually located between T8 and T12. It is rare in children.

For all posterior mediastinal lesions, after plain film detection of the lesion, MRI is the imaging modality of choice, especially with its multiplanar capabilities (Fig. 2-64). The classic "dumbbell" appearance of thoracic neuroblastoma is exquisitely demonstrated on MRI. MRI also has a definite advantage in postoperative, post–radiation therapy (follow-up) imaging protocols. CT is useful primarily to evaluate for calcifications and bony erosion (rib, neural foramen).

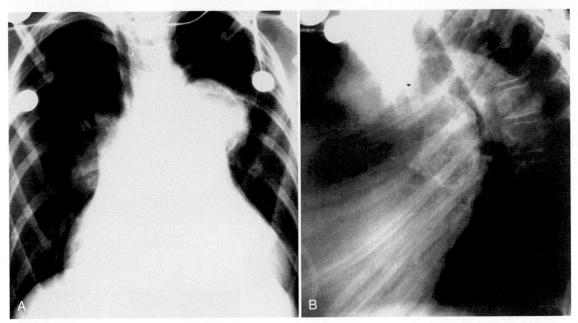

FIGURE 2-62. A 13-year-old patient with primary pulmonary hypertension. **A,** PA radiograph reveals peripheral artery "pruning." **B,** Lateral radiograph confirms enlarged pulmonary arteries with calcified wall.

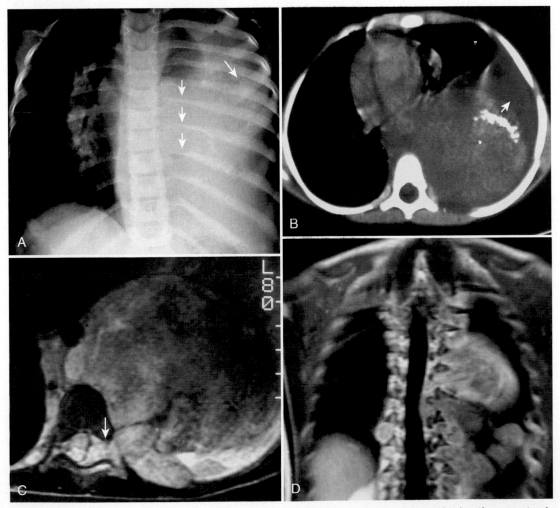

FIGURE 2-63. Neuroblastoma. **A,** Frontal radiograph reveals a large posterior mediastinal mass containing calcification *(long arrow)* and causing rib erosion *(short arrows)* and displacement of the mediastinum to the right. **B,** CT scan confirms radiographic findings and demonstrates an effusion *(arrow).* MR imaging defines the axial extent with "dumbbell" extension *(arrow)* of the lesion into the neural foramen **(C)** and coronal spinal canal extent **(D).**

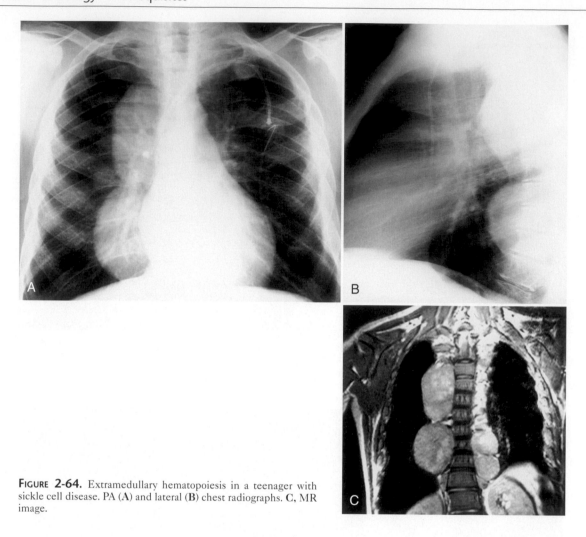

FIGURE 2-64. Extramedullary hematopoiesis in a teenager with sickle cell disease. PA (**A**) and lateral (**B**) chest radiographs. **C**, MR image.

▬ SUGGESTED READINGS

TEXTS

Carty H, Shaw D, Brunelle F, Kendall B (eds): Imaging Children, vol. 1. London, Elsevier, 2005, pp 1021-178 .

Lucaya J, Strife JL: Pediatric Chest Imaging. Berlin, Springer-Verlag, 2002, .

Kirks DR (ed): Practical Pediatric Imaging. Philadelphia, Lippincott-Raven, 1997, pp 619-820 .

Kuhn JP, Slovis TL, Haller JO (eds): Caffey's Pediatric X-Ray Diagnosis, ed 10, vol 1. Philadelphia, Elsevier, 2005, pp 767-1224 .

Sty JR, Wells RG, Starshak RJ, et al: Diagnostic Imaging of Infants and Children, vol 3. Gaithersburg, Md, Aspen, 1992, pp 105–232.

Swischuk LE: Imaging of the Newborn, Infant, and Young Child, ed 4. Baltimore, Williams & Wilkins, 1997, pp 1–158.

ARTICLES

Agrons GA, Courtney SE, Stocker JT, Markowitz RA: Lung disease in premature neonates: Radiologic-pathologic correlation. Radiographics 2005;25:1047-73.

Aquino SL, Kee ST, Warnock ML, et al: Pulmonary aspergillosis: Imaging findings with pathologic correlation. AJR 1994; 163:811-5.

Aquino SL, Schechter MS, Chiles C, et al: High-resolution inspiratory and expiratory CT in older children and adults with bronchopulmonary dysplasia. AJR 1999;173:963-7.

Bauman NM, Smith RJH: Recurrent respiratory papillomatosis. Pediatr Otolaryngol 1996; 43:1385-401.

Berdon WE, Baker DH: Vascular anomalies and the infant lung: Rings, slings and other things. Semin Roentgenol 1972;7:39-64.

Cleveland RH, Neish AS, Zurakowski D, et al: Cystic fibrosis: A system for assessing and predicting progression. AJR 1998;170:1067-72.

Donnelly LF, Strife JL, Bissett, GS III: The spectrum of extrinsic airway compression in children: MR imaging, AJR Am J Roentgenol 1997; 168:59-62.

Donnelly LF: Practical issues concerning imaging of pulmonary infection in children. J Thorac Imaging 2001; 16:238-50.

Frush DP, Donnelly LF, Chotas HG: Contemporary pediatric thoracic imaging, AJR 2000; 175:841-51.

Griscom NT: Diseases of the trachea, bronchi and smaller airways. Radiol Clin North Am 1993;31:605-615.

Griscom NT: Pneumonia in children and some of its variants. Radiology 1988; 167:297-302.

Harty MP, Kramer SS, Fellows KE: Current concepts on imaging of thoracic vascular abnormalities. Curr Opin Pediatr 2000;12:194-202.

Kirkpatrick JA: Pneumonia in children as it differs from adult pneumonia. Semin Roentgenol 1980;15:96-103.

Kuhn JP, Brody AS: High-resolution CT of pediatric lung disease. Radiol Clin North Am 2002;40:89-110.

Marks MJ, Haney PJ, McDermott MP, et al: Thoracic disease in children with AIDS, Radiographics 1996;16:1349-62.

Meuwly JY, Lepori D, Theumann N, et al: Multimodality imaging evaluation of the pediatric neck: Techniques and spectrum of findings. Radiographics 2005; 25:931-48.

Newman B, Congenital bronchopulmonary foregut malformations: Concepts and controversies. Pediatr Radiol 2006;36:773-91.

Northway WH Jr, Rosan RC: Radiographic features of pulmonary oxygen toxicity in the newborn: Bronchopulmonary dysplasia. Radiology 1968;91:49-58.

Norton KI, Kattan M, Rao JS, et al; P(2)C(2) HIV Study Group: Chronic radiographic lung changes in children with vertically transmitted HIV-1 infection. AJR 2001;176:1553-8.

Panicek DM, Heitzman ER, Randall PA, et al: The continuum of pulmonary developmental anomalies. Radiographics 1987;7:747-72.

Reid L: 1976 Edward B.D. Neuhauser lecture: The lung: Its growth and remodeling in health and disease. AJR Am J Roentgenol 1977;129:777-88.

Swischuk LE, Hayden CK: Viral versus bacterial pulmonary infections in children (is roentgenographic differentiation possible?). Pediatr Radiol 1986;16:278-84.

Swischuk LE, Shetty BP, John SD: The lungs in immature infants: How important is surfactant therapy in preventing chronic lung problems? Pediatr Radiol 1996; 26:508-11.

CHAPTER 3

Heart

Rajesh Krishnamurthy and Johan G. (Hans) Blickman

CONGENITAL HEART DISEASE

Congenital heart disease (CHD) occurs in about 1% of all live births. Approximately 25% of children with CHD become symptomatic in the first year of life, about 25% of patients with CHD eventually die of their disease, and approximately 25% of the deaths occur in the first month of life. Echocardiography plays a central role in the noninvasive delineation of congenital heart disease at all ages. Cardiac catheterization has traditionally been the diagnostic "gold standard," providing morphologic and functional information, including data on pulmonary vascular resistance and oxygen saturation within chambers and vessels. Computed tomography (CT) and magnetic resonance imaging (MRI) play increasingly important complementary roles in relation to echocardiography and catheterization in the delineation of CHD in the preoperative and postoperative periods.

Identification of Cardiac Chambers and Great Vessels

The first step in the analysis of CHD by cross-sectional imaging is accurate identification of the cardiac chambers and vessels. The *right atrium* (RA) is identified as the chamber that receives the insertion of the inferior vena cava and coronary sinus and by a broad-based triangular appendage with characteristic pectinate muscle morphology extending to the atrioventricular (AV) junction. The *left atrium* (LA) is identified by a narrow-based, tubular, finger-like appendage. The *right ventricle* (RV) is identified from the following features:
1. There is a muscular attachment between the free wall and the interventricular septum (moderator band).
2. The AV valve of the RV is more apically displaced than the AV valve of the left ventricle.
3. The presence of an infundibulum (conus) in the RV.

The *left ventricle* (LV) is identified from its smooth septal surface, which is devoid of any muscular attachments, and from the absence of a conus. The *pulmonary artery* (PA) is recognized as the vessel that supplies branches to the lungs, but not the systemic circulation. The *aorta* is identified as the vessel that supplies the coronary and systemic circulations.

Segmental Approach to Heart Disease

Any combination of atrial, ventricular, and great vessel morphology can occur in CHD. One must take a simple, logical, step-by-step approach in order to understand and describe the disease prior to determining treatment. The segmental approach to CHD described by Richard van Praagh consists of determining the following relationships:
1. The anatomic type of the three major cardiac segments: the viscero-atrial situs, ventricular looping, and relationship of the great arteries. For example, in corrected transposition of the great arteries (TGA), the atrial relationship is solitus (morphologic RA to the right of the morphologic LA), there is L-looping of the ventricles (morphologic RV to the left of the morphologic LV), and there is L-malposition of the great arteries (aorta lies anterior and to the left of the PA).
2. How each segment is connected to the adjacent segment. This determination involves analysis of the *atrioventricular canal*, which connects the atria to the ventricles, and the *conus (infundibulum)*, which connects the ventricles to the great

arteries. Potential AV connections are: concordant connection, discordant connection (ventricular inversion), common AV canal (CAVC), double inlet LV, unilateral AV valve atresia, straddling AV valve, and overriding AV valve. The options at the level of the conus are: normal connections, TGA, truncus arteriosus, double-outlet RV, double-outlet LV, anatomically corrected malposition, and outflow tract obstruction.
3. Associated malformations involving the atrial and ventricular septum, or the extracardiac vasculature. Examples are total anomalous pulmonary venous return (TAPVR), bilateral superior vena cava (SVC), coarctation, etc.
4. How the segmental combinations and connections, along with the associated malformations, function. For example, in Figure 3-1D, which shows a patient with mitral atresia, supracardiac TAPVR, double-outlet RV, and pulmonary stenosis, there is cyanosis with decreased pulmonary vasculature.

Accurate anatomical and physiologic diagnosis allows selection of therapeutic options, which may be medical, surgical, or both.

Physiologic Subgroups

Chest radiographs play an important role in determining the physiology of heart disease and palliative therapy at birth by distinguishing between lesions with increased pulmonary blood flow (left-to-right shunts, intermixing states with unobstructed pulmonary blood flow), decreased pulmonary vascularity (intermixing states with obstructed pulmonary blood flow), and lesions with pulmonary venous hypertension (left-sided obstruction) (see Fig. 3-1). Intermixing states are usually the result of a common atrial or ventricular chamber or a right-to-left shunt, and they cause cyanosis owing to mixing of deoxygenated blood with oxygenated blood before it enters the systemic circulation. After analysis of the chest radiographs and the physiologic information (murmurs, cyanosis etc.), a differential diagnosis can be assembled that is pertinent to determining palliative therapy at birth.

I. Increased pulmonary vascularity:
   A. Central left-to-right shunts (acyanotic):
      1. Ventricular septal defect (VSD).
      2. Atrial septal defect (ASD).
      3. AV septal defect (CAVC).
      4. Patent ductus arteriosus (PDA).
      5. Less common lesions: aortopulmonary window, coronary-cameral fistula, partial anomalous pulmonary venous return, etc.
   B. Peripheral left-to-right shunts:
      1. Vein of Galen malformation.
      2. Hepatic hemangioendothelioma.
      3. Large extremity AV malformations.
   C. Hyperdynamic states, such as thyrotoxicosis and anemia.
   D. Intermixing states without obstruction to pulmonary blood flow (cyanotic):
      1. TGA.
      2. Truncus arteriosus.
      3. Double-outlet RV.
      4. Single ventricle.
      5. TAPVR (unobstructed).
II. Decreased pulmonary vascularity:
   A. Intermixing states with obstructed pulmonary blood flow (cyanotic):

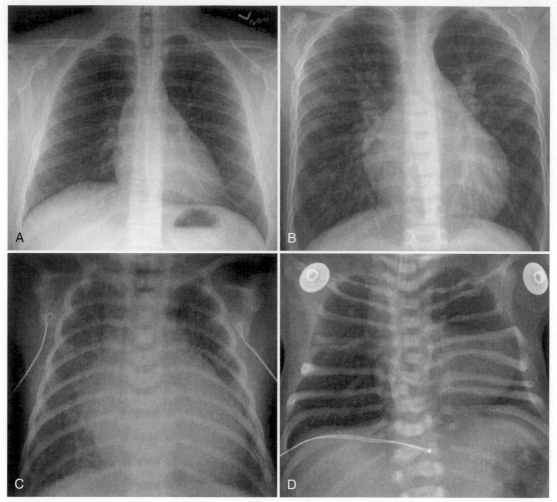

Figure 3-1. Patterns of pulmonary vascularity. **A** represents normal pulmonary vascularity. **B** is an example of increased pulmonary vascularity in a patient with an atrial septal defect. **C** is an example of pulmonary venous hypertension and interstitial pulmonary edema in a patient with severe coarctation. **D** represents diminished pulmonary vascularity in a patient with mitral atresia, double-outlet right ventricle, supracardiac total anomalous pulmonary venous return, and pulmonary stenosis.

1. Tetralogy of Fallot.
2. Pulmonary atresia with VSD.
3. TGA with pulmonary stenosis.
4. Truncus arteriosus with pulmonary stenosis.
5. Double-outlet RV with pulmonary stenosis/atresia.
III. Pulmonary venous hypertension and congestive heart failure:
   A. Left-sided obstructive lesions:
      1. Cor triatriatum.
      2. Hypoplastic left heart syndrome.
      3. Shone syndrome.
      4. Bicuspid aortic valve and aortic stenosis.
      5. Aortic coarctation.
   B. Hyperdynamic states.
   C. Severe left-to-right shunts.
IV. Normal pulmonary vascularity:
   A. Mild left-sided obstructive lesions.
   B. Intermixing states with balanced pulmonary blood flow.
   C. Right-sided obstructions without intermixing.

Treatment of Congenital Heart Disease

Immediate Palliation

The need for immediate palliative therapy of CHD at birth depends on the patient's clinical and hemodynamic status. The type of palliation is determined by echocardiographic and radiographic findings. In a patient with increased pulmonary vascularity, PA banding to diminish the amount of blood flow to the lungs may be considered. In a patient with decreased pulmonary vascularity, augmentation of pulmonary blood flow with a systemic arterial-to-pulmonary arterial shunt (such as a modified Blalock-Taussig shunt) is an option. Intermixing states are treated in the neonatal period through promotion of the extent of intermixing and optimization of pulmonary and systemic blood flow. Pulmonary venous hypertension due to left-sided obstruction is treated through relief of the cause of obstruction.

Permanent Palliation

After immediate palliation, decisions regarding permanent palliation are based on the number of functioning ventricles and the feasibility of separating deoxygenated and oxygenated blood flows. Conditions like tetralogy of Fallot, TGA, truncus arteriosus, and some forms of CAVC and double-outlet RV, for instance, are amenable to a two-ventricle repair, in which the anatomy is rearranged to restore physiologic venous return and unobstructed systemic and pulmonary arterial outflows, with two functional ventricles. When there is only one functioning ventricle, it is used as the systemic ventricle, with passive venous return to the lungs by means of cavopulmonary shunts; this is a *single ventricle repair*. Conditions that fall into the single ventricle pathway include unbalanced CAVC, tricuspid atresia, hypoplastic left heart syndrome, and double-inlet LV. Occasionally, conditions with two functioning ventricles may end up in the single ventricle pathway because of an inability to separate the deoxygenated and oxygenated circulations; examples are some forms of double-outlet RV, straddling AV valves, and Ebstein anomaly. A list of named surgical procedures is provided in the Appendix to this chapter.

Indications for Imaging by CT and MRI

In the preoperative period, CT and MRI are used to evaluate CHD when characterization of pathology by echocardiography is inadequate because of suboptimal acoustic windows. This typically involves the extracardiac vasculature, with examples being aortic coarctation, anomalous pulmonary venous return, scimitar syndrome, systemic venous anomalies, branch PA stenosis, and anomalous coronary artery origin. In the postoperative period, the goals of imaging change considerably, information about cardiac function and flow becoming more important than information about morphology. The goals of postoperative imaging are evaluation of ventricular function and valvular function, surveillance of grafts, conduits, and baffles, early detection of complications, and determination of the timing of surgical intervention. Examples are timing of pulmonary valve replacement in tetralogy of Fallot, determining the cause of cyanosis and prognosis after a Fontan procedure, evaluation of the systemic RV after intra-atrial repair of TGA, and screening evaluation prior to stage II and stage III Norwood procedures. The role of MRI increases in the postoperative period and in older patients when acoustic windows diminish.

▬ COMMON CONDITIONS

Left-to-Right Shunts

Acyanotic communications between the systemic and pulmonary circuits include intracardiac left-to-right shunts and large systemic AV connections. Common examples of the former are VSD, ASD, atrioventricular canal (AVC) defect, and PDA. Less common examples are partial anomalous pulmonary venous return, aortopulmonary window, and coronary-cameral fistula. Examples of peripheral left-to-right shunts are large systemic AV malformations like vein of Galen malformation, hepatic hemangioendothelioma, and Klippel-Trénaunay-Weber syndrome.

Ventricular Septal Defect

Excluding bicuspid aortic valve, VSD is the most common congenital intracardiac lesion in children, accounting for 20% to 30% of cases of CHD. Five percent of VSDs are associated with other lesions, particularly chromosomal abnormalities such as trisomies 13, 18, and 21. Many small VSDs close spontaneously, and classifying VSDs on the basis of size and location (Fig. 3-2) is important in deciding whether medical (expectant) or surgical treatment is indicated.

Muscular VSDs, which are defects in the muscular septum, are surrounded entirely by muscle. They may be described by their location in the septum (mid-muscular, apical muscular). "Swiss cheese septum" describes multiple muscular VSDs. *AV canal–type VSD* is a defect in the AV canal portion of the septum. Also known as *inlet VSD*, this condition is common in the setting of heterotaxy.

Conoventricular VSDs occur at the junction between the conal septum and the muscular septum/septal band. The strictest definition of a *membranous VSD* is a defect of only the membranous septum, which would result in a small defect. In day-to-day use, the term *perimembranous or paramembranous VSD* usually means that the defect includes the region of the membranous septum but also extends into the muscular septum, conal septum, or AV canal septum. Conoventricular defects may also exhibit *malalignment*, in which the conal septum is misplaced out of its expected plane, creating a substrate for outflow tract obstruction (tetralogy of Fallot = anterior malalignment; VSD with interrupted aortic arch = posterior malalignment).

Conal septal VSDs occur within the conal septum. These defects may be in close proximity to the semilunar valves and are also referred to as *subarterial VSD*. Clinically, it is important to evaluate for associated aortic valve prolapse and aortic regurgitation.

The classic presentation of a VSD consists of a prominent blowing pansystolic murmur at the lower sternal border. Affected patients can have congestive heart failure (CHF), repeated respiratory infections, or failure to thrive, and usually present after the first month of life when the pulmonary vascular resistance falls, with subsequent increase in the degree of shunting. In an older child, if pulmonary vascular resistance remains high, a large VSD may lead to pulmonary hypertension (see Fig. 3-2). In rare cases, pulmonary vascular obstructive disease develops with time and may even cause reversal of blood flow, leading to a right-to-left shunt across the septal defect (formerly known as "Eisenmenger physiology"). This condition may eventually lead to cyanosis. Most patients, however, will have undergone surgery to correct the VSD before pulmonary flow reversal occurs.

Conventional chest film findings are usually evident when the ratio of pulmonary to systemic blood flow is greater than 2:1. The pulmonary vascularity is increased, and there is biventricular enlargement and dilatation of the central pulmonary trunk (see Fig. 3-2). LA enlargement and resultant posterior displacement and elevation of the left mainstem bronchus are often also present. Radiographic signs of congestive failure may appear after the first month of life as the pulmonary vascular resistance falls.

Therapy for a VSD consists of surgical closure of the defect(s), although up to 50% of VSDs close spontaneously. Detachable catheter devices for closure of VSD are in development.

Atrial Septal Defect

ASD is the second most common cardiac anomaly in children, accounting for 10% of all cases of CHD. An ASD is the most common intracardiac shunt that persists into adulthood. It is classified according to its location in the atrial septum, as follows:

- A patent foramen ovale represents defective apposition of the septum secundum to the septum primum.
- An ostium secundum (II) ASD, which is most common (60% of cases), is located in the midseptum in the area of foramen ovale. It is usually an isolated anomaly.
- An ostium primum (I) ASD (30%) is situated low in the atrial septum, contiguous with the AV valves. *Partial AV canal defect* refers to a primum ASD associated with a cleft mitral valve.
- A sinus venosus ASD (5%) does not involve the interatrial septum and is a defect between the posterior wall of the RA and the right-sided pulmonary veins, usually near the entrance of the SVC. It is often associated with partial anomalous pulmonary venous drainage, usually from the right upper lobe pulmonary vein into the SVC.
- Coronary sinus septal defect (unroofed coronary sinus) occurs when the wall separating the coronary sinus from the LA is deficient. This is part of the Raghib syndrome, which includes a persistent LSVC to the unroofed coronary sinus.
- Common atrium is seen in association with the heterotaxy syndromes, and Ellis–van Creveld syndrome. The interatrial communication is very large, with deficiencies of both septum primum and septum secundum.

ASDs are found six to eight times more commonly in females than in males. The association of an ASD with mitral stenosis in rheumatic disease (rare today) is known as Lutembacher syndrome. An ostium secundum defect that is associated with conduction defects and skeletal abnormalities of the upper extremities (absence or hypoplasia of the thumb, hooked clavicles) is known as the Holt-Oram syndrome, an autosomal dominant entity.

Clinically, patients with ASDs are most often asymptomatic. When they enter adolescence or young adulthood, mild dyspnea or an asymptomatic heart murmur may be noted with a harsh systolic murmur along the high left sternal border. There is fixed

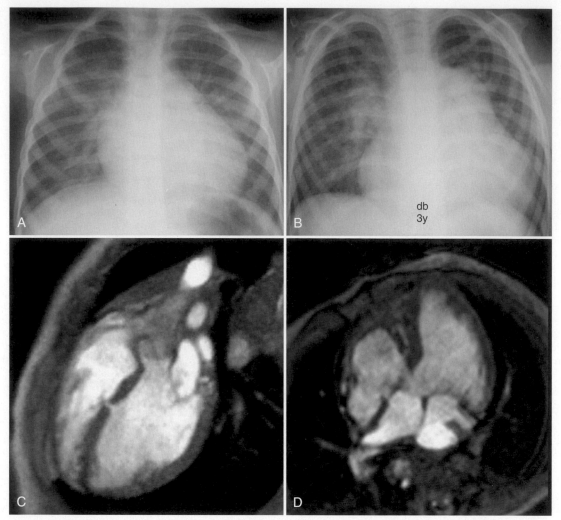

FIGURE 3-2. Ventricular septal defect (VSD). **A,** An example of VSD at birth, with cardiomegaly and increased pulmonary vascularity. **B,** The same patient at 3 years of life, with early changes of pulmonary arterial hypertension, including enlargement of the main pulmonary artery and proximal branch pulmonary arteries, and pruning of the peripheral pulmonary vasculature. **C,** Bright blood image from MRI showing an intramuscular VSD. **D,** Four-chamber view demonstrating an inlet (arteriovenous canal type) VSD. The patient also has an overriding tricuspid valve.

splitting of a loud second heat sound (S_2). A patient with an ostium primum ASD often has the blowing pansystolic murmur of mitral regurgitation.

Conventional chest radiographic findings are normal in infancy. Later in childhood, increased pulmonary vascularity appears with mild leftward rotation of the heart and the great vessels (Fig. 3-3). RA and RV dilatation may be significant. LA enlargement does not occur because of the immediate decompression of the greater volume of blood from the LA to the RA during both systole and diastole.

CT or MRI can be used to determine the site and size of the ASD prior to surgery or percutaneous closure (see Fig. 3-3) and to screen for the presence of anomalous pulmonary venous. In all forms of septal defects, quantification of shunt size (pulmonary-to-systemic flow ratio, otherwise known as the Qp:Qs ratio) by MR flow velocity mapping enables decision-making as to conservative therapy versus surgery (Fig. 3-4).

Treatment of an ASD usually consists of elective surgical closure, although percutaneous closure with a "clamshell" or wire-mesh device is becoming more routine.

Common Arteriovenous Canal

Endocardial cushion defect and *atrioventricular septal defect* are alternate terms for CAVC. The AV junction fails to develop normally into two distinct AV valves and complete the atrial septum and ventricular septum. *Common AV canal* therefore refers to a range of defects, from an isolated primum ASD with a cleft mitral valve (partial CAVC), to an isolated inlet VSD (incomplete CAVC), to a common AV valve with both a primum ASD and a VSD (complete CAVC). There are several systems of nomenclature to describe this defect, the Rastelli classification being the most used. It is based on the anatomy of the anterior bridging leaflet of the common AV valve. The common AV valve may be symmetrically located over both ventricles, resulting in a *balanced CAVC* in which both ventricles are of approximately equal size; *unbalanced CAVC* occurs when one ventricle is larger than the other.

Forty percent to 50% of patients with CAVC also have trisomy 21 (Down syndrome). Complete CAVC defects are often seen in patients with heterotaxy syndrome.

Conventional chest radiographs reflect enlargement on the right side (RA and ventricle) and large blood volumes (increased pulmonary flow) within the lungs. The *gooseneck deformity* is an angiographic finding referring to elongation and narrowing of the LV outflow tract by the anterior bridging leaflet of the common AV valve (Fig. 3-5). Corrective surgery involves patching of the ASD and VSD, and separation or resuspension of the valve leaflets.

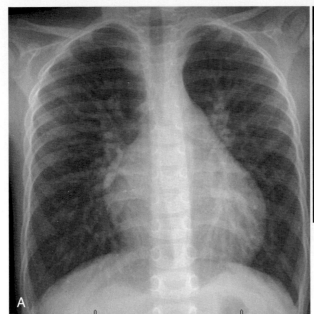

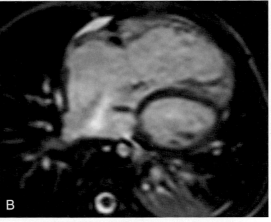

FIGURE 3-3. Atrial septal defect (ASD). **A** demonstrates increased pulmonary vascularity, enlargement of the right atrium, and prominence of the main pulmonary artery. **B** shows a large secundum ASD on a four-chamber view bright blood MRI sequence, and moderately severe dilatation of the right atrium and right ventricle.

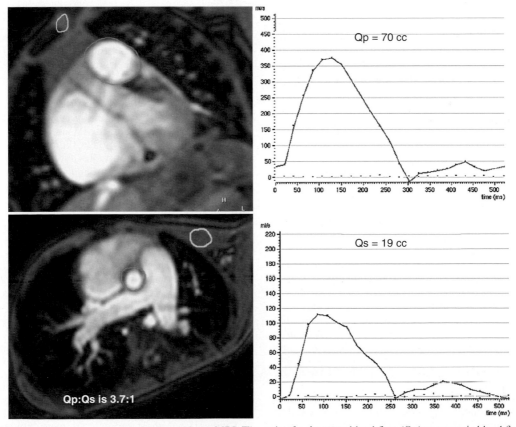

FIGURE 3-4. Calculation of pulmonary-to-systemic flow ratio on MRI. The ratio of pulmonary blood flow (Qp) to systemic blood flow (Qs) can be calculated by MR flow velocity mapping using a phase contrast sequence. Flow is measured across the main pulmonary artery and ascending aorta. In the patient shown in Figure 3-3, the Qp:Qs ratio is 3.7:1.

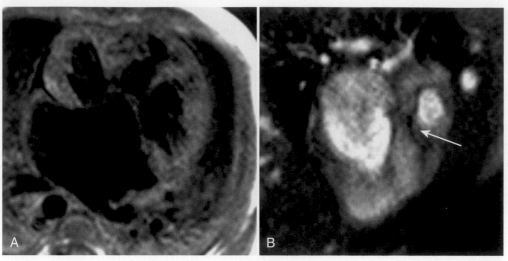

FIGURE 3-5. Common arteriovenous (AV) canal. **A,** Black blood image from MRI showing a common AV valve with an inlet ventricular septal defect and a functional common atrium. **B,** A left ventricular outflow tract view from a bright blood sequence shows gooseneck deformity of the left ventricular outflow tract *(arrow)* due to mass effect from the large anterior leaflet of the common AV valve.

Patent Ductus Arteriosus

A PDA is defined as a communication of the proximal descending aorta and the proximal PA due to persistence of the fetal ductus arteriosus, a remnant of the distal sixth aortic arch. The vessel may also connect to the subclavian or innominate artery. This entity constitutes 8% to 10% of CHD (occurring in 1 in 3000 term infants) and is more common in girls (2:1) and premature infants (50% of those weighing less than 1500 g). The communication functionally closes by 48 hours after birth; it is anatomically closed in 95% of infants by the third month of life. Low oxygen tension in the arterial blood flow and elevated fetal prostaglandin levels inhibit contraction and closure of the ductus.

A PDA is usually asymptomatic. The clinical presentation of a large PDA can range from a machinery-like murmur to frank CHF in infancy, depending on the degree of shunting. Surfactant deficiency disease in the premature infant may facilitate persistence of PDA in 25% of patients. Closure of the ductus is effected surgically (clip) or by medical therapy (indomethacin).

Conventional chest radiographs in the neonate with PDA may show increased pulmonary vascularity, pulmonary edema, or RA enlargement (Fig. 3-6). These findings may be difficult to evaluate if the changes of surfactant deficiency or bronchopulmonary dysplasia are also present. In the premature infant, interstitial edema (CHF) commonly occurs because there are fewer pulmonary arterioles to accommodate the increased flow. The classic patient with PDA is a premature infant in whom the radiographic signs of congestive heart failure develop at approximately 7 to 10 days of life, when the pulmonary vascular resistance starts to drop.

Radiographic evidence of a closed ductus may be evident as ligamentum calcification or as a surgical device (clip or "clamshell"). Partial closure of the ductus, which remains open at the aortic end, results in the ductus "bump" or ductus diverticulum, an incidental finding. It may occasionally enlarge to form a ductal aneurysm.

Partial Anomalous Pulmonary Venous Return

In partial anomalous pulmonary venous return, at least one but not all of the pulmonary veins return to the systemic veins or the RA, resulting in a left-to-right shunt. This classification includes the scimitar syndrome, in which the right lower lobe pulmonary vein or the entire right lung pulmonary venous return enters the IVC at the level of the diaphragm. It is associated with right lung hypoplasia, dextroposition of the heart (Fig. 3-7), and aortopulmonary collaterals from the abdominal aorta to the right lung. MRI is helpful to determine the presence and location of the pulmonary vein, the drainage area, the presence or absence of

associated obstruction, the degree of left-to-right shunting (Qp: Qs), and the presence or absence of associated anomalies like PA hypoplasia, aortopulmonary collaterals, and developmental lung anomalies, among others.

Intermixing States

The common anomalies in the category intermixing states are TGA, truncus arteriosus, and TAPVR. Less common anomalies are double-outlet right ventricle (DORV) and single ventricle.

Transposition of the Great Arteries

TGA is the most common form of cyanotic CHD (5% of cases). The origins of the aorta and the PA are from the "wrong" (discordant) ventricle; the aorta originates from the RA, whereas the PA arises from the RA. The aorta lies anterior and to the right of the PA. The atria, AV connections, and ventricles are normal. About 50% of infants have an intact ventricular septum; 25% have a conoventricular VSD; and the other 25% have VSD with pulmonary stenosis.

Dextro-TGA (D-TGA) results in the delivery of deoxygenated blood to the body that then returns to the RA, whereas oxygenated blood circulates from the heart to the lungs and back again. This parallel arrangement is incompatible with life unless there is a communication at the level of the atria, ventricle, or ductus arteriosus. This disorder commonly manifests as cyanosis in the first 24 hours of life. The incidence of D-TGA is 1 in 4000 live births and is higher in infants of diabetic mothers; affected boys outnumber affected girls 2.5:1.

The extent of pulmonary blood flow determines the level of cyanosis. Large volumes of pulmonary blood flow result in CHF and less cyanosis. Diminished pulmonary flow, in the setting of associated pulmonary stenosis, results in more intense cyanosis, which is evident on chest radiographs as slightly decreased pulmonary vascularity.

Conventional chest radiographs may demonstrate mild cardiomegaly, although a normal-size cardiac silhouette is the rule immediately after birth. A narrow mediastinal vascular contour is present owing to the parallel arrangement of the aorta and PA. There is hyperinflation and lack of a normal thymic contour (due to "stress"). This appearance has often been referred to as "egg on side" and "egg on a string" (Fig. 3-8).

Palliative therapy centers on creation of a large ASD to improve bidirectional flow, by means of catheter balloon septostomy

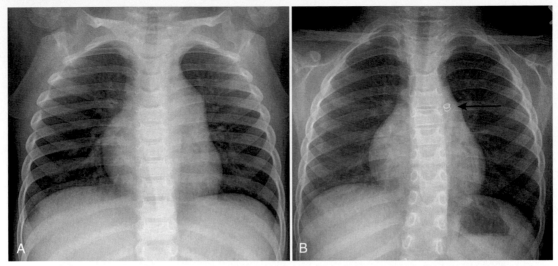

FIGURE 3-6. Patent ductus arteriosus (PDA). **A,** Preprocedure radiograph of a patient with PDA showing enlargement of the main pulmonary artery, increased pulmonary vascularity, and a mildly dilated ascending aorta forming the right cardiac margin. **B,** Postprocedure radiograph shows a PDA coil *(arrow),* resolution of main pulmonary artery dilatation, and normal pulmonary vascularity.

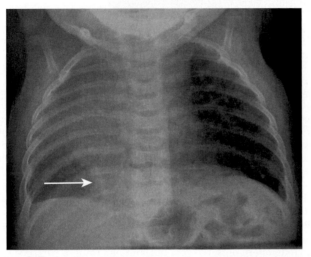

FIGURE 3-7. Scimitar syndrome showing hypoplasia of the right lung, dextroposition of the heart, and anomalous return of the right pulmonary vein to the inferior vena cava at the level of the diaphragm *(arrow).*

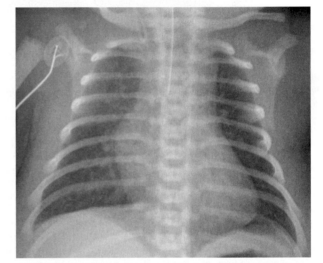

FIGURE 3-8. D-Transposition of the great arteries. An egg-on-side appearance of the cardiac silhouette is noted, with a narrow mediastinal vascular pedicle and increased pulmonary vascularity.

(Rashkind procedure). The goal of permanent palliation is to redirect blood flow in order to achieve deoxygenated systemic venous return into the PA and oxygenated pulmonary venous return into the aorta. There are two ways of accomplishing this goal: redirect blood at the atrial level (Mustard or Senning "atrial switch" procedure) and switch of the great arteries (Jatene "arterial switch" procedure). The arterial switch is the procedure of choice in the absence of a VSD. In the presence of a VSD, the LV is baffled to the aorta via the VSD, with continuity of the RV to the PA being established by a conduit. Complications after treatment include neo-aortic root dilatation (Fig. 3-9), branch PA stenosis, systemic venous thrombosis, and coronary artery kinking. MRI and CT play important roles in noninvasive monitoring and diagnosis of complications.

Corrected Transposition of the Great Arteries

This condition is not an intermixing state but is discussed in this section because of its anatomic similarity to D-TGA.

A congenitally corrected TGA, or levo-TGA (L-TGA), occurs when there is atrioventricular and ventriculo-arterial discordance. The condition consists of normal anatomy of the atria, inversion of the ventricles, and L-malposition of the great arteries. In situs solitus of the atria, the morphologic RV is located on the left, with blood reaching it from the LA, and leaving it through the aorta. The morphologic LV is on the right side, with blood reaching it from the RA and exiting through the PA. The aorta lies to the left of the PA. Coexisting lesions are the rule; they include VSD (in more than 50% of cases), tricuspid valve anomalies including incompetence, atresia, and Ebstein anomaly, and pulmonary stenosis.

Clinically, the findings depend on the severity of the associated intracardiac lesions. Conventional chest radiographs often appear normal but may show an abnormal fullness in the left upper heart border and mediastinum because the ascending aorta forms a border, arising from the left-sided RV. The pulmonary vascularity is often decreased because of the high incidence of pulmonary stenosis. Late RV failure is common, because the RV is not capable of sustaining a systemic workload for an entire lifespan. A "double switch" procedure is performed in early childhood at some centers for L-TGA; it consists of an atrial switch and an arterial switch, with the goal of making the LV the systemic ventricle. Long-term results of this procedure are still unknown. MRI plays

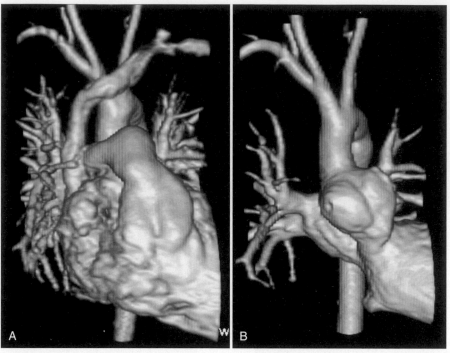

FIGURE 3-9. Arterial switch operation for D-transposition of the great arteries (D-TGA). Volume-rendered images from gadolinium-enhanced MR angiography. **A,** Typical changes following arterial switch operation for D-TGA, with the pulmonary arteries draped around the ascending aorta. **B,** Neo-aortic root dilatation is a common complication after the arterial switch operation.

an important role in the preoperative period in clarifying complex anatomy, such as criss-cross ventricles, and in monitoring the status of the systemic RV.

Persistent Truncus Arteriosus

Persistent truncus arteriosus is defined as a single artery arising from the base of the heart and giving rise to the coronary, systemic, and pulmonary circulations. It represents a failure of septation of the primitive truncus arteriosus into the aorta and PA. The resultant single trunk arises from a single semilunar valve possessing anywhere from two to six cusps. A VSD is usually present below the semilunar valve. Persistent truncus arteriosus accounts for approximately 1% to 4% of CHD. It is associated with right aortic arch in 21% to 36% of cases and with interrupted aortic arch in 11% of cases. Thirty percent to 35% of patients with persistent truncus arteriosus have 22q11 deletion (DiGeorge syndrome). It is classified according to the location of the pulmonary arteries and the presence or absence of a VSD and interrupted aortic arch (van Praagh).

Patients are presented early in infancy with cyanosis, failure to thrive, dyspnea, and CHF. Chest radiographs typically demonstrate cardiomegaly and increased pulmonary vascularity. A superiorly located proximal left PA may be present. A waterfall or hilar comma sign may be present, representing elevation of the pulmonary hilum on the side opposite to the aortic arch. CT and MRI are helpful in cases in which the PA anatomy cannot be determined by echocardiography.

Treatment consists of assigning the truncal valve to the LV, closure of the VSD, separation of the branch pulmonary arteries, and placement of a valved conduit between the RV and the neo-PA. The conduit may require revisions with somatic growth, and MRI plays an important role in determining timing of repeat surgery.

Total Anomalous Pulmonary Venous Return

In TAPVC, all pulmonary veins connect anomalously to the systemic venous circulation. The four forms of TAPVC (supracardiac, cardiac, infracardiac, and mixed) are named on the basis of the site of drainage of the pulmonary veins into the systemic venous circulation. Supracardiac TAPVC (Fig. 3-10) connects above the

heart, usually into the left innominate vein; it accounts for 40% of all cases of TAPVC and has a 50% chance of becoming obstructed. Cardiac TAPVC connects to the heart, either via the coronary sinus or directly into the atria; it accounts for 20% of cases and has a 20% chance of becoming obstructed. Infracardiac TAPVC connects below the heart; it accounts for 35% of cases and has a 95% chance of becoming obstructed. In mixed TAPVC, not all pulmonary veins connect to the same structure. Mixed forms account for 5% of cases and have a 75% chance of becoming obstructed.

Infants with TAPVC usually present in the first week of life. If there is high pulmonary flow and good admixture, cyanosis is mild. With greater severity of pulmonary venous obstruction, severe cyanosis and pulmonary edema supervene, and intervention is mandatory to preserve life. In about one third of patients with TAPVC, major associated conditions occur, such as heterotaxy, D-TGA, and hypoplastic left heart syndrome.

Classically, chest radiographs of patients with obstructed TAPVC show a normal-sized cardiac silhouette with severely congested pulmonary vessels and interstitial pulmonary edema. In chest radiographs of patients with TAPVC without obstruction, there is cardiomegaly (dilated RV and RA), an enlarged PA segment, and increased pulmonary flow. The classic "snowman" or "figure-of-eight" cardiac silhouette is seen in older patients with nonobstructive TAPVC and good intermixing, but not in infants and children. CT and MRI are useful to trace the entire course of the anomalous pulmonary vein, to exclude obstruction, and in the setting of mixed TAPVC. Treatment involves rerouting of the anomalous pulmonary vein to the LA and closure of the ASD. Recurrent pulmonary vein obstruction after TAPVC repair is an important indication for MRI in the postoperative setting and carries a poor prognosis.

Right-Sided Obstructive Lesions

The congenital lesions included in this group have a common denominator: right-sided obstruction of varying severity and the presence of a right-to-left shunt that results in cyanosis. Common examples are tetralogy of Fallot, tricuspid atresia, and Ebstein anomaly.

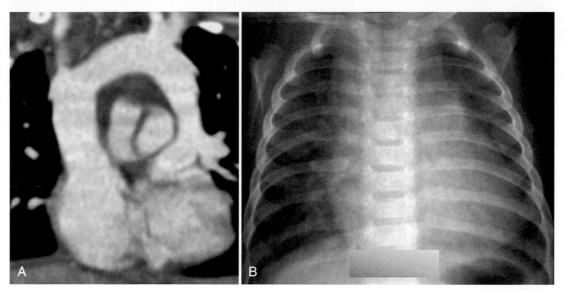

FIGURE 3-10. Total anomalous pulmonary venous return (TAPVR). **A** shows supracardiac TAPVR to the left innominate vein on CT angiography. **B,** This condition results in a snowman appearance on the corresponding chest radiograph, which also demonstrates increased pulmonary vascularity.

Tetralogy of Fallot

Tetralogy of Fallot is the most common cyanotic CHD of children and adults, accounting for 8% to 10% of cases. The pathologic substrate is anterior, cephalic, and leftward deviation of the conal septum, resulting in infundibular RV outflow tract obstruction, a conoventricular VSD, RV hypertrophy, and overriding of the VSD by the aorta. If the RV outflow tract obstruction is mild (one third of cases) and the VSD is large, the physiologic outcome is acyanosis in the infant, a so-called "pink tet." At the other end of the spectrum is a tetralogy of Fallot with pulmonary atresia, in which pulmonary blood flow depends on a patent ductus arteriosus, or major aortopulmonary collateral arteries (MAPCAs). Tetralogy of Fallot is associated with trisomy 21, tracheoesophageal fistula (TEF), and the VACTERL association (*v*ertebral abnormalities, *a*nal atresia, *c*ardiac abnormalities, *t*racheoesophageal fistula and/or *e*sophageal atresia, *r*enal agenesis and dysplasia, and *l*imb defects).

Radiographic findings in the chest are characterized by (1) decreased pulmonary flow, although the flow may be normal or even increased in patients with pink tet; (2) a cardiac waist that is notably narrow because of the absence of the pulmonary segment and thymic stress atrophy; and (3) RA hypertrophy, which rotates the heart and is evident as an upturned and prominent cardiac apex. This last feature explains the classic appearance of the coeur-en-sabot, or boot-shaped heart (Fig. 3-11). This particular cardiothymic contour is even more pronounced in the presence of a right-sided aortic arch, which occurs in 25% of patients.

The treatment for tetralogy of Fallot is surgical correction. Timing of surgery and procedures vary depending on the patient's anatomy and the physiology (severity and level of RV outflow tract obstruction, size of pulmonary arteries, presence of aortopulmonary collaterals, other associated cardiac defects). In the past, initial palliative procedures for pulmonary oligemia included central aortopulmonary shunts like the Potts, Waterston, and Blalock-Taussig shunts. The current treatment in most surgical centers is total correction in infancy, with closure of the VSD and enlargement of the RV outflow tract and PAs with a synthetic patch. In the setting of pulmonary atresia, a conduit is placed from the RV to the PA, typically a homograft (Rastelli procedure). A transannular patch repair leaves no functional pulmonary valve; therefore pulmonary regurgitation is the norm, with potential for RV volume overload, RV systolic and diastolic dysfunction, and arrhythmias.

MRI plays an important role in the postoperative period, in monitoring the RV and determining the optimal timing of pulmonary valve replacement. Patients with homografts require replacement procedures with continued growth; MRI and CT are helpful in screening such patients for stenosis as well as determining the optimal time for surgery (Fig. 3-12).

Tricuspid Atresia

Tricuspid atresia is complete absence of the tricuspid valve with no direct communication between the RA and RV. The RV is typically hypoplastic; the level of hypoplasia varies with the presence and size of associated VSDs. Infants who have an atretic tricuspid valve are cyanotic at birth and have an obligatory ASD, a VSD, and (rarely) a PDA in order to survive. The "RV" in tricuspid atresia is usually lacking the inflow portion and may consist only of the infundibulum or outlet chamber. If a VSD is present, it may also be termed the "bulboventricular foramen." Absence of the tricuspid valve is accompanied by transposition (D- or L-) of the great vessels in 30% of cases, and pulmonary stenosis (or, rarely, pulmonary atresia) in more than 50% of cases. The VSD may become restrictive over time, producing subpulmonary or subaortic stenosis.

Radiographs of the chest of a patient with tricuspid atresia show normal or decreased pulmonary flow, and a "rounded" cardiac apex caused by the RA enlargement. The RA contour is prominent, there may be a concave PA segment, and the aorta may be on the right side in 15% of children with tricuspid atresia. Initial palliation consists of maintaining pulmonary flow by keeping the PDA open with prostaglandins and by surgically creating a modified Blalock-Taussig shunt. Permanent palliation is accomplished by a single ventricle repair (Fig. 3-13). The survival rate is about 70% at 5 years.

Ebstein Anomaly

Ebstein anomaly is uncommon, constituting less than 1% of all cases of CHD. It is an abnormality of the tricuspid valve that consists of apical displacement of the annular attachments of the septal and posteroinferior leaflets. The anterior leaflet is usually attached at the normal position of the annulus, but is dysplastic and sail-like, resulting in severe tricuspid regurgitation. A portion of the RA becomes "atrialized" with a thin myocardium. An ASD is always present. Most infants are presented in the first month of life, although some survive to adolescence or even adulthood.

The radiographic findings in the chest depend on the extent of dilatation of the right side of the heart. The cardiac silhouette may resemble that of a pericardial effusion and be has been referred to as a "box-shaped heart" (Fig. 3-14). Pulmonary vascularity is often diminished, owing to right-to-left shunting at the atrial level. Treatment in the newborn may be palliative, consisting extracorporeal membrane oxygenation (ECMO) while the pulmonary vascular resistance is allowed to drop. The prognosis is variable; there is a 50% neonatal mortality rate by the first month for severe forms of Ebstein anomaly.

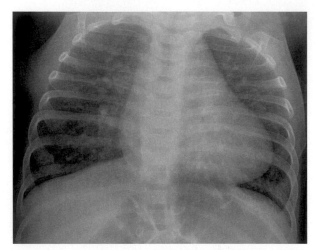

FIGURE 3-11. Tetralogy of Fallot. Typical boot-shaped heart with elevation of the cardiac apex in a patient with tetralogy of Fallot. This patient has relatively normal pulmonary vascularity because of the presence of only mild infundibular obstruction of the right ventricular outflow tract ("pink tet").

The differential diagnosis of the imaging findings also includes tricuspid insufficiency and Uhl anomaly. The latter consists of focal or complete absence of RV myocardium, resulting in a poorly functioning RV.

Left-Sided Obstructive Lesions

The most important left-sided obstructive lesions are (from proximal to distal) cor triatriatum, hypoplastic left heart syndrome, Shone syndrome, congenital aortic stenosis, and coarctation.

Hypoplastic Left Heart Syndrome

Hypoplastic left heart syndrome (HLHS), the most common cause of CHF in the neonate, manifests at birth. It is a spectrum of diseases in which the development of the left side of the heart is insufficient to sustain the systemic circulation. The major components of HLHS are hypoplasia or atresia of the aortic and mitral valves and varying degrees of hypoplasia of the left atrium, left ventricle, and ascending aorta (Fig. 3-15). There is an obligatory left-to-right shunt, most often at the atrial level. Chest radiographs show globular cardiomegaly with congestive changes in the lungs within 24 hours of birth.

The initial palliative surgery for HLHS is the stage I Norwood procedure, which comprises the following steps: The main PA is anastomosed to the ascending aorta, thereby making the RV the systemic ventricle (Damus-Kaye-Stansel procedure). An atrial septectomy is performed to redirect pulmonary venous return to the RV. The aortic arch is reconstructed to relieve the coarctation, and a Blalock-Taussig shunt is performed to provide pulmonary blood flow. The Stage II procedure is creation of the superior cavopulmonary shunt (bidirectional Glenn shunt in which the SVC is connected to the PA) and takedown of the Blalock Taussig shunt. Stage III consists of a total cavopulmonary shunt (Fontan procedure, in which the IVC is connected to the PA), which results in redirection of the entire systemic venous return passively to the lungs.

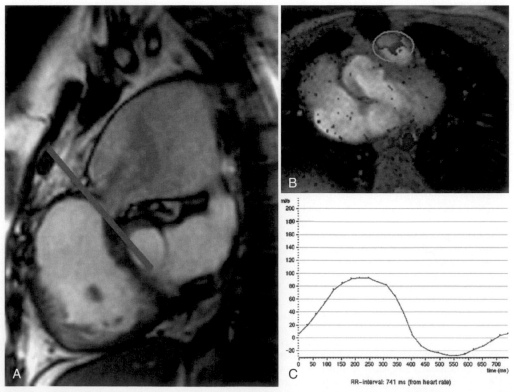

FIGURE 3-12. Postoperative MRI evaluation of tetralogy of Fallot. **A,** Recurrent right ventricular outflow tract (RVOT) obstruction with poststenotic dilatation of the main pulmonary artery demonstrated on a bright blood image. Flow-velocity mapping was performed across the RVOT in a plane marked by the *solid gray bar*, yielding a cross-sectional image of the RVOT as shown in **B**. A region of interest is drawn around the RVOT on the phase image to quantify the volume of forward flow and regurgitant flow within the RVOT, yielding a pulmonary regurgitant fraction of approximately 35%, as shown in **C**.

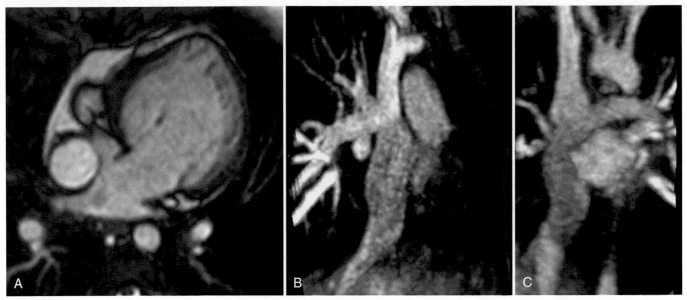

FIGURE 3-13. Tricuspid atresia. A, A long axis view of the heart on a bright blood MR image showing tricuspid valve replacement by atretic fatty, a normal mitral valve, and a functional single left ventricle. The patient has undergone palliation with a lateral tunnel Fontan procedure. B and C show the unobstructed superior and inferior cavopulmonary anastomoses, and the morphology of the branch pulmonary arteries on gadolinium-enhanced MR angiograms.

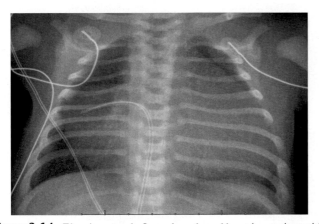

FIGURE 3-14. Ebstein anomaly. Large box-shaped heart in a patient with Ebstein anomaly, caused by a severely enlarged right atrium. There is associated reduced pulmonary vascularity.

The usual role of MRI in patients with HLHS is to clarify the status of the aortic arch prior to the stage I Norwood procedure and to determine the status of the branch pulmonary arteries, pulmonary veins, and systemic veins prior to the stage II and III procedures. This imaging modality is also helpful to monitor ventricular function, screen for thrombosis, and determine the cause of cyanosis after a Fontan procedure.

Shone Syndrome

Shone syndrome is a complex of four potentially obstructive anomalies of the left heart: supramitral ring, parachute mitral valve with a single papillary muscle of the LV, subaortic stenosis, and coarctation of the aorta. All four findings are not always present. It is considered a forme fruste of HLHS. An important decision in the neonatal period is whether the patient with Shone syndrome should undergo two-ventricle or single-ventricle palliation.

Cor Triatriatum

Cor triatriatum reflects the failure of the LA to incorporate the common pulmonary veins, resulting in a perforated pulmonary membrane that bisects the LA and impedes blood return from the lungs, akin to the physiology of mitral valve stenosis. Radiographs initially may show occasional interstitial edema with a normal-sized heart. When echocardiography findings are inconclusive, MRI is diagnostic, showing a membrane within the LA chamber that attaches proximal to the LA appendage.

Congenital Aortic Stenosis

Aortic valve abnormalities constitute the most common form of CHD. There are three types: most common is the valvular type, with a dysplastic, thickened, and frequently bicuspid aortic valve (70%) (Fig. 3-16). Subvalvular (fixed or dynamic) and supravalvular stenoses may also occur. The obstructive nature of the lesion eventually results in pressure overload of the RA. Subvalvular aortic stenosis may be fixed and discrete, caused by a fibromuscular ring, or may be dynamic and diffuse, often referred to as tunnel-type stenosis and related to idiopathic hypertrophic obstructive cardiomyopathy. The last entity may be familial in 35% of patients and has an equal gender incidence. Supravalvular stenosis may be sporadic or familial, or may be related to Williams syndrome (elfin facies, mental retardation, and neonatal hypercalcemia). In patients with Williams syndrome, associated findings include stenosis of the branch pulmonary arteries as well as the coronary arteries.

Patient age at presentation of aortic stenosis is inversely related to the severity of the obstruction; the clinical spectrum ranges from critical stenosis with CHF in the newborn to an asymptomatic murmur in children and adolescents. Valvular stenosis tends to be progressive with age and is characterized by a harsh systolic murmur at the upper right sternal border. Conventional chest radiographs most commonly show a normal heart size. The ascending aorta may be border forming on the right side of the mediastinum because of poststenotic dilatation (see Fig. 3-16). MRI helps delineate the location, extent, and nature of obstruction, especially in the setting of subvalvular or supravalvular stenosis.

Initial treatment of valvular aortic stenosis consists of balloon dilatation. If it is unsuccessful, an aortic valve commissurotomy is performed. Subvalvular and supravalvular stenoses are treated by resection of the obstructing segment, as follows:

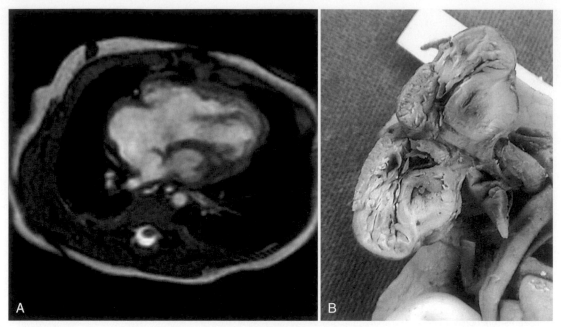

FIGURE 3-15. Hypoplastic left heart syndrome (HLHS). **A,** A four-chamber view from a bright blood MRI sequence showing severe hypoplasia of the left side of the heart. **B,** Postpartum image from a different patient with HLHS, showing mitral atresia and severe hypoplasia of the left ventricle.

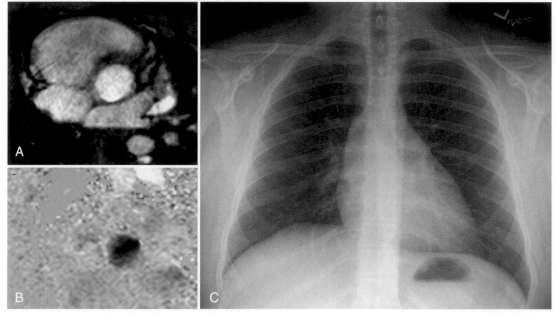

FIGURE 3-16. Congenital aortic valvular stenosis. Magnitude (**A**) and phase (**B**) images of a phase contrast MR sequence showing the characteristic appearance of a bicuspid aortic valve on cross-section. **C,** Chest radiograph demonstrating poststenotic dilatation of the ascending aorta secondary to congenital aortic valvular stenosis.

Konno procedure: For subvalvular aortic stenosis, the aortic annulus and RA outflow tract are enlarged through excision of a portion of the ventricular septum and insertion of a patch, followed by replacement of the aortic valve with a mechanical valve or homograft valve.

Ross procedure: For aortic valve insufficiency/stenosis, the aortic valve is removed, the pulmonary valve is "transplanted" ("autografted") to the aortic position, and a homograft is used to connect the RV to the MPA.

Coarctation of the Aorta

There are two types of coarctation, the discrete form, which involves the aortic isthmus, and the diffuse form, which involves the transverse aortic arch. Discrete coarctation occurs because of ductal tissue that is present in the aortic arch and involutes, resulting in narrowing of the arch. Most commonly occurring just distal to the origin of the left subclavian artery, discrete coarctation accounts for about 5% of all congenital heart lesions. Males are affected twice as often as females. The diffuse form is frequently associated with other proximal left-sided obstructive lesions, such as bicuspid aortic valve, aortic stenosis, Shone syndrome, and HLHS (Fig. 3-17). The presentation of the patient and timing of surgery depend on the severity of coarctation. Although most children with coarctation of the aorta are asymptomatic and are identified incidentally because of hypertension, some patients may present with CHF in the neonatal period.

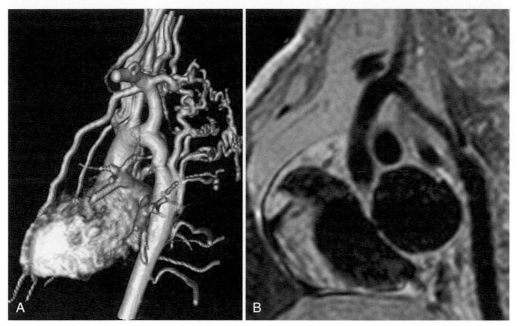

FIGURE 3-17. Types of aortic coarctation. **A,** A volume-rendered image from a gadolinium-enhanced three-dimensional MR angiogram showing discrete narrowing of the aortic isthmus with abundant collateral flow to the descending thoracic aorta. **B,** A black blood MR image showing diffuse hypoplasia and elongation of the transverse aortic arch.

The chest radiograph may show RA enlargement, especially on the lateral view, as well as poststenotic dilatation of the descending aorta. In contrast, the ascending aorta may be dilated and thus border forming on the right superior mediastinum because of turbulence caused by an associated bicuspid aortic valve. This combination of prestenotic and poststenotic bulging of the aortic arch has been described as the "figure-of-three" sign on the chest radiograph. The "reverse three," or "E," sign is the mirror image of these findings on an esophageal contrast study. Rib notching, which is rare in a child with coarctation of the aorta before 8 to 12 years of age, is typically located along the inferior aspects of ribs 3 through 8; it represents pressure erosion of hypertrophied intercostal arteries that are serving as collaterals. Rib notching is seen bilaterally unless an aberrant right subclavian artery is also present, in which case there is no notching on the right side.

The best estimate of the extent and severity of reduction in luminal caliber of the aorta is obtained from a high-resolution three-dimensional angiographic dataset with CT or MRI. The presence of RA hypertrophy with hyperdynamic systolic function correlates with systolic blood pressure and the pressure gradient across the coarctation. Reduction in LV systolic function in infancy is also an ominous sign of severe coarctation. The peak velocity distal to the coarctation, as determined by flow velocity mapping along the long axis of the descending thoracic aorta, is used to calculate the pressure gradient across the stenosis with the modified Bernouilli equation.

Treatment of coarctation of the aorta is coarctectomy with end-to-end anastomosis. The narrowed segment of the aorta is surgically excised, with or without patch augmentation.

▬ MISCELLANEOUS CONDITIONS
Pericardial Absence and Pericardial Cysts

Pericardial absence is classified as partial or complete, with partial left-sided defects being the most common. In one third of cases, it is associated with intracardiac defects such as PDA, ASD, and tetralogy of Fallot, or multisystem processes like pentalogy of Cantrell. The chest radiograph, in the setting of a small pericardial defect, shows an abnormal protuberance in the region of the LA appendage and main PA. Herniation of these structures through the defect is a rare complication. Partial pericardial

defect on the right side is very rare. In the setting of a large pericardial defect, the heart is rotated away from the sternum, causing an unusual cardiomediastinal contour with an elevated and rotated cardiac apex and a large retrosternal air gap. Fluoroscopy demonstrates abnormal mobility of the heart within the chest.

Pericardial cysts can be true or false. The true ones are located within the pericardial sac but have no communication with it; false cysts, or diverticula, are protrusions of parietal pericardium and consequently have direct communication with it. True cysts can occur anywhere on the pericardium but are found most often in the right costophrenic angle. They are clinically symptomatic in only a small number of cases and are usually diagnosed incidentally. If symptomatic, they are aspirated percutaneously or resected thoracoscopically.

Kawasaki Disease

Kawasaki disease is a mucocutaneous lymph node syndrome characterized by fever, rash, conjunctivitis, and cervical adenopathy. Its peak incidence is between 1 and 3 years of age. The symptoms are due to a generalized vasculitis, with involvement of the coronary arteries and myocardium being a characteristic feature. The coronary artery vasculitis may be complicated by aneurysm formation and stenoses of the proximal portions of both left and right coronary arteries, and may rarely be complicated by myocardial infarction, which is often clinically occult. Conventional chest radiographic findings are often normal, except for rare instances of cardiac enlargement in severe cases of myocarditis. MRI, which can accurately detect aneurysms of the coronaries and the systemic arteries, significant stenosis of the proximal coronaries, active vasculitis, and the presence of myocardial damage, is the preferred modality for follow-up of patients with Kawasaki disease (see Fig. 3-16). Aspirin and intravenous gamma-globulin administered early in the course of disease usually have an excellent outcome.

Rheumatic Heart Disease

Rheumatic heart disease is caused by acute rheumatic fever, which is a delayed complication of streptococcal disease, a throat infection with group A beta-hemolytic streptococci. It can cause long-term damage to the heart muscle or heart valves, especially in the setting of repeated and untreated episodes. Rheumatic heart disease is rare in the western world but is still a common affliction in developing countries. It is the most common cause of acquired valvular insufficiency and/or stenosis. Acute rheumatic fever may result in myocarditis, with valvular involvement of the mitral (85%) and aortic (55%) valves. If mitral stenosis or mitral regurgitation occurs, chest radiographs often show LA enlargement, as evidenced by an "atrial double density sign," and a prominence of the LA appendage. If pulmonary venous hypertension develops, there may be signs of congestive failure with Kerley B lines and interstitial edema. In children, treatment with appropriate antibiotics is often sufficient early in the course of the disease. In the setting of established rheumatic heart disease, however, surgery for the affected valves is required.

▬ APPENDIX

Cardiac Position

Levocardia: Heart in left chest, apex pointing leftward (normal position).

Mesocardia: Heart in the midline, apex pointing inferiorly.

Dextrocardia: Heart in the right chest, apex pointing rightward.

Ectopia cordis: Heart partially or completely outside the chest.

Dextroposition: Rightward displacement of the heart with apex pointing leftward, as may be seen in a left-sided tension pneumothorax.

Dextrorotation: Most commonly, the base of the heart is in the normal position, but the apex has rotated rightwards.

Dextroversion: An old term that has been replaced by *isolated dextrocardia*, which refers to dextrocardia in the setting of situs solitus.

"Isolated levocardia": Levocardia in the setting of situs inversus; there is a high incidence of CHD with isolated dextrocardia and isolated levocardia.

Visceral Situs and Atrial Situs

Situs refers to the position of the unpaired organs (liver, spleen, stomach) as well as the atria. There are three possibilities:

Situs solitus (S): Usual position; liver on right, spleen on left, RA on right, LA on left

Situs inversus (I): Mirror image of the usual position; liver on left, spleen on right, RA on left, LA on right

Situs ambiguus (A): Neither solitus nor inversus; midline liver, asplenia or polysplenia, common atrium or indeterminate morphologic right and left atria; also known as heterotaxy and frequently associated with complex CHD

Classic Radiographic Signs in Congenital Heart Disease

These signs are explained in the text:

Egg on a string: D-TGA.

Snowman sign: Supracardiac TAPVR to the left innominate vein.

Coeur-en-sabot or boot-shaped heart: Tetralogy of Fallot.

Box-shaped heart: Ebstein anomaly.

Scimitar sign: Partial anomalous pulmonary venous return of the right lung to the IVC.

Gooseneck deformity: Elongation of the LV outflow tract in the common AV canal.

Figure-of-three and reversed-three signs: Coarctation of the aorta.

"Named" Pediatric Cardiac Surgical Procedures

Aortopulmonary Shunts

The indication for these procedures is to increase pulmonary blood flow in lesions with inadequate pulmonary blood flow.

Blalock-Taussig shunt: The first palliative surgery for cyanotic heart disease. A classic Blalock-Taussig shunt consists of an end-to-side anastomosis of the subclavian artery to the PA. The modified version consists of interposition (side-to-side) of a polytetrafluoroethylene (PTFE; GORE-TEX) tube graft between the subclavian artery and the PA.

Central shunt: PTFE tube graft from the ascending aorta to the PA.

Potts shunt: Direct anastomosis of the descending aorta to the left PA.

Waterston (Cooley) shunt: Direct anastomosis of the ascending aorta to the right PA.

Procedures for Transposition of the Great Arteries

Blalock Hanlon atrial septectomy: A closed-heart procedure using clamps to isolate the posterior part of the atrial septum and cut it out; rarely used today.

Rashkind balloon atrial septostomy: A catheterization procedure using a stiff balloon pulled across the foramen ovale from the LA to the RA to rip the atrial septum and make a bigger ASD.

Arterial switch operation (ASO; Jatene procedure): The great arteries are divided and switched so that the aorta is connected to the LV, and the PA is connected to the RV. The coronaries are transferred to the neo-aortic root. The Lecompte maneuver refers to the repositioning of the pulmonary arteries in front of the neo-aorta from their original position behind the aorta.

Atrial switch procedures: Senning and Mustard: Also known as intra-atrial baffle procedures; the end physiology of these two operations is the same, but the procedures differ in the use of baffle material and placement. The native atrial septum is removed, and baffles are constructed to redirect the systemic venous return into the mitral valve, LV, and out the PA. The pulmonary venous return is directed into the tricuspid valve, RV, and out the aorta.

Rastelli procedure—for TGA with VSD and pulmonary stenosis: "Rastelli" is a term used for any RV to PA conduit, but the original operation was for TGA with a VSD and pulmonary stenosis. The VSD is closed in a way to connect the LV with the aorta, and a conduit is used to connect the RV with the PA.

Single Ventricle Palliations

Norwood procedure—stage I: Initially devised for HLHS, but also applied to any single ventricle lesion with systemic outflow obstruction. The first part is the Damus-Kaye-Stansel (DKS) procedure, in which the ascending aorta is connected to the main PA (with the result that the RV is used to pump systemic blood flow). The aortic arch is augmented. A modified Blalock-Taussig shunt is placed to provide pulmonary blood flow, and the atrial septum is excised to ensure free mixing of blood at the atrial level.

Bidirectional Glenn (BDG) stage II procedure: These procedures direct the systemic venous return from the upper body directly into the lungs by connecting the SVC to the pulmonary arteries.

Fontan–stage III procedure: The basic concept is to create a pathway for all venous blood to flow directly into the pulmonary arteries without passing through the heart. The *original Fontan* procedure connected the RA appendage to the pulmonary arteries. There was a high incidence of RA dilatation and atrial arrhythmias with this procedure, so the *lateral tunnel Fontan* procedure was developed to only utilize a portion of the atrium as a connection from the IVC to the pulmonary arteries. A fenestration (small hole) is usually left in the patch to provide a "popoff" for venous blood to return to the heart. There is still a high incidence of atrial arrhythmias with this variation, so the *extracardiac conduit Fontan* procedure was developed to involve less suturing in the atrium; a homograft is used to connect the IVC to the PA outside the heart.

Differential Diagnoses

Dilated PA:
- Valvular pulmonary stenosis
- Left-to-right shunts (VSD, ASD, PDA)
- Pulmonary arterial hypertension

Concave PA:
- Tetralogy of Fallot
- Pulmonary atresia
- TGA (secondary to rotation)

Dilated ascending aorta:
- Aortic valvular stenosis
- Bicuspid aortic valve
- Marfan syndrome
- PDA

Right aortic arch:
- Tetralogy of Fallot (25%)
- PDA (35%)
- Double-outlet RA (15%)
- D-TGA (10%)
- Tricuspid atresia (rarely)

▬ SUGGESTED READINGS

TEXTS

Araoz PA, Reddy GP, Higgins CB: Congenital heart disease: Morphology and function. In Higgins CB, de Roos A (editors): Cardiovascular MRI and MRA. Philadelphia, Lippincott Williams & Wilkins, 2002, pp 307-338.

Allen HD, Driscoll DJ, Shaddy RE, et al (eds): Moss and Adams' Heart Disease in Infants, Children, and Adolescents: Including the Fetus and Young Adults, ed 7. Philadelphia, Lippincott Williams & Wilkins, 2008.

Elliot LP (ed): Cardiac Imaging in Infants, Children and Adults. Philadelphia, Lippincott-Raven, 1991.

Krishnamurthy R, Chung T: Pediatric cardiac MRI. In Lucaya J, Strife JL (eds): Pediatric Chest Radiology: Chest Imaging in Infants and Children, ed 2 rev. (Medical Radiology/Diagnostic Imaging). Berlin, Springer-Verlag, 2007.

ARTICLES

Boechat MI, Ratib O, Williams PL, et al: Cardiac MR imaging and MR angiography for assessment of complex tetralogy of Fallot and pulmonary atresia. Radiographics 2005;25:1535-46.

Gaca AM, Jaggers JJ, Dudley LT, Bisset GS 3rd: Repair of congenital heart disease: A primer—part 1. Radiology 2008;247:617-31.

Gaca AM, Jaggers JJ, Dudley LT, Bisset GS 3rd: Repair of congenital heart disease: A primer—part 2. Radiology 2008;248:44-60.

Kellenberger CJ, Yoo SJ, Büchel ER: Cardiovascular MR imaging in neonates and infants with congenital heart disease. Radiographics 2007;27:5-18.

Krishnamurthy R: Pediatric cardiac MRI: Anatomy and function. Pediatr Radiol 2008;38:S192-9.

Rhodes JF, Hijazi ZM, Sommer RJ: Pathophysiology of congenital heart disease in the adult, part II: Simple obstructive lesions. Circulation 2008;117:1228-37.

Sommer RJ, Hijazi ZM, Rhodes JF Jr: Pathophysiology of congenital heart disease in the adult. Part I: Shunt lesions. Circulation 2008;26:117:1090-9.

Sommer RJ, Hijazi ZM, Rhodes JF: Pathophysiology of congenital heart disease in the adult. Part III: Complex congenital heart disease. Circulation 2008;117:1340-50.

Van Praagh R: Terminology of congenital heart disease: Glossary and commentary. Circulation 1977;56:139-43.

Van Praagh R: The segmental approach clarified. Cardiovasc Intervent Radiol 1984;7:320-5.

CHAPTER 4

Gastrointestinal Tract

Bruce R. Parker and Johan G. (Hans) Blickman

▬ IMAGING TECHNIQUES

Conventional Radiographs

In a child with abdominal symptoms, conventional radiographs of the abdomen are usually the recommended initial imaging evaluation. Most institutions now utilize computed radiographic or digital radiographic technology. Elaboration of these techniques' attendant artifacts is beyond the scope of this discussion, but they must be recognized by the radiologist.

Although many clinicians request ultrasound or computed tomography (CT) as the first imaging examination, conventional radiographs may provide useful information for tailoring the examination to the individual patient's problem. Abdominal radiographs are typically obtained in supine position and with a horizontal beam examination, preferably upright, although left decubitus views are obtained in newborns and ill or uncooperative patients. Single supine examinations may be obtained when the clinical suspicion is constipation or foreign body ingestion or if the examination is being performed for tube or catheter localization. On a cross-table lateral view it may be difficult to differentiate intraluminal air from extraluminal air, and decubitus or upright views are more useful.

There are pertinent points of difference between the abdominal radiograph of an adult and that of a child: the liver takes up a relatively larger space in the peritoneal cavity of a child. The spleen may not be visible and usually does not displace the gastric contour in a child. Likewise, the retroperitoneal fat "stripes" (psoas shadows) are frequently not seen on the radiograph of a child because of the relative paucity of fat in the infant's and small child's retroperitoneum. The lack of fat in the capsules of the solid organs makes evaluation of their size nearly impossible on radiographs. In contrast, the properitoneal fat stripes are visible from infancy. A soft tissue pseudomass in the abdomen may be the urinary bladder, the fluid-filled stomach or intestine, or an umbilical hernia (Fig. 4-1).

In the newborn there should be air in the stomach at birth. By 6 hours at the latest, the stomach and greater portion of the small bowel should be filled with air, and by 24 hours of life air should appear in the rectum, although rectal air is typically present much earlier. However, the appearance of air throughout the gastrointestinal (GI) tract is usually more rapid in normal newborns. Unlike adults, children up to the toddler age group typically have air throughout the entire GI tract. A variation in this sequence, such as absence of air in the stomach at 1 hour, should raise the possibility of an esophageal obstruction. However, the most common cause of a lack of intestinal air in the newborn is depression of crying and swallowing in ill babies, especially those with newborn lung disease. The neonate in whom an orogastric or nasogastric (NG) tube has been placed may have a relatively gasless abdomen without other underlying pathology. Other causes of a gasless abdomen are vomiting, medication that decreases peristalsis, and obstruction of a fluid-filled viscus. Peritoneal irritation (peritonitis) or ascites may also displace abdominal gas. Absence of meconium passage by 24 hours is abnormal, and abdominal distention or marked dilatation of any viscus in the first day of life should lead to further imaging evaluation.

Abnormal Gas Patterns

Abnormal gas patterns can be distinctive in the neonate and are described later, in the discussions of specific entities. In neonates and infants it is often impossible to differentiate small from large bowel, especially if the bowel becomes dilated. A prone film is frequently helpful because air rises into the rectum when obstruction is not present.

Adynamic Ileus

In infants and older children, adynamic ileus occurs after surgery, in cases of sepsis, or with gastroenteritis, or it can be associated with electrolyte disturbances such as dehydration and hypokalemia. In addition, drugs such as opiates and anticholinergics may cause ileus. Ileus should be suggested only when loops of intestine are dilated. Presence of air in normal-caliber large and small bowel is a common and normal finding in newborns and infants.

Dynamic Ileus

Dynamic (mechanical) ileus usually has an anatomic cause. The common causes of mechanical obstruction in the neonate are duodenal atresia and stenosis, and midgut malrotation with volvulus or obstructing peritoneal bands (Ladd bands). The differential diagnosis beyond the neonatal period, in descending order of likelihood, consists of (appendiceal) inflammation, intussusception, (inguinal) hernia, postoperative adhesions, post–necrotizing enterocolitis strictures, and midgut volvulus. Other causes of obstruction in childhood are quite uncommon (Fig. 4-2).

When it is difficult (if not impossible) to differentiate large from small bowel in the presence of bowel dilatation, determining the location and appearance of the distended loops often helps. In older children, valvulae conniventes and haustral markings distinguish small bowel and large bowel, respectively, and the distended colon is more peripheral in location than the more centrally located distended small bowel. These findings may not be applicable in the neonate or the child with midgut malrotation.

Pneumoperitoneum

Free air in the peritoneal cavity most commonly results from perforation of a hollow viscus. The causes are variable and are described in the individual sections later. Other causes of pneumoperitoneum are postoperative air and tracking of air from the mediastinum into the retroperitoneum and thence along the course of the mesenteric vessels, resulting in subserosal air, which can rupture into the peritoneal cavity. This latter phenomenon occurs in children who have pneumomediastinum and usually are undergoing pressure ventilation, but it has been described in asthmatic patients as well. This latter condition can be distinguished from visceral perforation by the lack of intraperitoneal air/fluid levels on horizontal beam radiographs.

Large amounts of free air are readily identifiable on supine abdominal radiographs, which may show the presence of Rigler sign, the rugby ball sign, and/or visualization of the falciform ligament. Small amounts of free air typically require a horizontal beam radiograph, either a decubitus or upright view. A cross-table lateral supine view may show a long colonic collection of air mimicking pneumoperitoneum. Perforation of a hollow viscus typically leads to intraperitoneal air/fluid levels as intraluminal fluid as well as air leaks into the peritoneal cavity.

Ascites

Ascites has many causes. In the neonate, ascites may be urinary in origin (25% to 30% of all cases) and secondary to obstruction, most commonly from posterior urethral valves and subsequent forniceal rupture of the collecting system. The second most common type of ascites is chylous ascites, which results from rupture

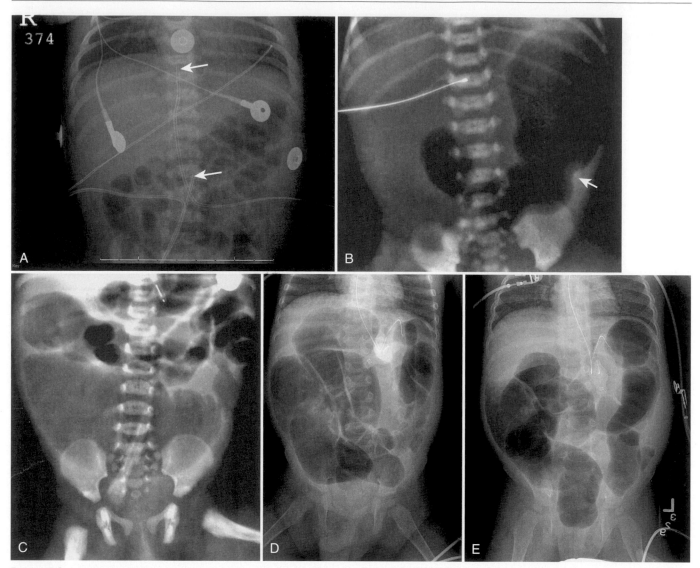

Figure 4-1. Value of "plain" radiographs. **A,** Correct positions of the umbilical venous *(upper arrow)* and arterial *(lower arrow)* catheters. **B,** Duodenal atresia. Abdominal radiograph showing air in the stomach and duodenal bulb, with a visualized peristaltic wave in the stomach *(arrow)* and no air distally. **C,** Ileal atresia. Markedly dilated loops of bowel with a transverse orientation in a 1-day-old child. **D,** Supine kidney-ureters-bladder (KUB) view shows multiple dilated loops of air filled bowel which could be adynamic ileus or low obstruction. **E,** Prone KUB view demonstrates air in the rectum denoting a nonobstructive ileus.

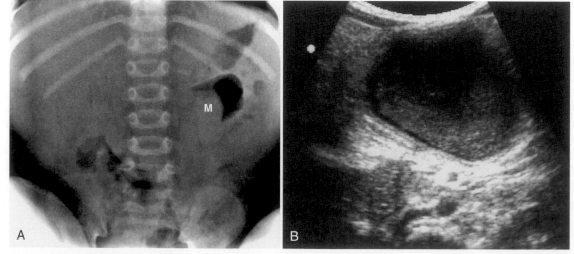

Figure 4-2. **A,** Abdominal radiograph in a 2-year-old child with abdominal pain suggests the intussusceptum (M) invaginating the intussuscipiens. **B,** Ultrasonogram depicts the lead point, an ileal duplication cyst.

of the lymphatic ducts due to either birth trauma or postoperative complications. Other causes of ascites are peritonitis due to bowel perforation (meconium peritonitis or necrotizing enterocolitis) or appendicitis, congestive heart disease, chronic liver or renal disease, and erythroblastosis fetalis.

Conventional abdominal imaging classically illustrates centralization of bowel loops on the supine examination (air rises!), blurring of the inferior hepatic edge, and obliteration of the properitoneal fat planes caused by fluid in the paracolic gutters. Ultrasound (US) is much more sensitive, as is CT, for detecting small amounts of fluid generally as well as in Morison's pouch or the pouch of Douglas long before they may be clinically suspected. Children with ascites are frequently quite ill, and bedside ultrasound provides excellent diagnostic information about the volume of ascites and may help diagnose the etiology of the fluid accumulation.

Calcifications

Structures that may contain calcifications include the peritoneal wall (meconium peritonitis) and viscera (appendicolith, torsion of an ovary) as well as the retroperitoneal organs (adrenal hemorrhage, neuroblastoma, Wilms tumor). The differential diagnosis of a calcified entity in the pediatric abdomen generally includes (infarcted or infected) mesenteric or duplication cysts, calcified thrombi secondary to arterial or venous line placement, nephrocalcinosis, and renal or gallbladder calculi. Liver and spleen calcifications occur in entities such as chronic granulomatous disease of childhood (CGDC), hemangiomas, hamartomas, hepatoblastomas, and some metastatic malignancies. Some of the medications used for cardiac surgery patients have been implicated in calcifications of intrahepatic vascular structures. Retroperitoneal calcifications may occur in the adrenal glands (neuroblastoma, resolved adrenal hematoma) or in the pancreas (pancreatitis, cystic fibrosis).

Tube and Catheter Positions

Most tubes and catheters are placed by the clinical team, but radiographs are typically used for confirmation of position. In the newborn, abdominal radiographs are commonly used to assess the positions of umbilical catheters, enteric tubes, and vascular access catheters.

Umbilical artery and vein catheters can be distinguished on the basis of their anatomic positions. The umbilical artery catheter enters one of the umbilical arteries and courses caudad to its junction with the internal iliac artery. It then turns cephalad, coursing through the iliac system to the abdominal aorta. The tip should be either in the thoracic descending aorta or, preferably, in the abdominal aorta below the origin of the great vessels and above the aortic bifurcation. The preferred position is below the superior endplate of L2 and above L4. The major complication is embolization of a great vessel or lower extremity artery by the thrombus that invariably forms at the tip of the umbilical artery catheter. The umbilical vein catheter courses from the umbilicus cephalad through the umbilical vein and ductus venosus into the inferior cavoatrial junction. Because the umbilical vein catheter shares sinusoids with the portal vein, it may enter the portal vein, the splenic vein, or the superior mesenteric vein (SMV) and should be replaced.

In older infants and children, venous access is often achieved through the iliac vein. The preferred position of the tip is in the inferior vena cava, although it is commonly left in the femoral vein. The major complication is venous thrombosis with the risk of subsequent pulmonary embolism. Perforation by a vascular catheter is fortunately quite rare but potentially fatal.

Orogastric tubes are more commonly used in the newborn, and NG tubes in older children. The tip of such a tube should reside in the stomach. Common complications of the use of orogastric or NG tubes are tracheal intubation, coiling of the tube in the pharynx or esophagus, and, rarely, perforation of the esophagus or stomach.

Contrast Examinations

Indications for contrast examinations of the GI tract are discussed subsequently in the appropriate sections.

Barium Compounds

There are two relative contraindications to using barium as a contrast agent, suspected bowel perforation and predisposition for pulmonary aspiration of barium. Neither one is an absolute contraindication. Barium in the retroperitoneum, mediastinum, or peritoneal cavity that is removed shortly after entering these spaces holds only a minimal risk for sequelae such as granuloma formation, adhesions, and peritonitis. However, successful removal is not always possible, and barium is generally contraindicated when the probability of perforation exists. Likewise, aspirated barium provokes a cough reflex. Thus, when routine care is taken, barium constitutes a most useful and safe contrast agent in the pediatric age group.

Water-Soluble Contrast Agents

The most commonly used of the water-soluble contrast agents are diatrizoate meglumine/sodium (Gastrografin or Gastroview) and, much less commonly these days, diatrizoate meglumine (Hypaque). Iothalamate meglumine (Conray; Cysto-Conray) is also used. These agents are hyperosmolar water-soluble media and should not be used routinely in the upper GI tract. There is a serious risk of pulmonary edema or death when these agents are aspirated, because the aspirated contrast medium causes a release of histamine or histamine-like substances in the lung. In addition, hyperosmolar agents may be toxic to the bowel mucosa, and their hydrophilic nature can result in massive fluid shifts, especially in neonates. These hyperosmolar contrast agents also draw fluid into the GI lumen, often resulting in their marked dilution, sometimes as early as the third portion of the duodenum, thus severely limiting their diagnostic use for the rest of the GI tract. In the large bowel, on the other hand, these agents can be used in an enema to exploit their hyperosmolar quality (e.g., to facilitate meconium plug evacuation by absorbing fluid into the bowel lumen, thus having a "lubricating" effect, especially when mixed with a wetting agent such as polysorbate 80). Through appropriate dilution of these agents, near isotonicity can be achieved. The package insert usually provides easy directions to accomplish this. A 3:1 solution is the most commonly used dilution formula.

Isotonic contrast agents are useful when perforation is suspected or when the anatomic integrity must be evaluated in the sick neonate. Indications include necrotizing enterocolitis (NEC) and bowel anastomoses after surgery.

Low-osmolar, water-soluble contrast agents have the advantages of not being diluted upon passage through the GI tract, of having virtually no effect on the lungs or peritoneum, and of not being absorbed into the tissues. Their major disadvantage is their cost, which is many times higher than that of conventional hyperosmolar agents.

Positive Contrast Studies

Positive contrast studies of the small and large bowel of a child do differ significantly from those of an adult, in that clinical circumstances to a large degree dictate which study is to be performed and in what fashion. Congenital abnormalities of the bowel, such as malrotation, occur more frequently in children, whereas inflammatory bowel disease (IBD) is uncommon in children younger than 10 years. It is therefore important that the radiologist be aware of the potential yield of an examination, its risks, and the effect of the examination on possible therapeutic regimens to follow.

In pediatric upper GI studies, the imager assesses the swallowing mechanism and for the presence or absence of nasopharyngeal reflux, laryngeal penetration, and tracheal aspiration. The contours and motility pattern of the esophagus and gastroesophageal junction, as well as the anatomic and functional integrity of the stomach, duodenum, and proximal jejunum, should be evaluated. The location of the duodenojejunal junction is paramount in assessment of normal rotation and positioning of the GI tract. Normally, the duodenojejunal junction is located to the left of the spine behind the stomach at the level of the duodenal bulb (Fig. 4-3). It may be located as medially as the left pedicle, or slightly lower than the level of the duodenal bulb. The ligament of Treitz forms properly when the duodenojejunal junction is appropriately located but is not present when midgut malrotation has occurred. The duodenal C-loop is usually smooth but may contain undulations (e.g., Z-loop). On occasion, especially in children younger than 1 year, the duodenal sweep is on a mesentery and is redundant, mimicking malrotation. Double-contrast views of the stomach and duodenum are worthwhile for evaluation of the mucosa but are not mandatory as they are in the adult population.

The radiographic evaluation of gastroesophageal reflux (GER) in children is controversial. There are some who assess the presence or absence of GER over 5 minutes while intermittently performing fluoroscopy, whereas others rely on an incidental observation of GER during the upper GI study. A pH probe study is the most reliable diagnostic tool for GER, but nuclear medicine evaluation (milk scan) may be used to evaluate GER. All infants younger than 9 to 12 months experience reflux from time to time, and imaging for GER often serves to objectify the subjective; in other words, therapy for symptoms possibly caused by GER should be guided by the clinical findings (e.g., visualized aspiration, recurrent pneumonias, or failure to thrive).

The contrast enema examination is performed in neonates primarily for anatomic evaluation of suspected "low" obstructions, neonatal small left colon syndrome, ileal atresia, or meconium plug. In infants and children it is used for suspected Hirschsprung disease and (rarely) for evaluation of lower GI bleeding. Rigorous preparatory cleansing of the colon, as is done in adults, is not usually necessary in children because intraluminal lesions (carcinoma, polyps) are less common. However, when the clinical concern is for polyps or tumors, double-contrast enemas can be successfully performed in patients of virtually any age. Particularly in the evaluation of Hirschsprung disease, there should be no preparation of the colon because it may preclude determination of a transition zone, especially in the rectum. For this reason, a straight-tipped nonbulbous catheter is often used to minimize disturbance of the anorectal anatomy. On the other hand, to evaluate the colonic mucosa in patients in whom IBD or polyps are suspected, adequate preparation is mandatory. The use of a balloon type enema tip is contraindicated in virtually all lower GI tract examinations in children. Proper taping into position of a soft, malleable, bulbous enema tip is sufficient and virtually atraumatic. Whether fluoroscopy should be performed with the patient in the prone or supine position is a personal preference; however, at the outset of the study, the patient should be in the (left) lateral position so that the presacral space as well as the puborectalis sling can be adequately evaluated. Spot films of the splenic and hepatic flexures and the sigmoid colon are necessary only in specific instances, especially in older teenaged boys with symptoms that may be caused by mucinous carcinomas of the colon.

A postevacuation film is mandatory, especially after reduction of intussusception, to check for recurrence, and after all other single-contrast enema examinations to evaluate for mucosal detail. The film can be omitted after double-contrast examinations. A 24-hour postevacuation film is no longer utilized because it can not differentiate Hirschsprung disease from other causes of prolonged retention of contrast material and stool.

Finally, throughout the entire small and large bowel, prominent lymphoid follicles, a normal finding that is particularly well seen in the terminal ileum, cecum, and ascending colon, should not be confused with pathology. This observation holds true for all children (Fig. 4-4), but is most prominent in patients with hypogammaglobulinemia.

Air

Air has been a useful contrast agent for decades. In pediatric imaging, air has been used with increasing frequency in the reduction of intussusception. Reluctance to use air has been attributed to its being more cumbersome to use. (It actually becomes easier to use with experience.) Additionally, there is reluctance to use air because the pressure of the insufflated air must be regulated, the absorbed radiation dose is somewhat higher, and the monitoring of the air column may be difficult. More important, the perforation rate with air has been noted to be as high as 2.5%, as opposed to 0.5% with positive contrast materials. Further discussion is presented later. On the other hand, air is very useful, although rarely needed, as a contrast agent in suspected esophageal atresia. One needs only a small amount administered through an esophageal tube to outline the atretic pouch, without the risk of aspiration that would be present if a positive contrast agent were used.

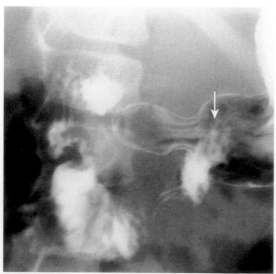

FIGURE 4-3. Normal ligament of Treitz. Note the duodenojejunal junction *(arrow)* behind the stomach at the level of the pylorus.

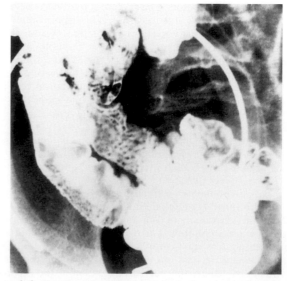

FIGURE 4-4. Prominent lymphoid follicles in the terminal ileum.

Ultrasound

US is the screening modality of choice in the child in whom an intra-abdominal or retroperitoneal mass, visceral calculi, pyloric stenosis, or intussusception is suspected. US is easy and quick to perform (can be done at the bedside and with minimal if any patient preparation), and uses no ionizing radiation. There is no known risk associated with the procedure, and the lack of fat in infants and children allows for better visualization of intra-abdominal and retroperitoneal structures than can be achieved in the adult.

In general, a directed approach (e.g., "right upper quadrant pain") leads to a higher diagnostic yield than one guided by vague symptoms (e.g., "abdominal pain"). High-resolution transducers should always be used. A variety of transducers is necessary to deal with children, who vary extensively in size. Color-flow Doppler US evaluation of all major vessels should be routine.

Computed Tomography

CT has proved to be an extremely accurate and fast imaging modality. Few children of any age require sedation when newer multidetector scanners (MDCT) are used. The different regimens used for sedation reflect personal radiologist preferences and are influenced by the availability of pediatric anesthesia monitoring. An abdominal CT scan should be performed with both oral and intravenous (IV) contrast agent, although a variety of protocols have been introduced to evaluate right lower quadrant pain. Box 4-1 outlines the requirements and suggestions for the pediatric age group with regard to oral and IV contrast administration as well as sedation.

The advantages of CT lie in the superior tissue plane resolution compared with that achieved with conventional radiographs. Multiplanar reconstructions and three-dimensional (3D) rendering have improved the diagnostic accuracy of CT in children as well as in adults. Disadvantages are relative. The radiation dose per slice from the average abdominal CT scan compares favorably with that of abdominal angiography and excretory urograms, especially given the amounts of information the modalities provide. However, publicly reported concerns about the long-term effects of radiation from CT have significantly and appropriately raised parent and physician apprehension. In all but the largest children, the radiation dose can be significantly reduced by decreasing both mAs and kV(p). Much of the potentially harmful radiation in children comes from the use of settings appropriate to adults. It is incumbent on the radiologist to assess the indication for the examination and the technical factors used.

Indications for the use of CT include the evaluation of intra-abdominal solid masses, abscesses, trauma, and hepatobiliary abnormalities as well as tumor staging. It is also helpful in the guidance of percutaneous biopsies, placement of drainage catheters, and establishment of radiation therapy portals.

Magnetic Resonance Imaging

Advantages of magnetic resonance imaging (MRI) are superior multiplanar capabilities, absence of ionizing radiation, excellent soft tissue contrast, and high-resolution imaging of the vasculature.

The disadvantages include the need for sedation in younger patients. Sedation of older patients is determined on a case-by-case basis (see Box 4-1). Motion artifacts related to breathing and bowel peristalsis also limit the use of MRI in this setting. The total scan time for MRI is typically considerably longer than that for CT (although the scan times are decreasing steadily with improving software applications). Claustrophobia is also an issue in the use of MRI with pediatric patients. MRI is usually more expensive than CT or US.

Protocols

The MRI protocols for evaluating gastrointestinal disorders in children are, for the most part, similar to those used for imaging the adult patient, with the following important caveats: (1) the need to adapt the sequences for free-breathing acquisition and (2) the requirement for higher spatial and temporal resolution due to the small size and rapid hemodynamic status of children. Following are some specific considerations for imaging pediatric patients:

Motion: Techniques used to minimize artifacts secondary to physiologic respiratory and cardiovascular motion include respiratory ordered-phase encoding, respiratory triggering, navigator respiratory gating, cardiac gating, gradient moment nulling ("flow comp"), and presaturation. Peristalsis may be temporarily halted by the intravenous administration of glucagon.

Spatial resolution: In order to achieve adequate resolution, the smallest coil that provides optimal coverage of the region of interest should be used. For infants and newborns, the head or shoulder coil can sometimes be used to image the abdomen. Small phased-array surface coils are an ideal choice in small children, providing excellent spatial resolution along with the ability to reduce scan time by means of parallel imaging. For larger children, phased-array coils with larger coverage (body coil) are optimal. The field of view, matrix, slice thickness, and slice spacing determine the spatial resolution of any given study and should be tailored to the specific demands of the clinical situation.

> ### *Box 4-1.* Suggestions for Contrast Agents and Sedation for Computed Tomography in Children
>
> **ORAL CONTRAST AGENTS**
> The contrast agent commonly used to opacify the GI tract is 5 mL of diatrizoate meglumine–diatrizoate sodium–iodine (Gastrografin) in 6 oz (180 mL) of orange juice. Orange juice is preferred because the taste of this agent in water is not pleasant.
>
> **Suggested Dosage According to Age**
> < 1 month: 1-1.5 oz
> 1 month-1 year: 3-4 oz
> 1-2 years: 4-5 oz
> 2-5 years: 6 oz
> 5-10 years: 8 oz
> 10-12 years: 10 oz
> 12-18 years: 12 oz
>
> **INTRAVENOUS CONTRAST AGENTS**
> *Note.* Requirement for informed consent with use of intravenous (IV) agents varies from institution to institution.
>
> It is strongly suggested that low-osmolar, water-soluble contrast agents (physician-administered or physician-supervised) be used because contrast reactions and discomfort in case of extravasation are much less with such agents than the reactions experienced with hyperosmolar water-soluble contrast agents. Power injection at 2 mL/kg is recommended. IV administration of contrast agents is not recommended for patients in sickle cell crisis.
>
> **SEDATION**
> *Note:* Informed consent is mandatory.
>
> Whenever possible, sedation should be administered by an anesthesiologist, a nurse anesthetist, or an intensive care unit physician who is also responsible for appropriate monitoring. If the radiologist provides the sedation, he/she is responsible for following the hospital's sedation guidelines

Contrast Agents

Oral Agents:

To opacify the bowel, children may be administered baby formula with ferrous sulfate 2 hours before imaging. The paramagnetic effect of iron results in a positive contrast effect within bowel. In order to create a negative contrast effect, diamagnetic substances like barium sulfate or a manganese-rich drink such as blueberry or pineapple juice or bismuth subsalicylate (Kaopectate) may be used. Negative contrast agents diminish artifacts related to peristalsis, thereby significantly improving the quality of studies like MR cholangiopancreatography. If a positive oral contrast agent is used, intravenous administration of glucagon prior to imaging is recommended to suspend peristalsis.

Intravenous Agents:

The usual pediatric dose and agent administered intravenously to children undergoing MRI of the abdomen is gadolinium-diethylene–triamine pentaacetic acid (Gd-DTPA), 0.05-0.1 mmol/kg.

Radionuclide Studies

Radioisotope examinations of the pediatric abdomen are studies for GER (milk scan) and gastric emptying, liver and spleen scans, and studies for ectopic gastric mucosa (Meckel diverticulum). These are reviewed in depth in *Nuclear Medicine: The Requisites*. Table 4-1 reviews the common procedures and isotope doses.

Miscellaneous Techniques

Placement of Tubes

A long tube can be placed either through the nose or through an existing gastrostomy, with or without the help of a guidewire. Placement of these tubes into the jejunum seldom leads to complications, although perforation has been reported. Fluoroscopic monitoring and alert, practical care are usually sufficient. The position of the tube should be checked before the procedure is ended, with contrast material injected through the line. A horizontal beam abdominal radiograph should also be obtained to ascertain whether or not perforation or aberrant positioning has occurred. Complications of gastrostomy tube placement include malposition, higher incidence of GER, and tube migration. All of these complications can be assessed by instillation of a few milliliters of isotonic contrast under fluoroscopic guidance. Gastrostomies, placement of gastroduodenal and gastrojejunal tubes, and cecostomies in children can be performed by experienced interventional radiologists.

TABLE 4-1. Common Pediatric Gastrointestinal Nuclear Medicine Procedures

Procedure	Radioisotope	Dose
Meckel scan	Technetium Tc 99m pertechnetate	1-5 mCi IV
Liver or spleen scan	Technetium Tc 99m sulfur colloid	0.5-5 mCi IV
Biliary scan	Technetium Tc 99m diisopropyl imino-diacetic acid	0.1-1 mCi IV
Milk scan	Technetium Tc 99m sulfur colloid	1 mCi PO or per NG tube
Gastric emptying study	Technetium Tc 99m sulfur colloid	< 1 mCi PO or per NG tube
	Indium In 111 diethylenetriamine pentaacetate	

IV, intravenous(ly); NG, nasogastric; PO, by mouth.

Esophageal foreign bodies—coins but not sharp objects—can be removed from the esophagus with the use of a Foley catheter passed orally beyond the coin followed by inflation of the balloon with air or non-ionic contrast agent. Under fluoroscopic control, the catheter is withdrawn, pulling with it the foreign body. The patient is usually prone, and the table is in Trendelenburg position. If the coin has been in position less than 24 hours (no soft tissue swelling of the esophagus around the object on lateral chest radiograph), this technique is highly successful. A postprocedural esophagram with a non-ionic contrast agent is necessary to check for perforation. More often than not, the passage of the tube pushes the coin into the stomach, also effectively treating the condition. This technique is controversial, both because there is a real but very small chance for aspiration of the coin and because the flexible pediatric endoscope is quicker and safer. It is no longer commonly performed.

Drainage of Fluid Collections

US is the most useful modality, followed by CT, to monitor drainage procedures. Informed consent must be obtained. Sedation is only occasionally necessary. Local anesthesia is sufficient for simple, quick biopsies of the liver or kidneys; difficult abscess drainages may necessitate conscious sedation.

After a needle has been inserted, guidewire exchange allows for insertion of (pigtail) catheters. The choice of biopsy needle is personal and is also influenced by the preference of the pathology department.

Potential complications include a pneumothorax if the pleural space has been violated, sepsis or bacteremia, and hemorrhage, either internally in the biopsied organ or around it. A follow-up US scan is usually sufficient to exclude and/or monitor these latter complications.

Stricture Dilatation

Esophageal strictures have been successfully dilated by balloon-catheter (Gruentzig) techniques. In children, narrowed blood vessels, the biliary tree, and post-NEC strictures are often better treated by surgical revision. However, with increasing numbers of well-trained pediatric interventional radiologists, these interventional procedures are being more commonly performed in children.

DEVELOPMENTAL ANATOMY

In the first 4 weeks of gestation, cephalocaudal growth of the embryo with lateral "folding" results in the formation of the primitive gut. There is free communication between the foregut and the amniotic sac at this stage. By 28 days the tracheobronchial diverticulum and the liver bud have started to develop. The foregut (from the oral cavity to just distal to the pancreatic ductal buds), the midgut (the distribution of the superior mesenteric artery [SMA]), and the hindgut (the distribution of the inferior mesenteric artery [IMA]) are thus recognizable by 6 weeks' gestation.

Normal positioning of the intestinal tract results after a process of herniation of the midgut into the yolk sac and its subsequent return with rotation of the midgut and subsequent fixation of the mesenteric structures to the posterior abdominal wall (Table 4-2). In the fifth week of gestation, the foregut (supplied by the celiac axis), hindgut (supplied by the IMA), and midgut (supplied by the SMA) are suspended from the posterior peritoneal wall. By the eighth week the midgut has rotated 90 degrees counterclockwise, allowing the stomach and proximal (prearterial) portion of the duodenum to be anterior to the SMA while the third and fourth (postarterial) portions of the duodenum and rest of the small and large bowel are located posterior to the SMA. This 90-degree rotation occurs with the entire GI tract outside the peritoneal cavity (extracoelomic). By the 10th week of gestation the midgut begins to return to the peritoneal cavity, a process that is complete by the 11th week, all the while undergoing an additional 90 degrees of

TABLE 4-2. Schematic Representation of Intestinal Rotation in the Fetus

Stage	Gestational Age (wk)	Duodenum Rotation (degrees)	Large Bowel Rotation (degrees)	Result If Rotation Does Not Occur
I	< 6	90	90	Nonrotation
II	6-10 (midgut into yolk sac)	90	0	"Reversed" rotation
III	> 10	90	180	Malrotation (midgut volvulus)
Total (degrees)		270	270	

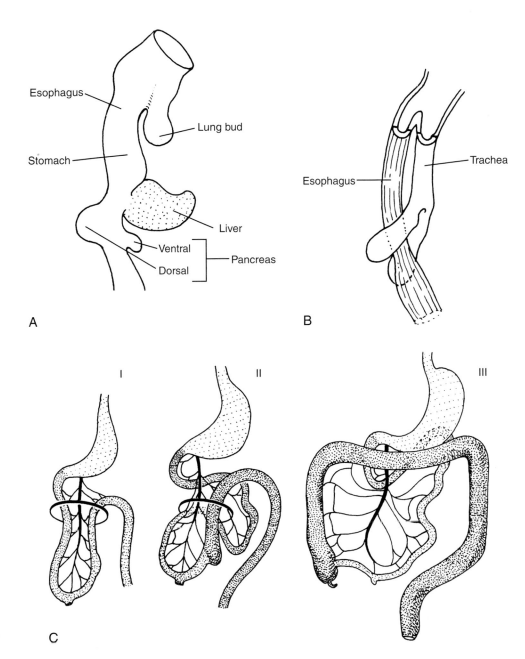

FIGURE 4-5. Diagrammatic representations of the embryo at 22 days' gestation (**A**) and at 5 to 6 weeks' gestation (**B**). **C,** Stages of rotation of the gastrointestinal tract in the fetus.

counterclockwise rotation. The total rotation is 270 degrees counterclockwise around the SMA (Fig. 4-5). The cecum then gradually descends into the right lower quadrant by 4 to 5 months' gestation. This "descent" may not be complete until after birth; for this reason, neonates and infants often have a "high-riding" cecum.

Once the cecum is fixed in the right lower quadrant, the normal small bowel mesentery has a broad "anchor," or base, extending from the region of the SMA to a position posterior to the cecum. This base prevents volvulus. Arrest of rotation and/or fixation may occur at any point in development, resulting in a narrower mesenteric "anchor" and thus predisposing the midgut to undergo volvulus. Occasionally the cecum is on a mesentery and is "mobile," but this situation rarely if ever leads to volvulus.

Internal hernias occur when there is protrusion of a normal viscus through a defect in the mesentery or other openings in the peritoneal cavity. Paraduodenal (left more often than right) hernias are most common. They account for about 2% of all intestinal obstructions.

Embryonic development of the rest of the GI tract and the accessory digestive organs is highlighted in subsequent individual sections.

GASTROINTESTINAL CONDITIONS REQUIRING PROMPT INTERVENTION

Necrotizing Enterocolitis

NEC occurs most commonly (85% of cases) in premature neonates who weigh less than 2500 g and are of less than 37 weeks' gestation. The clinical presentation is often at 3 to 5 days of life, although later presentations are not uncommon, with bloody diarrhea (25%) or abdominal distention, possibly signs of sepsis, and vomiting, apnea, or lethargy. The occurrence of NEC has been associated with hypoxia, stress, low blood pressure, and infection.

The cause of NEC is probably multifactorial; premature rupture of the membranes, preeclampsia, diabetes mellitus, multiparity, early feeding with (high-osmolar) formula, and placement of umbilical artery and venous catheters have all been identified as contributing to a higher risk for NEC.

The pathophysiology implicates bowel ischemia caused by decreased blood perfusion of the GI wall. Subsequent breakdown of the mucosal barrier allows for bacteria and/or air to enter the bowel wall. This may be either due to or facilitated by bowel wall necrosis or autolysis of intestinal flora. A viral role in this process is controversial. The interstitial bowel wall air may then enter the portal venous circulation, often accompanied by the development of metabolic acidosis and disseminated intravascular coagulation.

The most common site of occurrence of NEC is the distal ileum or the ascending colon, although any portion of the bowel, even the stomach, can be involved. Subsequent strictures are most common in the colon (80%), with the rest being in the small intestine. Strictures can occur in up to one third of all patients with NEC. Multiple strictures are not uncommon. The most common location of strictures is the splenic flexure. Strictures are noted as early as 30 to 60 days after an episode of NEC. Perforation occurs most often within the first 36 hours, most commonly in the ileocecal region.

Treatment for NEC involves bowel rest (no oral feedings), orogastric tube drainage, and antibiotics. If perforation does occur, surgical exploration is often performed. However, surgeons report excellent results with placement of a percutaneous drain in the right lower quadrant. This procedure can be performed at the bedside in these very ill infants. The predictive value of abdominal radiographs regarding perforation is controversial; some authorities believe that an acute change in orientation of the bowel loops heralds impending perforation, whereas others hold that a perforation may have occurred if a loop or loops remain unchanged on abdominal radiographs over time. Although death from NEC may occur, it is much less common with the aggressive therapy currently in vogue.

Abdominal radiographs obtained at the time of clinical presentation most commonly demonstrate a nonspecific adynamic ileus. However, they may reflect the friable and edematous qualities of the bowel wall, showing a "jumbled" pattern secondary to bowel wall edema that either compresses the lumen in some areas or causes an ileus appearance in other areas (Fig. 4-6A). Frequently, the two patterns coexist with or without pneumatosis.

The presence of air in the bowel wall manifests as either linear or bubbly pneumatosis. The air is most typically located in the submucosal layer and can be of a fleeting nature. It may reenter the GI tract or break through into the portal venous system. Subserosal air has also been reported.

Air in the portal venous system may distribute itself from the porta hepatis to the hepatic periphery. Portal venous air was formerly thought to be associated with increased mortality but is currently considered part of the overall clinical spectrum of NEC and does not appear to alter the morbidity or mortality (Fig. 4-6B).

If perforation is suspected either on clinical grounds or from physical examination, a left lateral decubitus film is preferred over the supine cross-table examination (Fig. 4-6C). Approximately two thirds of perforations are accompanied by free air, and in approximately one third, ascites develops. Free air may be identified on conventional radiographs from the rugby football sign, air outlining the falciform ligament, or air outlining both sides of the bowel wall (Rigler sign) (Fig. 4-7).

Contrast studies are rarely if ever indicated in the acute phase of NEC. Non-ionic contrast agents are preferred in such a setting. Evaluation for the presence of strictures, which are most frequently demonstrable 3 to 12 months after the acute stage of NEC, necessitates performance of a contrast enema study (Fig. 4-6D). Balloon dilatation of the strictures has been attempted but without consistent success.

Bowel wall thickening and ascites can be well demonstrated by US. Air can be identified within the portal vein. Attempts have also been made to use color-flow Doppler or duplex US to demonstrate air bubbles flowing through the portal vein and its tributaries. The waveform of these vessels may also be altered in NEC; the predictive value of this imaging finding is not yet clear.

Midgut Volvulus

Midgut volvulus can occur at any age but is most commonly seen in the neonate and infant. It represents a true emergency condition that can lead to necrosis of the twisted portion of intestine. The twisted portion rotates around the SMA. It can happen in utero but is most commonly (80% of cases) diagnosed in the first few days to weeks of life. Bilious vomiting, usually at 2 to 3 days of life, is the classic presenting symptom. Abdominal distention is not common.

The condition occurs because there is arrest of rotation or fixation of the GI tract (as previously described under "Developmental Anatomy"), with a resultant short mesenteric "anchor" that allows the small bowel to twist with the SMA as its fulcrum (axis). Midgut volvulus is an absolute emergency, and imaging is imperative so that surgical intervention can prevent vascular compromise of the bowel. Three and one-half turns around the SMA have been shown to be the critical point that leads to high mortality secondary to bowel necrosis; fewer turns may be less critical because they may cause only intermittent compromise of the venous and lymphatic drainage. Radiographically, however, this fact is irrelevant; one turn looks the same as three turns.

Conventional radiographs are suggestive in the majority of cases, showing disproportionate dilatation of the stomach and duodenal loop proximal to the volvulus in comparison with the distal small bowel (Fig. 4-8A). There may be edema of the involved bowel wall. These findings suggest a "high" obstruction with or without air-fluid levels. Static air-fluid levels may indicate bowel necrosis.

An oral contrast study is the initial examination of choice to demonstrate the volvulus. Barium is a safe contrast agent; a non-ionic agent is frequently used in a number of pediatric centers.

A classic "corkscrew" appearance of the second and third portions of the duodenum is seen in midgut volvulus, occurring to the right of the vertebral column (Fig. 4-8B). The ligament of Treitz does not develop because the duodenojejunal junction is malpositioned. The anatomic landmark of the duodenojejunal junction thus is not identifiable. A contrast enema study to diagnose malrotation is unreliable because a high-riding cecum is seen in 15% to 20% of normal neonates and infants. In fact, cecal position is not as reliable as the duodenojejunal junction to rule out malrotation.

US may show dilated and fluid-filled small bowel loops as well as reversal of the orientation of the SMV with regard to the SMA. This finding is helpful but not diagnostic for midgut volvulus because both false-positive and false-negative study results have been reported (Fig. 4-9). A "whirlpool" appearance may be present on US and is highly suggestive of volvulus on color-flow Doppler US.

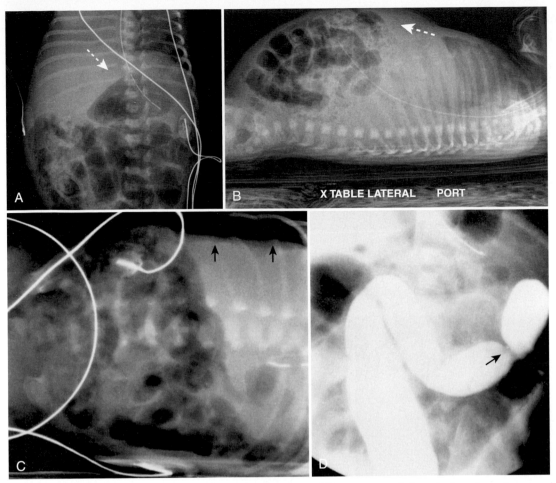

FIGURE 4-6. Necrotizing enterocolitis (NEC). **A,** Supine radiograph demonstrates diffuse pneumatosis intestinalis and portal venous air *(arrow)*. **B,** A cross-table lateral view shows the same findings to better advantage. **C,** Left lateral decubitus view demonstrates free intraperitoneal air between the liver and the abdominal wall *(arrows)*. **D,** Stricture in the descending colon *(arrow)* 3 months after NEC.

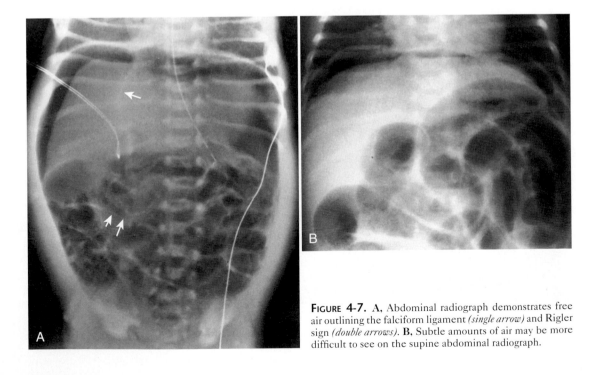

FIGURE 4-7. A, Abdominal radiograph demonstrates free air outlining the falciform ligament *(single arrow)* and Rigler sign *(double arrows)*. **B,** Subtle amounts of air may be more difficult to see on the supine abdominal radiograph.

Hypertrophic Pyloric Stenosis

Hypertrophic pyloric stenosis (HPS) is characterized by acquired hypertrophy of the circular pyloric muscles in the neonate and young infant; the longitudinal muscle is unaffected. Immature coordination between antral contractility and emptying may explain this affliction. Genetic (first-born male, familial incidence) or gastric (humoral: high gastrin levels) factors have been implicated. HPS usually manifests between 2 and 6 weeks after birth, but 20% of neonates have symptoms from birth. The symptoms are vomiting (projectile in 10% to 15% of cases) in association with dehydration, hypochloremic alkalosis, and jaundice. HPS is rare after 12 weeks of age.

The incidence of HPS is variable. Overall, it occurs in 1 in 500 live births in the United States, but in only 1 in 2000 in African Americans and 1 in 25 in Sweden. In addition, there is a seasonal variation in incidence, with HPS being more common in fall and winter. Boys outnumber girls 4:1. On physical examination, 10% to 40% of patients have either hyperperistaltic waves or a palpable pyloric "olive." The latter finding is rarely felt except by experienced observers. In such instances, imaging may not be indicated.

A conventional radiograph of the abdomen may show a distended stomach with or without an air-fluid level and relatively little bowel air distally in about 15% to 20% of cases. The gastric hyperperistalsis may be evident in a "caterpillar" configuration of the stomach (Fig. 4-10A).

The role and imaging characteristics of US and an upper GI evaluation are summarized and illustrated in Box 4-2. With US, a 5-MHz or 7.5-MHz linear transducer is most useful. True HPS presents no difficulty for the operator. A donut, or bull's-eye, should be readily apparent, with the infant slightly turned on the right side to take advantage of gastric contents in the antrum as a US "window" (Fig. 4-10B and C). For a positive diagnosis of HPS on US, the pyloric muscle thickness should be greater than 3 mm from mucosa to serosa, and the pyloric channel length should be more than 14 mm.

An upper GI examination is rarely necessary if US is available. It is performed with only a relatively small amount of contrast agent, which is either swallowed or, as preferred by some, administered through an NG tube. If the radiograph confirms the diagnosis, the contrast agent should be removed from the stomach before the infant leaves the imaging suite. The classic findings

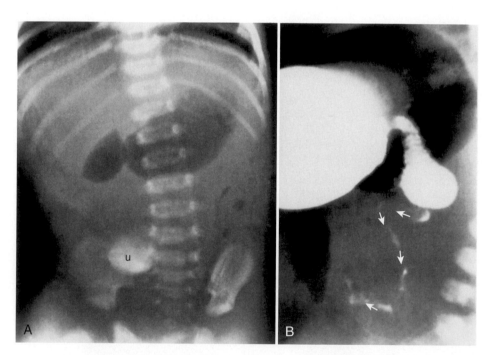

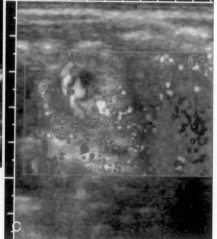

FIGURE 4-8. Midgut volvulus. **A,** Abdominal radiograph demonstrates air in the distended stomach and duodenal bulb with a few pockets of air distally. These findings remained unchanged over 6 hours. Note the umbilical hernia (u). **B,** Contrast study illustrates the "corkscrew" appearance of a midgut volvulus *(arrows).*

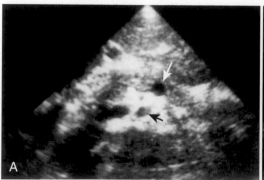

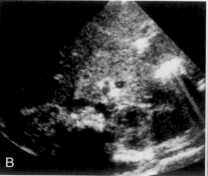

FIGURE 4-9. Transverse US images illustrate the superior mesenteric vein *(white arrow)* and superior mesenteric artery *(black arrow)* in the normal positions (**A**) and reversed in a 2-day-old neonate with midgut volvulus (**B**). **C,** Transverse color-flow Doppler US illustrates the "whirlpool" sign. See Plate 5 for color reproduction.

consist of hyperperistalsis of the stomach, the antral "teat," a "double-track" elongated pyloric channel, and an "umbrella" duodenal cap (Fig. 4-10D).

Pylorospasm, the main differential diagnostic alternative, is a controversial entity and can best be regarded as delayed gastric emptying. After a variable period (days to weeks), the symptoms of pylorospasm disappear. Whether or not pylorospasm represents a forme fruste of pyloric stenosis is not certain because adrenogenital syndrome, dehydration, and sepsis have also been implicated as causes. Severe pylorospasm may be seen in patients with organic brain disease. Finally, gastroenteritis, pyloric channel (stress) ulcer, and congenital abnormalities such as an antral web and gastric duplication may cause symptoms similar to those of HPS. However, US is usually successful in excluding HPS when one of these other conditions is present.

Intussusception

Intussusception is defined as the invagination of a portion of proximal bowel (intussusceptum) into a contiguous segment of distal bowel (intussuscipiens) (Fig. 4-11). It occurs in patients ranging in age from newborn to 18 years; the peak incidence (40%) is in patients between the ages of 5 and 9 months. Sixty percent of cases occur before the patients' first birthdays, and 90% before the second. Boys outnumber girls 3:2. The incidence varies according to season and geographic location, with intussusception occurring most commonly in winter and spring and in Australia and Europe.

Intussusception is most often idiopathic. A discernible lead point causing intussusception is uncommon (less than 5% of cases) and is more likely to occur in older children.

Idiopathic intussusception has been thought to be triggered by hypertrophy of lymphoid tissue (Peyer patches) in the terminal ileum that may be related to an antecedent (7 to 10 days prior) viral infection. Adenovirus has been isolated frequently in children with intussusception and has been thought to play a role in some cases by increasing motility of the bowel or producing hyperplasia of the lymphoid tissue.

Lead points that may cause intussusception include duplication cysts, Meckel diverticulum, lymphoma, polyps, hemorrhage into the wall of the bowel (such as Henoch-Schönlein purpura), appendiceal inflammation, and inspissated stool in patients with

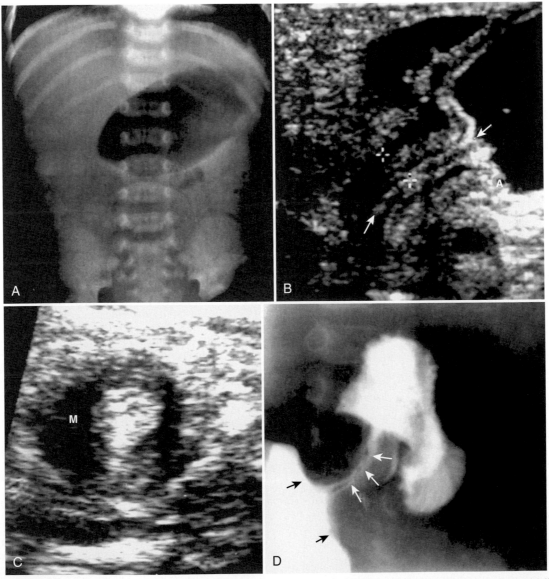

FIGURE 4-10. Hypertrophic pyloric stenosis (HPS). **A,** Supine abdominal radiograph demonstrates a dilated "contracting" stomach with little air distally. **B,** Longitudinal US scan depicts hypertrophied muscle *(markers)* and an elongated canal *(arrows).* "Shouldering" of the antrum (A) is also noted. **C,** Transverse US scan shows the thickened muscle (M) surrounding the echogenic pyloric channel (bull's eye). **D,** Upper GI study demonstrates the antral "teat;" shouldering *(black arrows)*; and the elongated, narrowed, double-tracked pyloric channel *(white arrows).*

Box 4-2. Diagnosis and Treatment of Suspected Pyloric Stenosis

Olive palpated?	→ Yes	→	Surgery
↓			
No			
↓			
Ultrasound			
↓			
Pyloric channel > 16 mm *and/or* pyloric muscle > 3 mm?	→ Yes	→	Surgery
↓			
No			
↓			
Upper gastrointestinal study if clinically indicated to evaluate other causes of vomiting			

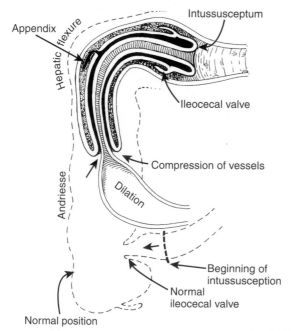

FIGURE 4-11. Schematic representation of an ileocolic intussusception.

cystic fibrosis. Lead points are most often present in neonates in the first month of life or in children older than 5 years. The most common lead point in patients older than 5 years is lymphoma; in infants, the most common lead point is a Meckel diverticulum.

With regard to location, approximately 90% of all intussusceptions are ileocolic; the remaining 10% are either ileoileal or colocolic. Ileoileal intussusceptions are most commonly seen in postoperative patients, in whom the mechanism is thought to be abnormal peristalsis during resolution of an ileus. Colocolic intussusceptions are very rare. Undetected ileoileal intussusception is often the lead point in patients with idiopathic ileocolic intussusception.

The most common clinical symptoms of intussusceptions are abdominal pain and vomiting (each occurring in more than 90% of cases) as well as blood per rectum and a palpable abdominal mass (each occurring in approximately 60% of cases). Approximately 20% of affected children have had an upper respiratory tract infection 2 weeks before presentation, and 10% have had diarrhea before the onset of symptoms. Fever is common. The typical "currant jelly" stools, consisting of blood and mucus mixed with stool, are seen in 15% to 20% of cases. They usually appear within 24 hours but may not appear until 2 days after the onset of symptoms. Lethargy is an ominous prognostic sign but does not preclude a careful diagnostic/therapeutic radiographic approach. Differential diagnostic considerations include viral gastroenteritis, peritonitis due to a ruptured viscus (appendix), and sepsis.

Conventional abdominal radiographs of the abdomen never rule out an intussusception but may confirm the presence of one by showing a mass or a colon devoid of contents. Emptying of the distal colon occurs because intussuscepted bowel leads to hyperperistalsis of the distal colonic segment, either in relation to the event itself (vagal?) or as a result of the cathartic properties of intraluminal blood. However, some patients with intussusception present with stool-filled colon. There may be signs of small bowel obstruction secondary to edema at the site of the intussusception.

Reduction of an intussusception can be achieved by surgical or nonsurgical means. Mortality associated with surgical reduction is currently estimated at about 0.1%; with properly performed hydrostatic or air reductions, no deaths have been reported. Hydrostatic or air pressure reduction is also advantageous because neither requires general anesthesia or laparotomy.

Current imaging in patients in whom intussusception is suspected consists of a preliminary radiographic examination of the abdomen followed by a therapeutic enema if the findings on plain films are suggestive (Fig. 4-12). US has extremely high sensitivity and specificity if a more definitive diagnostic test is desired. On color Doppler US, the absence of flow into the intussusception has been shown to be helpful in predicting reducibility. If results of diagnostic studies are positive and there are no contraindications, a therapeutic enema with water-soluble contrast material or air can be performed. Definitive reduction is assumed to have occurred when the contrast agent is seen on radiography to reflux freely into several feet of ileum (Fig. 4-13).

The only absolute contraindications to performing a therapeutic enema when intussusception is suspected are intestinal perforation and peritonitis. The duration of symptoms (more than 24 hours) need not be a contraindication, although a lower success rate of reduction has been noted in the presence of small bowel obstruction. The risk of perforation is higher when small bowel obstruction is present, although the mortality/morbidity of subsequent surgery is not.

The patient should be in satisfactory clinical condition before any form of treatment for intussusception is undertaken. Good hydration is especially important. IV fluids should be running during the therapeutic enema. The operating room staff and the surgical team should be notified, and the latter should be in the hospital if not in the imaging suite. Mild sedation before the enema, as well as immobilization, has been advocated by some. Other radiologists believe that the higher intra-abdominal pressure during crying may enhance the chance of a successful reduction.

The choice of contrast agent has been a frequent point of discussion. Air, water, and water-soluble agents have all been successfully used. Barium is not advised because the possibility of perforation is always present, although a rare event in experienced hands. When an enema is used, the height of the contrast column is traditionally 3 feet above the table top. Further elevation of the reservoir does not significantly alter the intraluminal pressure, but

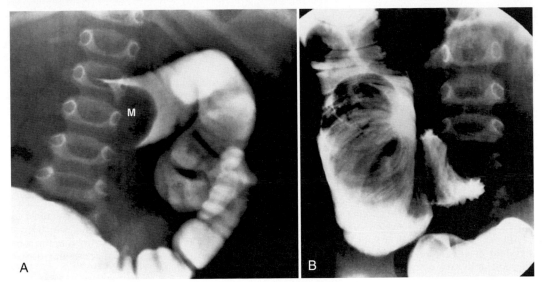

FIGURE 4-12. Intussusception. **A,** Diagnostic enema encounters the intussusceptum in the mid-transverse colon (M). **B,** The "coiled spring" appearance of an ileocolic intussusception: the contrast material has interdigitated between the intussusceptum and the intussuscipiens.

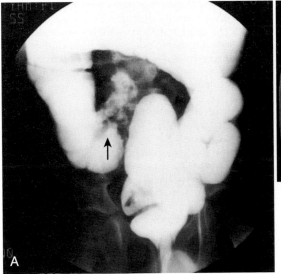

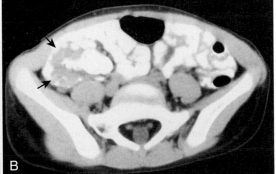

FIGURE 4-13. After contrast reduction. **A,** Postevacuation film: a "plump" ileocecal valve (*arrow*). **B,** CT confirmation of the same *(arrows).*

"the bag at eye level" is a convenient height. After insertion of the enema tip (a balloon is not used), the intussusception is identified. Monitoring is most easily done by fluoroscopy; as has been noted, US is also suggested by some. Three attempts should be made to reduce an intussusception. The end point of a successful reduction procedure consists of free flow of contrast agent into the distal and middle ileum. An air reduction attempt uses a balloon catheter and hand instillation of air or carbon dioxide. A pressure gauge and popoff mechanism must be present. The intraluminal pressure should not exceed 120 mm Hg. Care should be taken not to miss the presence of a residual ileoileal intussusception; likewise, an attempt should be made to identify a possible lead point.

A postevacuation film is of paramount importance because intussusception may recur during evacuation. A recurrence may be suspected when there is complete evacuation of the contrast agent out of the colon on the postevacuation film. Significant residual contrast agent in the colon is the rule after a successful reduction.

In addition, after successful reduction of intussusception, the ileocecal valve may remain enlarged for up to 24 hours, but this enlargement is not deemed pathologically significant. Perforation

does occur, but rarely (1 in 500). It is a surgical emergency. For patients in whom a liquid enema has been used, the major sequelae of perforation are peritonitis due to fecal contamination of the peritoneum, adhesions, and granuloma formation. Perforation during air reduction may cause a smaller tear and less fecal contamination.

The recurrence rate of intussusception varies between 1% and 15%, depending on the treatment after hydrostatic or surgical reduction, and most recurrences are seen within 24 to 48 hours. Another successful enema reduction is usually possible after one recurrence. A further recurrence requires surgical intervention.

Pneumoperitoneum

Free air within the peritoneal cavity may represent an emergency, depending on the patient's clinical history (Box 4-3). Air present in the peritoneum after surgery usually disappears by 3 days but may last as long as 1 or 2 weeks. If the air is diminishing in amount, it can be followed clinically; however, if the amount of air is increasing, a continuing connection between the peritoneum and an air-containing structure must be excluded. Pneumoperitoneum after insertion of a rectal thermometer or enema tip, or secondary to other iatrogenic procedures, can be a cause as well. The radiographic signs of pneumoperitoneum and their most common causes have been described previously.

Gastrointestinal Bleeding

GI bleeding is not as common in children as in adults. It is less useful in the pediatric age group to differentiate between upper and lower GI hemorrhage. The most common cause of GI bleeding is an anal fissure, followed by bleeding from a Meckel diverticulum, colonic polyps, or intussusception (Box 4-4). Infections and stress are seen most often in neonates and infants. In infants and children younger than 5 years, Meckel diverticulum, juvenile polyp, and intussusception should be considered. Clinically, in patients presented with brisk bleeding, a Meckel diverticulum or stress ulcer should be considered; in those presenting with melena or trace blood, a juvenile polyp, intussusception, or anal fissure is the likely cause. IBD may also manifest as chronic bleeding.

The diagnostic yield of conventional abdominal radiograph, US, or CT is unpredictable and often low for gastrointestinal bleeding. Contrast studies using barium may be useful to delineate underlying pathology. Double-contrast enema studies can be performed at virtually any age in the search for polyps. CT colonography is not yet practical in children.

A radionuclide study with technetium Tc 99m pertechnetate–labeled red blood cells can localize an actively bleeding site. Such a study sometimes helps visualize a Meckel diverticulum because of the ectopic gastric mucosa, the cells of which secrete the radiopharmaceutical. In skilled hands, endoscopy is the examination of choice.

▄ ESOPHAGUS

Anatomic and Developmental Anomalies
Pharynx and Esophagus
During the fourth and fifth weeks of gestation, lateral ridges appear in the foregut that fuse medially, separating the trachea and esophagus. The esophagus then elongates and becomes tubular, with anatomic features similar to those of the adult esophagus. The normal impressions of the aortic arch, left mainstem bronchus, and left atrium are consistently seen on a contrast study, and the stripping wave is usually quite prominent.

> ### Box 4-3. Differential Diagnosis of Free Air
>
> Gastric perforation in the newborn or after nasogastric intubation
> Necrotizing enterocolitis
> Visceral obstructions, such as in Hirschsprung disease and meconium-related conditions
> Dissection of air from a pneumomediastinum
> Perforated ulcer, Meckel diverticulum, and appendicitis

> ### Box 4-4. Common Causes of Gastrointestinal Hemorrhage
>
> **IN NEONATE**
> Necrotizing enterocolitis
> Infectious colitis
>
> **IN INFANT**
> Stress ulcer
> Meckel diverticulum
> Intussusception
>
> **IN CHILD**
> Polyp
> Inflammatory bowel disease

Intermittent sucking and swallowing of amniotic fluid, as well as mandibular movements, have been observed as early as 24 weeks' gestation on prenatal US. The swallowing mechanism matures rapidly after birth. Nasopharyngeal regurgitation is abnormal after 2 to 3 days of life. Small amounts of aspiration are usually followed by a clearing cough; this occurs occasionally in struggling or crying infants. Repeated aspiration of contrast agent during an upper GI study is a reason to terminate the study immediately and indicates possible respiratory problems. Video evaluation may provide diagnostic assistance in these disorders, because it clearly evaluates the tongue squeeze, elevation of the palate and pharynx, and contraction sequence of the swallowing mechanism.

Swallowing mechanism failure due to poor relaxation of the upper esophageal sphincter (cricopharyngeal spasm) or neuromuscular disorders such as cerebral palsy (most common), familial dysautonomia (Riley-Day syndrome, which occurs in Ashkenazi Jews), and other rare conditions affecting the esophagus (e.g., cranial nerve palsies, scleroderma, dermatomyositis) may all occur in children but are rare.

Branchial Cleft Anomalies
Five cartilaginous mesodermal ridges are present at about 5 weeks' gestation and are separated by branchial clefts, which are homologous to the gills of a fish. The ridges are opposed to five pharyngeal pouches from within the oral cavity. By the seventh week, these ridges have virtually disappeared, the second ridge having overgrown the third and fourth. Almost all branchial cleft anomalies arise from the second ridge; they constitute a spectrum of anomalies, ranging from a sinus to a cyst to a fistula. Mucoid drainage and a mass may be the presenting symptoms. CT is the imaging modality of choice after US characterization (see Fig. 2-10.)

Esophageal Atresia and Tracheoesophageal Fistula
Failure of differentiation, ridge formation, and elongation of the primitive foregut can result in various combinations of esophageal atresia (EA) and tracheoesophageal fistula (TEF) (Fig. 4-14). The incidence of these abnormalities varies between 1 in 2000 and 1 in 5000 live births, with a sporadic familial occurrence.

In one third of patients, a prenatal US scan obtained as early as 24 weeks' gestation can suggest the presence of these abnormalities if polyhydramnios is present. Coughing, choking, and cyanosis associated with the first feeding are the most common clinical presenting symptoms on the first day of life. There is a higher incidence of TEF in infants with Down syndrome. Clinically, about 30% of infants with EA/TEF are born prematurely. Inability to introduce an NG tube into a choking or drooling infant is a clue that EA may be present.

Imaging of EA/TEF with conventional radiographs may show (1) the air-distended esophageal atretic pouch, (2) the NG tube curled up in this pouch, or (3) excessive dilatation of stomach and/or small bowel as a result of a fistula communicating between the trachea and the distal esophagus (Fig. 4-15). EA coexisting with a gasless abdomen usually indicates that there is no coexisting distal fistula. In addition, conventional radiographs are useful to evaluate for associated abnormalities, most commonly the VACTERL association (*v*ertebral abnormalities, *a*nal atresia, *c*ardiac abnormalities, *t*racheoesophageal fistula and/or *e*sophageal atresia, *r*enal abnormalities, and *l*imb defects). Associated anomalies occur in about one third of patients with EA/TEF and may involve all organ systems (Box 4-5). Contrast evaluation is usually not necessary. Treatment consists of primary anastomosis of the proximal and distal esophagus when the infant has grown somewhat (a few months). Colonic interposition or gastric tube surgery may be needed if primary repair proves impossible. After repair, evaluation with a non-ionic contrast agent may be used to exclude postoperative leaks (occurring early in the postoperative phase) or stricture formation at the anastomotic site.

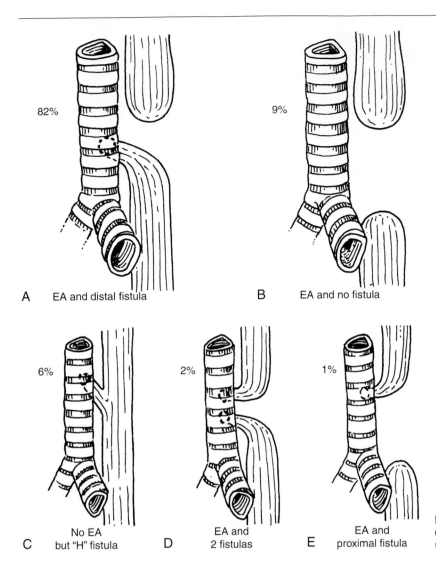

82%

A   EA and distal fistula

9%

B   EA and no fistula

6%

C   No EA but "H" fistula

2%

D   EA and 2 fistulas

1%

E   EA and proximal fistula

FIGURE 4-14. The common (**A** and **B**) and less common (**C** through **E**) combinations of esophageal atresia (EA) and tracheoesophageal fistula (TEF).

Noteworthy is that the distal esophageal segment exhibits disordered motility in more than 90% of infants after surgical repair of EA; the upper esophagus exhibits dysmotility in less than 10% of patients.

Rare anomalies of tracheal and esophageal separation are laryngotracheoesophageal cleft, tracheal agenesis (with or without a fistula), and an esophageal ("pig") bronchus.

Cystic Foregut Malformations

The spectrum of foregut malformations ranges from webs to duplications, with considerable overlap. In the chest, a foregut malformation may be visible on radiographs as a middle or posterior mediastinal mass. There may be associated malformations of the vertebral bodies, and the cysts themselves may contain respiratory (bronchogenic) mucosa, GI mucosa, or both. The secretory properties of the epithelia of these lesions may lead them to enlarge and thus cause symptoms.

Cystic foregut malformations can be divided into three broad categories: bronchogenic cysts, (neur)enteric cysts, and esophageal duplications. Bronchogenic cysts are discussed in Chapter 2. Enteric cysts tend to be more posterior than bronchogenic cysts, developing from the posterior part of the foregut. Enteric cysts present early in life, may hemorrhage or enlarge because of epithelial secretions, and may be associated with neurologic symptoms (paraplegia) secondary to cord compression. If they contain neural tissue, they are called *neurenteric cysts*. These are virtually always associated with vertebral anomalies (usually spinal segmentation anomalies). Esophageal duplications are half as common as ileal duplications (stomach

and duodenum rank next in incidence). Gender incidences are equal, and symptoms are usually related to obstruction. There is seldom communication between the duplication and the true lumen of the GI tract unless repeated inflammation has occurred.

Conventional radiographs may demonstrate a middle mediastinal soft tissue density, and a contrast examination may show a smooth submucosal lesion narrowing the esophageal lumen (Fig. 4-16). Vertebral lesions are usually obvious on conventional radiographs and may be associated with curvature of the spine.

CT may display the anatomic relationships to a better extent. MRI proves the presence of a cystic component on T2-weighted images and optimally delineates the boundaries.

Vascular Impressions on the Esophagus

In infants presenting with feeding disorders, spitting, or dyspnea, congenital vascular anomalies are high on the list of differential diagnostic possibilities. "Rings and slings" may manifest in the neonate with symptoms or as incidental findings at any stage. Their embryogenesis lies in six vascular arches present during fetal life that pass on either side of the developing foregut, within the ridges described earlier, to join posteriorly and form the descending aorta. The first two arches disappear. Normally, the fourth arch gives rise to the aortic arch, and the sixth arch gives rise to the pulmonary artery and the ductus arteriosus. The fifth arch fails to develop. Thus all congenital vascular rings and resultant impressions on foregut derivatives are ultimately determined by which portion of these paired ascending arches has persisted or degenerated during the developmental period.

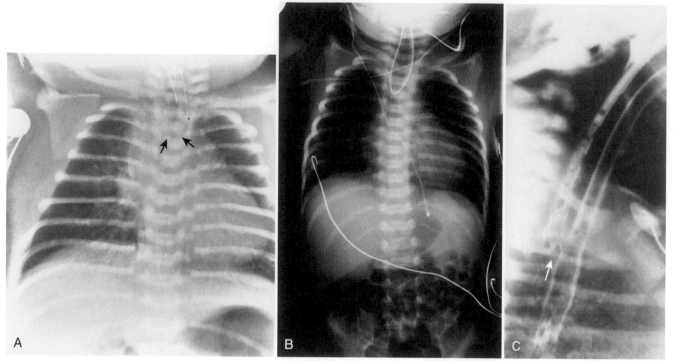

FIGURE 4-15. Esophageal atresia (EA) and tracheoesophageal fistula (TEF). **A,** Inability to pass a nasogastric (NG) tube and an air-distended proximal esophageal pouch *(arrows)* illustrated on an admission chest radiograph. Note the stomach bubble. **B,** NG tube is curled in the proximal pouch in another infant. **C,** Contrast study illustrates the proximal TEF *(arrow).* Contrast material is rarely needed to make the diagnosis except in cases of "H" type fistulas.

BOX 4-5. Anomalies Associated with Esophageal Atresia and Tracheoesophageal Fistula

CARDIAC ANOMALIES
Patent ductus arteriosus (Botallo)
Ventricular septal defect
Right-sided arch

GASTROINTESTINAL ANOMALIES
Duodenal atresia
Imperforate anus

GENITOURINARY ANOMALY
Renal agenesis (unilateral)

SKELETAL ANOMALIES
Vertebral anomalies
Down syndrome (10%)

Imaging by conventional radiographs, with or without the use of a contrast agent to outline the esophagus, may then show one of the four following common patterns (Fig. 4-17, shown *left to right*).
Concomitant posterior esophageal and anterior tracheal impressions: Concomitant posterior esophageal and anterior tracheal impressions are the result of a true vascular ring. The most common entity is a double aortic arch or a right aortic arch combined with an aberrant left subclavian artery. The ring in this instance is completed by the ductus remnant. If the ring is tight enough and causes tracheal compression, surgical treatment may be necessary. In 75% of cases of double aortic arch, the descending aorta is on the left, with the posterior arch more cephalad. The descending aorta is on the right in the remaining 25%, with the posterior arch more caudad. The posterior arch is the larger arch in the majority of cases. On conventional radiographs, the frontal projection demonstrates an indentation of the contrast-filled esophagus on both sides, usually with the right side

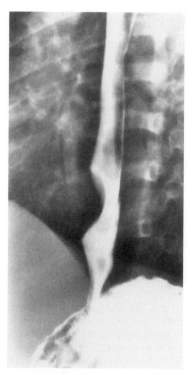

FIGURE 4-16. Esophageal duplication. Smooth submucosal lesion narrowing the distal esophageal lumen.

slightly higher than the left (Fig. 4-18). MRI gives exquisite detail if more advanced imaging is desired. The surgical treatment consists of dividing the smaller of the two arches.
Anterior tracheal impression: Anterior tracheal impression is caused when the innominate artery arises to the left of the trachea and ascends anteriorly. This impression is considered a normal

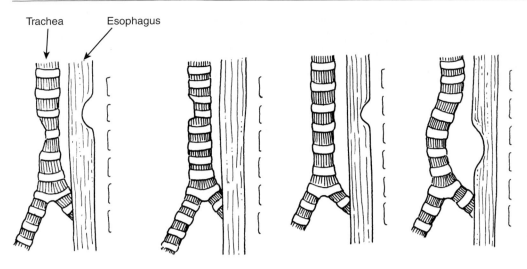

Trachea   Esophagus

FIGURE 4-17. Schematic diagram illustrates the four common tracheal and esophageal impressions. (See text for descriptions.)

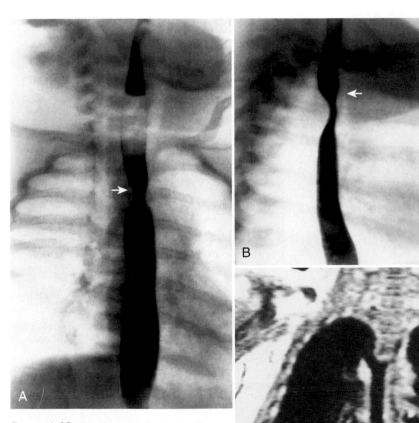

FIGURE 4-18. Double aortic arch. **A,** Frontal view shows an indentation on both sides of the contrast agent–filled esophagus, with the right side slightly more cephalad *(arrow).* **B,** Lateral view demonstrates the posterior esophageal impression and a subtle anterior tracheal narrowing *(arrow).* **C,** MRI confirmation on a coronal T1-weighted image.

finding unless accompanied by symptoms. Its presence can be proven with endoscopy or MRI. Symptoms of respiratory compromise may necessitate aortopexy (see Fig. 2-14.)

Posterior esophageal impression: Posterior esophageal impression is fairly common and is due to an aberrant right subclavian artery in cases of a left aortic arch; less commonly, it can be caused by an aberrant left subclavian artery with a right aortic arch. This condition is the result of the disappearance of the fourth arch during embryogenesis. Clinically, if it is not accompanied by symptoms, posterior esophageal impression is considered a normal variant and does not necessitate treatment. Dysphagia has rarely been reported. The position of the trachea is normal (Fig. 4-19).

Lesion between the esophagus and the trachea: A lesion between the esophagus and the trachea occurs when the left pulmonary artery arises from the right pulmonary artery and slings posteriorly and then to the left. It occurs because the sixth arch either becomes partially obliterated or fails to develop. Tracheomalacia secondary to diminution or absence of tracheal cartilage is frequently present. Tracheal compromise may manifest at birth as severe respiratory distress; correction of this abnormality is necessary to avoid continued respiratory problems. It may also manifest later in life. Conventional chest radiographs may

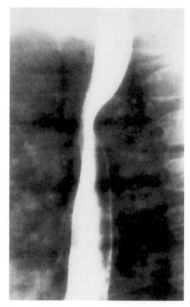

FIGURE 4-19. Aberrant right subclavian artery causing a posterior impression on the esophagus.

demonstrate the density between the trachea and the esophagus (Fig. 4-20) or may show air trapping in the right upper lobe. Even though lymph nodes and (rarely) a bronchogenic cyst can be considered in the differential diagnosis, they are usually more lateral in location. A rounded soft tissue density between the esophagus and the trachea thus represents a pathognomonic appearance of an aberrant left pulmonary artery. Normally the trachea is slightly deviated to the right because of the presence of the aortic arch, and it may be buckled anteriorly and to the right with respiration (on fluoroscopy) or flexion of the neck. Deviation of the trachea to the left should raise the possibility of an arch anomaly. MR angiography or CT angiography further delineates the anatomy in most cases.

A less common presentation of a vascular ring is profound bilateral symmetric air trapping when the vascular ring acts as a ball-valve obstruction. The diagnosis is easily made if passage of an endotracheal tube results in immediate relief of symptoms and resolution of the abnormal radiographic findings.

Acquired Conditions

Strictures

Although symptomatic narrowing of the esophagus can be congenital, it is usually acquired. In infants with rare congenital stenosis, there are two types of stricture. The most common form consists of a short stenosis at the junction of the middle and distal thirds of the esophagus. Symptoms usually do not occur until solid foods become part of the diet. The less common form of stricture is a long segment of narrowing anywhere along the esophagus. The cause of these congenital stenoses is unknown, although intramural tracheobronchial remnants and gastric or pancreatic tissue rests have been reported.

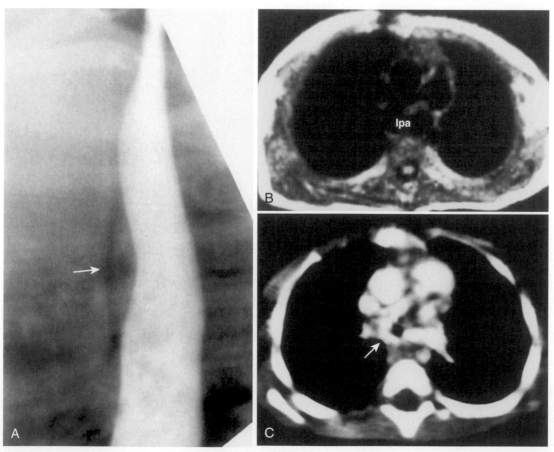

FIGURE 4-20. A, Lateral chest radiograph with contrast agent in the esophagus illustrates the aberrant left pulmonary artery between the esophagus and the trachea *(arrow).* **B,** MRI confirms the aberrant left pulmonary artery (lpa) between the esophagus and the trachea. **C,** CT scan does the same *(arrow).* (See also Figure 2-15.)

Box 4-6. Differential Diagnosis of Esophageal Stricture

Reflux esophagitis
Esophagitis after ingestion of a caustic substance
Previous repair of tracheoesophageal fistula
Radiation therapy (more than 4 months after therapy)
Barrett esophagus
Epidermolysis bullosa
Chronic granulomatous disease of childhood
Eosinophilic gastroenteritis

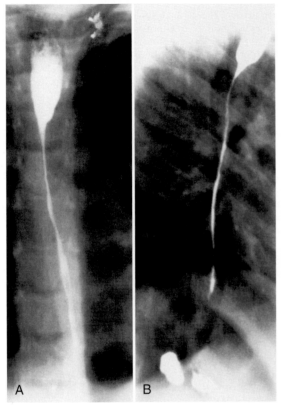

FIGURE 4-21. Anteroposterior (**A**) and lateral (**B**) views demonstrate an esophageal stricture caused by accidental lye ingestion.

Acquired esophageal stenosis is usually the sequela of GER, ingestion of caustic substances (lye), or candidal or viral esophagitis (Box 4-6).

GER can occur with or without a hiatal hernia, but it is most commonly seen in association with immaturity of the gastroesophageal junction. GER can be considered a normal finding in an infant up to 1 year of age unless the baby has repeated episodes of aspiration or failure to thrive, but longer-standing GER may cause inflammation of the distal esophageal mucosa. Inflammatory changes and subsequent strictures are best documented on contrast studies or endoscopy. Barrett esophagus (replacement of squamous epithelium by columnar epithelium because of GER) is rarely seen in children; if present, however, it may cause strictures and even carcinoma, typically in adulthood.

Lye (alkali) ingestion is the most common cause of a stricture (occurring in one third of patients who ingest lye). The caustic lye may lead to mucosal necrosis in 3 to 5 days and fibrous contraction by 3 to 5 weeks. Boys less than 3 years of age represent the majority of patients. The strictures may be long- or short-segment, most often occurring in the middle and lower thirds of the esophagus. These strictures often are amenable to balloon dilatation (Fig. 4-21).

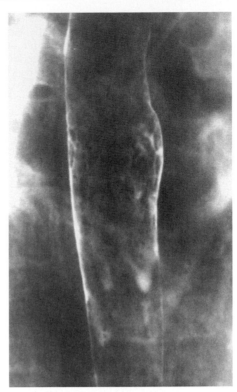

FIGURE 4-22. Esophagitis caused by cytomegalovirus in a 2-year-old child who has human immunodeficiency virus.

Esophagitis

The most common cause of esophagitis is GER. The most common infectious causes of esophagitis are *Candida* (in immunosuppressed patients or patients undergoing chemotherapy), herpes simplex virus type 1, and cytomegalovirus (common in patients with acquired immunodeficiency syndrome). Other types of noninfectious esophagitis are rare; they include epidermolysis bullosa, a congenital blistering disorder of the skin and mucous membranes that is inherited in an autosomal recessive pattern. The bullae can ulcerate and then progress to strictures. Eosinophilic gastroenteritis rarely affects the esophagus but can produce strictures and dysmotility, as can Crohn disease and graft-versus-host disease (GVHD). Iatrogenic causes of stricture formation, such as certain medications (antibiotics, anti-inflammatory drugs), prolonged intubation, and post–radiation therapy sclerosis (if the esophagus was included in the radiation portal) must be considered but are usually evident from clinical history.

Esophagitis can be suggested on conventional radiographs of the chest by a dilated, air-filled atonic esophagus. This appearance is rare, as are accompanying airspace changes in the lungs (suggesting aspiration). Esophagoscopy with biopsy is usually used to confirm the diagnosis of esophagitis. The extent of esophagitis can best be evaluated with the use of barium, to avoid possible extravasation from developing into mediastinitis or aspiration resulting in pulmonary edema. Disordered motility is the earliest radiographic finding in esophagitis, followed by mucosal ulceration and, eventually, stricture formation (Fig. 4-22).

Foreign Bodies

Infants and young children can and do swallow many types of foreign bodies, which may occasionally become impacted at any of the normal sites of relative narrowing in the esophagus. These sites are the thoracic inlet below the level of the cricopharyngeus muscle (75%), at the level where the aortic arch or the left mainstem bronchus crosses the esophagus (20%), and (rarely) at the level of the esophagogastric junction (5%). The patients are often acutely symptomatic. The risk of aspirating a foreign body or that it will perforate the bowel wall compels the clinician to remove it. If the foreign object can be propelled to the stomach, most often nature effects its removal. A useful rule of thumb is that 25% of objects larger than a U.S. quarter may not pass the ileocecal valve, which is the narrowest part of the GI tract. If the object remains lodged in the esophagus, it can be quite easily removed with a flexible endoscope. Removal with a Foley catheter under fluoroscopic guidance is somewhat controversial because of the risk of aspiration, but it has the advantage of not necessitating sedation. In experienced hands, it has a high success rate, although clinicians rarely refer these patients to radiologists any longer. If the object is not smooth or rounded and is lodged anywhere along the entire GI tract, surgical removal may be necessary.

Imaging should include an anteroposterior (AP) radiograph of the chest and abdomen (mouth to anus) and a lateral soft tissue examination of the neck (Fig. 4-23).

Coin-shaped foreign bodies have a distinctive plain film appearance in the upper esophagus. They are oriented en face on AP radiographs when lodged in the esophagus but are en face on lateral radiographs when located in the trachea. The presence of edema of the esophageal wall around the object suggests that a foreign body has been present for more than 24 hours. Perforation or fistula formation becomes more likely after the attempted removal, and nonsurgical removal should be avoided. Contrast studies with barium or non-ionic agents may be useful in the diagnosis of nonopaque foreign bodies, but the contrast agent may obscure small or minimally opaque foreign bodies.

If a foreign body is suspected to be in the airway and/or is not radiopaque, fluoroscopy is far superior to inspiration/expiration or decubitus radiographs. This imaging modality can be used to rule out air trapping through evaluation for mediastinal shift or can be used to assess for asymmetric hemidiaphragmatic motion.

Achalasia

Achalasia is rare in children, with only 3% of all cases occurring in children younger than 10 years. There is no gender predilection. This condition is caused by failure of the lower esophageal sphincter (LES) to relax in response to swallowing because of absence or destruction of the myenteric plexus. Radiographs of the chest often show pulmonary changes secondary to aspiration, an air-fluid level in a dilated esophagus, or a gasless stomach (70% of patients). A contrast study demonstrates the classic beaking as well as disordered peristalsis of the esophagus.

Neoplasms

Uncommon in children, benign tumors of the esophagus include leiomyomas, hamartomas (Peutz-Jeghers syndrome), and polyps.

Malignant tumors of esophagus are exceedingly rare in children. Lymphoma occurs more commonly in the pediatric patient and may involve the esophagus (extrinsic pressure). Esophageal carcinomas (secondary to esophagitis [lye ingestion]) occur very rarely.

As in adults, esophageal tumors are most often detected on a contrast (barium) study, characterized as filling defects. In carcinomas, there are acute angles to the wall, occasionally with ulceration. CT or MRI is then used to better characterize the extent of the lesion.

Diverticula

Rarely are diverticula congenital (posterior); they are almost always acquired. Most often, they occur after trauma (NG intubation in infants), after surgery (TEF repair), or as a result of pulsion (Zenker diverticulum) at the posterolateral weak spot in the esophagus, in the inferior constrictor muscle (Killian dehiscence). The congenital diverticulum may be seen as a forme fruste of esophageal duplication.

Varices

In the pediatric age group, varices are most commonly caused by portal hypertension. Endoscopy is usually necessary for confirmation, although often the lesions can be documented by US, CT, or MRI. Sclerotherapy is also easily accomplished using this technique.

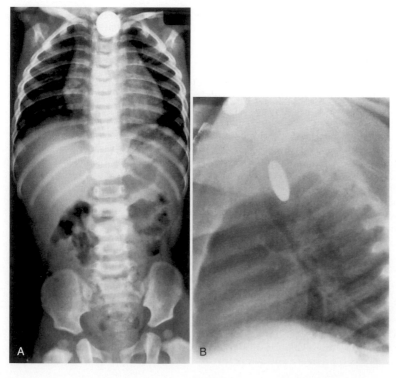

FIGURE 4-23. A, AP "mouth to anus" radiograph demonstrates a coin en face and, therefore, stuck in the esophagus. **B,** Lateral view confirms this position and suggests mild edema surrounding the coin, indicating that the coin has been lodged there for some time.

▬ STOMACH AND DIAPHRAGM

Anatomic and Developmental Anomalies

Embryogenesis and Variants

The embryogenesis of the diaphragm involves a ventral portion—formed from the septum transversum, which is located between the pericardial cavity and the coelomic cavity—and a posterior portion—formed from the pleuroperitoneal membrane, which develops striated muscle to form the muscular diaphragm. The pleuroperitoneal canals lie on either side of the esophagus and close by a membrane made up of pleura and peritoneum, thus forming the posterior portion of the diaphragm. If the striated muscle layer does not form, eventration of abdominal organs into the thoracic cavity occurs. Defective development of either portion results in hernia either anteriorly (Morgagni hernia) or posteriorly (Bochdalek hernia).

The stomach first appears as a fusiform dilatation of the foregut in the fifth gestational week. A 90-degree rotation about the longitudinal and AP axes and differential growth rates of the anterior (slower) and posterior (faster) walls of the foregut result in a relatively larger greater curvature, which rotates to its commonly occupied position. This process explains why the stomach is predominantly transverse in orientation during the first year of life (the "cascade" stomach). After gradual change in shape as the child grows (differential growth of the two sides), the stomach attains the adult shape by the early teen years.

Microgastria (small stomach) and agastria (absence of the stomach) are extremely rare conditions that manifest as massive GER. These conditions are usually associated with malrotation, asplenia, and aganglionosis of the GI tract.

Gastric duplication is the rarest (5%) form of GI tract duplication. This cystic lesion is almost always located on the (antral) greater curvature and does not communicate with gastric lumen. It may enlarge because of secretions, hemorrhage, or both and is more common in girls. The imaging (US) appearance of duplications is characteristic because of the echogenic appearance of the GI mucosa (Fig. 4-24). On conventional studies, a mass or mass effect may be noted, although duplications are also often diagnosed on prenatal US.

Both diverticula and webs are uncommon in children. The former are located posterolaterally in the fundus, the latter in the antrum. Diverticula usually occur in adults. If a web totally occludes the antral lumen, it may be associated with gastric or pyloric atresia, thus suggesting its origin most likely as an ischemic event rather than a failure of recanalization, because pyloric atresia may be associated with jejunal or ileal atresias (Fig. 4-25). An antral web may also be familial.

An abdominal film shows a large, air-distended stomach with little or no air in the bowel. The differential diagnosis includes midgut volvulus, annular pancreas, or duodenal atresia, depending on whether the web is complete or incomplete.

The stomach is fixed by ligaments connecting it to the liver, diaphragm, spleen, and colon. Rarely, laxity of these ligaments or deficient fixation may lead to volvulus of the stomach. Two types are described, mesenteroaxial and organoaxial (Fig. 4-26). In mesenteroaxial rotation, the axis of rotation is at right angles to the stomach and parallel to the mesentery. Mesenteroaxial rotation is the more common of the two types, often manifests acutely, is usually posttraumatic in origin, and is associated with a higher risk of vascular compromise and diaphragmatic herniation as a result of trauma to the diaphragm. The antrum is located in the region usually occupied by the fundus (Fig. 4-27). In organoaxial rotation, the axis of rotation is parallel to the long axis of the stomach, a condition rare in children. It is often associated with aerophagia.

Gastroesophageal Reflux

GER most often is an incidental abnormality in an otherwise normal child. It is defined as regurgitation of gastric contents into the esophagus. Lack of competency of the gastroesophageal junction is implicated, with or without the presence of a hiatal hernia. GER often disappears as the infant matures and begins standing. A hiatal hernia is probably caused by a pressure differential between the chest and abdomen. True hiatal hernias are relatively uncommon in otherwise normal children. The exact interplay between GER and a hiatal hernia in infants remains unclear.

The gastroesophageal junction contains the LES, which is in the process of maturation for up to 6 months after birth. The LES prevents GER from occurring because the LES normally only relaxes during swallowing in response to a peristaltic wave. The anatomic location of the LES is the junction of columnar epithelium and squamous epithelium, located below the diaphragm (about 4 cm long) in adults and at the diaphragm (about 1 cm long) in infants. This sphincter creates a 15– to 30–mm Hg barrier to regurgitation. In addition, the incident angle of the esophagus in relation to the cardia is less acute in infants than in

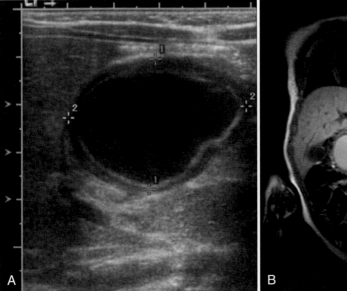

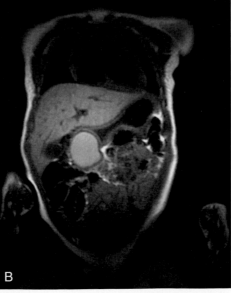

FIGURE 4-24. Gastric duplication cyst. **A,** US scan demonstrates the characteristic echographic "signature" of gastric mucosa lining the cyst. The mucosa is surrounded by an echolucent rim. **B,** Coronal MR image demonstrates the fluid-filled cyst and the bright mucosal lining.

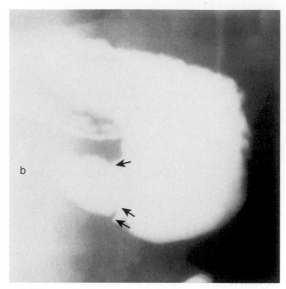

FIGURE 4-25. Antral web. A linear structure in the antrum *(arrows)* on upper GI examination in a vomiting child; b, duodenal bulb.

adults. This incident angle of the esophagogastric junction becomes more acute during the first year of life. During infancy, therefore, gastric contents may reflux into the esophagus (GER); this infantile GER is considered physiologic, and it should resolve by 9 to 12 months of age. GER is less likely to resolve when present after 1 year of age. GER can become clinically significant if the child vomits, aspiration occurs, esophagitis results, or the child fails to thrive. There is also a higher incidence of GER in association with Down syndrome, cystic fibrosis, and neurologically impaired states (cerebral palsy); the incidence is higher in males (3:1).

Conventional radiographs of the chest or abdomen do not detect GER itself but can suggest aspiration secondary to GER with airspace disease in infants, particularly in the upper lobes. In a supine patient, aspiration preferentially enters the dependent (upper lobe) region(s). The chest radiograph may also demonstrate the presence of a hiatal hernia with or without an air-fluid level.

US has shown reasonable correlation with the upper GI evaluation of GER using a contrast agent (barium). For both of these studies, sensitivity does not necessarily correlate with specificity. Because GER is an intermittent phenomenon and therefore may not be detected during intermittent imaging observation, a false-negative examination result is common. Some authorities observe the gastroesophageal junction under fluoroscopy for a

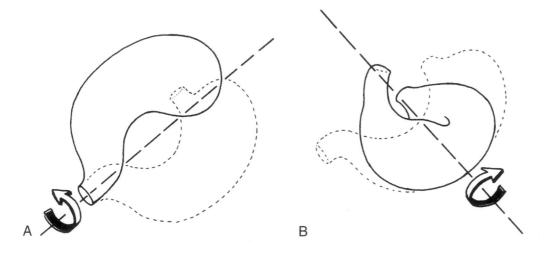

FIGURE 4-26. Schematic representations of an organoaxial volvulus (**A**) and a mesenteroaxial volvulus (**B**).

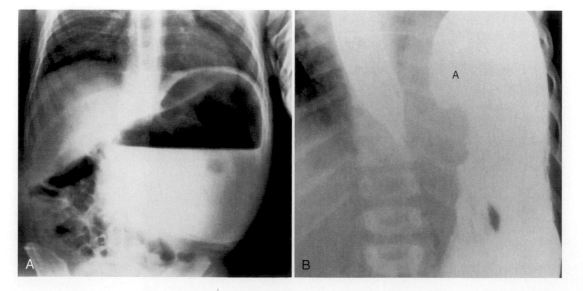

FIGURE 4-27. Mesenteroaxial gastric volvulus. **A,** Conventional radiograph shows a markedly dilated gastric contour with an air-fluid level. **B,** Contrast examination demonstrates the antrum (A) in the region of the fundus and a gastroesophageal junction in a lower than normal position.

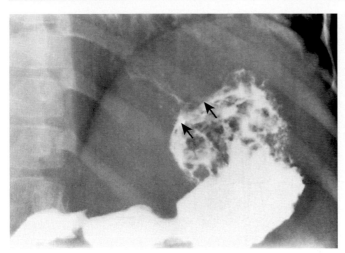

FIGURE 4-28. Radiograph obtained after Nissen fundoplication (antireflux measure), which resulted in a gastric cardia "pseudotumor" *(arrows)*.

period (5 minutes); others use a variety of GER-provoking maneuvers (e.g., gently applying pressure to the abdomen). Neither method is definitive or necessarily reproducible. Grading of GER is done at some institutions but, because of the intermittent nature of the condition, is of limited clinical use. GER is generally considered significant if the contrast agent reaches the level of the pulmonary hila or the clavicles. In short, the main use of the contrast examination is most often to verify normal anatomy and function of the gastroesophageal junction, stomach, gastric outlet, and proximal small bowel.

Nuclear medicine studies using technetium Tc 99m sulfur colloid in milk or food are easy and sensitive evaluations that allow for better quantification of GER but resolve little anatomic detail. However, the results correlate well with those of the pH probe test, an invasive test that necessitates hospitalization for passage of a pH probe catheter through the nose that is left in place for 24 hours. This test is currently considered the "gold standard." Treatment of GER is medical (thickened food) in infants, but if loss of weight, recurrent aspiration, or esophagitis (failure to thrive) supervenes, surgery is considered. Nissen fundoplication (an esophageal wrap using the gastric fundus) is the operative procedure often performed if GER persists after 18 months of age. Subsequent barium evaluation of this procedure shows the Nissen "pseudotumor" at the gastroesophageal junction (Fig. 4-28).

The complications of GER include esophagitis and stricture as well as a columnar epithelium–lined (Barrett) esophagus. These complications are more common in adults.

Diaphragmatic Hernia

The most common congenital diaphragmatic hernia is a herniation of peritoneal contents through the foramen of Bochdalek. It occurs in approximately 1 in 2000 live births and is much more frequent on the left side (75%). This left-side preference may result either because the pleuroperitoneal canal on the right closes earlier or because the liver "protects" against herniation on the right. Clinically, if the defect is large, the patient usually has severe respiratory distress, cyanosis, and a scaphoid abdomen at birth. Some infants present slightly later in the neonatal period with respiratory distress; in such instances the hernia is often smaller.

In the neonate, conventional radiographic examination of the abdomen and chest ("babygram") initially may demonstrate an opaque hemithorax with a paucity of bowel loops under the diaphragm. Air may enter the viscus after the infant swallows, and chest radiographs then become classically diagnostic (see Fig. 2-25).

Multiple radiolucencies in the affected hemithorax consistent with air-filled bowel loops are noted. Some loops of bowel may remain fluid-filled, but most become at least partially air-filled. There may be mediastinal shift to the other side, and a relative paucity of bowel gas remains in the abdomen. Occasionally a hydrothorax is present.

Contrast evaluation through an NG tube is diagnostic if conventional radiographs are not. Prenatal US and MRI studies often detect the herniation in utero, facilitating immediate postnatal intervention (Fig. 4-29). Successful fetal surgery is becoming more common, although intrauterine therapy still places the fetus at risk.

Because of the volume and concomitant mass effect of the herniated bowel on the ipsilateral lung, pulmonary hypoplasia results. The severity of pulmonary hypoplasia to a large extent determines morbidity and mortality, although the rates have remained overall at approximately 50% for decades. A significant mediastinal shift in utero may result in bilateral pulmonary hypoplasia. Malrotation of the GI tract is invariably present.

Treatment of a diaphragmatic hernia is surgical, often necessitating preoperative extracorporeal membrane oxygenation or high-frequency ventilation, depending on the severity of pulmonary hypoplasia. A rare form of diaphragmatic herniation occurs a few weeks after birth and, for unknown reasons (impaired diaphragmatic motion?), it becomes evident after (often streptococcal) pneumonia.

Acquired Conditions

Distention

Distention of a stomach by air may be caused by anxiety or crying (air swallowing), attempted NG or endotracheal intubation, or gastric outlet obstruction. The clinical history usually offers an explanation in these instances. Congenital lesions may, however, have to be ruled out if there is too much air (antral web or esophageal atresia with a distal fistula) or too little or no air (esophageal atresia or microgastria), all depending on the patient's age at presentation.

Causes of gastric outlet obstruction include hypertrophic pyloric stenosis, duodenal atresia/stenosis or web with or without annular pancreas, antral web (as discussed earlier), pylorospasm, and antropyloric inflammation. Benign gastric or duodenal ulceration in infants and children is usually stress related and is treated medically.

Inflammation

Gastritis can be of a primary or secondary nature. It is rare in adults, and even rarer in children. Primary causes include eosinophilic gastroenteritis, CGDC, and Crohn disease (predominantly involving the antrum), as well as Ménétrier disease (giant hypertrophic gastritis). Secondary causes include stress, trauma, burn, shock, medications (steroids and nonsteroidal anti-inflammatory agents), infection (in particular *Helicobacter pylori*, or *Candida* in immunosuppressed children), and accidental acid ingestion. Imaging (with barium) may reveal thickening of the rugae, mucosal nodularity, and decreased peristalsis (Fig. 4-30) as well as increased secretions. Antral narrowing is seen in eosinophilic gastritis and Crohn disease. US and CT are less useful for evaluation of gastric inflammatory lesions, although US demonstration of a thickened pyloric wall in an older child is virtually pathognomonic of chronic inflammation secondary to CGDC.

Ulceration

Gastric ulcers are rarely seen in children but manifest as pain and/or GI bleeding. They are very uncommon in children younger than 10 years, except for neonatal gastric ulcers, which are thought to be due to stress, possibly hypoxemic insult. Gastric ulcers are less common than duodenal ulcers, and in older children they

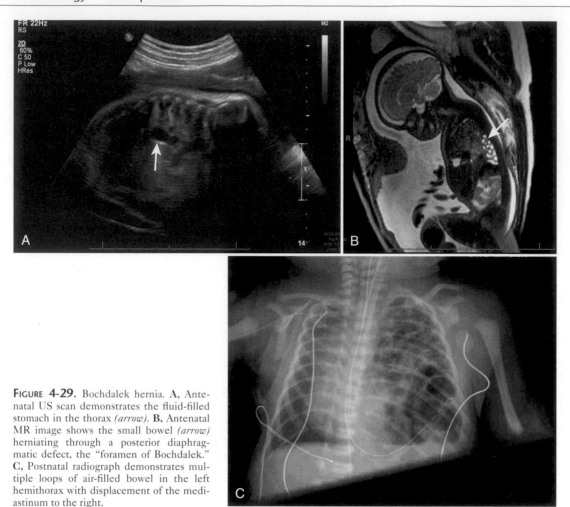

FIGURE 4-29. Bochdalek hernia. **A,** Antenatal US scan demonstrates the fluid-filled stomach in the thorax *(arrow)*. **B,** Antenatal MR image shows the small bowel *(arrow)* herniating through a posterior diaphragmatic defect, the "foramen of Bochdalek." **C,** Postnatal radiograph demonstrates multiple loops of air-filled bowel in the left hemithorax with displacement of the mediastinum to the right.

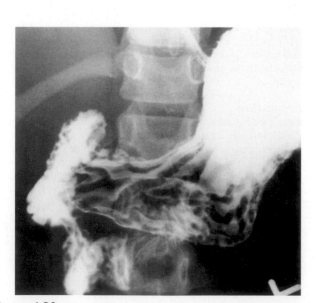

FIGURE 4-30. Eosinophilic gastroenteritis: nodular filling defects and thickened rugae.

mimic the symptoms of those occurring in adults. Gastric ulcers may be associated with aspirin ingestion, chronic pancreatitis, Zollinger-Ellison syndrome, cystic fibrosis, and multiple endocrine adenoma syndrome. Endoscopy is often diagnostic in patients older than 10 years.

Bezoars

Indigestible organic material can form a collection in the stomach called a bezoar. A bezoar can consist of hair (trichobezoar), vegetable matter (phytobezoar), or milk curd (lactobezoar). It manifests on conventional or barium evaluation as a solid, mobile mass that fails to exit the stomach. Trichobezoars and phytobezoars occur in (often emotionally troubled) children and adolescents, commonly with bad breath or an abdominal mass; they are frequently associated with anorexia and weight loss. The lactobezoar is seen in infants, probably as a result of having received formula that was mixed with insufficient water. Vomiting and the resultant dehydration constitute the clinical picture. Because of the current availability of better formula preparations, lactobezoars are seldom seen today.

Conventional radiographs of the abdomen are often characteristic and may be diagnostically sufficient. Plain radiographs of the abdomen show a soft tissue mass outlined by a rim of air in the upper abdomen. A contrast agent (barium) can be used to outline the (mobile) bezoar as well (Fig. 4-31). The treatment of choice consists of surgical (endoscopic) removal.

Neoplasms

Neoplasms in the pediatric stomach are rare. Benign lesions often occur as secondary gastric involvement in children with Gardner syndrome, Peutz-Jeghers syndrome, and familial polyposis. They consist of regenerative polypoid lesions located in the body and fundus. Benign lymphoid hyperplasia may be associated with immunoglobulin deficiency. Other rare, benign gastric

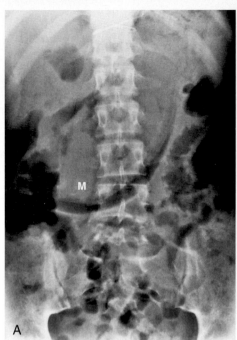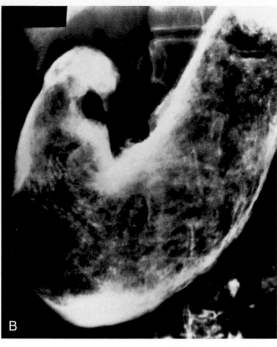

FIGURE 4-31. Bezoar. **A,** Conventional radiograph shows a mass (M) within the stomach outlined by gastric air. **B,** Contrast study confirms the trichobezoar.

tumors are mesenchymal in origin, including leiomyomas, teratomas, and lipomas. Aberrant (ectopic) pancreatic tissue is most often located along the greater curvature (antrum) and pylorus. It commonly contains a draining duct, seen as a dimple on contrast studies in 50% of cases, and it may grow to obstructive size. Endoscopy is often the definitive diagnostic tool.

Primary malignant tumors are exceptionally rare; they include gastric carcinoma (associated with Peutz-Jeghers syndrome) and leiomyosarcomas. Lymphoma may involve the stomach primarily or secondarily. A very rare, locally aggressive lesion with a benign course has also been described; called an inflammatory pseudotumor, it manifests as an epigastric mass in a teenager.

Although conventional radiographs can suggest masses or (rarely) calcifications (e.g., teratoma) of the stomach, a barium with air study most often best delineates the anatomy, particularly the mucosa. The extent of the tumor can be evaluated with US but is better assessed with CT using both peroral and IV contrast agent. Endoscopy is necessary to obtain a histologic diagnosis.

▬ SMALL AND LARGE BOWEL
Anatomic and Developmental Anomalies
Malrotation
Interference with the orderly sequence of rotation and fixation of the GI tract between 6 and 10 weeks' gestation may result in various severities of malrotation of the bowel. Subsequent malpositioning of the bowel may range from a "floppy cecum" to nonrotation of the entire GI tract. The explanation of this sequence of events is detailed in the following discussion and in the previous embryology section.

As the bowel returns to the peritoneal cavity during the process of extracoelomic rotation, there is interference with cecal descent if normal bowel rotation is not complete. This results in malpositioning of the bowel, with the mesentery attempting to "fix" the colon to the posterior peritoneal wall. This attempt is evident in fibrous peritoneal (Ladd) bands that are oriented diagonally across the abdomen and can obstruct the bowel lumen, most often the descending duodenum (Fig. 4-32). The extent of malrotation is further reflected in the length of the mesenteric attachment to the posterior peritoneal wall. A short mesentery allows the bowel to twist on itself, with the SMA as its fulcrum.

This twisting, up to three and one-half turns, either is asymptomatic or produces obstruction at the level of the third portion of the duodenum, resulting in lymphatic or vascular compromise that, if severe, may lead to bowel necrosis. The malposition may be totally asymptomatic or may manifest as vomiting and distention, depending on the degree of obstruction.

The majority of cases of midgut volvulus manifest in the neonate as bilious vomiting, which is often associated with peritoneal signs.

Imaging with conventional radiographs of the abdomen may show a "high" obstruction or abnormal position of bowel loops in cases of midgut volvulus. Partial duodenal obstruction is the most important finding (see previous discussion). A horizontal beam radiograph may be useful. Absence of small bowel air in the presence of peritoneal signs is an ominous finding. In the assessment for proper anatomic location of the small bowel, the most reliable indicator is the normal position of the duodenojejunal junction, not the position of the cecum. This is best demonstrated on an upper GI examination (Fig. 4-33). An upper GI study using barium or a nonionic contrast agent reveals the site of obstruction or an abnormal course of the second and third portions of the duodenum (see Fig. 4-8B).

A contrast enema study is not as reliable in excluding malrotation, because malrotation may be associated with a normal cecum in 10% to 15% of patients. US has been used to screen for malrotation through assessment of the normal location of the SMA to the left and lateral to the SMV. In malrotation this relationship has been observed to be reversed. However, patients with malrotation may have a normal SMA-SMV relationship, so the finding is not definitive (see Fig. 4-9).

Malrotation without volvulus represents an important diagnosis because many pediatric surgeons believe in prophylactic surgery to "tack down" the bowel and prevent volvulus. The diagnosis of midgut malrotation is easy when the previously described criteria are met. However, there is still disagreement among experts as to the diagnosis in ambiguous cases. Much of the ambiguity arises because of the common presence of a redundant duodenum on a mesentery, especially in neonates and infants. In these cases, it can be difficult to identify the duodenojejunal junction with assurance. Because the small intestine normally can be on either the left or right side of the

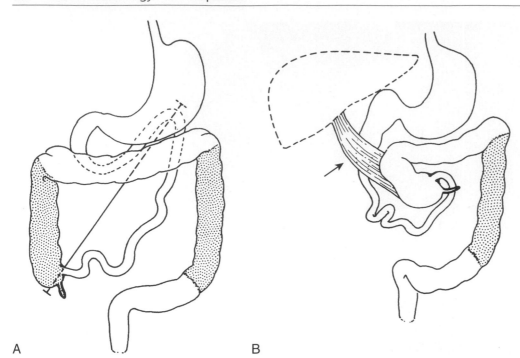

A B

Figure 4-32. Schematic representations of normal fixation (stippled) (**A**) and malpositioned intestinal tract (**B**). Note the Ladd bands *(arrow)*.

abdomen, its position is not helpful. With recognition of the possibility of false-positive and false-negative study results, the SMA-SMV relationship on US and the cecal position may provide supporting positive or negative evidence for the presence of malrotation.

Omphalocele

Total failure of the midgut to return to the peritoneal cavity during the tenth week of intrauterine life creates an exomphalos, or omphalocele. By definition, the interrupted rotation of the bowel results in malrotation. The liver and spleen may also be malpositioned. Thus an omphalocele's contents may vary from a single loop of bowel to the entire midgut and a solid organ. In rare cases, only the liver is contained in the omphalocele. An omphalocele can be differentiated from failed closure of the abdominal wall (gastroschisis) because an omphalocele is a midline structure, the herniated structures are covered by peritoneum and amnion, and the umbilical cord inserts at its apex; these features are well seen on prenatal US scans (Fig. 4-34A). Approximately 30% of patients with omphalocele are born prematurely; the incidence is 1 in 5000 live births, with a slight male preponderance. There may be associated cardiac anomalies. The kidneys are often located more cephalad than normal and may be found just under the diaphragm. An omphalocele may also occur in patients with Beckwith-Wiedemann syndrome. Conventional radiographs of the abdomen after birth may also show a large soft tissue mass protruding from the abdomen, occasionally demonstrating the umbilicus at its apex in association with an abnormal gas pattern (Fig. 4-34B). Surgery is mandatory and consists primarily of returning the omphalocele contents to the peritoneal cavity. A patch may be necessary to close the anterior abdominal wall.

Gastroschisis

The stomach, midgut, and, occasionally, portions of the urinary tract may protrude through a paraumbilical defect in the ventral abdominal wall lateral to or near the midline. This entity, gastroschisis, occurs twice as often as omphalocele. Because this (probably ischemic) rupture of the abdominal wall happens after the bowel has returned to the peritoneal cavity, the protruding viscera are not covered by peritoneum, and there is a normally positioned umbilicus. Malpositioning and shortening of bowel may be present, but

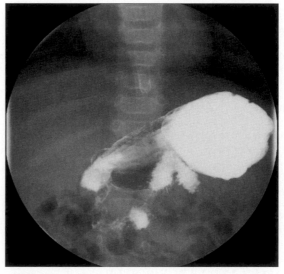

Figure 4-33. The duodenojejunal junction is in its proper place behind the stomach, to the left of the spine, and at about the level of the antropyloric region.

overall there is a low incidence of additional associated anomalies. The kidneys may be positioned more cephalad than normal. Children with gastroschisis are often born prematurely.

Imaging with US often allows the diagnosis to be made in utero, but on conventional abdominal radiographs, a soft tissue mass can occasionally be seen protruding paramedially; it can be confused with an omphalocele (Fig. 4-35). However, the umbilicus is normally located, the key differentiating point. Contrast studies may show poor peristalsis of the bowel, probably because it is in direct contact with amniotic fluid prenatally and resultant damage to the myenteric plexus leads to disordered motility.

Atresia and Stenosis

Duodenal atresia occurs in approximately 1 in 4000 live births. It is considered a failure of the recanalization process that occurs at 10 weeks' gestation. Total failure of recanalization resulting

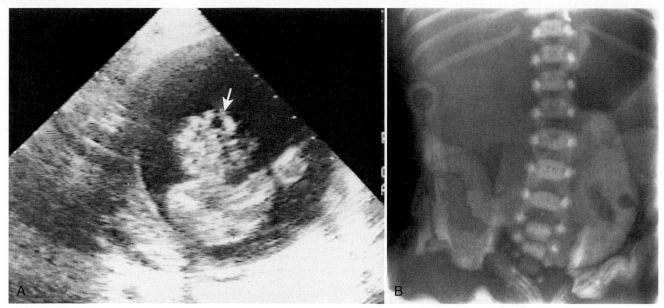

FIGURE 4-34. Omphalocele. **A,** Prenatal US scan shows the umbilicus coming off the dome of the soft tissue mass projecting anteriorly from the abdomen *(arrow)*. **B,** Conventional postnatal radiograph depicting the same.

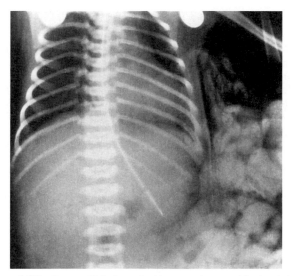

FIGURE 4-35. Gastroschisis. Intestinal loops project outside the abdominal cavity. A peritoneal lining is not present.

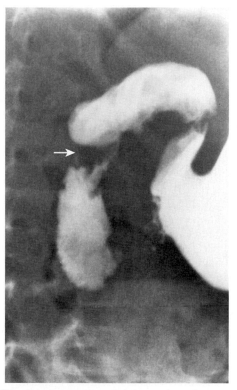

FIGURE 4-36. Annular pancreas. Persistent circumferential narrowing *(arrow)* in the proximal descending duodenum.

in obstruction accounts for most cases of duodenal obstruction. Partial failure of recanalization of the gut may result in duodenal stenosis, which is slightly more common than duodenal web. Duodenal stenosis may also be associated with either an annular pancreas, when the two anlagen of the pancreas fuse prematurely and encircle the descending duodenum (Fig. 4-36), or a preduodenal portal vein. A duodenal web (or diaphragm) may be stretched by peristalsis, resulting in an intraluminal diverticulum. The nearly constant location of these anomalies in immediate proximity to the ampulla of Vater lends further strength to an embryopathy as the cause. Twenty percent to 30% of patients with duodenal atresia have associated congenital heart disease, TEF, or imperforate anus. Down syndrome is found in up to 33% of patients with duodenal atresia, and malpositioning of the bowel in about 50%.

The degree of bowel obstruction determines the presence and severity of symptoms. Clinically, bile-stained vomiting within the first 24 hours of life is the hallmark of severe stenosis. An atretic lesion may be proximal to the ampulla of Vater, so the vomitus may not be bile stained. Minimal obstruction may have minimal symptoms. Prenatal US shows polyhydramnios in 50%, often proportional to the amount of obstruction to passage of bowel contents. Conventional radiographs may show the classic "double bubble" appearance (Fig. 4-37 and Box 4-7). In theory, this happens only if there is total atresia. If the duodenum is stenotic, a varying amount of air in the distal bowel is noted, according to the severity of stenosis. Upper GI findings also depend

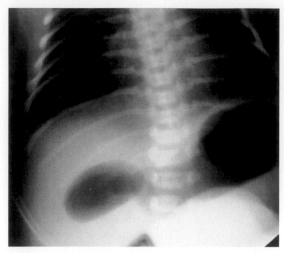

Figure 4-37. "Double bubble" appearance on a chest radiograph.

Colonic atresia is very rare (1 in 40,000 live births). The most common site of colonic atresia is near the anatomic splenic flexure, at or near the watershed between the parts of the colon supplied by the SMA and the IMA. This finding suggests an underlying vascular accident as the pathophysiologic pathway.

Treatment of all forms of atresia initially consists of an ileostomy or colostomy, followed by excision of the atretic (stenotic) segment and reanastomosis of the normal-caliber bowel segments.

Duplication Anomalies

Frequently discovered during infancy, duplication anomalies (incomplete recanalization around 8 weeks' gestation) can be spherical or tubular cystic lesions that are lined with intestinal mucosa and located on the mesenteric side of the GI tract, seldom on the antimesenteric side. They rarely communicate with the true lumen. At least 15% contain gastric mucosa. They arise most commonly in the ileum (35%), esophagus (20%), stomach, and duodenum; they may occur at multiple sites. Colonic duplication is very rare.

Clinically, a duplication most often manifests in the first year of life as an abdominal mass, which is palpable in one third of affected patients. Hemorrhage or intussusception is the presenting sign in 15% of patients. Vomiting due to obstruction is also common.

Conventional radiographs may show a mass, obstruction, or both, but findings are usually normal. Calcification is rare, and associated bony vertebral anomalies seldom occur. US shows a cyst lined by intestinal mucosa, an appearance that can be diagnostic (see Fig. 4-24). The differential diagnostic possibilities include omental cyst, choledochal cyst, mesenteric cyst, giant Meckel diverticulum, and ovarian cyst.

Meckel Diverticulum

After the extraperitoneal counterclockwise rotation of the midgut (6 weeks' gestation), the omphalomesenteric duct usually regresses and becomes the umbilicus. Failure of this obliteration can result in a fistula, sinus, omphalomesenteric duct cyst, or, most commonly, Meckel diverticulum (Fig. 4-39).

Meckel diverticula, which account for 90% of all omphalomesenteric duct abnormalities, are found in 2% of autopsies. They are situated about 2 feet from the ileocecal valve in the adult. Complications occur before age 2 years in 2% of all patients. Approximately 20% of Meckel diverticula contain ectopic gastric or pancreatic tissues that can ulcerate.

The diverticulum is located on the antimesenteric (omental) side of the ileum, contains gastrointestinal mucosa, and may be large. Clinically, GI hemorrhage is the most common presentation of a symptomatic diverticulum, and the amount of bleeding can vary from hematochezia to hemoccult levels. The cause of bleeding is ulcerating ectopic gastric mucosa, present in nearly 100% of cases with bleeding (Box 4-8). A Meckel diverticulum can be the lead point in intussusception or the focal point of a volvulus or obstruction.

Imaging with conventional abdominal radiographs may show obstruction, which—if it has led to volvulus and infarction—may be associated with air in the bowel wall or portal vein or even with free intraperitoneal air. Contrast studies, including techniques

on the extent of obstruction. They may range from total obstruction (atresia) or partial dilatation with a (circumferential) mass to (occasionally) the classic "wind sock" deformity, an intraluminal diverticulum. Upper GI evaluation is rarely necessary in patients with atresia or a tight stenosis because the distinction is unimportant to the surgical approach.

Atresia is much more common than stenosis. Distal atresia is twice as common in the small bowel as in the duodenum, where its occurrence is distributed equally between jejunum and ileum.

Jejunal or ileal atresia can be associated with other GI tract anomalies (malrotation or volvulus) in up to 25% of cases and virtually always manifests in the first 24 to 48 hours of life. About 10% of cases are associated with cystic fibrosis. The probable cause is a fetal vascular accident precipitated by embolus, volvulus, or intussusception. This possibility is corroborated by the presence of mesenteric defects at the site of atresia in many cases of jejunal or ileal atresia. Four types can be recognized. Type 1 atresia (least common) consists of a web occlusion of the lumen. Type 2 atresia consists of two blind-ending pouches connected by a fibrous cord (Fig. 4-38A and B). There is no gender predilection, and a quarter of patients with small bowel atresia are premature. Patients with duodenal atresia most commonly present with vomiting or a distended abdomen in the neonatal period.

There is a familial variant of jejunoileal atresia. In the "apple peel" small bowel type (type 3), the atresia is located near the duodenojejunal junction, with absence of the mesentery and SMA. This type is inherited as an autosomal recessive trait. Type 4 atresia consists of multiple small bowel atresias.

Prenatal US imaging may show polyhydramnios in 25% of affected infants, depending on how proximal the atresia is. The more proximal, the more succus entericus is produced distal to the obstructing lesion, so that polyhydramnios is absent or minimal. Conventional abdominal radiographs typically show dilated loops of small bowel proximal to the atretic or stenotic segment. Meconium peritonitis secondary to intrauterine perforation may be present. If a contrast enema study is performed, the colonic caliber depends on how proximal the stenosis is (Fig. 4-38C). With a more proximal (jejunal) atresia, sufficient succus entericus is produced to stimulate a normal-caliber colon; conversely, a more distal (ileal) atresia often results in a microcolon. The former occurs late in gestation, the latter early on. A hyperosmolar contrast agent should be used. Because both meconium ileus and meconium plug are differential diagnostic possibilities, the hydrophilic properties of this contrast agent can be therapeutic as well as diagnostic.

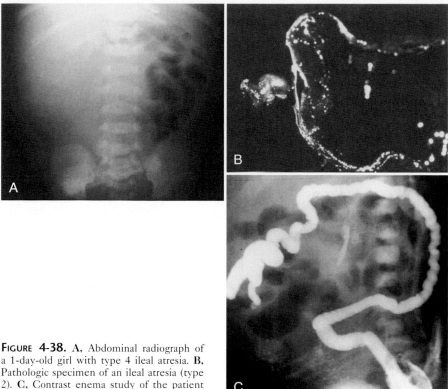

FIGURE 4-38. A, Abdominal radiograph of a 1-day-old girl with type 4 ileal atresia. **B,** Pathologic specimen of an ileal atresia (type 2). **C,** Contrast enema study of the patient represented in **A.**

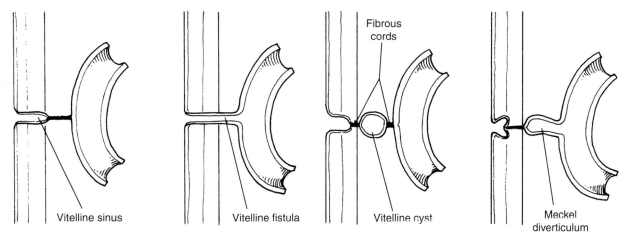

FIGURE 4-39. Fate of the omphalomesenteric (vitelline) duct.

such as enteroclysis, are of little use and are frequently only diagnostic in retrospect.

The most sensitive and specific imaging evaluation is a Meckel scan, using technetium Tc 99m pertechnetate. The result is positive only if gastric mucosa is present (in 20% of patients), in which case it has a greater than 95% sensitivity and specificity (Fig. 4-40). Angiography is rarely, if ever, indicated. In addition to necessitating anesthesia, detection by angiography requires a blood loss (flow) of at least 0.5 mL/min. If Meckel diverticulum is diagnosed, surgery is curative.

Meconium

Meconium consists of succus entericus that in turn is made up of bile salts, bile acids, and debris shed from the intestinal mucosa during intrauterine life. It is usually evacuated within 6 hours after birth or, because of perinatal stress, may be evacuated in utero, probably as the result of a vagal response. Normally meconium has a "mottled" appearance within the intestinal lumen on abdominal radiographs during the first 2 days of life.

Meconium Peritonitis

Meconium peritonitis occurs when there is antenatal bowel perforation and spillage of meconium into the perinatal cavity. It can occur as early as the second trimester. The meconium spillage causes a sterile chemical peritonitis, resulting in dystrophic calcifications that may be evident in as little as 24 hours. The perforation is often (in 50% of cases) the result of vascular accidents preceding obstructive lesions such as atresias and webs. The condition comes to clinical attention as an incidental finding on an abdominal radiograph or because of bowel obstruction caused by atresia or fibroadhesive

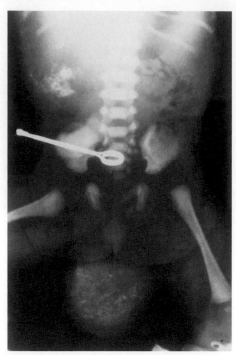

FIGURE 4-41. Meconium peritonitis. Flocculent calcification located in the right hemiabdomen as well as in the scrotum.

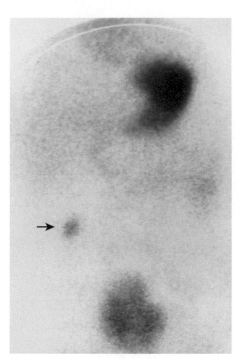

FIGURE 4-40. Meckel scan shows uptake of radionuclide in the right lower quadrant *(arrow)*, which indicates hemorrhaging gastric mucosa within the diverticulum.

bands resulting from the inflammatory peritoneal reaction. The bowel itself is commonly intact, the perforation having healed. Small amounts of spilled meconium frequently collect under the free edge of the liver, causing a linear calcification that parallels the liver edge. In a male, if the processus vaginalis testis is patent at the time the perforation occurs, there may be involvement of the scrotum by calcification or hernias. Ascites may also be present.

Conventional radiographs are most often diagnostic. There may be evidence of obstruction or ascites. Calcification can be of various shapes and configurations and may occur anywhere in the peritoneal cavity, including the diaphragm and the scrotum (most often on the right side) (Fig. 4-41). US may show ascites. The diagnosis is increasingly suggested on antenatal US.

Meconium Ileus

Meconium ileus occurs when meconium inspissates and obstructs the distal ileum, practically always (more than 99%) in patients with cystic fibrosis. Approximately 20% of infants with cystic fibrosis are found at birth to have meconium ileus. In the newborn infant, meconium ileus frequently manifests as vomiting and abdominal distention within hours.

Conventional abdominal radiographs show many dilated loops (often of different calibers) of bowel. Air-fluid levels are uncommon, unlike the findings in ileal atresia. Meconium in a dilated viscus is often seen.

A contrast enema with a hyperosmolar agent is diagnostic, and in 30% to 50% of cases of meconium ileus, the water-soluble contrast enema may be therapeutic. A microcolon is almost always present (Fig. 4-42A and B). US demonstrates multiple characteristic echogenic foci separate from the bowel wall both on prenatal and postnatal scans (Fig. 4-42C).

"Meconium Ileus Equivalent"

"Meconium ileus equivalent" is a misnomer. It is actually distal small bowel obstruction syndrome (DIOS) occurring in older children and adults. It has nothing to do with meconium, yet the stool on the abdominal radiograph looks like meconium because of the digestive abnormalities in patients lacking normal pancreatic enzymes. In 15% of adolescents and adults with cystic fibrosis, abnormally viscous bowel contents become impacted in the distal small bowel. An enema with hyperosmolar contrast material mixed with a wetting agent may be therapeutic, but only if reflux into the impacted distal ileum can be achieved.

Recurrent bowel obstruction (often correlated with poor therapeutic compliance in patients with cystic fibrosis), evident as recurrent colicky abdominal (right upper quadrant) pain, is the most common clinical presentation. On radiographs, mottled stool (which mimics meconium) is seen in dilated loops of small bowel (Fig. 4-43).

Meconium Plug Syndrome

"Functional colonic obstruction in the full-term neonate" is another name for meconium plug syndrome. A (long) plug of thick meconium lodges in the (distal) colon, probably caused by poor peristalsis as a result of neuronal underdevelopment (bowel innervation matures in a craniocaudad progression). Affected children are usually full term and present at 2 or 3 days of life with clinical signs, including abdominal distention, failure to pass meconium, and vomiting.

Conventional radiographs of the abdomen may show "low" obstruction with distention of the bowel. Contrast enemas using a water-soluble contrast agent usually show a normal-caliber left colon

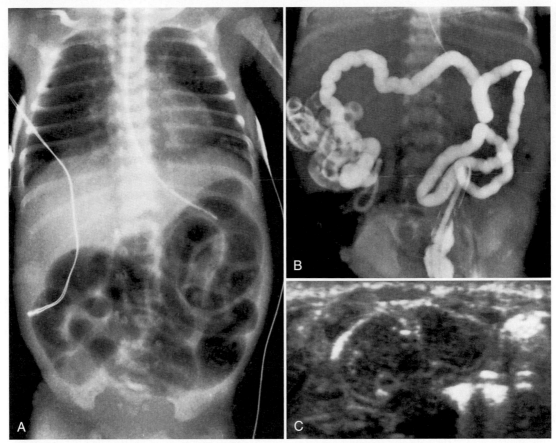

FIGURE 4-42. Meconium ileus. **A,** Conventional radiograph shows a "low" bowel obstruction. **B,** Contrast enema study demonstrates microcolon as well as loops of ileum filled with meconium. **C,** US scan shows multiple echogenic foci within the dilated bowel lumen.

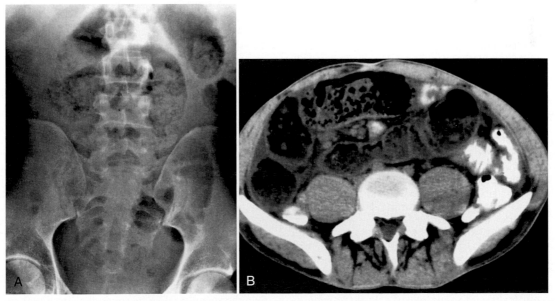

FIGURE 4-43. Distal intestinal obstruction syndrome ("meconium ileus equivalent"). **A,** Small bowel stool impaction in a 16-year-old patient with cystic fibrosis. **B,** CT scan confirms stool within dilated loops of small bowel with a normal-caliber colon.

with distention of the transverse colon and, occasionally, right colon as well as the meconium plug. A poorly understood variant, known as *neonatal small left colon syndrome*, mimics Hirschsprung disease in that there is a plug and an apparent zone of transition in the proximal descending colon (Fig. 4-44). This variant is typically found in infants born of diabetic mothers and resolves with time.

Functional immaturity of the colon occurs often in very premature infants, especially in infants of diabetic mothers. In addition, the functional obstruction may be exacerbated because of inspissation of the feedings. This latter complication is most often seen in premature infants who are fed powdered milk formulas, but it can be the result of the entry of any food into hypoperistaltic bowel.

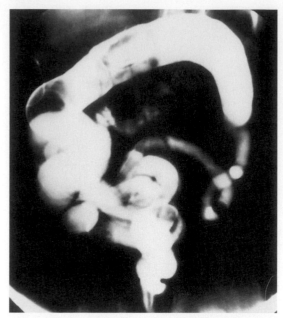

FIGURE 4-44. Small left colon syndrome. Small-caliber descending colon with normal-caliber transverse and ascending colon. This appearance can look similar to that of Hirschsprung disease (see Fig. 4-46), although the normal-caliber sigmoid leads to the correct diagnosis.

A contrast enema study usually demonstrates microcolon. This condition resolves spontaneously with the passage of several stools. It may be difficult, on radiographs, to distinguish functional immaturity of the colon from long-segment Hirschsprung disease.

The differential diagnosis of "low" bowel obstruction includes Hirschsprung disease, described in the following discussion, as well as the megacystis–microcolon–intestinal hypoperistalsis syndrome, which manifests as dilated bladder, microcolon, and hypoperistalsis of the colon. This latter entity is occasionally familial; it occurs in girls but is very rare.

Hirschsprung Disease

Hirschsprung disease, or colonic aganglionosis, occurs in 1 in 4500 live births. It is characterized by an absence of ganglion cells in the myenteric plexus, probably caused by failure of craniocaudal migration of neuroblasts between the 7th and 12th weeks of gestation. In 85% of cases, the aganglionosis involves the distal sigmoid and rectum, whereas in the remainder, the colon lacks ganglion cells proximal to the splenic flexure (Fig. 4-45). The disease occurs four times more often in boys, and there is a higher incidence of Hirschsprung disease in children with Down syndrome. Involvement of the entire colon and sometimes the terminal ileum (total aganglionosis) occurs equally in males and females, occasionally with a family history. Aganglionosis rarely, if ever, occurs in patients with a history of prematurity.

Clinically, the diagnosis is often made within the first month of life (80%). Usually (90%) a newborn with Hirschsprung disease presents with failure to pass meconium within 24 hours; abdominal distention is common. In 15% of patients there may be development of enterocolitis, which manifests as explosive watery stools, fever, and sometimes shock; these patients have a mortality rate of 20% to 30% unless prompt treatment is instituted.

In the newborn, imaging with conventional abdominal radiographs typically shows "low" obstruction with multiple air-fluid levels and distention of the bowel. In older children, there may be abundant stool in a distended colon. In neonates whose conventional radiographs show "low" bowel obstruction, the differential diagnosis includes meconium ileus, meconium plug syndrome, and atresia or stenosis of small bowel (or rarely colon) (Box 4-9).

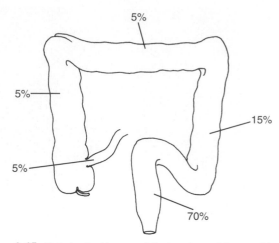

FIGURE 4-45. Relative incidences of the locations of the transition zone in Hirschsprung disease.

Box 4-9. Differential Diagnosis of "Low" Intestinal Obstruction with Many Dilated Loops

Imperforate anus
Colonic atresia
Hirschsprung disease
Meconium plug syndrome
Ileal atresia
Meconium ileus

Contrast examination of the colon is a common screening test for Hirschsprung disease, although its value may be limited in the first month of life. Its sensitivity increases with advancing age, and the examination is very useful in patients older than 6 months. A straight catheter should be used and prepared so that no more than 1 to 1.5 cm of it enters into the rectum. Otherwise, a very low transition zone may be missed. Delayed radiographs (24 hours) in contrast examinations are no longer deemed necessary because they show retained contrast agent and stool regardless of the cause of constipation.

The transition zone is best identified on the initial lateral rectal view taken during early filling (Fig. 4-46A and B). It may be abrupt or gradual but often is not identified at all, either because of fecal or enema distention or because some patients do not have a transition zone. If a transition zone is identified, there is no need to continue the contrast enema, because doing so might in fact present a risk for retention of contrast material. Retention is of less concern when a water-soluble contrast agent is used. A useful sign is the presence or absence of the rectal shelf. The rectum normally sits on the puborectalis muscle, courses perpendicular to the sacrum, and then ascends in the curve of the sacrum. Patients with aganglionosis often have a conical rectum with increased presacral space. This finding is not observed in neonates and is increasingly positive with advancing age.

The rectosigmoid index can also be used to evaluate for a transition zone. In the normal patient, the rectum is usually wider than the sigmoid colon; however, the opposite is true in patients with Hirschsprung disease. A rectosigmoid ratio greater than 0.9 excludes the diagnosis of rectosigmoid Hirschsprung disease. However, this index is reliable only when a transition zone is identified. Finally, irregular, spiculated contractions may be noted in the aganglionic segment, a finding that needs to be differentiated from enterocolitis (Fig. 4-46C). Patients with enterocolitis are desperately ill. Spiculations are caused by the uncontrolled muscle contractions of the denervated rectum. The sign is virtually pathognomonic but occurs in no more than 20% of patients with Hirschsprung disease.

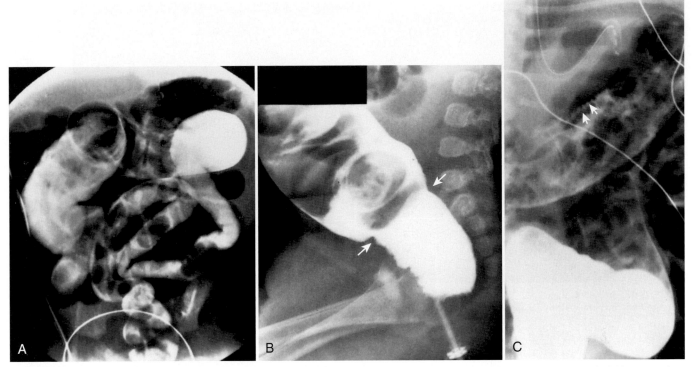

FIGURE 4-46. Hirschsprung disease. **A,** Neonatal Hirschsprung disease with a transition zone in the proximal descending colon mimicking meconium plug (see Fig. 4-44). **B,** Lateral radiograph demonstrating a rectosigmoid transition zone *(arrows).* **C,** Hirschsprung colitis as evidenced by spiculated edematous transverse colonic mucosa *(arrows).*

The imaging evaluation, if inconclusive, is followed by rectal manometry and suction biopsy. If this procedure does not establish the diagnosis, a full-thickness biopsy specimen is taken at least 2 to 3 cm above the dentate line.

Surgical management of Hirschsprung disease initially consists of construction of a defunctionalizing colostomy. Subsequently, there are three possible surgical interventions for definitive treatment.

- The Soavé pull-through procedure consists of permanent intussusception of the normal colon through the aganglionic segment. The radiographic appearance on contrast enema study eventually returns to normal. This method is used most often.

Two other techniques have been performed in the past.

- An often-used technique was developed by Duhamel, in which an end-to-side anastomosis is performed just above the rectum. This method preserves extrinsic innervation of the rectum but creates a rectal reservoir that often causes postoperative complications. It is easier to perform than the Swenson operation.
- The more difficult Swenson technique consists of formation of an end-to-end anastomosis after removal of the aganglionic segment. This procedure sometimes leads to a higher incidence of fecal and urinary incontinence.

Variants of Hirschsprung disease include total colonic aganglionosis and neuronal intestinal dysplasia. The former commonly manifests in the first week of life, but a number of infants (35%) may present after 1 month of age. All patients have vomiting and abdominal distention. Imaging may reveal a normal colon (75%) or microcolon (25%). A variable finding is unusual ease of reflux into the distal ileum, which may be slightly dilated if it is not itself aganglionic.

In neuronal intestinal dysplasia, hyperplasia of neuronal plexuses results in a megacolon that mimics Hirschsprung disease (pseudo-obstruction). It may be an isolated condition or may form in association with neurofibromatosis type 1 or multiple endocrine neoplasia type II.

Anorectal Malformations

Major anomalies of anorectal structures occur in 1 in 5000 live births and are slightly more common in boys. Most common are an imperforate anus and anal atresia, both manifesting as low obstruction with marked dilatation of the bowel in the neonate. The underlying cause most likely involves abnormal separation of the genitourinary and hindgut structures (the urogenital septum or perineal body) during fetal development.

Classification of these malformations as high (a supralevator position), intermediate (partially at the level of the levator muscle) and low (fully through the level of the levator muscle) is based on the location of the patent portion of the rectum in relation to the puborectalis muscle. As illustrated in Figure 4-47A, in most infants with a high or intermediate imperforate anus the rectum may develop fistulas into the neighboring structures: the urethra and bladder in males, the vagina in females, or the perineum in either. High lesions are treated with a colostomy at birth; the anorectal anomalies are repaired later after some somatic growth has occurred. Low malformations may also develop fistulas to the perineum. Fistulas occur more often in girls (90%) than in boys (70%). Low lesions can be primarily repaired through a perineal approach, usually by anoplasty.

The role of imaging is to delineate the level of the pouch and evaluate for the presence of fistulas and associated anomalies. Anomalies of the lower spinal cord, typically in patients with high lesions, are found in 30% to 40% of patients (tethering of the cord), thus necessitating US screening of the spine.

Urinary tract abnormalities are seen in 25% of patients with a low malformation and in 40% of patients with a high malformation. A voiding cystourethrogram is thus recommended as the initial modality to delineate this portion of the anatomy.

On the abdominal radiograph, calcification may be noted in the GI tract. This is the result of urine and meconium mixing because of the fistula between the colon and urinary system. US may demonstrate this calcification as well. US may also be used to delineate the distance from the anal dimple to the pouch via a transperineal approach (Fig. 4-47B). MRI is reserved primarily for

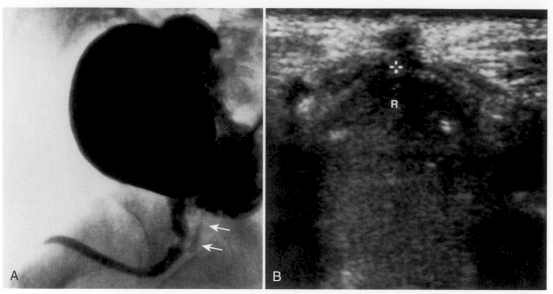

FIGURE 4-47. Imperforate anus. **A,** Communication between the posterior urethra and the rectum *(arrows)*. **B,** Transperineal US scan illustrates the distance from the pouch (R) to the anal dimple *(marker)* as well as calcific densities within the meconium in the rectal pouch.

better delineation of the anatomy, both before and after the pull-through operation and for associated spinal canal abnormalities.

Acquired Conditions

Gastroenteritis

Gastroenteritis is a very common condition affecting children and can be bacterial, viral, or parasitic in origin. The viral cause is human rotavirus in almost half the cases of diarrhea between the ages of 2 and 6 years. Adenovirus and other viruses have also been implicated.

Bacterial gastroenteritis (occurring in approximately 10% to 15% of North American patients with diarrhea) is most commonly caused by *Salmonella, Shigella, Escherichia coli, Yersinia,* and *Campylobacter.*

Parasitic gastroenteritis, most commonly caused by *Ascaris* (roundworm), *Strongyloides* and *Trichuris trichiura* (whipworm), is seen less frequently. Giardiasis, caused by the protozoon *Giardia lamblia,* is especially common in children with dysgammaglobulinemia and is a frequent cause of malabsorption.

Conventional supine and upright abdominal radiographs may have normal findings or may show air-fluid levels in small and large bowel that can mimic obstruction or ileus (Fig. 4-48). These are all manifestations of the diarrhea that patients with gastroenteritis most frequently present with.

Contrast (barium) studies may show longer transit time, nodular or thickened folds, or dilution of the contrast agent ("wet") while it passes through the small bowel. However, these are nonspecific findings, and their differential diagnosis is detailed in Box 4-10 and Box 4-11.

Crohn Disease

Regional enteritis has no known cause, although infection, altered immunity, and stress have been implicated. It is characterized by segmental full-thickness granulomatous involvement with inflammation of the bowel wall. Bowel stenoses (the "string sign") are less common in children than in adults.

The incidence is 6 per 100,000 children. In children younger than 10 years, the disease is rare (3.5% of childhood cases). Peak incidence is between ages 20 and 40 years; 20% of cases are diagnosed in childhood. There is a familial tendency, and clinically the disease often manifests as failure to

thrive, symptoms similar to those of appendicitis, or recurrent vague abdominal pain. There is often diarrhea and bleeding per rectum, and perirectal fistulae may occur. In 10% of children, sacroiliitis or arthritis of large joints may be present. The most common skin manifestation, although rare, is erythema nodosum.

Imaging hallmarks include skip lesions, irregular stenoses with loss of normal mucosal landmarks, increased separation of bowel loops secondary to mesenteric thickening, and fistula formation (Fig. 4-49).

Conventional radiographs can be suggestive of IBD in three fourths of patients. There may be obstruction, bowel wall edema simulating the "thumbprinting" of mural hemorrhage, or bowel wall thickening. A mass and ascites may be present.

US may illustrate thickening of the terminal ileal wall, but this modality is more useful in excluding appendicitis, ovarian pathology, and ascites from the differential diagnosis.

Contrast evaluation of the small bowel determines whether there is terminal ileum involvement, fistulae, "cobblestoning" (transverse ulcerating fissures), or a mass. Unfortunately, the terminal ileum is normal in 15% of children with Crohn disease. The colon may be similarly involved on contrast enema on which normal areas alternate with involved areas ("skip lesions"). Contrast colon examinations are less common now, because gastroenterologists prefer endoscopy.

CT is useful to look for recurrence of disease and to better assess for extraluminal involvement (mesenteric thickening, phlegmon, fistula, abscess) (Fig. 4-49C and D).

Surgery is avoided as long as possible in patients with Crohn disease because the procedure may exacerbate the disorder. Recurrences have been related to stress (e.g., during school examination periods, onset of menses, or pregnancy).

Ulcerative Colitis

Ulcerative colitis (UC) is an idiopathic mucosal disease that occurs more commonly in adults (30 to 60 years of age). In 15% of cases, the disorder is diagnosed in childhood, manifesting as diarrhea, abdominal pain, and rectal bleeding. In fewer than 5% of all patients with UC, these symptoms develop before age 10 years. There is an increased incidence of UC in first-degree relatives of affected patients and in patients with HLA-B27 antigen.

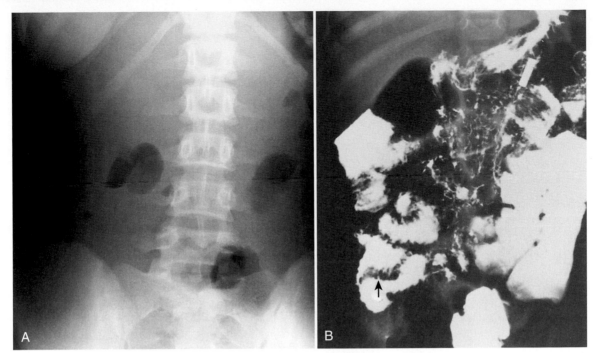

FIGURE 4-48. **A,** Air-fluid levels in small bowel and large bowel representing the excessive intraluminal fluid secretion of gastroenteritis. **B,** Thickened *(arrow)* and "wet" small bowel loops in a contrast examination of a patient with protein-losing enteropathy.

Box 4-10. **Differential Diagnosis of Thickened, "Wet" Small Bowel Loops**

Enteric infections:
  Yersinia
  Campylobacter
  Salmonella
  Shigella
  Escherichia coli
  Parasites (*Ascaris lumbricoides*)
Protein-losing enteropathy (with or without peripheral eosinophilia)
Celiac disease (gluten enteropathy):
  Most common chronic malabsorptive syndrome in children
  Onset at about 1 year of age with diarrhea
  Thickening of the valvulae conniventes is variable; the lumen is always dilated
Graft-versus-host disease:
  Develops in almost 50% of bone marrow transplant recipients between 2 weeks and 2 months after transplantation
Henoch-Schönlein purpura:
  Characterized by isolated submucosal hematomas that occur in children with anaphylactoid purpura
  Caused by angiitis of capillaries or small arterioles
  Similar findings occur in hemophilia
Lymphangiectasia:
  Primary (congenital) or secondary caused by obstruction of lymphatics (e.g., inflammatory lesion or malrotation)
  The protein loss causes diarrhea

Box 4-11. **Differential Diagnosis of Nodular Fold Thickening of the Small Bowel**

Nodular lymphoid hyperplasia (see Fig. 4-4)
Lymphoma
Polyposes syndromes
Amyloidosis, chronic granulomatous disease, cystic fibrosis, Crohn disease
Infections (e.g., *Yersinia, Giardia, Candida*)

The most common clinical feature in children is diarrhea, often accompanied by rectal bleeding. The latter can be copious and acute in 30% of patients. Failure to thrive is the presenting symptom in 15% of patients. Common adult clinical presentations, such as stomal aphthae, arthritis, uveitis, and toxic megacolon, are rare in children. In one third of patients there may be abnormal liver function test results, and fatty infiltration of the liver may be seen on US or CT. Toxic dilatation of the (transverse) colon occurs in 1% to 3% of children with UC (megacolon).

Imaging by conventional abdominal radiographs may show bowel wall thickening or loss of the normal haustral pattern. If a toxic megacolon is noted, contrast enema evaluation is contraindicated. In all other cases, the imaging method of choice after a plain film is a double-contrast barium enema. Diagnostic findings early in the disease include granularity of the mucosa, beginning at the rectum and extending proximally to a variable extent. More severe disease is heralded by punctate ulceration progressing to submucosal tracking ("collar button" ulcer). UC is confined to the rectosigmoid area in 25% of patients and extends to the transverse and left colon in another 50%. The entire colon is involved in the remaining 25% of patients. Backwash ileitis is seen in 10% of patients. As the disease progresses, ulceration becomes more obvious. Areas of regenerating colonic mucosa and focally spared mucosal islands result in the appearance of pseudopolyps. Postinflammatory (filiform) polyps are seen in the healing phase. Chronic disease may result in fibrosis and foreshortening of the colon, which appears ahaustral (Fig. 4-50).

The overall death rate can be as high as 2% per year after the first 10 years (a factor 20 times the normal incidence), and there is a higher incidence of adenocarcinoma of the colon in patients with UC than in the general population. For these reasons, total colectomy is often the treatment of end-stage disease.

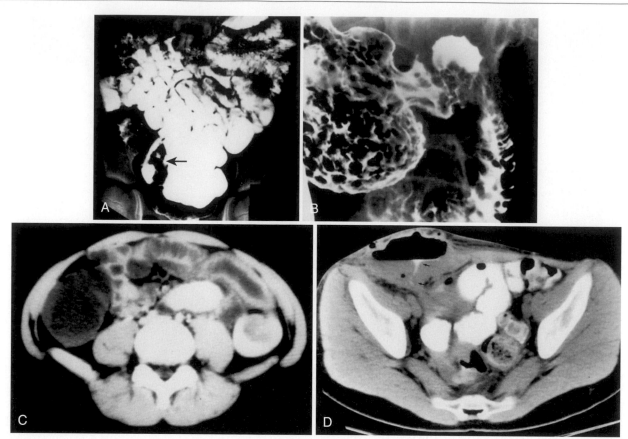

FIGURE 4-49. Crohn disease. **A,** Thickened, fixed terminal ileum and cecum *(arrow)* on upper GI study. **B,** Edematous antral wall and duodenal folds with "cobblestoning." **C,** CT scan confirming the findings of **A. D,** CT scan demonstrates an abscess with a fistulous tract.

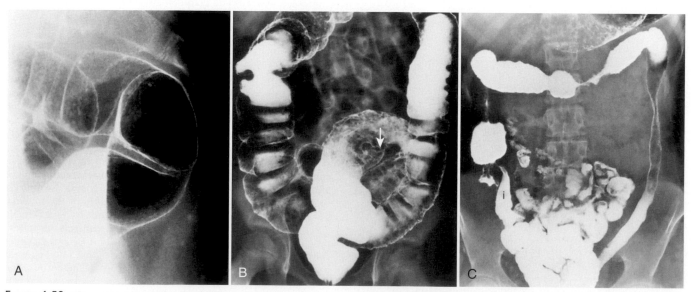

FIGURE 4-50. Ulcerative colitis (UC). **A,** Double-contrast view of the lateral rectum reveals fine granularity of the mucosa. **B,** Postinflammatory (filiform) polyps in the sigmoid *(arrow)*. **C,** An ahaustral left colon, "backwash" ileitis (i), and generalized colonic foreshortening in chronic UC.

The differential diagnosis includes infectious causes, as noted in the next section. A unique additional consideration in children is the hemolytic-uremic syndrome, which has been closely linked to *Shigella* and *E. coli* infections. It manifests as hemolytic anemia, renal failure, and thrombocytopenia. Bowel involvement is not common, but a prodromal colitis is seen in 80% of patients up to weeks before the renal symptoms appear (Fig. 4-51).

Other Colitides

A variety of organisms (*E. coli, Salmonella, Shigella, Yersinia, Campylobacter,* and *Entamoeba histolytica*), as well as cytomegalovirus in immunosuppressed patients, can cause colitis and cause diarrhea and abdominal pain with or without bleeding. Conventional radiographs often show air-fluid levels and dilated bowel loops. Barium enema findings mimic those in patients with IBD and colitis

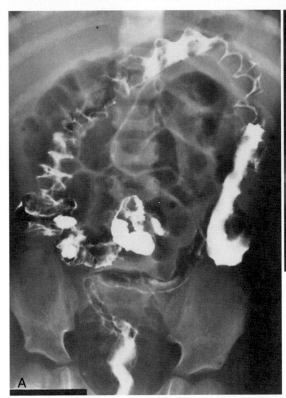

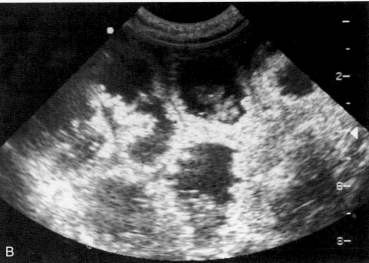

FIGURE 4-51. Hemolytic-uremic syndrome. **A,** Barium enema shows thickened colonic wall that is consistent with colitis 7 days before renal symptoms appeared. **B,** US scan demonstrates thickened bowel wall.

caused by *Campylobacter* and *Yersinia* as well as findings of Crohn disease in patients with amoebic or cytomegalovirus colitis.

Pseudomembranous colitis occurs in patients who have received a course of antibiotics. Alteration of normal flora by the antibiotic results in colonization by *Clostridium difficile*. Symptoms typically begin with severe diarrhea 4 to 10 days after institution of antibiotic therapy. A similar infection may occur in infants without previous exposure to antibiotics.

Conventional radiographs of the abdomen demonstrate dilatation and air-fluid levels in the colon. A contrast enema is contraindicated in severe cases; endoscopy is diagnostic (Fig. 4-52A). CT may be useful in screening septic immunosuppressed children (Fig. 4-52B).

Typhlitis (from the Greek word *typhlon*, meaning cecum) is a necrotizing colitis in young adults who are neutropenic. The more commonly used term theses days is *neutropenic colitis*. The disorder is usually associated with acute lymphoblastic leukemia, lymphoma, or aplastic anemia. *Pseudomonas*, cytomegalovirus, and *Candida* are the most common associated organisms.

Conventional or abdominal radiographs may show a small bowel obstruction or ileus or, occasionally, pneumatosis. Contrast enema examination is contraindicated. US findings are frequently suggestive, demonstrating a thickened cecal wall and cecal wall hyperemia. CT is diagnostic, providing exquisite delineation of the cecal wall thickening (Fig. 4-53).

Epidemic cholera is found in third world countries, but imaging studies are rarely performed.

Appendicitis

Appendicitis, which may be difficult to diagnose, is the entity most commonly necessitating abdominal surgery in the pediatric age group. Inflammation causes obstruction of the appendiceal lumen, which in turn causes retention of secretions, bacterial invasion, and vascular compromise. Appendicitis is less common in children younger than 7 years but has been reported even in neonates; the peak ages of incidence are the teen years. Perforation

at the tip of the appendix occurs in one third to one half of infants and young children, often leading to abscess formation. In older children, the omentum is thought to prevent abscess formation from occurring as frequently. However, earlier diagnosis is possible in older children, which is probably also a factor in their lower incidence of perforation.

Clinically, there may be abdominal tenderness migrating around McBurney point. "McBurney sign," consisting of tenderness over the inflamed appendix, is often elicited on US examination. Nausea, vomiting, fever, leukocytosis, and diarrhea also frequently occur. However, younger children commonly do not have typical presenting symptoms, making clinical diagnosis more difficult. The younger the child, the less likely he or she is to have high-grade fever or significant leukocytosis.

Conventional abdominal radiographs may show ileus localized to the right lower quadrant (70%), small bowel obstruction (43%), splinting of the lumbosacral spine, a mass (25%), obliteration of the psoas shadow (15%), or an appendicolith (10%). An appendicolith is presumably caused by postinflammatory precipitation of calcium salts in inspissated feces. If an appendicolith is noted on an abdominal radiograph, prophylactic laparotomy is advocated by some surgeons. Air in the appendix, especially if it is retrocecal, has been thought to indicate appendicitis but may in fact be a normal finding.

US evaluation may demonstrate the inflamed appendix (wall thickness greater than 6 mm and noncompressible). This technique is highly accurate (93%), with a specificity and sensitivity of 95%. A 5- or 7-MHz linear transducer with color-flow Doppler US capabilities demonstrates the hypervascularity of an inflamed appendix. Resistive indices range from 0.8 to 0.95 in normal appendices, with a mean of 0.54 noted in the inflamed appendix. US also rules out other causes of right lower quadrant symptoms, such as ovarian cyst, IBD, and endometriosis.

CT is now more widely used than US for the suspected diagnosis of appendicitis. Although the two examinations may be comparable in accuracy, US is highly operator dependent. Radiologists and US technologists with limited experience do not approach

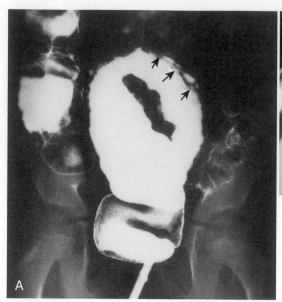

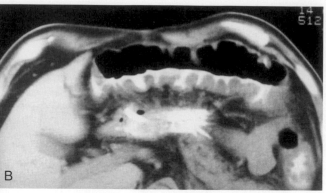

FIGURE 4-52. A, Pseudomembranous colitis. A pseudomembrane is illustrated in the sigmoid colon *(arrows).* **B,** CT scan confirms thickened "accordion pattern" of the colonic wall.

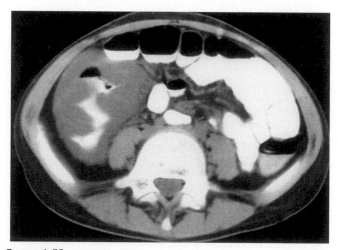

FIGURE 4-53. Typhlitis. CT scan shows cecal wall thickening in a patient treated for acute lymphoblastic leukemia.

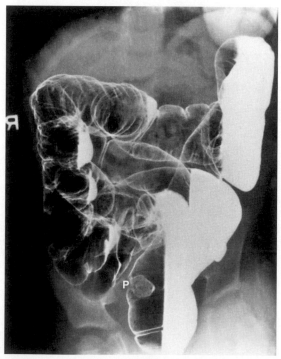

FIGURE 4-55. Juvenile polyp. Air contrast enema study demonstrates a juvenile polyp in the rectosigmoid (P).

the level of accuracy that is obtained in experienced hands. For this reason, in the United States, CT is usually the examination of choice in all but the largest pediatric centers. In some children's hospitals, US is preferred in children younger than 9 to 12 years and/or in very thin patients, whereas CT is the first examination in older children and overweight children.

CT should always be the modality of choice in complex cases, for demonstrating the presence or extent of an abscess (Fig. 4-54). US can identify phlegmon formation and abscesses, but the enhanced definition of CT provides more information. CT is more sensitive in identifying multiple interloop abscesses. Both CT and US are used for percutaneous drainage of an abscess.

Contrast (barium) enema study is now seldom used for suspicion of appendicitis, as a result of the experience gained in

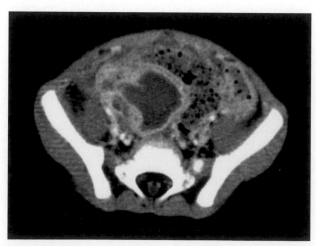

FIGURE 4-54. CT scan demonstrates a thick-walled abscess after appendiceal perforation.

TABLE 4-3. Polyposis Syndromes

Syndrome	Type	Location	Inheritance	Malignancy?
Juvenile polyposis	Juvenile	Colon (100%)	AD	No
Familial polyposis	Adenoma	Colon (100%) Small bowel Stomach (70%)	AD	Yes
Gardner syndrome	Adenoma	Colon (100%) Small bowel Stomach (70%)	AD	Yes
Turcot syndrome	Adenoma	Colon	AR	Yes
Peutz-Jeghers syndrome	Hamartoma	Small bowel (95%) Stomach (30%)	AD	Maybe

AD, Autosomal dominant; AR, autosomal recessive.

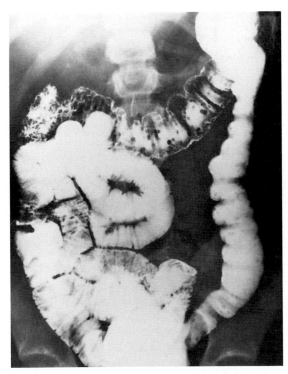

FIGURE 4-56. Familial polyposis with polyps throughout the colon and distal small bowel, a veritable "carpet."

diagnosing appendicitis by US and CT and because it often was noncontributory. Nonfilling of the appendix by barium may be seen in up to 30% of normal children.

Even with excellent clinical skills and optimal imaging, there is a 15% to 20% chance that laparotomy will result in removal of a normal appendix. Nonetheless, because rupture of the inflamed appendix occurs in more than 35% of patients, early diagnosis is important.

Neoplasms

Except for the premalignant polyposis syndromes, such as Gardner syndrome and Peutz-Jeghers syndrome, a malignant lesion of the small or large bowel in children is extremely rare. The non-Hodgkin lymphomas, including Burkitt lymphoma, are the most common primary malignancies of small bowel in the pediatric age group, with patients younger than 8 years most at risk. This entity most commonly involves the terminal ileum at first and frequently manifests as intussusception or hematochezia. Adenocarcinoma is the next most common cause, but it is extremely rare and occurs in the teen years. Because most colon carcinomas in children are of the mucinous variety, speckled calcification in the tumor or in liver metastases may be seen on plain radiographs. The appearances on contrast enema examination and CT scan are the same as those in adults. Carcinoid lesions do occur in children, and most are benign.

The most common benign lesions are juvenile polyps. Most common between 2 and 6 years of age, they probably originate from a primary hamartomatous process. Eighty percent are located in the rectosigmoid, and they are often solitary (25% multiple); there is a slight male preponderance. Juvenile polyps have no inheritance or malignant potential (Fig. 4-55). Other benign lesions are neurofibromas, hemangiomas (Osler-Weber-Rendu disease), lipomas, and leiomyomas.

The polyposis syndromes, all more common in adults, are summarized in Table 4-3. Familial polyposis occurs in 1 in 8000 live births; two thirds of affected patients have a family history and usually present by the teen years. Commonly, sheets of small polyps cover the entire colon; they occur in the stomach in 70% of patients but less commonly in the rest of the small bowel (Fig. 4-56). Familial polyposis is frequently premalignant.

Siblings of patients with familial polyposis coli should undergo yearly colonoscopic surveillance from 10 to 50 years of age.

Only 20% of patients with Gardner syndrome have the triad of soft tissue hamartomas and osteomas of the mandible and facial bones. Mesenteric fibromatosis (desmoid tumor) occurs in 5% of patients; it is avascular and may lead to adhesions.

Peutz-Jeghers syndrome is the most common small bowel polyposis syndrome, but only 15% of patients present before reaching their twenties. There is accompanying pigmentation of all mucocutaneous surfaces, especially the lips and buccal mucosa. Approximately 50% of patients have a family history of the syndrome.

SUGGESTED READINGS

TEXTS

Carty H, Shaw D, Brunelle F, Kendall B (eds): Imaging Children, vol 1. London, Churchill Livingstone, 1994, pp 249-560.

Kirks DR (ed): Practical Pediatric Imaging, ed 3. Philadelphia, Lippincott-Raven, 1997, pp 821-953.

Siegel MJ (ed): Pediatric Sonography, ed 3. Philadelphia, Lippincott Williams & Wilkins, 2002, pp 337-384.

Skandalakis JE, Gray SW (eds): Embryology for Surgeons, ed 2. Baltimore, Williams & Wilkins, 1994, pp 17-404.

Slovis TL (ed): Caffey's Pediatric Diagnostic Imaging, ed 11, vol 2. Philadelphia, Elsevier, 2008, pp 139-271, 1759-221, 2464-2476.

Stringer DA: Pediatric Gastrointestinal Imaging. Philadelphia, Mosby–Year Book, 1991.

Sty JR, Wells RG, Starshak RJ, et al: Diagnostic Imaging of Infants and Children, vol 1. Gaithersburg, Md, Aspen, 1992, pp 139-246.

Summer TE, Auringer ST (eds): Pediatric Gastrointestinal Radiology. Radiology Clinics of North America vol. 34, issue 4. Philadelphia, WB Saunders, 1996, pp 701-15.

Swischuk LE: Imaging of the Newborn, Infant and Young Child, ed 4, Baltimore, Williams & Wilkins, 1997, pp 353-486, 530-564.

ARTICLES

Alison M, Keniche A, Azoulay R, et al: Ultrasonography of Crohn disease in children. Pediatr Radiol 2007;37:1071-82.

d'Almeida M, Jose J, Oneto J, et al: Bowel wall thickening in children: CT findings. Radiographics 2008;28:727-46.

Berdon WE, Slovis TK, Campbell RB, et al: Neonatal small left colon syndrome: Its relationship to aganglionosis and meconium plug syndrome. Radiology 1977;125:457-62.

Blumhagen JD, Maclin L, Krauter D, et al: Sonographic diagnosis of hypertrophic pyloric stenosis. AJR Am J Roentgenol 1988;150:1367-70.

Daneman A, Alton DJ: Intussusception: Issues and controversies related to diagnosis and reduction. Radiol Clin North Am 1996;34:743-56.

Daneman A, Navarro O: Intussusception. Part I: A review of diagnostic approaches. Pediatr Radiol 2003;33:79-85.

Eklöf O, Hugosson C: [Post-evacuation findings in barium enema treated intussusceptions]. Ann Radiol (Paris) 1976;19:133-9.

Hayden CK Jr: Ultrasonography of the gastrointestinal tract in children. Abdom Imaging 1996;21:9-20.

Hernanz-Schulman M: Infantile hypertrophic pyloric stenosis. Radiology 2003;227:319-31.

Hernanz-Schulman M, Ambrosino MM, Freeman PC, Quinn CB: Common bile duct in children: Sonographic dimensions. Radiology 1995;195:193-5.

Hur J, Yoon C-S, Kim M-J, et al: Imaging features of gastrointestinal tract duplications in infants and children: From oesophagus to rectum. Pediatr Radiol 2007;37:691-9.

Jabra AA, Fishman EK, Taylor GA: CT findings in inflammatory bowel disease in children. AJR Am J Roentgenol 1994;162:975-9.

Kharbanda AB, Taylor JA, Bachur RG: Suspected appendicitis in children: Rectal and intravenous contrast-enhanced versus intravenous contrast-enhanced CT imaging. Radiology 2007;243:520-6.

Kirks DR, Caron KH, Bisset GS III: CT of blunt abdominal trauma in children: An anatomic "snapshot in time." Radiology 1992;182:631-2.

MacPherson RI: Gastrointestinal tract duplications: Clinical, pathologic, etiologic and radiologic considerations. Radiographics 1993;13:1063-80.

Markowitz RI, Meyer JS: Pneumatic versus hydrostatic reduction of intussusception. Radiology 1992;183:623-4.

McAlister WH, Kronemer KA: Emergency gastrointestinal radiology of the newborn. Radiol Clin North Am 1996;34:819-44.

Oh SK, Han BK, Levin TL, et al: Gastric volvulus in children: The twists and turns of an unusual entity. Pediatr Radiol 2008;38:297-304.

Sivit CJ, Newman KD, Boenning DA, et al: Appendicitis: Usefulness of US in diagnosis in a pediatric population. Radiology 1992;185:549-52.

Sizemore AW, Rabbani KZ, Ladd A, et al: Diagnostic performance of the upper gastrointestinal series in the evaluation of children with clinically suspected malrotation. Pediatr Radiol 2008;38:518-28.

Strouse PJ: Disorders of intestinal rotation and fixation ("malrotation"). Pediatr Radiol 2004;34:837-51.

Taylor GA, Eichelberger MR, O'Donnell R, et al: Indications for computed tomography in children with blunt abdominal trauma. Ann Surg 1991;213:212-8.

Toma P, Granata C, Magnano G, et al: CT and MRI of paediatric Crohn disease. Pediatr Radiol 2007;37:1083-92.

CHAPTER 5

Accessory Organs of Digestion

Bruce R. Parker and Johan G. (Hans) Blickman

▬ LIVER AND BILIARY TREE

Anatomy and Developmental Anomalies

The liver, gallbladder, and biliary tree originate from endodermal cells that form a diverticulum arising from the duodenal region of the primitive embryonic gut between 4 and 10 weeks' gestation. The larger cranial division (pars hepatica) gives rise to the liver, whereas the smaller, caudal part (pars cystica) develops into the gallbladder and cystic duct. The intrahepatic and extrahepatic components of the biliary tree develop independently and then unite by 12 weeks' gestation. At birth, the liver represents about 5% of total body weight (200 g). Bile secretion commences between 12 and 16 weeks' gestation. Hematopoiesis occurs only in the fetal liver and will have ceased by age 6 weeks in normal infants.

Although the liver is usually located in the right upper quadrant (the left upper quadrant in cases of situs inversus totalis), it may be midline and more symmetric in patients with heterotaxy syndromes than in normal patients. This may occur in approximately 80% of patients with asplenia and in about 50% of cases of patients with polysplenia (Fig. 5-1).

Between 70% and 80% of the blood supply to the liver is through the portal venous system. The portal venous branches, hepatic arterial branches, and biliary radicles run parallel to one another in the center of hepatic segments, the so-called triad arrangement.

Absence of either the right or left hepatic lobe has been reported but is extremely unusual, as is absence of the gallbladder.

Accessory lobes of the liver are rare. Caudal elongation of the right lobe of the liver, known as a Riedel lobe, is a normal variation.

Biliary Atresia

Biliary atresia enters the differential diagnosis spectrum when cholestatic jaundice persists beyond 4 weeks of age. Neonatal jaundice may be due to sepsis, hemolysis, infection (cytomegalovirus, hepatitis A and B, rubella), and metabolic abnormalities (e.g., α_1-antitrypsin deficiency, cystic fibrosis [CF]). When these other causes for jaundice have been excluded, neonatal hepatitis or biliary atresia accounts for more than two thirds of remaining cases of conjugated hyperbilirubinemia in the neonate. It is postulated that both biliary atresia and neonatal hepatitis are part of the same clinical spectrum of cholestatic jaundice and hepatomegaly. This theory might explain the variations encountered in the types of biliary atresia, as well as the fact that surgical results to repair biliary atresia are significantly better before 2 months of age—suggesting that early intervention may slow the progression of the disease (Fig. 5-2). Finally, approximately 10% of children with biliary atresia have noncardiac polysplenia syndrome. This complex consists of some or all of the following anomalies: polysplenia, bilateral bilobed lungs, azygous continuation of the inferior vena cava (IVC), preduodenal portal vein, and anomalous origin of hepatic artery.

The differentiation between biliary atresia and neonatal hepatitis depends to a large and significant extent on imaging. This differentiation is important because surgery is the treatment for the former but not the latter, and because liver biopsy results are falsely negative in up to 40% of cases for either condition. This latter fact is further suggestive proof that these entities are parts of the same cholangiopathy.

Imaging evaluation by ultrasound (US) can reveal either a normal liver or an inhomogeneous parenchymal pattern in both entities, and a 1.5- to 2-cm-long gallbladder is visualized (present) in up to 20% of patients with biliary atresia. The presence or absence of the gallbladder is thus not diagnostic but merely suggestive; absence of the gallbladder suggests biliary atresia, and presence of the gallbladder makes hepatitis more likely. Evidence of biliary duct dilatation is characteristic of biliary atresia, because the biliary tree does not dilate in hepatitis. Periportal fibrosis may be seen early in biliary atresia, evident on US as increased periportal echogenicity. Practically speaking, US serves primarily to exclude choledochal cysts, choledocholithiasis, and other liver lesions.

Nuclear scintigraphy using technetium Tc 99m iminodiacetic acid (IDA) derivatives is more reliable in differentiating the two entities. Visualization of the radionuclide in the duodenum essentially excludes biliary atresia. The diagnosis of biliary atresia may be entertained if the radionuclide (1) is not visualized in the gallbladder at 15 minutes or (2) is not visualized in the proximal small bowel at 30 minutes and (3) disappears from the liver by 6 hours with a significant concomitant increase in renal excretion; with these findings, delayed imaging is considered useful. The sensitivity of radionuclide studies to detect biliary obstruction is 100%, and the specificity about 80%. Phenobarbital premedication is essential. In contrast, the hallmark of neonatal hepatitis is normal hepatic uptake of the radionuclide but significantly delayed clearance of it from the liver (longer than 12 hours) (Fig. 5-3).

After radionuclide imaging confirms the diagnosis of biliary atresia, further imaging of the biliary tree is performed at laparotomy, because a preoperative percutaneous cholangiogram is difficult to perform in neonates and infants and requires anesthesia. An intraoperative cholangiogram is therefore performed to identify the anatomy in order to assess whether primary anastomosis of the biliary tree, which is feasible in 10% to 15% of patients with biliary atresia, should be attempted. The main right and left hepatic ducts must be of normal caliber at least down to their junction for a Roux-en-Y anastomosis to be successful (see Fig. 5-2).

The Kasai hepatic portoenterostomy is a technique used when this favorable anatomy is not present. The jejunum is anastomosed to the undersurface of the liver, allowing bile to drain into it. Operative success depends on the presence of microscopic biliary structures at the liver hilus. The rate of success is also inversely proportional to the age of the patient. Liver transplantation is an option when the Kasai operation fails or if progressive neonatal hepatitis has resulted in cirrhosis.

Choledochal Cysts

Choledochal cysts are rare and occur four times more frequently in girls than in boys. They are more common in Asians. Fifty percent of patients have symptoms before age 10, including abdominal pain (50%), fever, obstructive jaundice (80%), and a mass (50%). The classic triad— episodic abdominal pain, jaundice, and a right upper quadrant mass on the right side—is present in 15% to 20% of cases.

These cysts are considered cystic malformations of the biliary tree. Their cause has been ascribed to an obstruction at the sphincter of Oddi or to abnormal insertion of the common bile duct (CBD) into the pancreatic duct. Another theory is that biliary atresia, choledochal cysts, and neonatal hepatitis have a common viral cause. Finally, a congenital weakness in the wall of the biliary tree has also been suggested as a cause. Thus the choledochal cyst in the neonate is most likely congenital, whereas the pathogenesis of the choledochal cyst in the older child is thought to be secondary to anomalous (pancreatic) biliary drainage.

The four types of choledochal cysts are as follows; the first type has two suptypes (Fig. 5-4):

Type IA: Fusiform or concentric dilatation of the CBD *below the cystic duct.*

Type IB: Fusiform dilatation of the CBD *above the cystic duct.*

Type II: Eccentric diverticulum of the CBD.

Type III: Dilatation of the CBD at the level of the sphincter of Oddi (choledochocele); rarest form.

Type IV: Multiple fusiform dilatations of the intrahepatic bile duct (Caroli disease) without evidence of obstruction; very rare.

Type IV may in fact be a distinct entity, an autosomal recessive inherited disorder. Some authorities then divide it into two forms: the pure form, type 1, consisting of intrahepatic biliary dilatation, and type 2, associated with hepatic fibrosis. The former manifests as stone formation, the latter as portal hypertension and varices.

The differential diagnosis of a right upper quadrant cyst includes hydrops of the gallbladder, pancreatic pseudocyst, renal cyst, enteric duplication cyst, omental cyst, and ovarian cyst.

Conventional radiographs, as well as contrast (barium) studies, may show evidence of a mass, but the findings are usually normal.

US provides information about the size, contour, position, and character of choledochal cysts. Calculi and wall calcification are rare. Hepatic fibrosis is uncommon, and associated renal cysts seldom occur.

Endoscopic retrograde studies can further delineate the degree and extent of the dilatation.

The appearance on computed tomography (CT) is often specific in cases of choledochocele and clearly demonstrates the other types of choledochal cysts and their complications (Fig. 5-5).

Radionuclide studies using the Tc 99m IDA derivatives may also be useful, particularly when US or CT does not clarify whether there is communication between the cyst and the biliary tree. These studies may occasionally show delayed accumulation of the radionuclide in the cyst in these cases.

The treatment of choledochal cysts consists of total excision with direct enteric drainage of the biliary tree. Treatment delay may result in cirrhosis, portal hypertension, cholangitis, or pancreatitis. There is a 20-fold higher risk of biliary tract carcinoma in patients with choledochal cyst than in the normal population.

Cystic Liver Disease

Polycystic liver disease is often associated with polycystic disease of the kidneys and is also accompanied by varying extents of periportal fibrosis. In patients with the infantile and juvenile forms of autosomal recessive polycystic kidney disease (ARPKD), imaging findings consist of hepatomegaly, dilatation of the biliary radicles, and fibrous replacement of liver parenchyma. The last leads progressively to symptomatic portal hypertension.

The size of the cysts and the extent of intrahepatic fibrosis and biliary obstruction determine the clinical presentation and prognosis. US shows multiple round noncommunicating cysts of varying sizes; the diagnosis is confirmed when enlarged hyperechogenic kidneys are demonstrated at the same time. There is usually no need to perform CT or magnetic resonance imaging (MRI) to clinch the diagnosis; liver scintigraphy often shows areas of photopenia with normal excretion of the radionuclide into the gastrointestinal (GI) tract (Fig. 5-6).

Congenital Hepatic Cysts

Congenital hepatic cysts, which are occasionally multilocular, are extremely rare and are often round or ovoid. They occur more commonly in the right lobe of the liver and probably arise from

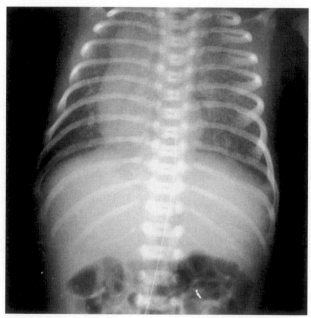

FIGURE 5-1. Abdominal radiograph illustrating a midline liver in heterotaxy syndrome.

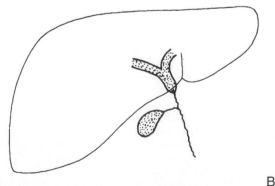
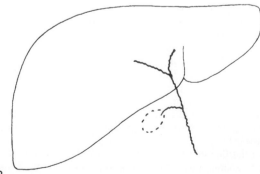

FIGURE 5-2. Biliary atresia. The main right and left hepatic ducts down to their junction may be normal (**A**) or abnormal (**B**), with many variations possible. The former appearance accounts for 10% to 15% of all cases and is correctable; the latter is not.

aberrant biliary radicles. In addition, they may be completely or partially within the liver, or may even be pedunculated.

Imaging is no different from that required in polycystic liver disease, yet the differential diagnosis must include cystic abdominal masses seen in infants, such as duplication cysts, mesenteric cysts, and ovarian cysts.

Acquired Conditions

Hepatitis
Viral Infection
In the newborn, cytomegalovirus and hepatitis B virus are the most common etiologic agents that produce chronic inflammatory change, fibrosis, and eventual cirrhosis (Fig. 5-7). In older children, an often self-limited acute hepatitis may be caused by the following viruses: hepatic A, B, or C, herpes simplex, Epstein-Barr, by mumps, varicella, and coxsackievirus. Any viral infection, but most commonly the hepatitis B virus, can lead to a chronic carrier state with persistent hepatitis or chronic active hepatitis. This may be dormant for years or may become fulminant; occasionally it may be followed by the development of hepatocellular carcinoma.

Scintigraphy confirms the mild to moderate hepatomegaly, but the findings are otherwise nonspecific. Imaging findings with US, CT, or MRI are often normal, yet occasionally there may be parenchymal inhomogeneity and increased echogenicity.

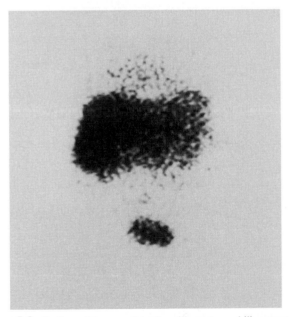

FIGURE 5-3. Radionuclide scan of the liver illustrates no biliary excretion in a patient with biliary atresia at 45 minutes.

Bacterial Infection
Perinatally, liver infections are most often caused by *Escherichia coli*, although *Streptococcus* and *Listeria* have also been implicated. In the neonate, an umbilical venous catheterization can also be the cause of hepatitis. In older children, bacterial infection most often develops in an immunosuppressed host. The infection then takes the form of a bacteremia, with multiple microabscesses that may or may not become larger by coalescing. Nuclear scintigraphy often demonstrates inhomogeneous radionuclide accumulation and may identify the microabscesses along with hepatomegaly. Single-photon emission computed tomography (SPECT) improves the sensitivity and localization of liver abscesses; gallium and indium scintigraphy can sometimes be useful as well. Hepatic abscesses may be demonstrated on US or CT as lesions that may be smaller than 1 cm in diameter; these can be ill-defined, hypoechogenic, or of low attenuation, and they rarely contain air. A low-attenuation or hypoechogenic rim may surround the microabscesses.

Fungal Infection
Fungal infections almost always occur in immunocompromised hosts. *Candida* is the most common etiologic agent, followed by *Aspergillus*, mucormycosis, and *Cryptococcus*. Imaging with scintigraphy, US, or MRI is not specific enough to differentiate fungal from viral or bacterial infection.

Parasitic Disease
Hydatid disease occurs in the liver in 80% of cases, in the lungs in 15%, and in other areas of the body in 5%. The disease is rare in the United States, but it is seen more often today because of expanding travel opportunities. The cysts, occasionally with some debris, contain clear fluid. They develop about 5 to 6 months after ingestion of the larvae of *Echinococcus granulosis* (occasionally *Echinococcus multilocularis*), and the cysts eventually may become multiloculated. Symptoms include an abdominal mass, pain, and jaundice, the latter two often associated with rupture of a cyst. US and CT may demonstrate one or more large (expanding) cystic lesions with daughter cysts (Fig. 5-8). There may be calcifications in the cyst wall. MRI has shown a low-intensity rim surrounding the cysts. The cysts may rupture into the containing pericyst, into the biliary tree, or into the pleural or periportal spaces. On US the appearance of the fluid becomes more echogenic.

Amebiasis
Entamoeba histolytica is a protozoon that disseminates via the portal venous system and leads to multiple hepatic abscesses, most often in children younger than 3 years. These children present with fever, hepatomegaly, and diarrhea; jaundice is unusual. Cysts are seen on US and CT that are often contiguous with the liver capsule; these have a poorly defined hypoechoic rim, and there may be a peripheral halo. Scintigraphy may show one or more photopenic defects in a normal-size liver; MRI shows a well-defined heterogeneous mass that is usually hypo-intense on

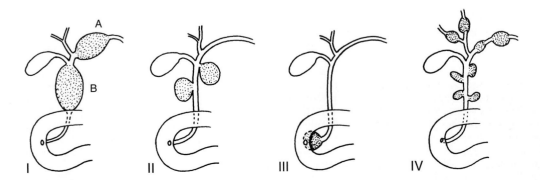

FIGURE 5-4. Types of cystic malformations of the biliary tree. See text for explanation.

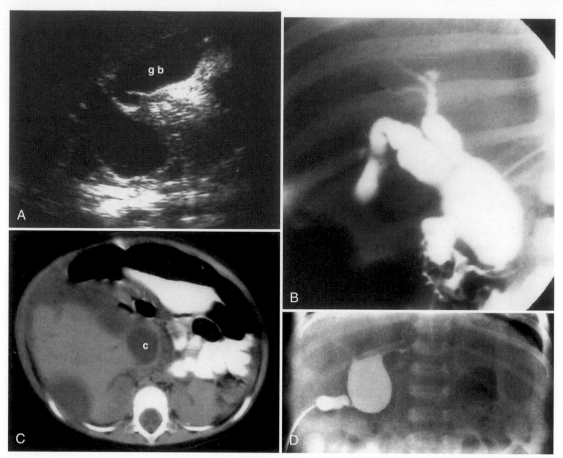

FIGURE 5-5. Choledochal cyst. **A,** US evaluation demonstrates a cystic structure communicating with the gallbladder (gb). **B,** Endoscopic retrograde cholangiopancreatogram confirms the fusiform dilatation of the distal common bile duct. **C,** CT scan confirms the choledochal cyst (C) and the biliary ascites with which the patient presented. **D,** Contrast study demonstrates a choledochal cyst and biliary atresia.

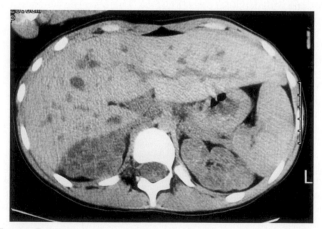

FIGURE 5-6. CT in an 8-year-old with autosomal recessive polycystic kidney disease shows multiple cysts.

T1-weighted images and hyperintense on T2-weighted images in comparison with normal liver.

Cholecystitis

Acute *calculous* cholecystitis represents inflammation of the gallbladder, with gallstones present that obstruct the cystic duct. An organism is seldom recovered, and the condition is more common in adolescent girls. Repeated self-limited episodes of calculous cholecystitis may lead to chronic cholecystitis (Fig. 5-9).

Acute acalculous cholecystitis occurs in the absence of gallstones, possibly secondary to greater bile viscosity, as seen in children receiving total parenteral nutrition and having suffered trauma. Viral and bacterial organisms have rarely been isolated. Right upper quadrant pain, jaundice (40% of patients), and nausea are the most common clinical symptoms.

Chronic cholecystitis is most often associated with gallstones or infection by *Salmonella typhi* and *Clonorchis* organisms. Symptoms are normally less severe than in the acute entities.

US demonstration of an anechoic gallbladder with a thickened (greater than 3 mm), often hyperreflective irregular gallbladder wall or occasionally with sludge or gallstones, as in the adult, signifies cholecystitis. A hypoechoic halo around the gallbladder is often present. However, this finding can also be seen in ascites or hypoalbuminemia and after a recent meal (Fig. 5-9A).

In chronic cholecystitis, US findings may be normal. Biliary scintigraphy illustrates obstruction of the cystic duct, with nonvisualization of the gallbladder (by 4 hours; normally visualization occurs by 1 hour), yet normal uptake of the radionuclide in the liver with prompt excretion into the bile ducts and GI tract.

Hydrops of the Gallbladder

Hydrops of the gallbladder is thought to be due to a transient obstruction of bile flow, because of either adenopathy or vasculitis, leading to cholestasis. Multiple infectious causes (e.g., generalized sepsis, scarlet fever, ascariasis) and total parenteral nutrition have been implicated. Mucocutaneous lymph node syndrome (Kawasaki disease) also may manifest as enlarged, dilated gallbladder with a normal wall thickness and occasional sludge. The gallbladder is often longer than the right kidney. Clinically, abdominal pain, a right upper quadrant mass, and mild elevation of the hepatic enzymes may be noted.

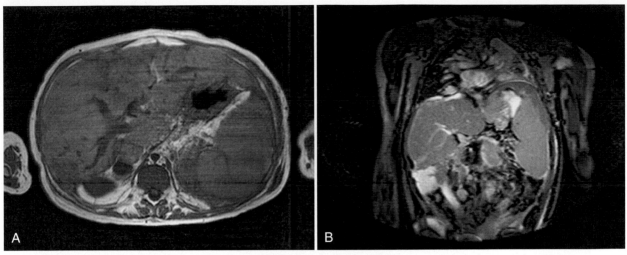

FIGURE 5-7. A and B, MR images demonstrating a nodular liver and splenomegaly in a patient with cirrhosis after viral hepatitis.

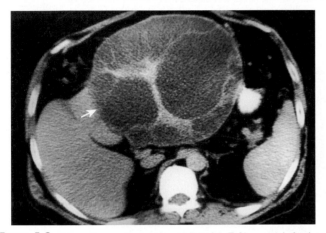

FIGURE 5-8. Liver abscess *(arrow)* in a child with *Echinococcus* infection.

Calcifications

Intrahepatic Calcifications

The differential diagnosis for intrahepatic calcifications includes primary tuberculosis or histoplasmosis, hemangiomas, hamartomas, neoplasms, biliary calculi secondary to furosemide therapy, and chronic granulomatous disease of childhood. Intrahepatic calcifications have occasionally been detected prenatally.

Cholelithiasis

Cholelithiasis is often idiopathic but may have nonhemolytic or hemolytic causes. Girls are more commonly affected than boys. Familial incidence, obesity, estrogen therapy, and diabetes may predispose a child to the formation of gallstones.

In infants, immature physiologic mechanisms that predispose to gallstones and sludge formation include the lower secretory rate of bile acids as compared with that of adults (approximately 50% of the adult rate); the immature biliary conjugation pathways; and lack of oral feeding and diuretic therapy (furosemide [Lasix]) in premature infants. These stones are often pigment stones. Prenatal gallstones are extremely rare.

Hemolytic diseases, such as sickle cell disease, thalassemia, and hereditary spherocytosis, as well as sepsis may lead to gallstone formation secondary to cholestasis.

Conventional abdominal radiographs may demonstrate up to 50% of these gallstones. US imaging, on the other hand, is almost always sufficient for diagnostic purposes (95% accuracy).

In the spectrum of gallstone formation, sludge, sludge balls, and echogenic densities that change position with gravity are all well demonstrated by US. In patients receiving total parenteral nutrition, sludge develops in 10 to 14 days. Biliary duct dilatation (cholestasis) can be assessed reliably by US as well. The upper limits of the normal dimension of the CBD are 4 mm in teenagers and as much as 7 mm in older patients.

In approximately 40% of older children, cholelithiasis is idiopathic. A hemolytic cause (sickle cell disease, thalassemia), as well as Wilson disease, is responsible for about 30% more of the cases. Abnormal enterohepatic circulation is the proposed cause in inflammatory bowel disease affecting the ileum; CF, obesity, and short gut syndrome (after GI surgery) have also been associated with gallstone formation secondary to the interrupted enterohepatic circulation.

In contradistinction to the infant, an older child with cholelithiasis is often symptomatic, having right upper quadrant pain, nausea, and vomiting. The differential diagnosis of a right upper quadrant calcific density should include (in addition to biliary causes) renal, appendiceal, and ovarian entities. Treatment for gallstones is cholecystectomy. Extracorporeal shockwave lithotripsy in children remains under study.

Infiltrative Lesions

Metabolic Diseases

Several hereditary metabolic diseases may manifest as neonatal hepatocellular and renal tubular dysfunction; they are tyrosinemia, glycogen storage disease (type I), galactosemia, and fructosemia.

Glycogen storage disease type I (von Gierke disease) is an autosomal recessive trait that results from a defect of glucose-6-phosphatase enzyme with subsequent accumulation of glycogen in liver, kidney, and intestine. The disease may manifest in infancy as hypoglycemia, hepatomegaly, and renomegaly. Hepatic adenomas and hepatocellular carcinoma have been described.

Tyrosinemia is another autosomal recessive inborn error of metabolism. It is due to a deficiency in the enzyme fumarylacetoacetase, which is the final step in the catabolic pathway of tyrosine. The result is abnormal accumulation of tyrosine, primarily in the liver and kidney. An infant or child presenting with evidence of hepatic dysfunction, rickets, and renal disease should be suspected of having tyrosinemia (Fig. 5-10).

Imaging methods such as US and CT most commonly show hepatomegaly and heterogeneous architecture. Rarely occurring nodules may be hyperdense or hypodense on CT.

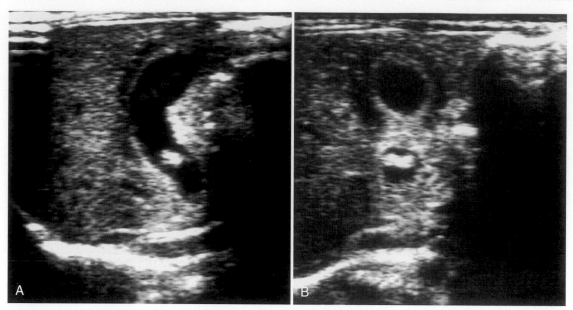

FIGURE 5-9. A, US scan shows gallstones and a possibly thickened gallbladder wall. **B,** Transverse scan of the gallbladder confirms a thick wall and identifies a common bile duct stone.

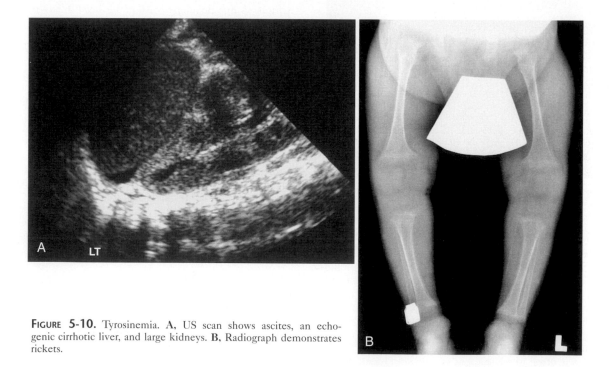

FIGURE 5-10. Tyrosinemia. **A,** US scan shows ascites, an echogenic cirrhotic liver, and large kidneys. **B,** Radiograph demonstrates rickets.

Fatty Infiltration of the Liver

The differential diagnosis for fatty infiltration of the liver includes CF, malnutrition or hyperalimentation, glycogen storage disease, and steroid therapy.

Although conventional radiographs may suggest fatty infiltration, CT or MRI is diagnostic (Fig. 5-11).

Air over the Liver

The differential diagnosis of *portal venous air* includes necrotizing enterocolitis, bowel obstruction, sepsis, and iatrogenic causes (e.g., umbilical catheterization) (see Fig. 4-6). The differential diagnosis of *air in the biliary tree* includes fistulae, trauma, and infection. Conventional radiographs are often diagnostic. US with Doppler is sensitive to air bubbles in the portal vein, but it lacks specificity.

Neoplasms

Benign Lesions

Infantile Hemangioendothelioma

Infantile hemangioendothelioma (IH) is a benign vascular tumor that reportedly accounts for between 13% and 22% of all liver tumors in children. IH is the most common liver tumor in the first 6 months of life, with nearly 50% of cases manifesting in the first month of life. Girls are affected more often than boys.

Depending on the size of the lesion, presenting symptoms include hepatic enlargement, respiratory compromise, and congestive heart failure (CHF). Arteriovenous shunting in the lesion produces CHF in 25% of the cases.

Thrombocytopenia and consumptive coagulopathy (Kasabach-Merritt syndrome) are caused by platelet sequestration and are usually associated with giant or multiple lesions. Hemoperitoneum is occasionally seen as a result of rupture of the lesion. Cutaneous hemangiomas may occur in up to 40% of these cases. Other sites of vascular lesions are the lung, GI tract, pancreas, thymus, and brain.

Histologically, the lesion is composed of vascular channels lined by endothelial cells. Connective tissue, which serves as a supporting stroma, separates the channels. The lesions may be multiple and diffuse (multinodular) or, less commonly, a single, spongy mass ranging in size from 0.2 to 15 cm. Areas of hemorrhage, infarction, and dystrophic calcification are often present. The extent of fibrosis increases with the duration of the tumor.

It has been suggested that hemangioendotheliomas and capillary and cavernous hemangiomas in infancy may each represent a phase in the tumor's life cycle, because there is an early proliferative stage and a later involutional stage. Endothelial hyperplasia decreases, and fibrosis occurs between the vascular spaces during involution. Tumors with numerous capillary elements may eventually assume a more cavernous appearance as the tumor involutes.

The sonographic features of IH are varied. A complex mass with enlargement of the celiac and hepatic arteries with a decreased aortic caliber distal to the origin of the hepatic artery is strongly suggestive of the diagnosis.

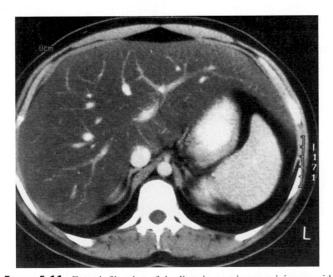

FIGURE 5-11. Fatty infiltration of the liver in a patient receiving steroid therapy. Note the normal spleen.

On CT, the typical pattern of contrast enhancement after bolus injection of contrast agent and serial imaging at one level is early centripetal enhancement with delayed central enhancement over time. If the center of the tumor is fibrosed or thrombosed, this pattern of enhancement is not seen (Fig. 5-12).

On MRI the tumor is most commonly heterogeneous and multinodular in appearance, with varying hyperintensity on T_2-weighted images. As the tumor involutes and fibrotic replacement occurs, there is decreasing signal intensity on T_2-weighted images.

Although infrequently used, a technetium Tc 99m–labeled red blood cell scan is a highly specific examination. Its main use has been to confirm the diagnosis of infantile hemangioma and to detect other hemangiomas that were unsuspected. In the typical case of IH, the scan shows the lesions with a blood pool higher than the normal surrounding hepatic parenchyma.

Mesenchymal Hamartoma

Mesenchymal hamartoma is a rare benign lesion that likely represents a developmental anomaly rather than a malignancy. Typically it consists of a multicystic mass histologically resembling a mixture of mesenchyma, bile ducts, hepatocytes, and inflammatory and hematopoietic cells.

Gross examination shows a solitary mass with varying size cysts separated by septa. The cysts are filled with gelatinous or clear fluid. In 75% of cases, the mass arises in the right hepatic lobe. On occasion, the left or both lobes are affected. Rarely, the mass is pedunculated or solid.

The median patient age at presentation is 11 months, with the majority of children presenting before age 2. There is a slight male preponderance. As is the case with hepatoblastoma, the most common presenting sign is an abdominal mass.

Plain radiographs of mesenchymal hamartoma usually demonstrate a large mass in the right upper quadrant of the abdomen. Calcification is unusual. The US, CT, and MRI appearances depend on the predominance of cysts or stroma (mesenchymal elements) (Fig. 5-13). Rim enhancement is explained by the angiographic appearance.

Because the serum α-fetoprotein concentration is not elevated in mesenchymal hamartoma, knowledge of its value is particularly helpful in distinguishing this disorder from hepatocellular carcinoma and hepatoblastoma.

Focal Nodular Hyperplasia

Focal nodular hyperplasia (FNH) is uncommon in the pediatric age group. It most frequently occurs in adults, but 8% of affected patients are younger than 15 years. The female-to-male ratio is as high as 4:1 in the pediatric age group. Although FNH typically manifests as a solitary lesion, multicentricity has been described

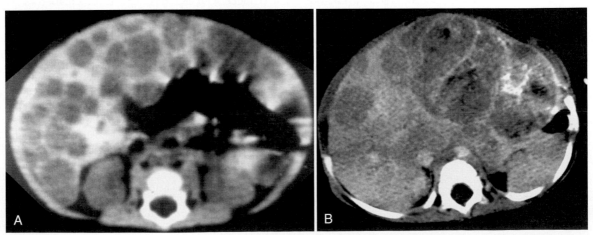

FIGURE 5-12. Hemangioendothelioma. **A,** Unenhanced CT scan shows multiple low-attenuation lesions. **B,** Contrast-enhanced CT scan in a different patient demonstrates an enlarged heterogeneous liver with areas of enhancement and necrosis.

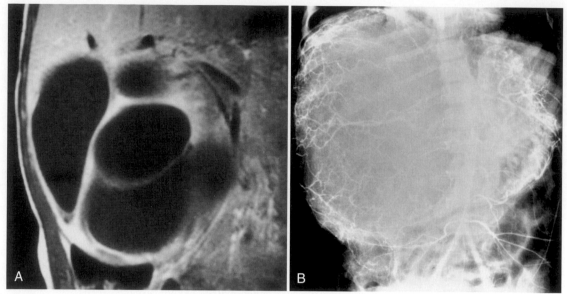

FIGURE 5-13. Multiple cysts in the liver: mesenchymal hamartoma. **A,** MR image. **B,** Angiogram.

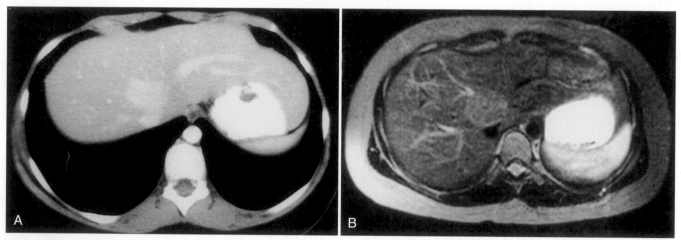

FIGURE 5-14. Focal nodular hyperplasia. **A,** CT scan shows a mildly enhancing lesion anterior to the inferior vena cava. **B,** MR image confirms the lesion.

in 20% of adult cases and in a higher number of pediatric cases. A relationship to oral contraceptives has been postulated.

Grossly, the lesion is usually subcapsular, but it may be a pedunculated, grayish white, solid mass that is not encapsulated. A stellate band of fibrosis is seen centrally. Histologic examination demonstrates ectatic vessels in the central scar, and benign lobules of hyperplastic hepatocytes containing bile ducts surround the scar.

Peripheral uptake of radioisotope in Kupffer cells around a central scar is diagnostic. Results from CT, US, or MRI often are difficult to interpret because the lesion blends into the normal surrounding liver tissue.

MRI appearance of FNH on T_1- and T_2-weighted images is variable, but the lesion may be isointense to liver. The central scar, if present, is isointense to hypointense on T_1-weighted images and hyperintense on T_2-weighted images. Prompt enhancement of the lesion is seen after administration of intravenous gadopentetate dimeglumine (Fig. 5-14).

Malignant Lesions

Hepatoblastoma

Primary hepatic tumors are relatively uncommon lesions accounting for 0.5% to 2% of all pediatric neoplasms. Malignant lesions are more common (75%) than benign lesions. Of

the primary hepatic tumors in childhood, hepatoblastoma occurs most frequently. Most hepatoblastomas manifest in children younger than 5 years; the majority of children are 2 years old or younger, with the mean age at presentation being about 16 months. The male-to-female ratio has been reported to be as high as 2:1. Many associated conditions and predisposing factors in development of hepatoblastoma have been reported, including Beckwith-Wiedemann syndrome, maternal use of clomiphene citrate (Pergonal), familial adenomatous polyposis (polyposis coli), occurrence in siblings, and trisomy 18. There is a higher incidence in infants whose mothers have been exposed to paints, petroleum products, and metals. Hepatoblastoma has no definite association with chronic liver disease.

Presenting features include an enlarging abdomen, anorexia, and weight loss. Less frequently, nausea, vomiting, and abdominal discomfort are present.

Some hepatoblastomas produce human chorionic gonadotropin, which causes precocious puberty in males. Other conditions caused by the tumor's production of hormones are hypoglycemia, hyperlipidemia, osteomalacia, hypercalcemia, polycythemia, and thrombocytosis. Elevated serum concentrations of α-fetoprotein, sometimes marked, may be found. Hepatoblastomas tend to be single masses with a right hepatic lobe predominance (right, 58%;

bilateral, 27%; left, 15%). Histologic classification can be subtyped on the basis of the epithelial and mesenchymal components of the tumor. Subtypes include epithelial, mixed (mesenchymal and epithelial), and anaplastic variants. Further subdivision of the epithelial type depends on the relative proportions of fetal and embryonal cell types present. The mixed cell type contains osteoid, which correlates with the presence of calcifications seen on radiographs. The lung is the most common site of metastases (10% at presentation), followed by abdominal lymph nodes (portal or periaortic). Bone, bone marrow, and brain are other uncommon sites of metastatic spread.

Resectability of hepatoblastomas seems to be the single most important prognosticator, regardless of cell type. To this end, preoperative imaging evaluation plays a critical role in determining resectability and evaluating for metastasis.

US is the ideal screening modality for suspected hepatic tumors; it is highly sensitive, yet not that specific. The US appearance of a hepatoblastoma is quite variable indeed. Often, a heterogeneous mass, more typically echogenic with either well-defined or poorly defined margins, can be seen. Color-flow Doppler US is extremely useful in the evaluation of hepatic vessels, to assess for tumor invasion. Pulsed Doppler examination may show high-peak systolic frequency shifts and antegrade diastolic flow in hepatoblastoma; however, this pattern has also been observed in infantile hepatic hemangioma.

On pre-contrast CT scans of the abdomen, attenuation is lower in the mass than it is in surrounding liver. Areas of inhomogeneity, related to hemorrhage or necrosis, may be noted. Calcifications are frequently evident and are usually coarse and stippled. On postcontrast scans, a hepatoblastoma enhances less than normal liver.

MRI may offer an advantage over CT in predicting tumor resectability. As is the case with most hepatic tumors, these lesions are of low signal intensity on T1-weighted images and of increased signal intensity on T2-weighted images. The MRI appearance varies with the histology: epithelial tumors are generally homogeneous, whereas the mixed cell type is heterogeneous with fibrotic septations that are hypointense on both T1- and T2-weighted images (Fig. 5-15A and B).

After diagnosis, the recommended evaluation for the staging of hepatoblastoma includes CT scan of the chest and abdomen and technetium Tc 99m methylene diphosphonate bone scan for (rare) metastatic disease.

Hepatocellular Carcinoma

After hepatoblastoma, hepatocellular carcinoma (HCC) is the most commonly occurring hepatic tumor in childhood. HCC is usually seen in patients ranging from 5 to 15 years of age. There is a slight male preponderance. HCC has a definite association with chronic liver diseases, most notably cirrhosis, biliary atresia, hereditary tyrosinemia, glycogen storage disease, and chronic hepatitis.

The gross appearance of HCC is quite variable, being solitary, multicentric, or diffuse. The tumor may be surrounded by a fibrous capsule.

Microscopically, HCC has either narrow or broad trabeculae of variable-appearing malignant hepatocytes. With central necrosis of the larger trabeculae, a pseudoglandular pattern is produced. A solid pattern results when the trabeculae grow together. If the malignant hepatocytes are well differentiated, bile may be produced. Vascular invasion is common, whereas biliary invasion is not. The most common presenting sign is an abdominal mass, followed by local pain or discomfort. Jaundice is an unusual presenting feature. A serum α-fetoprotein elevation is found in about half of patients with HCC.

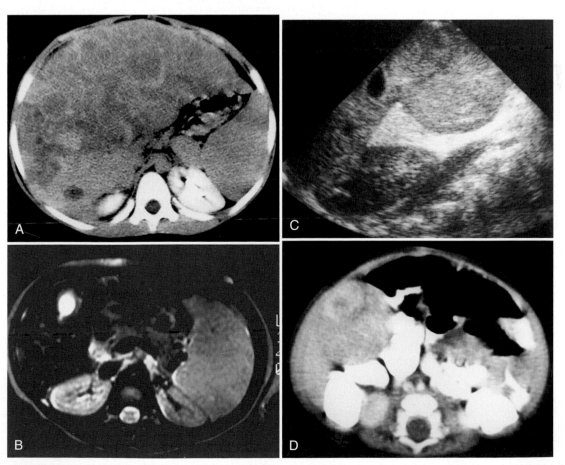

FIGURE 5-15. Hepatoblastoma: **A,** Contrast-enhanced CT scan; **B,** MR image. Hepatocellular carcinoma can look identical: **C,** US appearance; **D,** CT scan with contrast agent.

The ability of US, CT, or MRI to accurately distinguish hepatoblastoma from HCC is quite limited. In patients older than 5 years, the presence of intercurrent liver disease and imaging studies showing local vein invasion are both clues to the diagnosis of HCC. The imaging appearance of HCC also depends on the tumor's growth pattern. Solitary or multifocal lesions may be relatively easy to detect, whereas diffuse involvement may be difficult (Fig. 5-15C and D).

Fibrolamellar HCC, occurring primarily in young adults, is histologically distinct from HCC. The tumor is composed of deeply eosinophilic hepatocytes and abundant lamellated parallel fibrous bands. It may contain dystrophic calcifications, but a central scar with multiple fibrous septa, hemorrhage, and necrosis are not features of fibromellar HCC. Elevation of the serum α-fetoprotein concentration is unusual.

MRI most commonly shows a well-demarcated mass, slightly hypointense on T1-weighted images. The lesion may be isointense to slightly hyperintense on T2-weighted images. The classic central scar fibrosis is seen as a hypointense region on both T1- and T2-weighted images.

Rhabdomyosarcoma

Rhabdomyosarcoma of the biliary tree is a rare lesion that manifests as jaundice in children younger than 5 years. Most rhabdomyosarcomas occur in the urogenital or skeletal systems. In the liver, this lesion is most commonly associated with bile duct dilatation. It occurs equally in males and females, with a uniformly poor prognosis.

US and CT illustrate the dilatation of the biliary tree and may define the mass. Differentiation from other hepatic tumors is almost impossible. The mass often resembles Swiss cheese on US. On cholangiography, the botryoidal (grapelike) quality of the tumor is most evident.

Undifferentiated Embryonal Cell Sarcoma

Undifferentiated embryonal cell sarcoma is a highly malignant lesion that occurs primarily in older children. A slight female preponderance is seen. An abdominal mass with or without pain is noted in 90% of patients. The serum α-fetoprotein concentration is rarely elevated.

Histologically, the lesion is composed of spindle-shaped cells with a myxoid stroma. Occasionally, a pseudocapsule of dense fibrous connective tissue separates the compressed normal liver from the lesion. The tumors are predominantly cystic in nature. Hemorrhage and necrosis occur.

US and CT reflect the cystic and solid features of undifferentiated embryonal cell sarcoma. On MRI, the lesion is predominantly hypointense on T1-weighted images and hyperintense on T2-weighted images. If a pseudocapsule is present, it is of low signal intensity on both T1- and T2-weighted images.

Metastatic Lesions

A variety of neoplasms can invade the liver parenchyma. The differential diagnosis includes neuroblastoma (particularly stage IV-S in children younger than 1 year), Wilms tumor, and lymphoma or leukemia. US is the screening modality of choice, although it has a 15% to 20% false-negative rate for metastatic lesions. CT is the more sensitive modality to delineate the number and is valuable for determination of the extent of the lesions. MRI can be highly sensitive, showing metastases as hyperintense lesions on T2-weighted images (Fig. 5-16).

Benign Teratoma

Benign teratoma, a rarely occurring lesion of the liver, deserves mention because it may be confused histologically with the mixed type of hepatoblastoma with teratoid features. This tumor is composed of mesoderm, ectoderm, and endoderm. Most cases occur within the first year of life, manifesting as an abdominal mass. The serum α-fetoprotein may be elevated. The presence

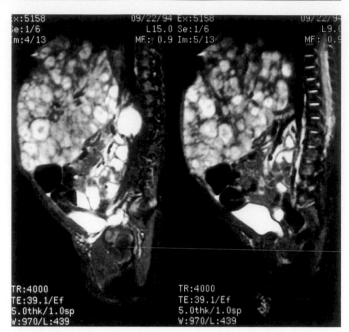

FIGURE 5-16. MRI appearance of metastatic neuroblastoma.

of embryonal or fetal hepatoblastoma cells eliminates teratoma as a diagnostic consideration.

Transplantation

Although a variety of diseases may lead to liver transplantation, biliary atresia accounts for more than half of the patients undergoing the procedure. Most patients have undergone a Kasai procedure in infancy, allowing them to grow to a size and age at which a more successful transplantation can be performed.

Preoperative evaluation consists primarily of assessment of liver anatomy as well as of the status and patency of the hepatic and portal venous vascular systems, and discovery of any unexpected complications that may preclude a successful transplantation. Abdominal US with Doppler imaging of the vessels remains the primary imaging modality for these evaluations. CT adds more anatomic information, and MRI provides both anatomic and vascular information. For most patients, however, appropriate US results obviate the need for advanced preoperative imaging.

Postoperative imaging also relies heavily on Doppler US imaging to evaluate the patency of the vascular anastomoses, which are prone to asymptomatic occlusion. Complications discovered by US or from the development of patient symptoms may require advanced imaging techniques, especially if intervention is contemplated. Infection is a common complication and may need CT assessment, in particular for evaluation of possible abscess formation or intraperitoneal fluid collections. CT or MR angiography may provide added information in the patient with vascular complications or biliary leakage.

■ PANCREAS

Anatomy and Developmental Anomalies

By week 7, the main pancreatic duct of Wirsung and the accessory duct of Santorini fuse in direct apposition in the wall of the duodenum in more than two thirds of patients. In about 20% of patients, however, the accessory duct does not reach the lumen, and in 10%, the two ductal systems do not connect at all, resulting in "pancreas divisum": the main pancreatic duct and accessory pancreatic duct have two separate openings on the medial aspect of the duodenal sweep, the accessory duct being the more proximal. The higher incidence of pancreatitis probably occurs because the duct of Santorini may be too small to allow proper drainage for pancreatic secretions. When the two anlagen of the dorsal and ventral pancreas fuse during week 6—that is, during the rotational phase of the organ formation of the pancreas—an annular pancreas is the result. This annular pancreas effectively encircles the descending duodenum and may therefore obstruct the antegrade flow of bowel contents. Anomalies associated with an annular pancreas include esophageal atresia, tracheoesophageal fistula, duodenal stenosis or atresia, and trisomy 21 as well as malrotation.

Ectopic pancreatic tissue may be found along the entire GI tract. It is most commonly seen in the stomach (in three fourths of patients) and duodenum, and in a Meckel diverticulum. The greater antral curve is the most common location.

Aplasia or hypoplasia of the pancreas is a very rare anomaly associated with the patient's early demise. The critical event in the development of the pancreas is thus the rotation and fusion of the primordia. At birth, the endocrine and exocrine functions are histologically present.

Congenital Pancreatic Malformations

Agenesis of the pancreas describes complete absence of the pancreas with the anticipated clinical presentation of diabetes mellitus and malabsorption in infancy. It is extremely rare.

A congenitally short pancreas occurs when there is failure of development of either the ventral or dorsal primordium. The dorsal bud gives rise to portions of the pancreatic head, body, and tail, whereas the ventral bud forms a portion of the pancreatic head and the uncinate process (Fig. 5-17). The associations of congenital short pancreas with polysplenia alone and of congenital short pancreas with polysplenia, bilobed lungs, malrotation, and congenital heart disease have been described. The development of both the pancreas and spleen in the mesogastrium is postulated as the reason that anomalies often occur in both organs in the same patient.

Most patients with congenital short pancreas and normal situs have diabetes mellitus, and all occasionally have pancreatitis. Neither diabetes mellitus nor pancreatitis is typical in patients with congenital short pancreas and polysplenia.

Pancreatic enlargement has been described in a number of entities. Infants with Beckwith-Wiedemann syndrome may present with macroglossia, omphalocele, visceromegaly, and macrosomia. About one half of the infants have hypoglycemia secondary to the hyperinsulinemia caused by islet cell hyperplasia. Although the hypoglycemia is transient, the islet cell hyperplasia may persist. Beckwith-Wiedemann syndrome has been associated with development of neoplasms in the pancreas, liver, adrenal glands, and especially the kidney.

Immune and nonimmune hydrops, another cause of pancreatic enlargement, is secondary to extramedullary hematopoiesis.

Congenital syphilis is associated with enlargement of the pancreas, which is due to inflammation and extensive fibrosis.

Massive enlargement of the pancreas may be seen secondary to leukemic infiltration. In children, metastatic disease to the pancreas is more common than a primary pancreatic neoplasm. Burkitt lymphoma is the most common metastasis to the pancreas. Diffuse glandular infiltration by solitary or multiple discrete lesions may be seen. On US, the masses usually appear hypoechoic relative to the normal pancreas.

Nesidioblastosis is a term used to describe diffuse neoproliferation of pancreatic cells, or nesidioblasts, that differentiate from ductal epithelium. Nesidioblastosis may manifest during infancy or in older children as a cause of hyperinsulinemic hypoglycemia. The loss of normal islet cell architecture is thought to lead to loss of appropriate digestive regulation. The US appearance of the pancreas with nesidioblastosis varies from normal to increased size, either of which is accompanied by greater echogenicity. CT confirms the finding (Fig. 5-18).

Acquired Lesions

Acute Pancreatitis

The most common cause of acute pancreatitis in children is blunt trauma, whether major or minor, which in turn may lead to pseudocyst formation. Nontraumatic pancreatitis may be caused by medication (steroid drugs), systemic illnesses such as hemolytic uremic syndrome, sepsis, CBD obstruction, or hereditary pancreatitis.

Upper abdominal pain, often associated with nausea and vomiting, is the most common symptom; fever is uncommon. Elevated amylase and lipase values are useful laboratory features.

Imaging features in pancreatitis are nonspecific on conventional radiographs of the abdomen, unless there is a mass due to a pseudocyst. A local ileus might be present, the so-called sentinel loop. US and CT may show focal enlargement or change in attenuation or echotexture of the pancreas, and there may be surrounding fluid or the beginning of a pseudocyst. Other cystic lesions in the pancreas may be seen in autosomal dominant polycystic kidney disease, and imaging of the kidneys may confirm this finding. Dilatation of the pancreatic duct and peripancreatic fluid collection are well documented by either modality (Fig. 5-19A).

Chronic Pancreatitis

Unusual in children, chronic pancreatitis is most likely caused by autosomal dominant, familial hereditary pancreatitis. Pancreatic calcifications are noted in more than half of affected patients; pseudocysts may occur as well. Ductal dilatation is almost always present (see Fig. 5-19).

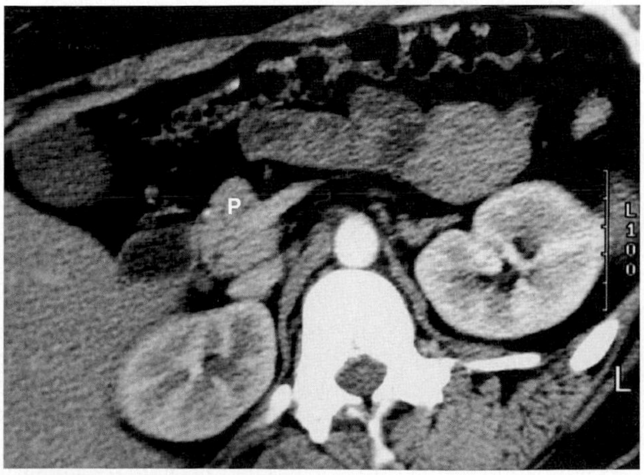

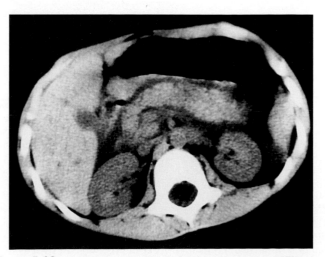

FIGURE 5-17. Congenital short pancreas (P).

FIGURE 5-18. Nesidioblastosis: enlarged dense pancreas on a CT scan.

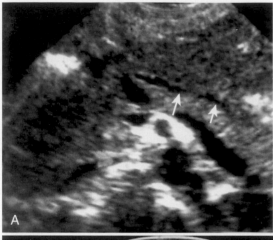

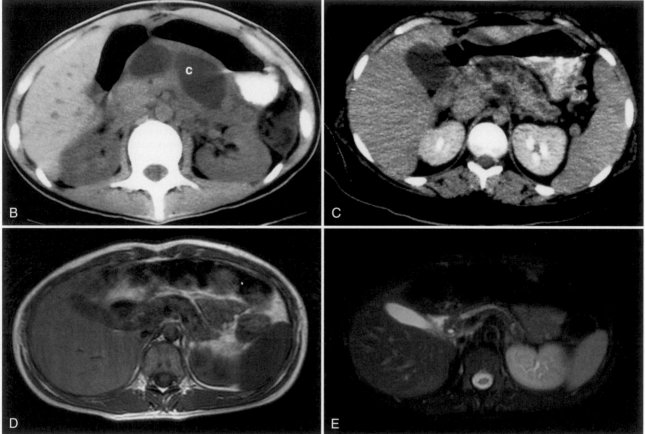

FIGURE 5-19. Pancreatitis. **A,** Transverse abdominal US scan shows diffuse enlargement of the pancreas with a dilated pancreatic duct *(arrows)*. **B,** CT scan demonstrates a multiloculated pseudocyst (c). **C,** Contrast-enhanced CT scan of chronic pancreatitis with areas of necrosis. **D** and **E,** MR images demonstrating a shrunken nodular pancreas and pancreatic ductal dilatation.

Cystic Fibrosis

Pancreatic insufficiency is the hallmark of more than 80% of cases of CF. The pancreatic ducts are obstructed by thick tenacious secretions, over time leading to fibrosis and atrophy of the pancreas. Fatty replacements and calcifications may be noted as well. On US, the pancreas is often echogenic because of fatty infiltration. It may be slightly enlarged early on, but eventually it reflects the size of the atrophic gland.

Pancreatic Cysts

Congenital pancreatic cysts are considered true cysts lined by glandular epithelium. They may be solitary, multiple, unilocular, or multilocular. Cysts may occur in other organs, such as the liver and kidney. The cysts may be seen as a component of other malformation syndromes, as in polycystic kidney disease, Meckel-Gruber syndrome, Jeune asphyxiating thoracic dystrophy, trisomy 9, von Hippel–Lindau disease, and tuberous sclerosis. The cause of these congenital cysts is likely anomalous pancreatic ductal system development. US and CT may demonstrate a cystic lesion, which may be simple or multilocular with interspersed septae.

Other cystic pancreatic lesions reported in children are dermoid cysts, teratomas, and intestinal duplications. The intestinal duplications must communicate with the pancreatic duct, because the duplication cysts are occasionally found within the pancreas itself.

Cyst formation within the pancreas may occur in patients with CF, in whom the spectrum of pancreatic involvement is highly variable. Eventually, the majority of patients with CF progress to pancreatic insufficiency. The pancreas in CF may contain multiple microcysts or macrocysts of varying sizes. These are true cysts lined by ductal epithelium. Inspissated secretions are thought to cause obstruction and ductal ectasia with the development of cysts. *Pancreatic cystosis* is a term used to describe complete cystic transformation of the pancreas. At birth, the pancreas appears normal, but in time fibrosis and atrophy may ensue. The sonographic appearance of the pancreas may vary from normal to that of increased echogenicity with decreased glandular size.

Pancreatic pseudocysts are sequelae of repeated pancreatic infections or trauma. The resultant secretions incite an inflammatory reaction, which may become encapsulated. Once a thick, mature rind is demonstrated on US or CT, the pseudocyst may be drained either surgically or percutaneously (Fig. 5-19B).

Pancreatic Tumors

Primary pancreatic tumors are exceedingly rare in childhood. The tumors are classified as either epithelial cell or non–epithelial cell in origin. Epithelial tumors are ductal, acinar, or endocrine. In adults, most pancreatic tumors originate from ductal cells (adenocarcinoma), whereas in children, most arise from the acinar cell, resulting in pancreaticoblastoma. Non–epithelial cell tumors of the pancreas include sarcoma and lymphoma.

Adenomas of the pancreas represent aggregates of endocrine cells that may or may not be secretory. Usually, one cell type predominates in an adenoma. Classification of endocrine tumors is based on hormone production of insulin, gastrin, active peptides, somatostatin, and glucagon. Insulin-secreting tumors (insulinoma) tend to manifest early, with symptoms secondary to the hormone production—seizures or unexplained hypoglycemia possibly occurring shortly after birth. These tumors are frequently small and difficult to detect. Of the endocrine tumors in childhood, insulinomas and gastrinomas are the most common, whereas glucagonomas almost never occur. Insulinomas are more likely to be benign (more than 90%), whereas gastrinomas are less likely to be benign than the others listed (50%).

If the lesions are detected by US at all, they tend to be small, well-defined lesions that are hypoechoic in comparison with the surrounding pancreas. On CT, after contrast administration, the lesion often enhances and is well defined. The MRI characteristics have been described in adults; for instance, islet cell tumors may show as hypointense lesions in the background of hyperintense pancreas on a T_1-weighted image using fat-suppression and spin-echo techniques. Because these lesions are frequently hypervascular, they appear more hyperintense and conspicuous on dynamic, contrast-enhanced MRI than normal pancreas.

Pancreaticoblastoma, or infantile adenocarcinoma, can occur at any age. The mean age at presentation is 4.5 years, with a male preponderance. Definite malignant potential exists, with the most common sites of metastases being the liver and abdominal lymph nodes. Elevated serum α-fetoprotein concentration has been reported. Pancreaticoblastoma has also been described in association with Beckwith-Wiedemann syndrome.

US often demonstrates a well-defined mass with hyperechoic solid areas and hypoechoic cystic areas. CT usually shows a well-defined mixed attenuating mass. Fine calcifications may be seen.

The biologic behavior of adenocarcinoma of the pancreas in children is similar to that in adults, with local metastasis and early demise of the patient a frequent occurrence. US generally demonstrates an anechoic, complex mass with local spread at the time of presentation.

■ SPLEEN

Anatomy and Developmental Anomalies

The spleen develops around the fifth week of gestation as a mesenchymal bulge of the mesogastrium. Congenital variations of the spleen include differences in shape, size, and number (accessory spleens occur in 10% to 15% of the population) as well as ectopic spleen, asplenia, and polysplenia. The last two entities are part of the heterotaxy syndrome. By the third month of gestation, the spleen has organized into white and red pulp (cords), the former containing lymphocytes, the latter macrophages and red blood cell elements, and the organ has attained its adult shape. Weighing at birth about 20 g, it functions to filter the blood stream, although in utero erythropoiesis also occurs in the spleen. This erythropoiesis is maximal at about 20 weeks' gestation and is nonexistent shortly after birth. The spleen is attached to the left upper quadrant by ligaments attached to the stomach, diaphragm, and left kidney. Spleen ectopia, which is due to absence of the lienorenal ligament, may be associated with a diaphragmatic hernia. A "wandering" spleen may undergo torsion and infarction. Accessory splenic tissue may result from abnormal budding of the mesenchymal bulge. Seen in 10% to 15% of children, accessory splenic tissue is usually located in the hilum (Fig. 5-20).

Radioisotope scanning with technetium Tc 99m sulfur colloid is useful to assess splenic anatomy and function, and it will demonstrate accessory splenules. US is the screening modality of choice for size and texture; however, it may be difficult to image the entire spleen on US, and splenic measurements using this modality are not very reliable. If the tip of the spleen reaches lower than the lower pole of the left kidney on US, splenomegaly can

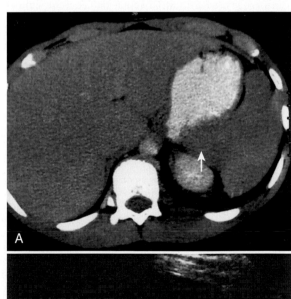

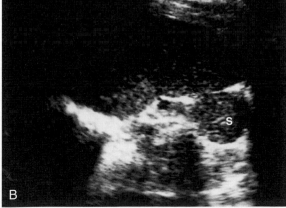

FIGURE 5-20. The spleen. **A,** CT scan demonstrates the medial lobe of the spleen *(arrow)*. **B,** US demonstration of a splenule (s).

be strongly suggested (Box 5-1). On CT and T_1-weighted MRI, the attenuation and texture of the spleen are almost identical to those of the liver; the spleen is hyperintense on T_2-weighted images.

Asplenia

Asplenia (bilateral right-sidedness) is associated with bilateral, trilobed ("right") lungs and eparterial bronchi. In addition, GI anomalies such as situs inversus and a centrally located symmetric liver can be found (see Fig. 5-1). Severe congenital cardiac abnormalities (e.g., atrial septal defect, atrioventricular canal, transposition, total anomalous pulmonary venous return) are associated as well. Most affected infants are male; asplenia results in greater susceptibility to infection, and most infants die before 1 year of age.

Polysplenia

Polysplenia (bilateral left-sidedness) is associated with bilateral, bilobed ("left") lungs and hyparterial bronchi. The GI anomalies are similar in incidence to those in asplenia, but the cardiac anomalies are less severe (atrial septal defect, ventriculoseptal defect). Interruption of the hepatic portion of the IVC with azygous continuation occurs in 60% to 70% of patients. Most affected patients are girls, and CHF is the most common clinical finding.

Infection or Abscess

Infection of the spleen is usually associated with a predisposing cause, such as an immune deficiency state, otitis media, endocarditis, or sickle cell disease. The imaging appearance, depending on the type of infection, ranges from that of diffuse involvement to that of abscess formation.

Often, microabscesses form as a complication of systemic sepsis, parasites, or disseminated disease (e.g., tuberculosis), most commonly in immunocompromised hosts (leukemia or acquired immunodeficiency syndrome). Fungal infections or *Pneumocystis carinii* infection in patients with AIDS is well described. Often microscopic in size, these cystic lesions must be larger than 1 cm to be identified on CT. Most splenic abscesses, however, are multiple and small and thus may be difficult to image. Current linear-array US transducers resolve microabscesses as small as 2 mm. *Candida* infection of the spleen may occasionally have a typical "Swiss cheese" appearance, as may *Salmonella* infection of the spleen in patients with sickle cell disease (Fig. 5-21).

Neoplasms

Malignant Lesions

Lymphoma and leukemia most frequently affect the spleen primarily; the lesion in such diseases may be nodular or diffuse in character. Metastatic disease from many primary causes can involve the spleen, most commonly the lymphoma/leukemia group. Often, these lesions are microscopic and therefore often diagnosed only at autopsy.

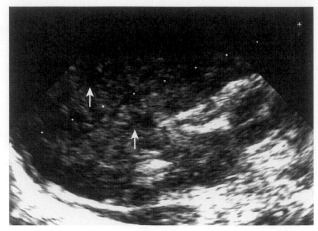

FIGURE 5-21. Microabscesses in the spleen *(arrows)* in a patient with sickle cell disease; infection was with *Salmonella*.

Benign Lesions

Cysts

True splenic cysts are rare. Splenic cysts can be divided into true epidermoid cysts (lined by epithelium) and secondary cysts resulting from hemorrhage, infection (hydatid disease), or infarction.

The most common cause of a splenic cyst is trauma, followed by hydatid disease (Fig. 5-22). Other cystic lesions, such as lymphangiomas and hamartomas, are rare.

CT and US can both identify the cysts as anechoic lesions; if there is flow on Doppler US, "flow" lesions may be considered. Such lesions include lymphangiomas, either single or multiple, and abscesses. Splenic hamartomas are rare, as are hemangiomas.

Percutaneous drainage of benign splenic cysts is usually not successful because of a high rate of recurrence. Injection (sclerosis) of such a cyst may be curative.

▬ TRAUMA

General Considerations

Traditionally, peritoneal lavage was the method that, in addition to physical examination, assessed whether intraperitoneal bleeding had occurred after trauma. False-negative results were few and were probably caused by the retroperitoneal location of the injuries. False-positive results studies were probably the result of traumatic insertion of the trocar. It is important that peritoneal lavage, if it is performed at all, should not precede CT, because retained lavage fluid may simulate intraperitoneal fluid on a CT scan, and air may suggest visceral perforation. Peritoneal lavage is seldom used in children today.

In the pediatric patient, CT is currently the initial imaging method most in use in the United States. Level I trauma centers frequently have a CT scanner in or adjacent to the emergency department and a CT technologist available in the hospital on a 24-hour basis. CT is at least as accurate as scintigraphy and US, and in many instances, it is more accurate. In Europe, US is more commonly utilized as the initial imaging modality.

CT can be performed safely and accurately in the severely injured child; it therefore does not delay the diagnostic process but rather speeds it along if done properly and if a multidetector scanner is used. Anatomic detail is superior to that provided by scintigraphy and US: the extent of injury is imaged more completely by CT, and associated injuries are illustrated better than by US or excretory urography. Multiplanar reconstructions may provide additional diagnostic information. A negative abdominal CT scan result, however, does not mean absence of injury, and it also should not preclude additional tests when these are deemed clinically necessary.

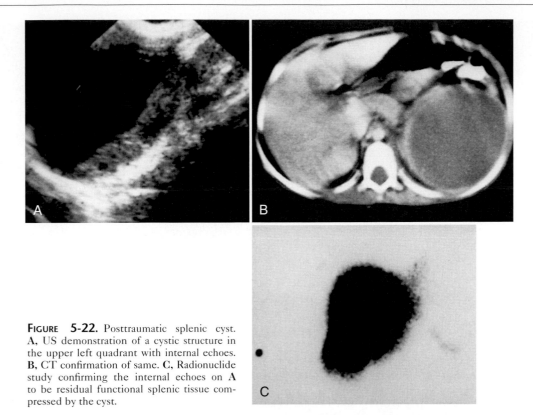

FIGURE 5-22. Posttraumatic splenic cyst. **A,** US demonstration of a cystic structure in the upper left quadrant with internal echoes. **B,** CT confirmation of same. **C,** Radionuclide study confirming the internal echoes on **A** to be residual functional splenic tissue compressed by the cyst.

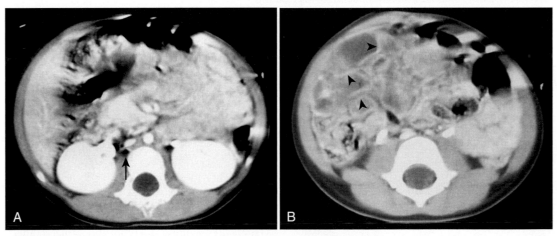

FIGURE 5-23. Appearance of "shock" on a CT scan obtained in a patient with trauma. **A,** Small-caliber inferior vena cava *(arrow)* contrasted to the normal-size aorta. **B,** Enhancing bowel loops *(arrowheads).*

Prompt evaluation with CT determines the presence or absence of intraperitoneal or retroperitoneal hemorrhage and the integrity of the major solid organs. Furthermore, CT may detect a bleeding source, and contusions or superficial lacerations of the solid organs (as well as the bowel) may be demonstrated. A small-caliber IVC and enhancement of the bowel wall together suggest volume depletion and impending shock (Fig. 5-23).

Only about 8% to 10% of pediatric patients with abdominal trauma require surgery, so imaging is necessary particularly to identify those who require surgical intervention. Certain appearances, including significant perihilar fluid tracking (13% mortality), a large hemoperitoneum (30% requiring surgery), and large areas of poor perfusion in solid organs, strongly suggest that surgical intervention is needed.

Scintigraphy has had an advantage over CT in that it is affected less by patient motion, does not necessitate sedation, and does not require contrast media. Conversely, the procedure of scintigraphy takes as long as or longer than CT, and its radiation dose to the patient is higher; also, scintigraphy may not be available on an emergency basis outside routine working hours. However, the modality is quite specific to liver and spleen. On the other hand, CT scanning using a multidetector scanner has eliminated most disadvantages of CT imaging except the use of contrast material, which carries a very minimal risk in well-hydrated children.

Imaging should be postponed or tailored if significant hypoxemia or clinical instability necessitates immediate laparotomy.

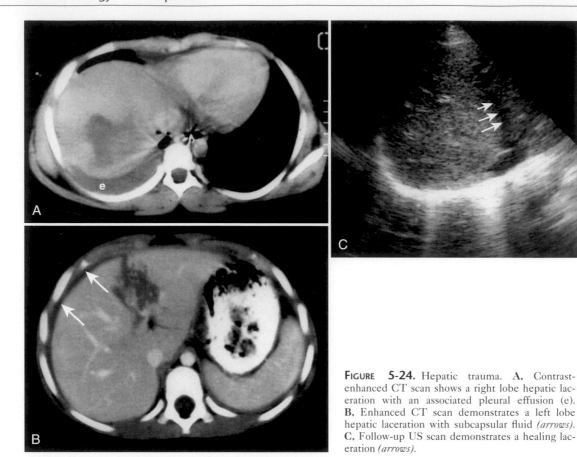

FIGURE 5-24. Hepatic trauma. **A,** Contrast-enhanced CT scan shows a right lobe hepatic laceration with an associated pleural effusion (e). **B,** Enhanced CT scan demonstrates a left lobe hepatic laceration with subcapsular fluid *(arrows)*. **C,** Follow-up US scan demonstrates a healing laceration *(arrows)*.

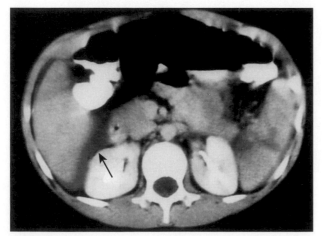

FIGURE 5-25. Splenic trauma. Enhanced CT scan shows splenic laceration with fluid in Morison pouch *(arrow)*.

Liver

The appearance of the typical hepatic laceration is a low-attenuation lesion that is focal, peripheral, and most commonly located in the right lobe. It is often associated with a right pleural effusion and possibly contusion in the right lung with or without rib fractures. Acute hepatic hemorrhage may be hyperdense because of the high protein content of the retracted clot or fractionated blood, whereas bile collections (bilomas) have lower attenuation. The evolution of healing in hepatic trauma can be exquisitely demonstrated on CT, obviating other studies. CT therefore is the imaging modality of choice, and its use contributes to the trend

to more nonoperative management of this injury in the child (Fig. 5-24).

Rarely, trauma is associated with a biloma and hematobilia and, over time, with pseudoaneurysms of the hepatic artery as well as bile duct disruption.

Left lobe lesions are more severe and harder to detect and are often associated with trauma to the pancreas and duodenum. The caudate lobe, because of its posterior location, is only rarely involved in trauma.

Hepatobiliary

Gallbladder injuries from blunt abdominal trauma are extremely rare. When the clinical course is stable, a follow-up scan in 7 to 10 days is most useful to assess the evolution of the injury, either with CT or US, regardless of the initial imaging modality used.

Spleen

In 10% to 20% of patients, the diagnosis of splenic injury is not obvious. Other injuries may overshadow its symptoms, and the finding of splenic rupture can be delayed (48 to 72 hours after trauma). In addition, US and radionuclide evaluation both have false-positive rates of about 7% and false-negative rates of about 2% for splenic trauma. Over the last few decades splenic trauma has been treated conservatively in children; it is therefore important that the modality used to evaluate the spleen have a high sensitivity.

The sensitivity of CT in splenic abnormalities is assessed at near 100%. The ability to image the rest of the intra-abdominal structures concurrently is a further distinct advantage of CT over organ-specific imaging, such as radionuclide imaging or US. Intravenous

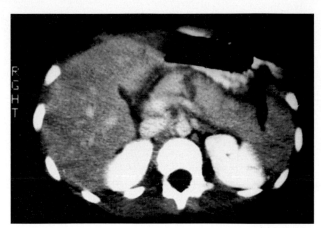

FIGURE 5-26. Pancreatic trauma. Enhanced CT scan demonstrates a transverse fracture of the body of the pancreas.

contrast administration is essential for the detection of subcapsular hematomas and lacerations. Most splenic injuries are associated with a "sentinel clot" and a hemoperitoneum (Fig. 5-25). In addition, one must be familiar with the variants of splenic anatomy because they may contribute to false-positive interpretation by the unwary (see Fig. 5-20). Streak artifacts from ribs and inhomogeneous enhancement by contrast medium may further hinder the correct interpretation of imaging findings. Grading systems for extent of trauma have met with limited success in pediatric liver and spleen trauma. Long-term sequelae of splenic trauma include splenosis and pseudocyst formation.

Pancreas

Pancreatic injuries often escape early detection in children. In early childhood, trauma is the most common cause of pancreatitis, which may be complicated by sepsis, shock, and the later development of pseudocysts.

In children, the CT delineation of the pancreatic outline may be difficult to determine without meticulous oral and intravenous contrast enhancement because of the lack of retroperitoneal fat. It is unusual to see the slightly obliquely situated gland in the upper abdomen on one CT slice. The measurements of pancreas size, which depend on the age of the patient, are not very practical.

CT can demonstrate transection of the pancreas and pancreatitis (Fig. 5-26). Posttraumatic pancreatic pseudocysts can be detected within 72 hours. CT is the recommended initial study in complex cases.

US is a useful screening modality for the pancreas. It can demonstrate peripancreatic fluid; it can also assess the other solid organs and identify pseudocysts, although with less sensitivity and specificity than CT using a multidetector scanner. Overlying dressings and/or air may be a limiting factor. Endoscopic retrograde or magnetic resonance cholangiopancreatography may be needed to confirm the integrity of the pancreatic duct.

Bowel and Mesentery

Trauma to the bowel and its mesentery can involve any part of the colon or small bowel. Specific injuries can be detected on CT, but with difficulty and often only retrospectively. The lacerated viscus is only rarely identified on CT; pneumoperitoneum is seen only in one third of patients, and the amount does not correlate

with severity. An intramural hematoma is identified in only about 50% of patients; bowel wall thickening is also a useful sign of injury.

Summary

CT is highly effective in demonstrating the presence, extent, and severity of intra-abdominal trauma, with the information contributing most significantly to the high level of monitoring required by affected patients.

CT is particularly effective for the following types of pediatric patients:
1. The severely injured but stable patient in whom injuries to multiple intra-abdominal organ systems is suspected.
2. The patient with an abdomen that cannot be examined with US, because of open wounds, extensive dressings, or extreme abdominal tenderness.
3. The unstable patients or the patient with severe head trauma who needs evaluation of the abdomen that is not complete on physical examination.
4. The patient with abdominal trauma in whom the results of other modalities either are equivocal or do not fit the clinical impression.

▬ SUGGESTED READINGS

TEXTS

Kirks DR (ed): Practical Pediatric Imaging, ed 3. Philadelphia, Lippincott-Raven, 1997, pp 954-1008.
Skandalakis JE, Gray SW (eds): Embryology for Surgeons, ed 2. Baltimore, Williams & Wilkins, 1994.
Slovis TL (ed): Caffey's Pediatric Diagnostic Imaging, ed 11. Philadelphia, Mosby Elsevier, 2008.
Swischuk LE: Imaging of the Newborn Infant, and Young Child, ed 4. Baltimore, Williams & Wilkins, 1997, pp 487–529.

ARTICLES

Abramson SJ, Berdon WE: Biliary atresia and noncardiac polysplenic syndrome: US and surgical considerations. Radiology 1987;163:377-9.
Berrocal T, Prieto C: Sonography of pancreatic disease in infants and children. Radiographics 1995;15:301-13.
Delaney L, Applegate KE, Karmazyn B, et al: MR cholangiopancreatography in children: Feasibility, safety, and initial experience. Pediatr Radiol 2008;38:64-75.
Haller JO: Sonography of the biliary tract in infants and children. AJR Am J Roentgenol 1991;157:1051-8.
Hernanz-Shulman M, Ambrosino MM, Freeman PC, et al: Common bile duct in children: Sonographic dimensions. Radiology 1995;195:193-5.
Kasai M, et al: Surgical limitations for biliary atresia: Indications for liver transplantation. J Pediatr Surg 1989;24:851-4.
King LR, Siegel MJ, Balfa D: Acute pancreatitis in children: CT findings of intra- and extrapancreatic fluid collections. Radiology 1995;195:196-200.
Kirks DR, Caron KH, Bissett GS III: CT of blunt abdominal trauma in children: An anatomic "snapshot in time". Radiology 1992;182:631-2.
Mergo PJ, Ros PR, Bueton PC, et al: Diffuse disease of the liver: Radiologic and pathologic correlation. Radiographics 1994;14:1291-307.
Powers C, Ros PR, Stoupis C, et al: Primary liver neoplasms: MR imaging with pathologic correlation. Radiographics 1994;14:459-82.
Roebuck DJ, Aronson D, Clapuyt P, et al: 2005 PRETEXT: A revised staging system for primary malignant liver tumours of childhood developed by the SIOPEL group. Pediatr Radiol 2007;37:123-132.
Sivit CJ, Taylor GA, Bulas D, et al: Post-traumatic shock in children: CT findings associated with hemodynamic instability. Radiology 1992;182:723-6.
Stein B, Bromley B, Michlewitz H, et al: Fetal liver calcifications: Sonographic appearance and postnatal outcome. Radiology 1993;197:489-92.
Taylor GA: Imaging of pediatric blunt abdominal trauma: What have we decided in the past decade? Radiology 1995;195:600-1.
Taylor GA, Kaufman RA: ER US in the initial evaluation of blunt abdominal imaging in children. Pediatr Radiol 1993;23:161-3.
Zamboni GA, Pedrosa I, Kruskal JB, et al: Multimodality postoperative imaging of liver transplantation. Eur Radiol 2008;18:882-91.

CHAPTER *6*

Genitourinary Tract

Johan G. (Hans) Blickman and Carla Boetes

▬ IMAGING TECHNIQUES

Voiding Cystourethrography

Voiding cystourethrography (VCUG) is the most commonly used as well as the optimal method to evaluate for vesicoureteral reflux (VUR), assess bladder anatomy and function, and judge urethral anatomy.

Urinary tract infection (UTI) is the most common indication for a VCUG, followed by further delineation of dilatation of the renal collecting system (hydronephrosis), detected either prenatally or postnatally by ultrasound (US). In addition, because genitourinary (GU) tract anomalies may be associated with anorectal malformations, myelodysplasia, and prune-belly (Eagle-Barrett) syndrome, a VCUG is needed in these instances to delineate anatomic and functional relationships. Voiding dysfunction and enuresis in boys are also common indications.

There are no real contraindications to performing VCUG. Labial adhesions are considered a relative contraindication because VCUG is usually performed after medical or surgical release of such adhesions. The usual contrast medium, chosen because it is least irritating to the bladder wall, is a 17% water-soluble contrast agent. Sterile catheterization of the bladder (by 5 or 8 Fr pediatric feeding tube) is a benign procedure because complications, such as re-infection and the creation of a false passage, are extremely rare.

After catheterization of the bladder, the contrast medium is preferentially dripped in by gravity, with the reservoir suspended approximately 3 feet above the tabletop. Cessation of flow heralds a full bladder and the beginning of the imaging sequence. In neonates, hand injection of the contrast agent is used as well. The rule of thumb for estimated bladder volume (in milliliters) for children younger than 6 years can be estimated either as the sum of the child's age (years) plus 2, multiplied by 30, or as the child's weight (kg) multiplied by 7 (Fig. 6-1). Particularly in neonates, who void frequently, cyclic filling may be necessary. There is no need to instill the contrast material under pressure.

A routine, tailored VCUG (Box 6-1) entails seven exposures in girls (eight in boys), resulting in approximately 25 mrad of gonadal radiation exposure (about 50% less radiation exposure if digital or pulsed fluoroscopic fluoroscopy is used). Contrary to earlier thought, it is not necessary to remove the catheter for optimal visualization of the posterior urethra in boys.

Video-urodynamics, a combination of a VCUG with pressure, flow, and electrophysiologic data, is the standard for lower tract assessment of neurogenic bladder and nonneurogenic functional disorders.

Excretory Urography

Excretory urography (EU) denotes visualization of the entire urinary tract by means of intravenously administered contrast agent that is subsequently excreted by the kidneys. This modality demonstrates anatomic detail and enables a semiquantitative estimate of renal function.

Indications for EU have all but disappeared, except for evaluation of posturologic (anatomic) complications. Dehydration and shock are absolute contraindications to performing an EU. Knowledge of previous allergic reactions to contrast agents or shellfish may constitute a relative contraindication.

In the neonatal age group, the glomerular filtration rate (GFR) increases from about 20% of the adult GFR value at birth to 50% of the adult value at 10 days of age. The GFR reaches adult levels by 18 months of age. The contrast media used ionic (1200 to 1400 mosm/L), non-ionic, and low-osmolar (600 to 700 mosm/L) compounds. The advantages of the latter include less irritation (pain) to the extravascular soft tissues (in case of extravasation) and a much lower incidence of adverse reactions (less than one tenth the incidence than that for ionic contrast agents). For children younger than 10 years, approximately 1 mL/lb is a reliable contrast dose for intravenous (IV) enhancement, with the maximum dose being 50 mL (Box 6-2). A prone 1- to 2-minute image of the renal beds followed by a 15-minute full-length abdominal image usually suffices. A higher GFR will result in a more diagnostic EU.

Ultrasonography

The main advantages of US are that it provides exquisite delineation of renal and (retro)vesical anatomy without the use of ionizing radiation and that it is available at the bedside; the relative disadvantages are that US does not give functional information and is fairly operator dependent. Duplex Doppler and color-flow Doppler US methods allow for the evaluation of the extent of vascularity, particularly in hypertension, for neoplastic screening, and in renal transplant patients. Determination of resistive indices has not yet proved to be clinically reliable in evaluating for either rejection of renal transplants or renal obstruction. Harmonic imaging, extended field-of-view US, echo-enhanced US, and three-dimensional US have great promise but have not been prospectively tested to see whether they are reliable, cost-effective, and efficient, especially for evaluation of the ureters and the functional aspect of the dilated collecting system.

Prenatal US has significantly influenced the indications for postnatal screening because hydronephrosis, infravesical obstruction, and the anatomy of the kidneys can be detected and analyzed in the fetus from 18 weeks' gestation onward. Mild to moderate prenatal hydronephrosis has resolved in more than 95% of neonates at birth; moderate to severe hydronephrosis must be reevaluated postnatally. VUR, multicystic dysplastic kidney (MCDK), and ureteropelvic junction (UPJ) obstruction are the most common underlying conditions for moderate to severe hydronephrosis. Aside from the follow-up indications, postnatal real-time US is the screening method of choice in the infant or neonate with urosepsis and an abdominal mass, and in children at high risk for renal anomalies and tumors, ambiguous genitalia, and genital tract anomalies. The younger the infant, and the higher (7.5-15 MHz) the resolution of the probe, the better the anatomic detail afforded by US.

The normal US appearance of the kidney changes with increasing age (Fig. 6-2). In the vast majority of infants the renal cortex and liver parenchyma are of equal echogenicity. The current explanation is that more glomeruli occupy the renal cortical volume in infants up to 6 months of age. In addition, the renal pyramids are very prominent because of their hypoechoic character. This hypoechogenicity is attributed to a relatively larger medullary fluid volume (more loops of Henle), with little supporting stroma. This US feature may persist for up to 18 months. Fetal lobulation may remain apparent up to 1 year of age. A unique embryologic remnant, the interrenicular septum (junctional defect), is seen

121

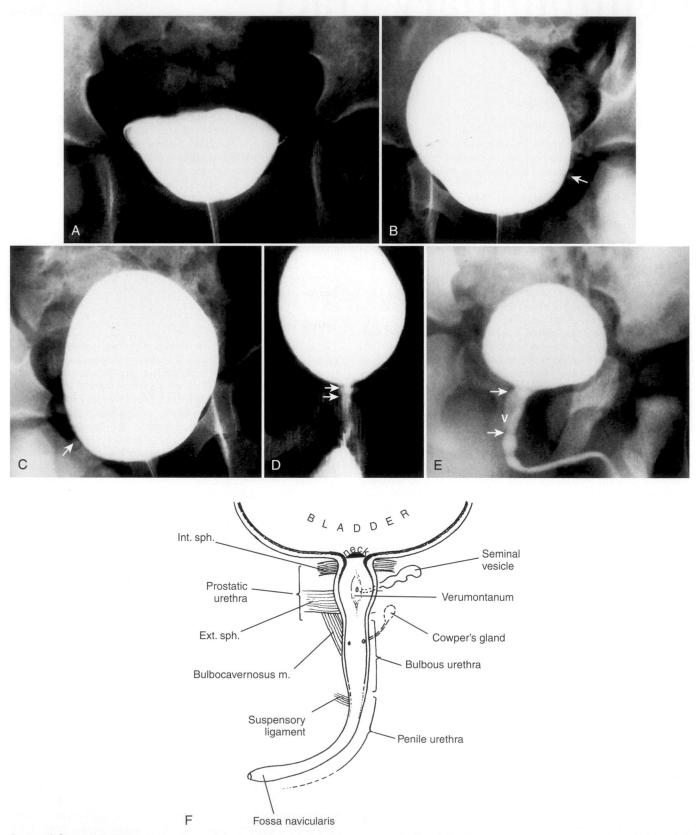

FIGURE 6-1. A, Early filling film verifies catheter position and excludes a ureterocele. **B** and **C,** Oblique views to evaluate ureterovesical junction *(arrows).* **D,** Normal female urethra: internal and external sphincters *(arrows).* **E,** Normal male urethra internal and external sphincters *(arrows);* v, verumontanum. **F,** Schematic representation of the male urethra; ext. sph., external sphincter; int. sph., internal sphincter.

more often on the right side and anterosuperiorly. It is believed to represent the site of fusion of metanephric reniculi. It can be confused with a renal scar. A renal US evaluation should contain at least two views of the bladder, and the retrovesical structures in a girl.

There are no contraindications to US evaluation of the urinary tract, and sedation is seldom (if ever) needed or used.

Nuclear Scintigraphy

Several radiopharmaceuticals are available for GU imaging. They are divided into glomerular agents (for which glomerular filtration is the main mechanism of renal uptake) and tubular agents (for which tubular secretion is the main mechanism of renal uptake). The most clinically important agent in the former group is diethylenetriamine pentaacetic acid (DTPA). Tubular agents are preferred because of the lower GFR in the neonate and these agents' higher first-pass extraction rate.

Technetium Tc 99m (^{99m}Tc) DTPA is neither absorbed nor excreted by the collecting tubules in the kidney, thus making it an ideal compound to evaluate prerenal blood flow, (differential) renal function (GFR), and postrenal collecting system integrity. After an initial flow phase (perfusion), a second functional phase with time activity curves identifies and quantifies lesions such as UPJ obstruction and ureterovesical junction (UVJ) obstruction. A rough estimate of renal size and shape may also be obtained. Depending on the clinical circumstance, a diuretic may help elucidate certain aspects of a radionuclide renogram. In the obstructed system, the radioisotope does not wash out (Fig. 6-3) readily, allowing the grading of an obstructive uropathy.

The agents classically used for evaluation of collecting tubules contained methenamine (Hippuran) for the evaluation of renal plasma flow, but currently they consist mainly of mercaptoacetyltriglycerine (MAG$_3$) compounds. ^{99m}Tc MAG$_3$ results in better image quality and a lower absorbed radiation dose. The cortical imaging agents include dimercaptosuccinic acid (DMSA) and glucoheptonate. ^{99m}Tc DMSA and ^{99m}Tc glucoheptonate are concentrated by the tubular cells and therefore are frequently used for better assessment of renal morphology, as in assessment for scars, malfunctioning of kidneys, the column of Bertin, or a local inflammatory process. At 2 to 4 hours after injection, maximum cortical binding (40% to 50%) of these compounds occurs, allowing for pinhole camera and single-photon emission computed tomography (SPECT) evaluation of scars or masses. Glucoheptonate is seldom used today.

To evaluate for VUR, ^{99m}Tc pertechnetate is used as a contrast agent. The study is performed in the same fashion as the conventional VCUG: The radioisotope is instilled into the bladder by catheter, and the renal beds and ureteral course are imaged by gamma camera for 20 minutes. Compared with a conventional VCUG, the radiation dose to the gonads and bone marrow is much less with scintigraphy (5%), and the sensitivity for VUR is much higher. On the other hand, the specificity of scintigraphy for lower urinary tract anatomic abnormalities is significantly lower than of a conventional VCUG.

There are no contraindications to GU scintigraphy. Allergic reactions are virtually unknown. Sedation may occasionally be needed because the study takes longer than EU/VCUG or US. (The time needed to perform renal nuclear medicine studies, in addition to the lower organ specificity, limits their usefulness in trauma settings.)

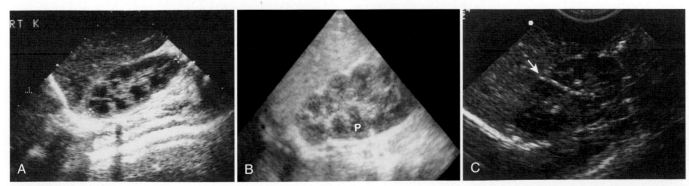

FIGURE 6-2. **A,** Premature infant's kidney shows relatively echogenic cortex, virtually equal to the liver. **B,** Neonatal kidney reveals lobulations and the relatively echo-free renal pyramids (p). **C,** Interrenicular septum *(arrow)*.

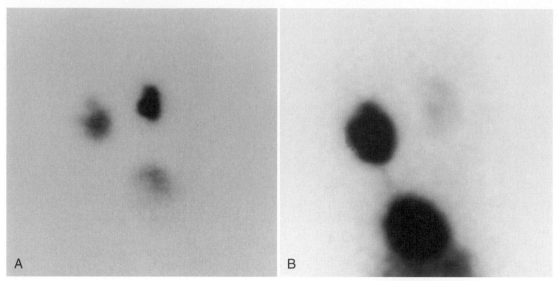

FIGURE 6-3. **A,** Radionuclide renogram (anteroposterior view) showing poorly functioning right kidney. **B,** After administration of furosemide (Lasix), ureteropelvic junction obstruction is shown on the right, and normal washout on the left.

Computed Tomography

The strength of CT lies in its cross-sectional depiction of anatomy without the image being adversely affected by gastrointestinal (GI) air, bone, or extracorporeal bandages or casts. It amplifies information gathered on US or EU, especially after the administration of an IV contrast agent; therefore it is especially useful in special circumstances, such as trauma or tumor staging. CT is particularly useful in assessing renal injury and the extent of trauma to the other intra-abdominal structures. The spiral or helical acquisition of CT data has shortened the examination time drastically and has rendered the EU or renogram virtually obsolete, especially in the trauma setting.

The recommended dose of IV contrast agent is the same as for an EU (1 mL/lb up to 50 mL in a child up to 10 years of age), and the contraindications (dehydration and shock) are also identical. In a trauma setting, if intracranial hemorrhage is noted on the cranial CT, IV contrast agent should not be administered, so as to avoid the reported increased incidence of seizure activity caused by the agent's distribution through a disruption of the blood-brain barrier.

The advent of multiple-slice CT has also had a great impact on pediatric urinary tract imaging. Acquisition of near isotropic data allows exquisite three-dimensional anatomic reconstruction, and its speed of acquisition has almost eliminated the need for sedation. This modality still requires intravenous contrast administration, and the ionizing radiation dose is increased. Indications include the evaluation of (ad)renal masses, vascular involvement, and adenopathy. If renal US findings are inconclusive, the renal stone CT protocol can be used, but nephrolithiasis in children is not as common as in adults and the radiation dose is significant (Fig 6-4).

The timing of imaging (delay) after intravenous contrast agent administration is earlier than in adults because children have a faster circulation time. CT in blunt abdominal trauma should always be performed with intravenous contrast medium, and scanning must start about 10 seconds later. Delayed images may be useful to rule out laceration, perinephric hematoma, or urinoma. The optimal delay is about 8 minutes. A radiation reducing protocol should always be used.

Magnetic Resonance Imaging

In the GU tract, the main advantage of magnetic resonance imaging (MRI) over CT lies in better resolution of anatomic information and its multiplanar capabilities. One disadvantage of MRI in

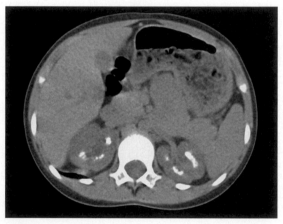

FIGURE 6-4. CT renal stone protocol scan demonstrates multiple calcific densities in the renal pyramids.

children is the occasional need for sedation because of long data acquisition times and occasional anxiety because of claustrophobia.

Magnetic resonance urography (MRU) is a new and exciting way to evaluate the urinary tract, taking advantage of the MRI capabilities to reformat flow in a tube (ureters) with T2-weighted 3D inversion recovery turbospin pulse sequences. MRI of the urinary tract provides a unique soft tissue contrast, and rapid acquisition times bypass the motion artifacts that in former days posed the limitation to abdominal MRI by using dynamic T1-weighted 2D gradient echo sequences after contrast enhancement and diuretic push (Fig. 6-5).

MR angiography (MRA) is the method of choice for the evaluation of the (renal) vessels. Although the spatial resolution of MRI is lower than subtraction angiography, it is much safer and avoids the use of ionizing radiation. Coronal three-dimensional imaging is the fundamental technique for MR angiography of the renal arteries. MR angiography with a high spatial resolution, a small field of view, and axial three-dimensional contrast-enhanced views should be performed to evaluate the renal arteries. The contrast medium given is gadolinium-containing medium in a dose of 0.1 mmol/kg body weight; it should be administered at a rate of 2 mL/sec.

Cost, availability of equipment, and the need for sedation are limiting factors for implementation of MRI in general use.

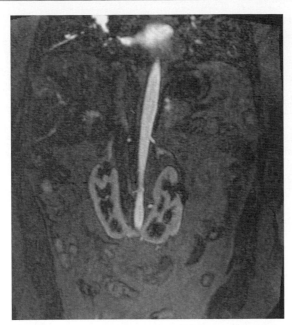

FIGURE 6-5. T2-weighted half-Fourier acquisition single-shot turbo spin-echo (HASTE) MR urogram depicts a horseshoe kidney on the left.

■ NORMAL ANATOMY

Upper Urinary Tract

The development of the kidneys differs from that of the viscera. Organs such as the liver and pancreas evolve by a direct, continuous process beginning with and incorporating the primordium. In the case of the kidneys, three sets of structures appear successively, and only the last one differentiates into the full-grown organ.

The set of structures that appears in the first two embryonic weeks is called the *pronephros*.

The *mesonephros* is formed overlapping the caudal part of the *pronephros*. The *metanephros* develops from the ureteric bud and the *metanephrogenic blastema*. The ureteric bud forms the primitive ureter of the metanephric kidney and dilates at its upper end to become the renal pelvis, enveloped by the metanephrogenic cap. Once this occurs, calyceal branches subdivide and form minor calyces and collecting tubules. This process is completed toward the end of the fifth month of gestation. The metanephrogenic cap forms Bowman's capsule, the proximal and distal convoluted tubules, and the loop of Henle. This development is intimately intertwined with the development of the ureteric bud; the end result is that each new tubule has its own cap of mesoderm. This can be appreciated in the fetal kidney that is lobulated (developing units are visible). The kidney then smoothes out until the lobulations disappear by 4 to 6 months after birth (see Fig. 6-2B).

There are usually seven anterior and seven posterior lobes, which are separated by a fibrous longitudinal band that may be visible as the interrenicular septum or, if it is incomplete, the junctional parenchymal defect. This "band" is identified for most of the first year of life (more often on the right side; 3:1) (see Fig. 6-2C).

As the "renal ascent" progresses, the nephrogenic mass starts its 90-degree medial rotation into the renal fossa. This so-called ascent up the posterior abdominal wall is not only a result of the renal ascent. It is also the result of the growth of the lumbar and sacral regions of the body and the straightening of its curvature. Concomitantly, the ureter elongates.

Renal blood supply is provided by successively higher levels of splanchnic arteries off the aorta. The venous drainage is, in large part, derived from the supracardinal anastomoses.

There are thus three critical events in the development of the normal kidney: (1) the appearance of the ureteric bud at the end of the fifth week; (2) the invagination by the ureteric bud of the nephrogenic blastema during the sixth week; and (3) the ascent of the kidney during the sixth and seventh weeks. Failure of proper development at either of the first two stages results in absence, aplasia, or hypoplasia of the kidney. Splitting of the ureteric bud results in various forms of duplication of the kidney and the ureter. Failure or arrest of the ascent results in ectopia of the kidney.

Lower Urinary Tract

In contradistinction to upper tract structures, which are formed from mesoderm, the structures of the lower urinary tract are formed from endoderm. The development of these latter structures is intimately tied to that of the anus, rectum, and lower reproductive tract.

At about the 13th day of development, the future bladder can first be identified as the allantois, a ventral outgrowth of the hindgut. The mesonephric (wolffian) ducts enter the bladder laterally, just caudal to the allantoic stalk. The urorectal septum then starts to divide the cloaca in a coronal plane. The cloacal membrane ruptures, resulting in the formation of the anal and urogenital orifices. The ventral aspect of the cloaca then elongates and forms the following structures in the male: (1) the prostatic and membranous part of the urethra (formed from the pelvic portion of the urogenital sinus); (2) the distal or phallic part of the urethra; and (3) the urachus. In the female, the pelvic portion of the urogenital sinus develops into the urethra.

The urachus descends into the pelvis to become the bladder. The tract of descent becomes a fibrous remnant at term, which may be identifiable in the adult as the medial umbilical ligament. Failure of this descent results in a patent urachus. Obliteration of the allantoic stalk at the ventral and dorsal ends only results in a urachal cyst, whereas incomplete fusion may leave a urachal remnant at the dome of the bladder. If the cloacal membrane does not form correctly, the formation of the bladder is affected. The spectrum of anomalies ranges from the severe form, classic bladder exstrophy, to the mildest form, epispadias.

Pseudodiverticula of the bladder (so-called bladder ears) may occur, in which the bladder protrudes into the still soft and patent internal os of the inguinal canal. As the infant grows, the inguinal canal solidifies. These bladder ears are not visible upon full distention of the bladder (Fig. 6-6). True diverticula of the bladder are congenital (described by Hutch), in that they arise at the UVJ with herniation of the bladder mucosa through a bladder wall muscular defect. They may cause secondary VUR as they distort the UVJ, and they may also predispose to infection and stone formation. Only 5% of bladder diverticula in children are acquired. Small Hutch diverticula may be seen only after voiding; larger ones may be associated with Menkes (kinky-hair) syndrome, Ehlers-Danlos (cutis laxa) syndrome, and Eagle-Barrett (prune-belly) syndrome (Fig. 6-7).

The ureteric bud of each side arises near the termination of the corresponding mesonephric duct. With the development and growth of the bladder, the ureters migrate laterally and cranially to open at the lateral angles of the trigone, while the mesonephric (wolffian) ducts remain midline and migrate distally. In the male, they regress; in the female, they become the uterus and oviducts (fallopian tubes).

In the male, the remaining mesonephric duct forms the epididymis, vas deferens, and common ejaculatory duct. In the female, the duct totally involutes (Table 6-1).

The gonads initially appear as a genital tubercle, a slight midline protuberance just cephalad to the distal end of the cloaca. Cloacal folds located on both sides evolve into a labioscrotal swelling with a central phallus. In the absence of stimulation by androgens, this complex forms the female external genitalia. However, under the influence of androgens, the labioscrotal folds swell and fuse to form the scrotum. The ridges of urethral folds fuse to form the bulbous urethra by 12 to 14 weeks of gestation.

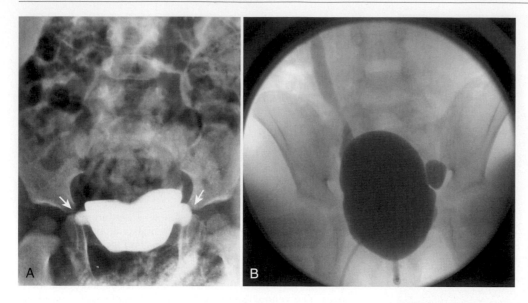

FIGURE 6-6. **A,** EU shows pseudo-diverticula, or "bladder ears" *(arrows)*. **B,** A true bladder diverticulum causing contralateral vesicoureteral reflux.

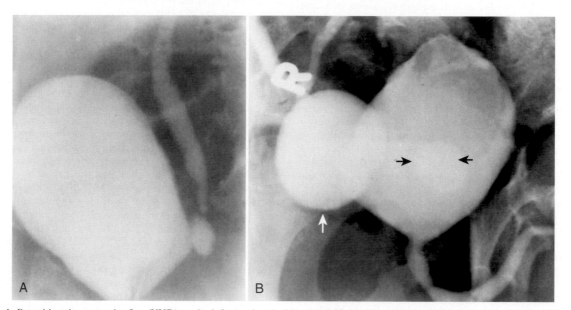

FIGURE 6-7. **A,** Prevoid vesicoureteral reflux (VUR) on the left associated with a small Hutch diverticulum. **B,** During voiding, a large Hutch diverticulum on the right side *(arrow)* associated with VUR is noted in addition to a smaller Hutch diverticulum on the left side *(small arrows)*.

TABLE 6-1. Fate of Mesonephric Structures

	Male	Female
Tubules	Epididymis	Mesosalpinx
	Efferent ductules of testes	
Ducts	Vas deferens	Complete involution
	Seminal vesicles	
	Ejaculatory ducts	

Adrenal Gland

At birth, the fetal adrenal cortex is responsible for the large aspect of the adrenal, which is up to one third the size of the adjoining kidney. It takes its characteristic shape partly because it "sits" on the upper pole. Likewise, if the kidney is not present, the adrenal assumes a discoid or "straight" shape (Fig. 6-8); this latter appearance should prompt one to search for the ipsilateral kidney.

Congenital adrenal hyperplasia is caused by an enzymatic deficiency (21-hydroxylase in > 90% of cases) in the cortisol biosynthesis, is inherited as an autosomal recessive trait, occurs more commonly in girls than boys, manifests as either genital ambiguity or salt-losing symptoms, and is diagnosed on US. Adrenal limb width greater than 4 mm, undulating gland surface (like that of brain), and replacement of the central hyperechogenic stripe by a stippled pattern are the three criteria for congenital adrenal hyperplasia; the presence of two criteria, preferably the latter two, is diagnostic.

▬ CONGENITAL ANOMALIES
Renal Agenesis

Bilateral renal agenesis is incompatible with life. It occurs in 1 in 8000 births, with a male-to-female ratio of 3:1. The characteristic clinical presentation consists of oligohydramnios, prematurity, and Potter facies—low-set, floppy ears, prominent epicanthal folds, and micrognathia. Concomitant pulmonary hypoplasia may be associated with a pneumothorax. Prenatal US often establishes the diagnosis.

Unilateral renal agenesis is a fairly common congenital anomaly, occurring in approximately 1 in 500 births. It may be caused by a lack of development or a disappearance of the ureteric bud or the nephrogenic blastema. The ipsilateral adrenal gland is present in 85% of case and is discoid. The ipsilateral hemitrigone and ureter are absent. The solitary (contralateral) kidney usually undergoes compensatory hypertrophy after birth. The anatomic splenic flexure of the colon may occupy the renal fossa

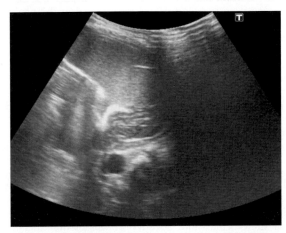

FIGURE 6-8. US of a discoid adrenal gland showing cortex and echogenic medulla.

in patients with left renal agenesis (or ectopia), or the duodenum may relocate into the empty right renal fossa (Fig. 6-9). Renal agenesis may be seen associated with genital malformations; in girls these malformations include vaginal atresia and vaginal septum sometimes resulting in hydrometrocolpos. The association of unilateral agenesis and müllerian abnormalities (absence of the uterus) is known as the Mayer-Rokitansky-Küster-Hauser syndrome. In boys, genital abnormalities associated with unilateral renal agenesis include cryptorchidism, hypospadias, and absence of the testes.

Renal Hypoplasia

Renal hypoplasia may manifest as focal, global, unilateral, or bilateral hypoplasia. If all renal structures (i.e., a reduced number of calyces, pyramids, and lobes) are smaller than normal, a "miniature" kidney results. If the hypoplasia is segmental, the reduced number of calyces may result in cortical loss; for example, an Ask-Upmark kidney contains a unilateral or bilateral characteristic area of parenchymal thinning, usually at the poles but occasionally in the midportion. This can be identified as a groove in the capsule. A groove caused by gross parenchymal thinning is also seen in association with VUR: focal reflux nephropathy (Fig. 6-10).

Renal Ectopia

Renal ectopia denotes an abnormal position of the kidney. It occurs more often in boys. The spectrum of renal ectopia ranges from a kidney that may have "ascended" too far cranially (a thoracic kidney), to the more common, not completely ascended kidney, which comes to rest anywhere from the pelvis to the renal fossa

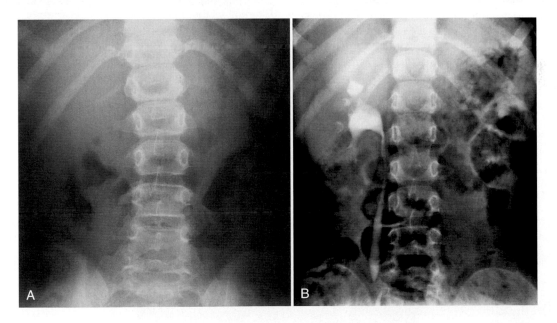

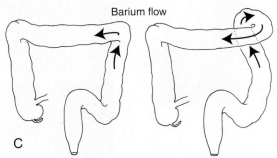

FIGURE 6-9. **A,** Normal abdominal radiograph. Note the position of the splenic flexure. **B,** EU showing the "empty" left renal fossa. Note the compensatory enlargement of the solitary right kidney. **C,** Schematic diagram of the normal splenic flexure anatomy *(left),* and anatomy occurring in left renal agenesis or ectopia with the GI tract (duodenum) "dropping" in *(right).*

Barium flow

(Fig. 6-11). One kidney (or both) may have crossed the midline and may be located on the other side of the abdomen. In these cases the crossed ectopic kidney is almost always fused to the orthotopic kidney (crossed-fused ectopia). More commonly (1 in 500 newborns), during ascent the renal *anlagen* "touch," or fuse, and a "horseshoe" kidney results (Fig. 6-12). In more than 90% of these cases, the lower poles are fused across the midline, creating an isthmus composed of renal tissue, fibrous tissue, or a mixture of both. Any kidney that is ectopic in location fails to undergo the 90-degree rotation along its longitudinal axis that is necessary for the renal pelvis to have its normal anteromedial orientation. This anteriorly oriented, often extrarenal, pelvicalyceal system can cause relative obstruction to efflux of urine.

This condition may lead to a hydronephrotic appearance and stasis of urine, which in turn may predispose to stone formation and infection. In addition, there is the arterial supply and venous drainage pattern are often anomalous. On US, an ectopic kidney usually loses the characteristic central echo complex

and demonstrates an extrarenal collecting system. In a horseshoe kidney, Wilms and transitional cell tumors are more common; hypertension develops more often in anomalously positioned kidneys as well.

US may demonstrate an ectopic kidney, but radionuclide studies or CT/MR may be necessary to confirm the location, structure, and function of renal ectopia.

Renal Dysplasia

Duplex Systems

Different forms of renal duplication occur in about 1 in 5 patients, and the spectrum ranges from a bifid renal pelvis to complete duplication of kidney and ureter to the level of the bladder. In the latter instance, the ureters enter the bladder through separate orifices: One is the "correct" trigonal location (orthotopic); the other is an ectopic location. Duplication is the result of premature branching of the metanephric duct and is the most common abnormality of the upper tracts. It occurs more often unilaterally (5 times as common) and is more often incomplete. It occurs four to five times more frequently in girls. When duplication is complete, the Weigert-Meyer rule applies: The ureter draining the lower pole moiety, usually larger, inserts in its normal trigonal position (orthotopically) (Fig. 6-13A). The ureteral orifice of the upper pole moiety inserts medially and caudal to this location (ectopically) in the bladder, or (less often) into the uterus, vagina, epididymis, or urethra (Fig. 6-13B). The portion of the upper pole kidney associated with the ectopically inserting moiety (the upper pole) is often obstructed and is almost always associated with a ureterocele. The severity of obstruction dictates the amount of "drooping" of the "lily" (Fig. 6-14).

The incidence of VUR in the normally located ureter is the same as in the general population; it may be higher if there is distortion of the ureteric orifice by the nearby insertion of the ectopic ureter. US may demonstrate a dilated (obstructed) upper pole and may suggest an unobstructed duplex system if the central echo complex of the medulla is "split."

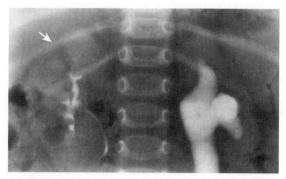

FIGURE 6-10. Reflux nephropathy. VCUG demonstrates focal scarring caused by vesicoureteral reflux on the right *(arrow)*. Global renal hypoplasia is seen on the left.

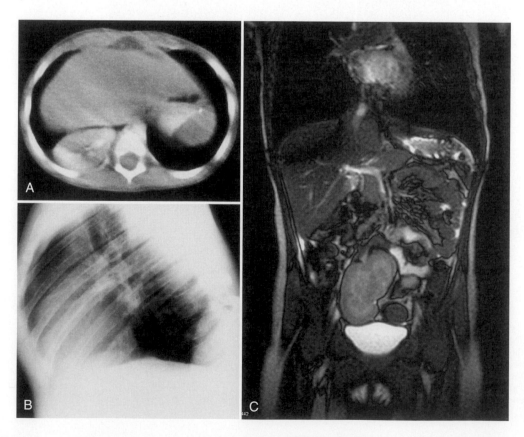

FIGURE 6-11. Renal ectopia. **A,** CT demonstrates (thoracic) ectopic kidney. **B,** Lateral chest radiograph in the same patient. **C,** Pelvic kidney shown on coronal T2 MR image.

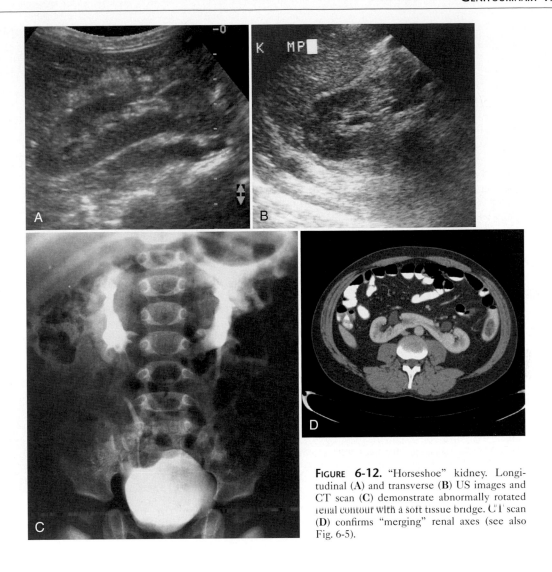

FIGURE 6-12. "Horseshoe" kidney. Longitudinal (**A**) and transverse (**B**) US images and CT scan (**C**) demonstrate abnormally rotated renal contour with a soft tissue bridge. CT scan (**D**) confirms "merging" renal axes (see also Fig. 6-5).

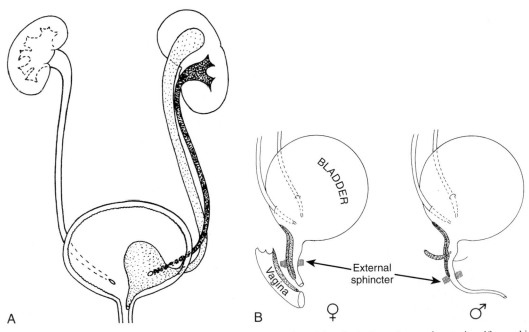

FIGURE 6-13. **A,** Weigert-Meyer rule. The upper pole ureter inserts medially and caudal to the ipsilateral normal ureteric orifice and is often associated with a ureterocele. **B,** Diagram of possible ectopic ureterocele orifice locations *(shaded areas).*

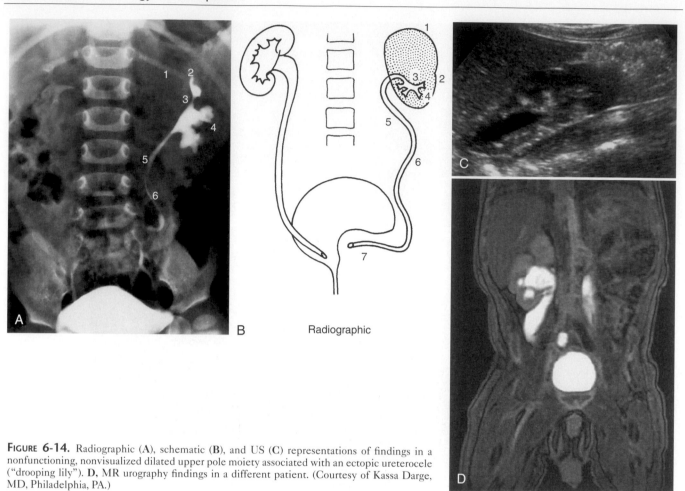

FIGURE 6-14. Radiographic (**A**), schematic (**B**), and US (**C**) representations of findings in a nonfunctioning, nonvisualized dilated upper pole moiety associated with an ectopic ureterocele ("drooping lily"). **D,** MR urography findings in a different patient. (Courtesy of Kassa Darge, MD, Philadelphia, PA.)

Multicystic Dysplastic Kidney

Next to hydronephrosis, MCDK is the most frequent cystic abdominal mass in the neonate. It is usually discovered on the first day of life or on prenatal US (Fig. 6-15). There is no evidence that MCDK is inherited. The incidence is about 0.03% at autopsy, and the cause is thought to be atresia at the UPJ. There is an equal gender incidence. Two forms are recognized:

Pelvo-infundibular MCDK: Most common; involves atresia of ureter and pelvis, resulting in multiple cysts.

Hydronephrotic MCDK: Occurs less frequently; there is a dominant cyst in the region of the renal pelvis.

A small, hypoplastic renal artery is present in both types, along with total absence of functioning renal tissue. In about 15% to 20% of cases of unilateral MCDK, there is a contralateral abnormality, most commonly a UPJ obstruction. Approximately 50% of affected patients have congenital heart disease and facial anomalies.

MCDK was previously thought to be premalignant and was therefore surgically removed. Current opinion suggests that there is little or no need to remove an asymptomatic MCDK. US criteria supporting this clinical decision include no enlargement of the lesion during the 3 years of follow-up (at 6-month intervals) after diagnosis, decrease in size and eventual disappearance of all recognizable renal (cystic) tissue, and absence of clinical hypertension and sepsis.

If US does not show cysts of variable size and absence of renal parenchyma, radionuclide scanning should confirm the absence of function on the affected side. If the lesion grows, CT must be performed to exclude a cystic renal (Wilms) tumor.

Hydronephrosis

The most common cause of a neonatal abdominal mass is hydronephrosis. Overall, underlying UPJ obstruction, posterior urethral valve, and ectopic ureterocele are each responsible about 20% of the time. Eagle-Barrett (prune-belly) syndrome and UVJ obstruction account for another 20%. Obstruction is not the only cause of hydronephrosis, however. VUR accounts for the remaining 20%, and polyuria and urinary sepsis may also cause dilatation of the urinary tract. Hydronephrosis often is diagnosed prenatally. If the ureteropelvic dilatation is moderate to severe, it may persist after birth and necessitate further evaluation (by VCUG). In mild cases, prenatal hydronephrosis disappears, probably in relation to the child's emergence from the special environment of the uterus (perhaps from gravity or improved GFR). Evaluation and follow-up by US are usually sufficient for a month or two; after such time, a VCUG may be needed to exclude VUR as the underlying cause.

Ureteropelvic Junction Obstruction

It is thought that the cause of obstruction of the UPJ, the most common site of obstruction of the urinary tract, may be either intrinsic (abnormal musculature) or extrinsic (increased fibrosis), resulting from the mechanical compression of either an aberrant vessel or a fibrous band (vascular remnant) or a postinflammatory stricture. The majority of UPJ obstructions are on the left side, with the incidence of contralateral UPJ obstruction being approximately 15% to 20%. The severity of a UPJ obstruction ranges from a mild holdup of flow to a full-blown obstruction (Fig. 6-16).

Most neonates with UPJ obstruction present with an abdominal mass. US can delineate a hydronephrotic renal pelvis with or without associated dilatation of the calyces that is of a lesser severity than the pelvic dilatation. Renal scintigraphy can further substantiate the diagnosis. Obtaining a VCUG is also necessary to exclude VUR as the cause of hydronephrosis, because VUR of grade IV or grade V can certainly simulate, and also exacerbate, an existing UPJ obstruction. This possible coexistence of VUR and UPJ obstruction, although rare, must be excluded because therapy is severely affected. VUR must be treated first. Mild holdup of flow at the UPJ is often treated expectantly by follow-up US in the first 6 months of life. Significant UPJ obstruction is treated by surgical excision of the narrowed segment and subsequent reanastomosis of the renal pelvis and ureter (a "dismembered" pyeloplasty).

In young children, a UPJ obstruction often manifests as gross hematuria because a dilated renal pelvis is more prone to trauma. In these cases, in addition to US evaluation of the kidneys, a look at the retrovesical region is mandatory to exclude primary megaureter or ectopic ureterocele as the underlying cause.

Variants of calyceal dilatation can take several forms, as follows:

• Calyceal diverticula or pyelogenic cysts may be 1 cm or more in diameter and are incidental findings. Congenital outpouchings of the collecting system that rarely necessitate surgical intervention, they may become infected.

• Fraley syndrome is a rare condition characterized by upper pole calyceal dilatation due to compression of the infundibulum by vascular structures.

• Congenital megacalyces, which are very uncommon, are characterized by caliectasis due to underdevelopment of medullary pyramids. They are often 20 to 25 in number and occur in boys more often than in girls. Renal function is not affected. The imaging appearance can be confused with severe obstructive hydronephrosis with dilated, flat calyces. In the case of congenital megacalyces, however, normal function is preserved, and the condition occurs unilaterally.

Primary Megaureter

A primary megaureter is dilated because it has a short juxtavesical segment that is normal in caliber but aperistaltic and therefore functionally obstructed. It is one of the major causes of obstructive hydronephrosis in children, although it is less common than UPJ obstruction and is probably due to fibrosis of the distal ureteral segment. The fact that the aperistaltic segment does contain ganglion cells refutes the notion that this lesion is the urinary tract equivalent of Hirschsprung disease. It is more common in boys than in girls (2.4:1), varies in severity, is found at all ages,

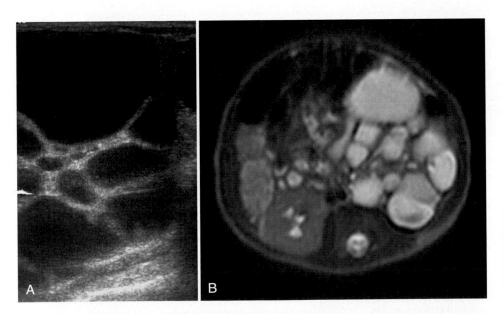

FIGURE 6-15. Multicystic dysplastic kidney (MCDK). **A,** US demonstrates multiple nonconnected cysts of varying size in a 1-day-old neonate with an abdominal mass. **B,** Transverse T_2-weighted half-Fourier acquisition single-shot turbo spin-echo (HASTE) MR image of a normal right kidney, with MCDK on the left.

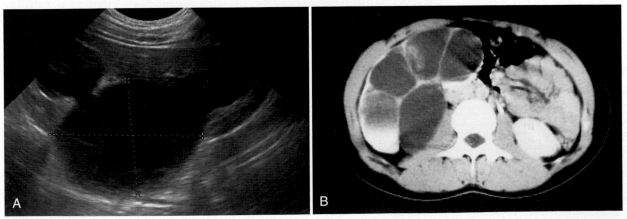

FIGURE 6-16. Ureteropelvic junction (UPJ) obstruction. **A,** US demonstrates marked obstruction at the UPJ. **B,** CT scan shows the dilated right pelvi-calyceal system with dependent layering of the contrast agent.

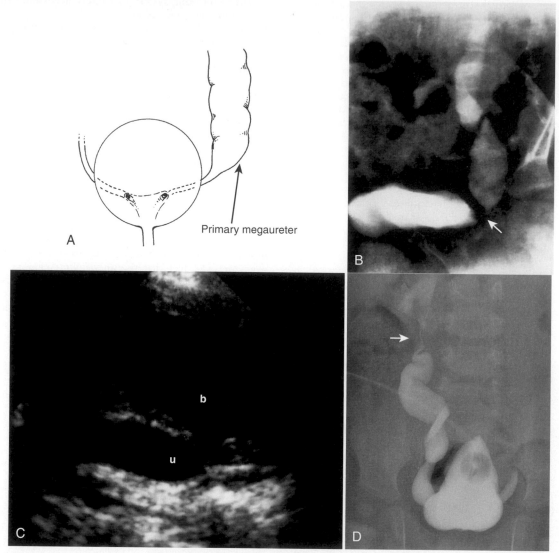

Figure 6-17. Primary megaureter. **A,** Schematic diagram. **B,** Oblique bladder view on EU shows "rat-tail" appearance *(arrow)*. **C,** Longitudinal US scan demonstrates the dilated ureter (u) adjacent to the bladder (b). **D,** Suprapubic cystogram best illustrates the nonperistaltic juxtavesical segment and the classic discrepancy in dilatation of the ureter and renal pelvis *(arrow)*.

and tends to be stable when uncomplicated. It is more common on the left side and is bilateral in 20% of patients. The aperistaltic segment may also be demonstrated on EU, VCUG, and US, which may also illustrate ureteric peristaltic waves. Because the UVJ itself is normal, VUR may coexist and is demonstrable on VCUG (in approximately 10% of cases). Imaging by MR urography shows columnization and dilatation but no tortuosity of the ureter proximal to a normal distal juxtavesical segment (Fig. 6-17). Treatment is either expectant or surgical. Surgery consists of excision of the distal aperistaltic segment and reimplantation of the ureter. The dilated ureter and pelvicalyceal system often return to normal caliber after a successful operation.

Ureterocele

A *ureterocele* is defined as a congenital dilatation of the intramucosal portion of the ureter; it is thought to be caused by delayed rupture of Chwalle's membrane during embryogenesis. Ureteroceles are divided into ectopic and single varieties.

Ectopic Ureterocele

Ectopic ureteroceles are invariably associated with the upper moiety of a duplex system and are usually unilateral. They are far more common in girls than in boys (5:1) and usually cause

obstruction of the upper pole collecting system and ureter. An ectopic ureterocele may, because of its size and location, cause VUR into the ipsilateral lower pole ureter by distorting the angle and length of the UVJ. An ectopic ureterocele is associated with a contralateral ureterocele in up to one third to one half of patients. An ectopic ureterocele often manifests as UTI or hematuria in a child younger than 2 years, but it may be signaled prenatally by the detection of hydronephrosis. Ectopic ureters without ureterocele can occur and may manifest as epididymitis or hydronephrosis in boys or as constant wetting or UTI in girls. These different presentations reflect the different embryology of the ectopic orifice in girls, in whom the ectopic ureter may empty distal to the external bladder sphincter and therefore anywhere along the uterus, vagina, and broad ligaments. In boys the ureter must drain proximal to the distal bladder sphincter but may terminate in the epididymis, vas, or spermatic cord (see Fig. 6-13B).

Imaging with VCUG may not demonstrate the ectopic ureterocele because the lesion may be flattened and even everted by the intravesical pressure of the contrast medium. To avoid this possible false-negative result, an early filling film is part of the routine on VCUG. Otherwise, a filling defect in the bladder is characteristic on early filling films (see Fig. 6-18B) for duplex systems.

Simple Ureterocele

Simple ureteroceles are located entirely within the bladder and are primarily adult lesions. They are much less common than ectopic ureteroceles and occur equally in males and females. The ureteral orifice is usually normally located, and the orifice is stenotic, either congenitally or post-traumatically. The lesion may be either unilateral or bilateral. Its characteristic appearance is that of a radiolucent filling defect in the bladder on VCUG. If an intravenous contrast agent is used, contrast material within the ureterocele is surrounded by a radiolucent halo; bilateral ureteroceles demonstrate the so-called cobra-head appearance. On US, the ureterocele is often clearly delineated in the urine-containing bladder (Fig. 6-18).

Eagle-Barrett (Prune-Belly) Syndrome

The classic triad of prune-belly syndrome consists of hypoplasia (absence) of the abdominal musculature, cryptorchidism, and marked dilatation of the urinary tract. The cause is either primary nondevelopment of the anterior abdominal musculature or hypoplasia of the abdominal musculature secondary to the marked dilatation of the urinary tract. It occurs almost exclusively in males, has a frequency of about 1 in 40,000 live births, and may have several associated clinical abnormalities (Box 6-3). About 20% of affected patients die in infancy.

VCUG may reveal a hypertrophied bladder, often with a urachal remnant (diverticulum). Severe VUR occurs in about 75% of patients, leading to tortuous, dilated, and poorly peristaltic ureters. The massive VUR may impede diaphragmatic motion and therefore lead to pulmonary hypoplasia; it may result in cystic dysplasia of the kidneys. There is marked dilatation of the posterior urethra and, often, filling of a utricle (vagina masculina) (Fig. 6-19). There may be a (mild) form of urethral atresia. Preoperative CT or radionuclide renography can assess renal size, shape, position as well as residual renal function.

Posterior Urethral Valve

Immediately distal to the verumontanum is the inferior urethral crest, which terminates in several plicae (folds) that are oriented caudally and encircle the urethra. When these folds are too prominent, they "become" membranous and may resemble a valve.

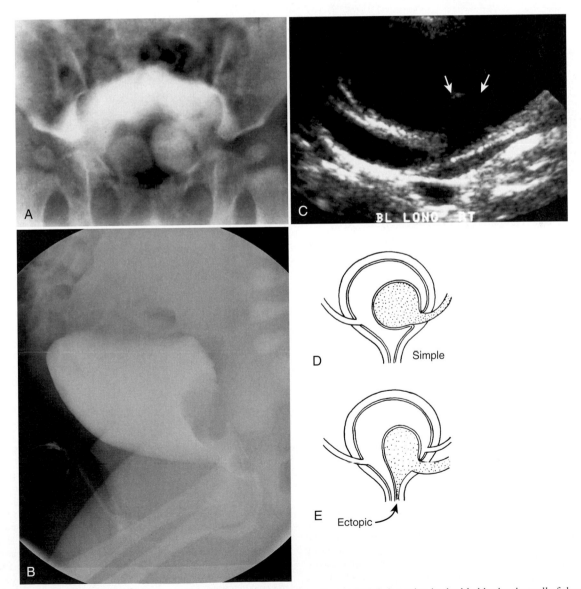

FIGURE 6-18. A, Contrast-laden urine within the ureteroceles is separated from the contrast-laden urine in the bladder by the wall of the ureteroceles (the classic "cobra head"). **B,** VCUG reveals a filling defect in the bladder. **C,** US representation of the ectopic ureterocele *(arrows)*. **D,** Schematic diagram of **A. E,** Schematic diagram of **C.**

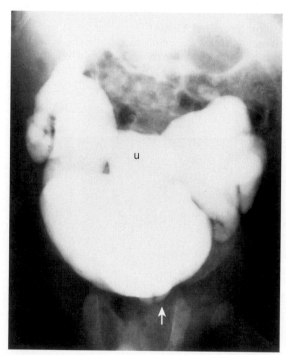

FIGURE 6-19. Prune-belly (Eagle-Barrett) syndrome. VCUG demonstrates an enlarged bladder with a urachus (u) and massive bilateral VUR. Reflux into the utricle *(arrow)* is also shown.

This posterior urethral valve occurs in about 1 in 5000 to 1 in 8000 boys. The following three types are classically described:

Type I (most common): Fusion of the anterior margins of the normal plicae collicularis. The resulting membrane circumferentially obstructs the antegrade flow of urine.

Type II (rarest): Mucosal folds extend cranially from the verumontanum to the bladder neck.

Type III (rare): Consists of a disk-like membrane just distal to the verumontanum.

Many physicians now believe that there is only one type of valve (type I), with several anatomic yet minor variations.

Clinically, patients with posterior urethral valve may have difficulty voiding, an abdominal mass (distended bladder), UTI (urosepsis), or prenatal US demonstration of hydronephrosis or oligohydramnios. About 50% of patients with posterior urethral valve present in the first 3 months of life. VCUG is the modality of choice to diagnose a posterior urethral valve because the valves are invisible to retrograde examination by both imaging and endoscopy. Imaging findings on VCUG are characterized by dilatation and elongation of the posterior urethra. There is a distinct caliber change between the normal anterior urethra, and the abnormal posterior urethra, caused by the obstructing valve. There may be associated VUR (30%), trabeculation, enlargement

of the bladder, and urinary ascites (Fig. 6-20). If the obstruction is severe, the neonate may have pulmonary hypoplasia (and a pneumothorax) as a consequence of oligohydramnios. Treatment consists of fulguration of the valve, and the prognosis depends on the severity and duration of existing urinary obstruction and subsequent renal impairment.

Anterior Urethral Valve

An anterior urethral valve is a semilunar fold, often the anterior lip of a urethral diverticulum, that occurs in the floor of the urethra near the penoscrotal junction. It is rare but accounts for the second most common obstructive urethral lesion in boys. This diverticulum may balloon with urine to such an extent that it obstructs the antegrade flow of urine or becomes infected. VCUG delineates this lesion best; US has also been useful (Fig. 6-21).

Congenital Abnormalities of the Lower Genitourinary Tract

Epispadias and Cloacal Exstrophy

Epispadias and cloacal exstrophy together constitute a rare spectrum of conditions caused by failure of the urogenital septum to induce fusion of the anterior abdominal wall. Normally, the urorectal septum divides the GU and GI tracts. The cloacal membrane ruptures when it touches this urorectal septum, thus forming the normal GU (urethral) and GI (rectal) orifices. Failure of the septum to touch the cloacal membrane results in persistence of the cloaca as a communal receptacle of body waste. The failure of the cloacal membrane to regress prevents the normal closure of the anterior abdominal and pelvic walls and produces the entity known as cloacal exstrophy. Cloacal exstrophy is the most severe part of this spectrum; epispadias is the mildest form.

The epispadias/exstrophy complex can be suspected radiographically if there is separation of the pubic symphysis (greater than 1 cm); there may be an association with spinal dysraphism or intestinal malrotation (omphalocele) (Fig. 6-22). The upper urinary tracts are usually normal. Clinically, the umbilicus is noted to be in lower than normal position. In male epispadias, the urethral meatus may be located anywhere along the dorsum of the penis. Urinary continence is frequently preserved. Female epispadias, which is very rare, is characterized by a divided clitoris and a short urethra with absence of the bladder neck.

Bladder exstrophy, although rare in itself (incidence is 1 in 30,000 births), is the most common anomaly of the previously mentioned spectrum; it affects boys more than twice as often as girls (2.5:1). Because the bladder is not fused anteriorly, the trigone and urethral openings are exposed. The margins of the everted bladder are continuous with the anterior abdominal wall. A septate vagina or short upward-curving penis (dorsal chordee) may be evident. Unilateral or bilateral cryptorchidism is often present. Upper tract abnormalities are rare.

On the other hand, cloacal exstrophy is very rare (incidence is 1 in 200,000 births) with a slight male predominance. The underlying cause is thought to be a primary defect of mesodermal migration in the anterior abdominal wall, with the end result being that the cloaca becomes exstrophied. In boys, there is a hypoplastic, paired penis. In girls, the vagina may be septate. About 50% of children with cloacal exstrophy have a myelomeningocele or an omphalocele. Renal dysgenesis is frequently present. The affected infant is often delivered prematurely.

Cloacal malformation occurs in girls only and is characterized by convergence of the rectum and GU tract at different levels in the perineum and subsequent emptying through a small cloacal opening.

Imaging by VCUG and catheterization of the skin orifices most often confirm physical findings. Cross-sectional imaging (MRI) may be necessary to plan surgical reconstruction of the bladder and (temporary) ureteric diversion. A US scan or renal scan verifies mostly normal upper tracts.

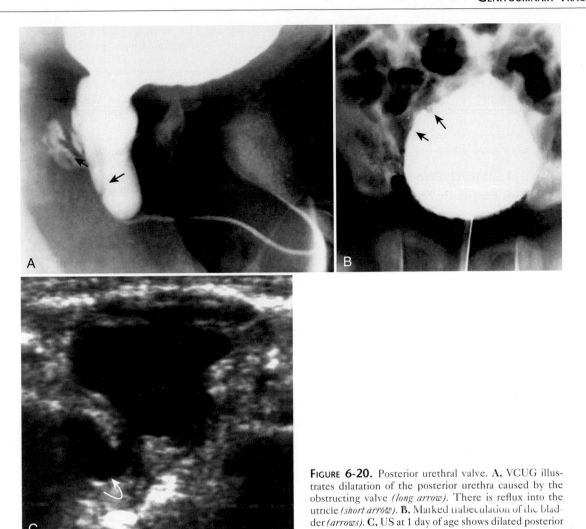

FIGURE 6-20. Posterior urethral valve. **A,** VCUG illustrates dilatation of the posterior urethra caused by the obstructing valve *(long arrow)*. There is reflux into the utricle *(short arrow)*. **B,** Marked trabeculation of the bladder *(arrows)*. **C,** US at 1 day of age shows dilated posterior urethra *(curved arrow)*.

FIGURE 6-21. Antegrade urine flow (VCUG) demonstrates an anterior urethral valve.

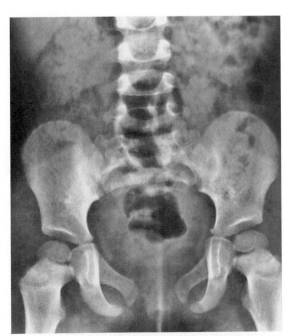

FIGURE 6-22. Exstrophy. Conventional radiograph shows separation of the pubic symphysis and possible absence of the sacrum (which was proven at surgery).

Hypospadias

Hypospadias in males is characterized by abnormal termination of the urethra on the ventral aspect of the penis. The glandular and coronal types account for 85% of these cases, and a horseshoe kidney may be associated. "Female" hypospadias is often seen on VCUG in girls up to age 4 years. Its hallmark, vaginal reflux, may occur because of (1) failure of complete descent of the urogenital septum, (2) plump labia, or (3) negative intrapelvic pressure during the voiding process. No matter what the cause, it resolves spontaneously in time (Fig. 6-23).

▬ CYSTS AND CALCIFICATIONS

Autosomal Recessive Polycystic Kidney Disease

"Infantile polycystic disease" and "adult polycystic disease" are no longer considered useful terms because there is no clear-cut separation between the two entities. Division along inheritance lines is considered more appropriate. In infants and children with autosomal recessive polycystic kidney disease (ARPKD), the relative severity of renal and hepatic involvement results in a spectrum of clinical presentations. The majority of infants with ARPKD die shortly after birth, but some children survive for several years, even into adolescence, with slowly progressing renal insufficiency. The ARPKD gene locus has been mapped to chromosome 6; the incidence of this disorder is about 1 in 40,000 live births. The underlying defect consists of medullary ductal ectasia with associated cellular hypoplasia. The

involvement may vary in severity. These cellular changes lead to loss of concentrating ability, tubular atrophy, and, eventually, systemic hypertension. There may be concomitant biliary duct hyperplasia and portal fibrosis, which may eventually lead to portal hypertension. The various forms of ARPKD are listed in Box 6-4. The renal changes in ARPKD may be thought of as inversely proportional to liver and biliary ductal hyperplasia and portal triad fibrosis.

US, the imaging modality of choice, demonstrates nephromegaly with an increased and occasionally inhomogeneous echotexture, leading to virtual "obliteration" of the central echo complex. Overall function depends on the extent of tubular involvement (Fig. 6-24). Stone formation, demonstrable on US or CT, may occur.

Autosomal Dominant Polycystic Kidney Disease

Autosomal dominant polycystic kidney disease (ADPKD) is inherited as an autosomal dominant trait with variable penetrance. Incidence is about 1 in 1000 live births. It results from mutations in one of at least three distinct genetic loci: PKD1 on chromosome 16, PKD2 on chromosome 4, and a third that is neither PKD1 nor PKD2. ADPKD usually manifests in late childhood or in adulthood, quite consistently among the members of one family. The cysts are located anywhere along the nephron (glomerular, ductal, tubular); when they enlarge, they compress and destroy normal renal tissue, with concomitant obstruction of

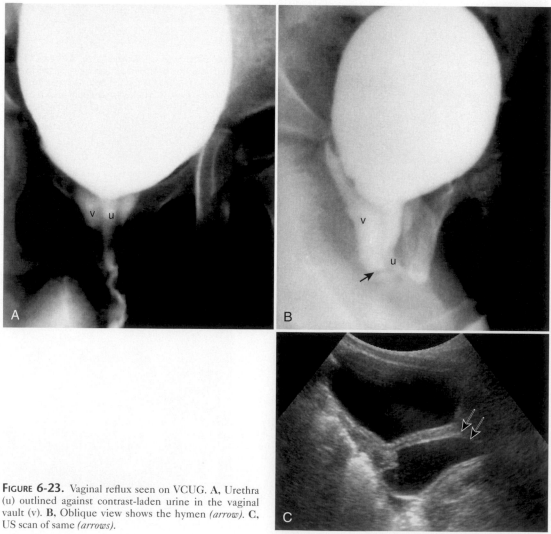

FIGURE 6-23. Vaginal reflux seen on VCUG. **A,** Urethra (u) outlined against contrast-laden urine in the vaginal vault (v). **B,** Oblique view shows the hymen *(arrow)*. **C,** US scan of same *(arrows)*.

the collecting system. The underlying fibrosis is notably absent. Cysts may also be noted in the spleen, ovaries or testes, pancreas, and lungs. Intracranial berry aneurysms are present in approximately 20% of adult patients.

The US appearance of ADPKD may be identical to that of ARPKD: nephromegaly with increased echotexture. Macroscopic

cysts may be noted, and their suggested cause is defects in production of polycystins 1 and 2. Hepatic cysts occur in about one third of patients but can be of varying size (Fig. 6-25). In neonates and young children with ADPKD, the imaging findings are often initially normal.

Simple Cysts

Simple cysts in children are seen with increasing frequency (2% to 4%) and must be differentiated from renal cystic disease (Box 6-5). They must meet the US criteria for simple cysts; otherwise, further evaluation to exclude pathology is mandatory (Fig. 6-26). Simple cysts are not familial and are seldom associated with other urinary tract anomalies.

Medullary Cystic Disease

Medullary Sponge Kidney

Medullary sponge kidney (precalyceal canalicular ectasia) is unusual in the pediatric age group. Microscopically, the anomaly consists of dilated (ectatic) collecting tubules. On US, echotexture is often normal, with occasional increased echogenicity in the renal pyramids, the result of renal stone formation.

Juvenile Nephronophthisis

Juvenile nephronophthisis (autosomal recessive) is the juvenile-onset form of medullary cystic disease. The cysts are detected microscopically, and the child is presented with polyuria or polydipsia and decreased concentrating ability. In the adult-onset form of renal medullary cystic disease (autosomal dominant), these cysts can be seen macroscopically. The juvenile form is the most common cause of idiopathic renal failure in adolescents. Boys and girls are affected equally. Pathologically, the condition is characterized by medullary cysts that

---

> **Box 6-4.** Classification of Autosomal Recessive Polycystic Kidney Disease
>
> **PERINATAL FORM**
> Most affected infants die within the first month of life. Presentation at birth with nephromegaly, with 90% of renal tubules involved along with *some hyperplasia of the biliary ducts.*
>
> **NEONATAL FORM**
> Most affected infants die at 2 to 8 months of life. Presentation with nephromegaly at birth, with about one half of the renal tubules involved and *mild hepatic fibrosis, in addition to biliary ductal hyperplasia.*
>
> **INFANTILE FORM**
> Renal and hepatic failure is not evident until 5 to 10 years of age, although the nephromegaly may be diagnosed as early as 1 year of age. Only about one quarter of the renal tubules are involved, but there is *moderate hepatic fibrosis and biliary ductal hyperplasia. Portal hypertension often develops.*
>
> **JUVENILE FORM**
> Hepatomegaly and portal hypertension are diagnosed in the first year of life, but nephromegaly is seldom present because less than 10% of the renal tubules are involved.

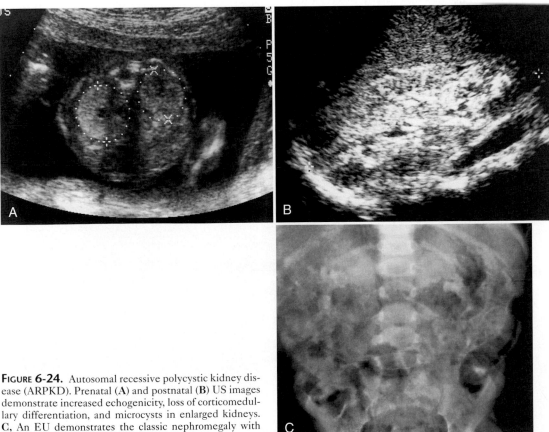

FIGURE 6-24. Autosomal recessive polycystic kidney disease (ARPKD). Prenatal (**A**) and postnatal (**B**) US images demonstrate increased echogenicity, loss of corticomedullary differentiation, and microcysts in enlarged kidneys. **C,** An EU demonstrates the classic nephromegaly with poor excretory function, or "puddling."

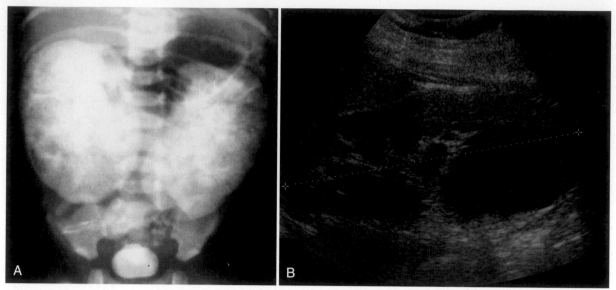

FIGURE 6-25. Autosomal dominant polycystic kidney disease (ADPKD). **A,** EU demonstrates brushlike appearance of the collecting systems and bilaterally enlarged kidneys with good function. **B,** Renal US shows multiple macrocysts of different sizes.

Box 6-5. Syndromes with Renal Cysts

**SYNDROMES IN WHICH RENAL CYSTS
MAY BE PRESENT**
Tuberous sclerosis
von Hippel–Lindau disease
Ehlers-Danlos syndrome
Jeune asphyxiating thoracic dystrophy
Zellweger (cerebrohepatorenal) syndrome

SYNDROMES WITH MICROCYSTS IN THE KIDNEY
Congenital cutis laxa syndrome
DiGeorge syndrome
Noonan syndrome
Turner syndrome
Ivemark syndrome
Goldenhar syndrome

---

are associated with interstitial nephritis, which in turn leads to small, scarred kidneys. These pathologic changes, characterized best on US, consist of a mildly echogenic cortex and medullary echogenic changes with cysts in bilaterally small kidneys. In the adult form, the condition manifests as similar imaging findings and may be associated with renal or retinal dysplasia and cone-shaped epiphyses (retinitis pigmentosa and the Mindsner-Saldino syndrome).

Calcifications

The two main categories of urinary tract calcifications are nephrocalcinosis (increased calcium content of the kidney) and nephrolithiasis, distinct entities that may coexist.

Nephrocalcinosis

In general, deposition of calcium within the pyramids or parenchyma is uncommon in children. *Nephrocalcinosis* is defined as

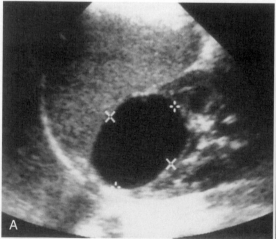
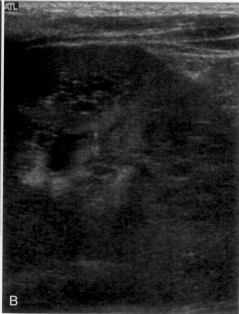

FIGURE 6-26. A, Simple cyst. US demonstrates upper pole cyst with no internal echoes, posterior wall enhancement, and "beaking" of the renal cortex. **B,** Eccentric (upper pole) microcyst location, rest of renal parenchyma still sonographically normal.

medullary deposition of fine, occasionally coarse, calcifications in the wall and lumen of the distal collecting tubules. They seldom appear as shadows on US. This process of calcium deposition in the renal pyramids has been called the Anderson-Carr-Randall progression. The most common causes include renal (distal) tubular acidosis, hypercalciuria or hypercalcemia of a chronic nature, renal tissue damage (e.g., by chemotherapy), and hyperoxaluria (e.g., due to short bowel syndrome) (Box 6-6). Truly opaque calcium stones account for 70% of all stones; magnesium–ammonium phosphate (struvite) stones account for 20% and may be moderately opaque.

Imaging traditionally consists of conventional radiographs of the abdomen. Early detection of calcium, however, depends on the density of the calcification. Early treatment may arrest the pathologic process and prevent renal damage. US exquisitely demonstrates the Anderson-Carr-Randall progression of calcium deposition in the renal pyramids (Fig. 6-27).

Urolithiasis

Calcific foci within the urinary tract are usually idiopathic (30%). Other causes are chronic UTI, urinary stasis, proximal renal tubular acidosis, and enteric causes such as interruption of the enteropathic circulation (oxalate stones) and excessive enteric loss

---

> **Box 6-6.** Common Causes of Nephrocalcinosis
>
> **HYPERCALCIURIA OR HYPERCALCEMIA**
> Renal tubular acidosis (distal)
> Drugs (diuretics)
> Immobilization, primary hyperparathyroidism
> Milk-alkali syndrome
> Hereditary hyperoxaluria
> Cushing syndrome
>
> **TISSUE DAMAGE**
> Renal cortical necrosis
> Renal papillary necrosis
> Medullary sponge kidney
> Chronic pyelo(glomerulo)nephritis

of fluid (diarrhea) leading to uric acid stones. In premature neonates, prolonged furosemide therapy for hyaline membrane disease (IRDS or surfactant deficiency disease) is a well-recognized cause (Fig. 6-28A).

US may demonstrate renal calculi, especially if they cast acoustic shadows (Fig. 6-28B). Conventional abdominal radiographs

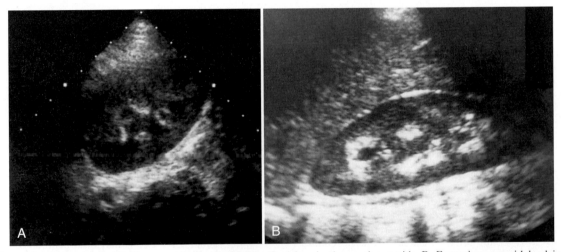

FIGURE 6-27. Nephrocalcinosis. **A,** US illustrates rimlike deposition of calcium in the renal pyramids. **B,** Extensive pyramidal calcium deposition (Anderson-Carr progression).

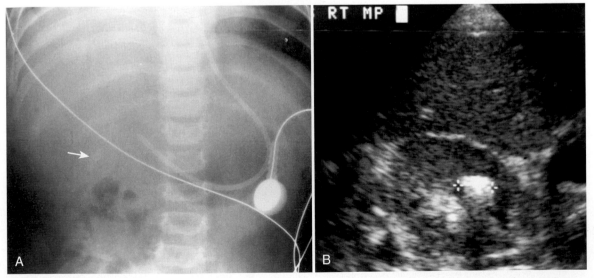

FIGURE 6-28. A, Renal stones noted on an abdominal radiograph in a premature neonate receiving furosemide therapy *(arrow)*. **B,** Stone resolution is monitored on US.

may also be diagnostic although in only a relatively small percentage (30%).

For imaging or the acute sequelae of urolithiasis, nonenhanced CT is the preferred modality because it identifies the location of calculi and shows early obstruction of the renal pelvis and ureters (columnization) more reliably and earlier than US. The radiation dose of nonenhanced CT for nephrolithiasis is of concern, however, estimations of a 1-in-1000 lifetime risk for development of cancer being reported. A modified, low-dose technique is a partial solution. US is useful for the follow-up of hydronephrosis but is limited in visualizing the entire urinary tract.

Bladder stones are rare but may be seen in patients with neurogenic or hypotonic bladder or secondary to an intravesical foreign body. These stones are usually laminated and as such can be differentiated from phleboliths.

▬ NEOPLASMS
Renal Masses
Mesoblastic Nephroma

Mesoblastic nephroma (fetal renal hamartoma) is the most common neonatal mesenchymal neoplasm. It arises from the metanephric blastema, like nephroblastomatosis and Wilms tumor. A solid renal lesion occasionally diagnosed by prenatal US, mesoblastic nephroma manifests as a large nontender abdominal mass in the neonate younger than 3 months. In the past, mesoblastic nephroma was considered an early form of Wilms tumor. Currently, it is considered a benign entity. There is no gender predilection. The lesion is therefore characterized by a benign course without the appearance of metastatic lesions.

On US, there is evidence of a large, solid, hypoechoic homogeneous mass replacing most, if not all, of the renal parenchyma (Fig. 6-29). Cystic change may occur but is rare. Further imaging (i.e., MRI, CT) cannot differentiate this lesion from the (rare) neonatal Wilms tumor. Therefore treatment is by surgical excision.

Column of Bertin

A normal variant, a column of Bertin is defined as normal renal cortical parenchyma that can be seen extending into the renal medulla, embryologically considered an infolding of the cortical renal tissue between adjacent renal pyramids. It may cause splaying of the calyces and thus simulate a renal mass. US confirms a mass of renal-like echogenicity most commonly between the upper and middle poles. Traditionally, renal scintigraphy was used to show normal uptake in that area. MRI clinches the diagnosis. This entity is of no clinical significance once it has been differentiated from a neoplastic lesion or cyst.

Multilocular Cystic Nephroma

Multilocular cystic nephroma (cystadenoma) is a benign unilateral, often solitary lesion occurring in both young children (2 to 5 years of age) and young adults (18 years and older). Boys are more often affected than girls, and women more often than men. Multilocular cystic nephroma represents 2% to 3% of all primary renal lesions and manifests as an abdominal mass. CT, MRI, and US show multiple noncommunicating cysts of variable size that are difficult to differentiate from a cystic Wilms tumor or MCDK (Fig. 6-30). Consequently, nephrectomy provides the definitive diagnosis of the pathologic specimen and is unfortunately the only definitive therapy.

Angiomyolipoma

An angiomyolipoma is a solitary yet rare tumor; however, it can be seen in up to 50% of patients with tuberous sclerosis. In these patients, the tumors occur bilaterally and are often asymptomatic. There is equal gender incidence. Renal angiomyolipomas not associated with tuberous sclerosis occur most commonly in middle age, with a 4:1 female preponderance, and are unilateral. Whether sporadic or associated with tuberous sclerosis, most angiomyolipomas become symptomatic because of hemorrhage within them. The lesions are extremely vascular and contain both muscle and fat, the latter making imaging by CT with IV contrast characteristic. On US the lesion is hyperechogenic also because of the fatty content. About 20% of angiomyolipomas are locally invasive (Fig. 6-31).

Nephroblastomatosis

Nephroblastomatosis is considered a precursor to Wilms tumor. The lesion consists of immature metanephric tissue (nephrogenic rests) that can be identified as subcapsular nodules in the renal cortex. These are often identified as microscopic cysts (in 1%) of autopsies in neonates, whereas more massive subcapsular involvement is most often seen in children in the first 2 years of life. The risk for development into Wilms tumor varies. Nephroblastomatosis lesions may disappear; however, if they are

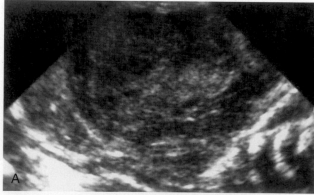
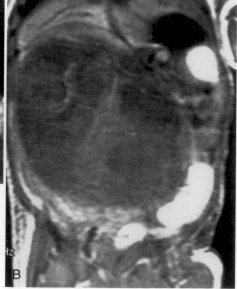

Figure 6-29. Mesoblastic nephroma. **A,** US demonstration of a right upper quadrant, inhomogeneous renal mass in a 2-month-old infant. **B,** MR image confirms extent and character of the lesion.

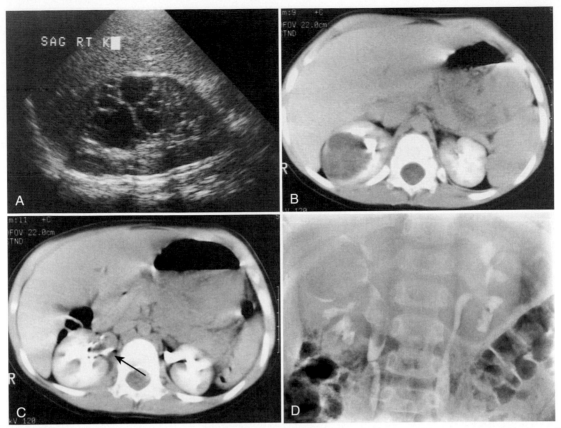

FIGURE 6-30. Multilocular cystic nephroma. **A,** US scan demonstrates a multicystic lesion. **B** and **C,** CT scans with contrast show the lesion with pelvicalyceal extension (*arrow*). **D,** EU appearance of the lesion.

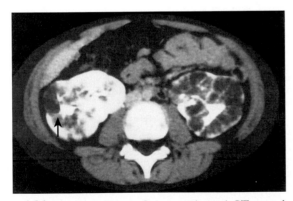

FIGURE 6-31. Angiomyolipoma. Contrast-enhanced CT scan demonstrates multiple lesions containing fat (*arrow*) in a patient with tuberous sclerosis.

present in a kidney removed for Wilms tumor, the patient has a 20% risk for development of a Wilms tumor in the other kidney. Nephroblastomatosis is commonly associated with trisomies 13 and 18 and with Beckwith-Wiedemann and Drash syndromes. Imaging demonstrates enlarged kidneys with multifocal parenchymal masses of abnormal echogenicity on US (Box 6-7). CT confirms the irregular outline and the masses (Fig. 6-32). It may be difficult to differentiate this entity from ARPKD except for the poor renal function in the latter. Chemotherapy for nephroblastomatosis is controversial.

Wilms Tumor

Wilms tumor accounts for about 10% of all childhood malignancies. It is the most common renal malignancy, with a peak incidence between 4 months and 4 years of age; 80% of cases occur in children between 1 and 5 years of age. Males slightly outnumber females (1.2:1); about 500 new cases occur each year in the United States. There is a 1% familial incidence. Associated congenital abnormalities occur in 15% of all children with Wilms tumor (Box 6-8).

Approximately 1% of all patients with Wilms tumor have sporadic aniridia, and there may be a chromosomal basis with deletion of the short arm of chromosome 11. Other associated

---

Box 6-7. Differential Diagnosis of Bilaterally Enlarged Kidneys on Ultrasound

Beckwith-Wiedemann syndrome (5%)
Hemihypertrophy
Male pseudohermaphroditism and nephritis (Drash syndrome)
Sporadic nonfamilial aniridia
Neurofibromatosis type 1
Cerebral gigantism (Sotos syndrome)
Nephroblastomatosis
Nephrotic syndrome, glomerulonephritis, pyelonephritis
Polycystic kidney disease
Glycogen storage disease
Lymphoma/leukemia

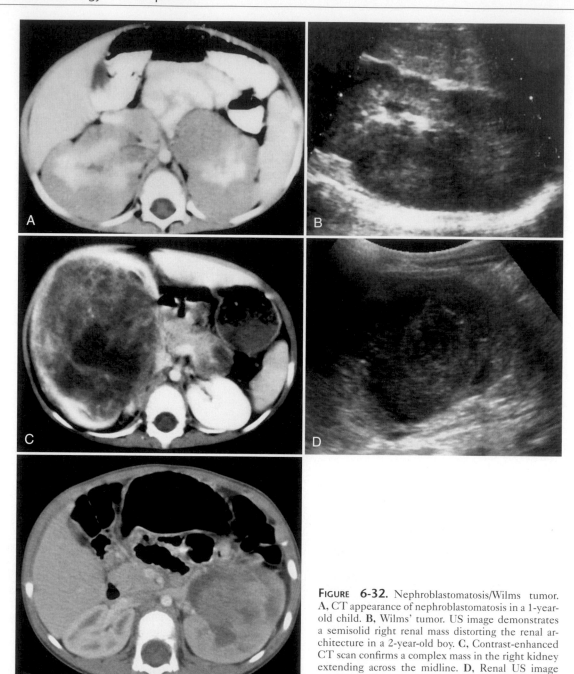

FIGURE 6-32. Nephroblastomatosis/Wilms tumor. **A,** CT appearance of nephroblastomatosis in a 1-year-old child. **B,** Wilms' tumor. US image demonstrates a semisolid right renal mass distorting the renal architecture in a 2-year-old boy. **C,** Contrast-enhanced CT scan confirms a complex mass in the right kidney extending across the midline. **D,** Renal US image reveals a solid mass in the left kidney; **E,** CT scan confirms the mass's renal origin.

Box 6-8. Malformations in which Wilms Tumor Has a Tendency to Occur More Frequently

Beckwith-Wiedmann syndrome (5%)
Hemihypertrophy
Male pseudohermaphroditism and nephritis (Drash syndrome)
Sporadic nonfamilial aniridia
Neurofibromatosis type 1
Cerebral gigantism (Sotos syndrome)

chromosomal abnormalities are various trisomies, chromosome translocations, and 45X.

Most children are well at the time the abdominal mass is noted. The tumor often enlarges suddenly and dramatically because of hemorrhage. Hematuria and hypertension are common,

and bilateral tumor lesions occur in about 5% of cases. Metastatic disease preferentially occurs locally, then spreads to the lungs and liver.

Imaging is initially accomplished by US, which reveals an often large, echogenic intrarenal lesion (see Fig. 6-32). It usually is sharply marginated and can be separated from the liver by its equal or slightly higher echogenicity. Necrosis and hemorrhage may result in mixed hypoechoic and hyperechoic areas within the tumor. The major advantage of US lies in Doppler imaging evaluation of the vena cava. The tumor or clot may extend into the renal vein and inferior vena cava in 15% of patients, but this feature may be difficult to assess on US if the tumor is large and bulky and compresses the vena cava.

CT defines the location and extent of the intrarenal and extrarenal components of the tumor better than US. Calcifications are demonstrated in about 15% of patients, and there is excellent delineation of necrosis or hemorrhage. CT is also the optimal

TABLE 6-2. Anatomic Staging of Wilms Tumor

Stage	Description	Two-Year Survival Rate (%)*
I	Confined to the kidney and totally resectable	95
II	Tumor extending beyond the kidney but totally resectable	90
III	Residual tumor but no hematogenous spread	85
IV	Hematogenous metastases to lung, liver, bone, or brain	55
V	Bilateral synchronous renal involvement	Individual stage dependent

*When two lesions appear at different times, there is a 40% survival rate.

modality to evaluate the contralateral kidney, which contains metachronous Wilms tumor in 5% to 10% of patients. CT of the chest demonstrates pulmonary metastases in about 10% of patients at the time of initial diagnosis. On MRI, Wilms tumor has prolonged T_1 and T_2 relaxation times. The appearance may be highly variable because of necrosis or hemorrhage. The main advantage of MRI lies in its excellent tissue resolution (allowing for multiplanar staging) and its exquisite visualization of the major abdominal vessels. Staging of Wilms tumor is summarized in Table 6-2.

There are two major types of Wilms tumor, one with favorable histology (90% survival rate) and the other with unfavorable histology (54% survival rate; contains many anaplastic cells). The type with sarcomatous histology occurs in about 10% of patients. Liver metastases are present in about 10% of patients, and bone metastases occur in another 5% and are osteolytic. Surgical excision is achieved through a flank incision if no interior vena caval involvement is documented, or through transabdominal incision if there is tumor spread.

Renal Cell Carcinoma
Less than 1% of renal cell carcinomas occur in the pediatric population, and their occurrence is extremely rare before age 5 years. The lesion is most often part of the von Hippel–Lindau syndrome, in which the renal carcinoma develops in the (bilateral) cysts.

Metastatic Disease to the Kidney
The most common lesions metastasizing to the kidneys are neuroblastoma and leukemia/lymphoma. In 75% of patients with lymphoma, renal involvement is noted that may be either nodular (masses) or (more often) diffuse in character (Fig. 6-33). In 50% of patients with leukemia, the infiltrative process in the kidneys is bilateral and diffuse. US and CT illustrate nephromegaly and occasional nodules; US shows increased echogenicity of the cortex. There may be some advantage to the use of IV contrast enhancement. Regional lymphadenopathy is better illustrated with CT.

Neonatal Adrenal Hemorrhage
Neonatal adrenal hemorrhage is a relatively common abnormality. It may manifest as anemia or jaundice, occurs on the right side 70% of the time, and may be bilateral in 10% of infants. Birth trauma, stress, anoxia, and/or dehydration have been implicated as causes. US is the modality of choice for demonstrating the adrenal glands and hemorrhage (Fig. 6-34). Hemorrhage most often manifests as a suprarenal echogenic mass that may be slightly inhomogeneous. It is difficult to differentiate this lesion from neuroblastoma unless there is decreasing size or central liquefaction of the enlarged gland in 3 to 5 days. To differentiate hemorrhage from an adrenal neoplasm, clot lysis and calcifications can be demonstrated over time as signs of a benign lesion. Doppler evaluation may be useful in showing the relative hypovascularity of neonatal adrenal hemorrhage. Neuroblastoma is usually more vascular and may have coexisting renal vein thrombosis. Absence of VMA (vanillylmandelic acid) in the blood clinches the diagnosis.

Neuroblastoma
Neuroblastoma is, like Wilms tumor, the third most common malignancy of childhood after leukemia and primary brain neoplasms. It accounts for 8% to 10% of all pediatric neoplasms. There are about 500 new cases each year in the United States, with an incidence of 1 in 10,000 children. The tumor arises from primitive neuroblasts in the neural crest of sympathetic ganglia and can originate anywhere from the cervical region to the pelvis. Approximately two thirds of neuroblastomas are located in the abdomen—with two thirds of these located in the adrenal gland. Of the remaining one third, 20% are located in the chest; the rest are located in the head and neck region.

In two thirds of cases, neuroblastoma manifests as an incidental abdominal mass. Likewise, two thirds of patients with this lesion

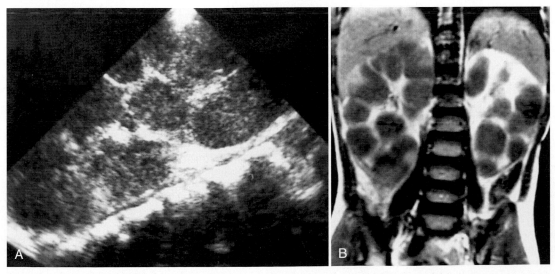

FIGURE 6-33. Leukemia/lymphoma. **A,** Renal US scan demonstrates multiple solid nodules. **B,** MR image of the same.

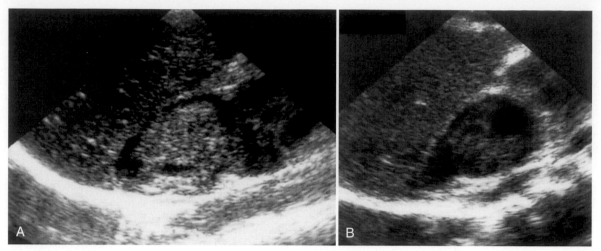

FIGURE 6-34. Adrenal hemorrhage. **A,** US scan at day 1 of life reveals an echogenic suprarenal mass. **B,** After 5 days, liquefaction and fragmentation of the clot can be seen.

are younger than 4 years, with the majority between 2 months and 2 years. The tumor is slightly more common in boys than in girls, with a familial incidence reported. At least two thirds of patients have disseminated disease at the time of presentation, with metastatic involvement of the skeleton, bone marrow, liver, lymph nodes, and skin reported. "Dumbbell" extradural extension is common in the chest but is unusual in the abdomen.

Neuroblastoma is unique among malignant pediatric lesions because it can spontaneously transform into the more benign ganglioneuro(blasto)ma. Syndromes associated with neuroblastoma include Beckwith-Wiedemann, Klippel-Feil, and fetal alcohol. Hirschsprung disease also has a reported association. Neuroblastoma is clinically silent until it invades adjacent structures. Symptoms then include (bone) pain, fever, weight loss, and anemia. Approximately 10% of children are presented with hypertension. Two thirds demonstrate excess urinary catecholamine excretion and therefore may initially have flushing, sweating, and irritability.

Two paraneoplastic syndromes may occur in children with neuroblastoma. *Opsoclonus/myoclonus*, or "dancing eyes and dancing feet" and cerebellar ataxia, occurs in about 2% of patients with neuroblastoma. Up to 50% of patients with myoclonic encephalopathy of infants are thought to have associated neuroblastoma. In children with myoclonic encephalopathy of infants and neuroblastoma, there is an equal gender incidence, a higher frequency of thoracic lesions, and a better prognosis (greater than 90% survival) than for those with neuroblastoma alone. *Watery diarrhea with hypokalemia syndrome* is caused by excess secretion of vasoactive intestinal peptides and catecholamines. It occurs in 7% of patients with neuroblastoma. Occasionally, there may be periorbital tumor deposition, which resembles what has clinically been called "raccoon eyes."

The staging of neuroblastoma and survival rates are summarized in Table 6-3. The overall survival rate is 72% for patients younger than 1 year, 28% for patients 1 to 2 years old, and 12% for patients older than 2 years.

Imaging by conventional radiographs may show a mass that in two thirds of patients contains calcification, which may be stippled, diffuse, or amorphous. Metastatic lesions to bone are often lytic and permeative, often located in the metaphyses. EU, which classically showed displacement but not distortion of the pelvicalyceal system by the tumor, has been virtually replaced by US, CT, and MRI. US, particularly when used as the screening modality for suspected abdominal pathology, most often demonstrates a suprarenal mass; it may reveal the inhomogeneous echotexture of both the mass and the often hypoechoic metastatic disease to the liver as well as tumor encasement of vessels.

TABLE 6-3. Staging of Neuroblastoma and Survival Rates

Stage	Description	Two-year survival rate (%)
I	Tumor confined to organ of origin with complete surgical removal (15%)	75
II	Tumor extension beyond the organ of origin; nodes may be positive; no crossing of the midline (10%)	75
III	Tumor crosses the midline (5%)	25
IV	Distant metastases (50%)	25
V (or 4S)	Metastatic disease confined to liver, skin, and bone marrow, with the primary tumor stage I or II (20%)	75

CT is superior to US in defining the extent and retroperitoneal spread of the primary tumor (Fig. 6-35). It is almost 100% sensitive and reveals calcifications in 85% of patients.

MRI has an advantage over CT in that it can demonstrate vertebral canal extension without the need for intrathecal contrast administration. MRI also nicely shows bone marrow involvement by metastatic lesions, often depicting a straight line of demarcation between normal and abnormal marrow. Encasement of the superior mesenteric artery and other vessels is appreciated to a greater extent because of the superior resolution of MRI and the capability for multiplanar imaging. The tumor usually has prolonged T_1 and T_2 relaxation times and may be quite inhomogeneous as a result of tumor necrosis.

Pheochromocytoma

A pheochromocytoma arises from catechol-secreting (chromaffin) neural crest cells and is usually a benign lesion. About 5% of these lesions occur in childhood, about 5% are malignant, and 5% are bilateral. Two thirds arise in the adrenal medulla. There may be a familial incidence, especially with an associated disorder. The associated syndromes, which occur in about 10% of patients with pheochromocytoma, include the multiple endocrine neoplasia syndrome (higher likelihood of malignant lesions) and the phakomatoses (von Hippel–Lindau disease, Sturge-Weber syndrome,

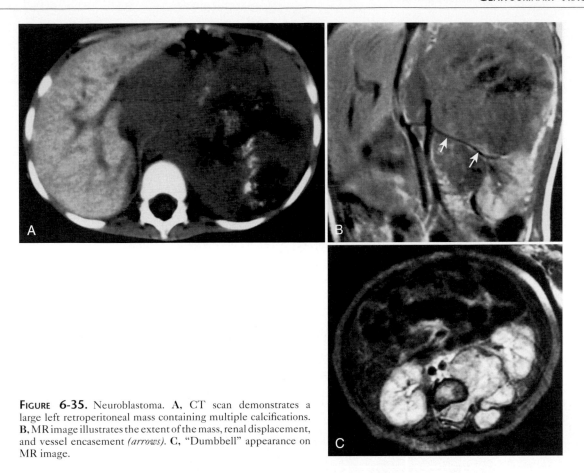

FIGURE 6-35. Neuroblastoma. **A,** CT scan demonstrates a large left retroperitoneal mass containing multiple calcifications. **B,** MR image illustrates the extent of the mass, renal displacement, and vessel encasement *(arrows)*. **C,** "Dumbbell" appearance on MR image.

and neurofibromatosis type 1). Affected patients come to clinical attention with signs of sympathetic overstimulation (flushing, tachycardia) or during an evaluation for hypertension. Eighty percent of patients with pheochromocytoma have hypertension, although only 10% of pediatric patients who have hypertension have an underlying pheochromocytoma.

CT with IV contrast should be used only after premedication of the patient with a blocking agent to avoid a hypertensive crisis. Scintigraphy and MRI are currently under investigation as screening examinations for pheochromocytoma (Fig. 6-36).

Wolman Disease
Wolman disease is a rapidly fatal, inherited disorder of lipid metabolism. The classic imaging finding on an abdominal radiograph consists of calcification of both adrenal glands at birth.

Bladder Masses

Thickening of the bladder wall may be difficult to assess because it may be hard to fully distend a child's bladder. Asymmetric thickening should be carefully evaluated (Fig. 6-37). Both benign and malignant bladder lesions are rare in children.

Benign Lesions
Benign bladder entities seen in children include hemangiomas and neurofibromas in patients with neurofibromatosis type 1. In half of these patients the mass is palpable. Other hemangiomas are found in about 40% of patients with hemangiomas of the bladder. Bladder involvement by neurofibroma constitutes a pathognomonic finding for neurofibromatosis.

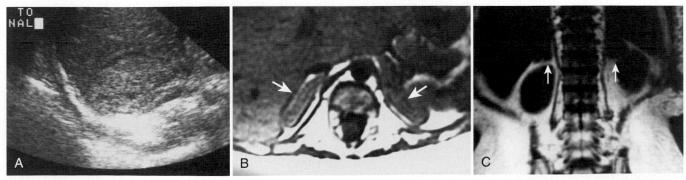

FIGURE 6-36. **A,** US scan showing suprarenal mass. **B,** T2-weighted MR image demonstrates a bilateral pheochromocytoma *(arrows)*. **C,** Coronal T1-weighted MR image of the same *(arrows)*.

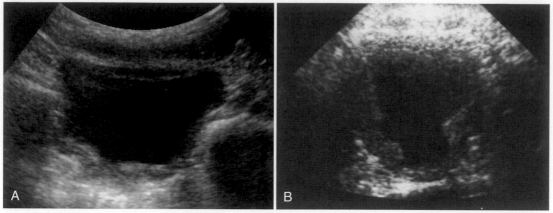

FIGURE 6-37. **A,** Normal bladder wall thickness on transverse US scan. **B,** US scan of a bladder showing cystitis.

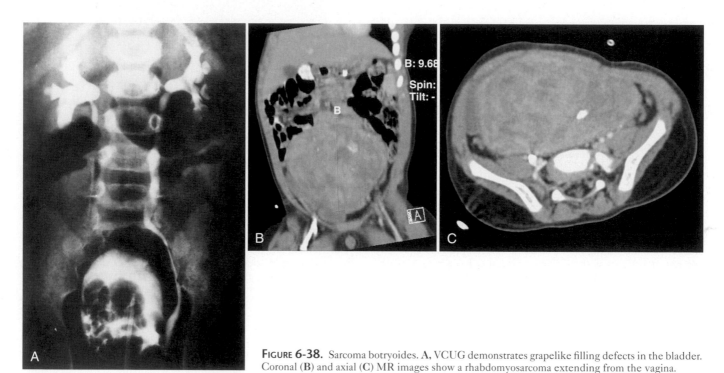

FIGURE 6-38. Sarcoma botryoides. **A,** VCUG demonstrates grapelike filling defects in the bladder. Coronal (**B**) and axial (**C**) MR images show a rhabdomyosarcoma extending from the vagina.

Malignant Lesions

The most common malignant bladder lesion is rhabdomyosarcoma. Twenty percent of all rhabdomyosarcomas occur in the lower urinary tract, especially the bladder (trigone) and prostate. Of the non-GU tumors, 40% occur in the head and neck and 20% in the extremities. Age at presentation usually is less than 5 years, with boys more commonly affected than girls, and African Americans affected four times as often as whites. Overall survival rate is around 75%, with metastatic disease occurring to the lungs and liver. VCUG may show a classic sarcoma botryoid (grapelike) pattern or a mass projecting from the dome in 25% of cases. US may demonstrate nodularity and bladder wall thickening, and both CT and MRI are useful for staging the pelvic extent of the tumor (Fig. 6-38).

Metastatic disease to the bladder is uncommon but is seen in leukemia/lymphoma. A thickened bladder wall is the most common finding.

▬ URINARY TRACT INFECTION

Urinary Tract Infection and Vesicoureteral Reflux

UTI is the second most common infection in childhood after upper respiratory tract infection. There is an incidence of 3% to 5%, which translates to 1.7 per 1000 boys and 3.1 per 1000 girls annually presented with a UTI. A UTI is a further indicator of an anatomic and/or functional urinary tract disorder in 35% to 50% of children younger than 6 years. VUR is present in 30% to 35% of patients, but it is present in 85% of children with evidence of renal scarring. This scarring, in turn, is responsible for 20% to 40% of cases of end-stage renal failure in patients younger than 40 years.

There are many misconceptions concerning VUR and UTI—UTI causes reflux, VUR causes UTI, VUR is secondary to distal obstruction, cystoscopy is necessary in UTI, US is sufficient to rule out VUR. These are all *false:* VUR is a primary abnormality of

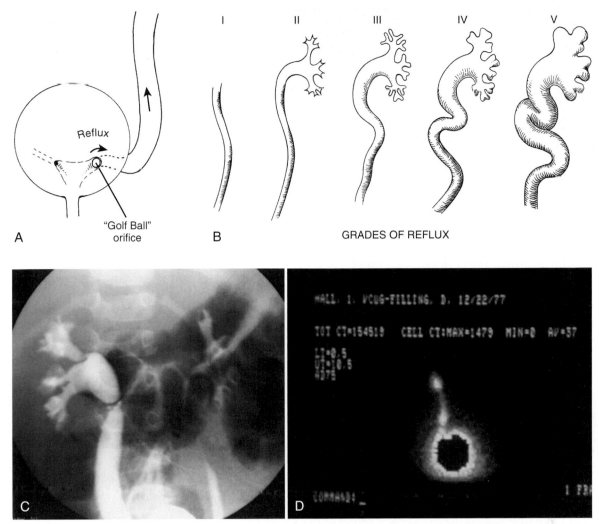

FIGURE 6-39. Vesicoureteral reflux (VUR). **A,** Schematic diagram of primary VUR. **B,** Grading of VUR according to the International Reflux Study Committee. **C,** Grade II VUR on the left; grade III VUR on the right. **D,** Radionuclide cystogram to evaluate for the persistence of VUR after medical therapy.

the ureteric mucosal tunnel, and it most often manifests as UTI. Imaging of only the upper tract is insufficient, and cystoscopy is outdated.

The objective of early diagnosis and treatment of VUR is prevention of damage and subsequent scarring of renal parenchyma. The younger the child, the greater the risk for hypertension (20%) or renal failure (12% of adults younger than 50 years); the resultant incidence of scarring is estimated at about 1% for boys and 0.5% for girls.

The key imaging questions therefore are as follows:

1. After a documented UTI, is there an underlying anatomic abnormality (e.g., VUR, UPJ or UVJ obstruction, ureteroceles, posterior urethral valve)?
2. How should the imaging evaluation be structured to be most effective?

Any child younger than 5 years who has a well-documented UTI should be evaluated with both VCUG and an upper tract study. A US suffices if the VCUG is normal, and a RN renogram is appropriate if the VCUG shows VUR or other anatomic abnormality. A ^{99m}Tc MAG$_3$ scan, particularly in children younger than 2 years, is sensitive to detect scarring.

"Abnormal" imaging findings in a patient with a documented history of UTI most often consists of the demonstration of VUR, next most commonly UPJ or UVJ obstruction, then a ureterocele or posterior urethral valve. VUR can be *primary*, in which

case it is caused by a congenitally ineffective valve mechanism (short tunnel, abnormal insertion angle) at the UVJ (Fig. 6-39A), or *secondary*, in which the submucosal "valve" mechanism is distorted by adjacent anatomic abnormalities (Hutch diverticulum, ureterocele, or cystitis). Primary VUR spontaneously disappears by age 6 years in 95% of cases (rule of thumb: 25% per 2-year period), with lower grades disappearing more spontaneously than higher grades.

Grading of VUR is illustrated in Figure 6-39B and C. VUR occurring during bladder filling is called low-pressure VUR. VUR that occurs only during voiding is called high-pressure VUR. There is a well-established association between VUR and renal scarring. This scarring can be caused by sterile VUR alone but is virtually always associated with UTI. It has been established that intrarenal reflux is necessary to cause scarring. Intrarenal reflux occurs most often in the compound calyces that are found in the renal poles (Fig. 6-40).

For older children or adolescents presented with UTI, US is the screening modality of choice. A small, scarred, or hydronephrotic kidney is then further evaluated with VCUG and/or radionuclide renography.

Medical management for VUR usually consists of low-dose chemoprophylaxis, which aims to maintain sterile urine while anticipating that the VUR will disappear with age. Follow-up, preferentially with radionuclide cystography (see Fig. 6-39D)

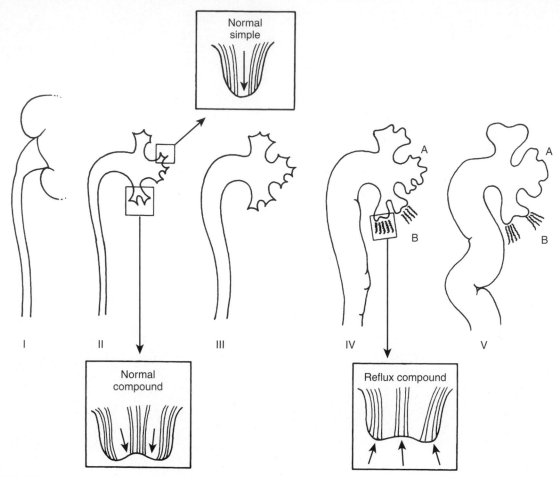

Figure 6-40. Grading of reflux and illustration of its effect on simple and compound calyces. The orientation of the collecting tubules is oblique, preventing reflux into simple calyces.

or VCUG and US or renal scans are usually scheduled at 6- to 12-month intervals to monitor this progress. After treatment for VUR, a radionuclide study (^{99m}Tc MAG$_3$ or ^{99m}Tc DMSA) and US are the preferred modalities to monitor scarring or to ensure its arrest. Surgical management of VUR is currently re-served for patients who have severe VUR (grades IV and V) in the presence of scarring or in whom the VUR is resistant to medical therapy. Urodynamic evaluation may also be necessary in such patients to rule out bladder-sphincter dyssynergia; if this condition is documented, anticholinergic medication can be of help.

Pyelonephritis

Acute Pyelonephritis

Acute pyelonephritis is an ascending infection that occurs in both the presence and the absence of VUR, although it is more severe in the presence of VUR. The acute infection is caused most often by *Escherichia coli*, *Proteus*, or *Staphylococcus aureus* and manifests as flank pain in 80% of cases. It is blood borne in neonates and in patients with endocarditis. The kidney may be edematous and/or contain an inflammatory cellular infiltrate.

There is a paucity of imaging findings in acute pyelonephri-tis (Fig. 6-41). Nuclear medicine studies are most useful. Scin-tigraphic evaluation with ^{99m}Tc MAG$_3$ (^{99m}Tc DMSA involves a higher radiation dose to the kidneys) is the most reliable modal-ity to demonstrate acute bacterial infection of the kidneys. It is more accurate than US, but it is less accurate than CT with regard to suspected perirenal infection. Ultrasonographic clues to acute

pyelonephritis are (1) an indistinct corticomedullary junction in part or all of an enlarged kidney that may show either increased or decreased echogenicity; (2) impaired renal movement with respi-ration; and (3) a size discrepancy of more than 1 cm in comparison with the contralateral, normal kidney. In a child with pyelone-phritis, complications such as perinephric abscess, pyonephrosis, and a renal carbuncle (most commonly caused by *S. aureus*) may occur. A focal area of pyelonephritis, also called lobar nephro-nia, may progress to a carbuncle (a spherical mass of increased echotexture) that then rarely progresses to the findings of an ab-scess with central necrosis.

Pyonephrosis

Pyonephrosis refers to an infected, obstructed urinary tract. Best imaged by US but may need further delineation by CT, this con-dition is initially treated best by percutaneous drainage.

Xanthogranulomatous Pyelonephritis

Xanthogranulomatous pyelonephritis (XPN) is extremely rare in children and may be associated with obstructing renal stones and resultant UTI. It is almost always unilateral, occurs more frequently in girls, and has the potential for extension into the perirenal space. In children, the localized form of XPN is more common than the generalized form. It may be detectable on US, but CT is better suited to evaluate the perirenal structures. Both modalities may show a mass and destruction of normal architecture with nonfunction, which in association with a positive gallium scan confirms the diagnosis of XPN. Surgical nephrectomy is the treatment of choice.

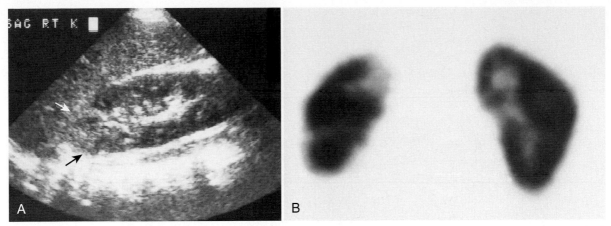

FIGURE 6-41. A, US scan showing acute pyelonephritis of the right upper pole with loss of corticomedullary differentiation and increased echogenicity *(arrow).* **B,** ^{99m}Tc DMSA renogram confirms a right upper pole defect.

Glomerulonephritis

The majority of patients who present with glomerular disease have either nephritic syndrome or nephrotic syndrome.

Acute Nephritic Syndrome

Acute nephritic syndrome is defined as abrupt onset of hypertension, oliguria, azotemia, hematuria, and proteinuria; it is usually caused by streptococcal glomerulonephritis. The pathophysiology is immune complex–related and is more common in boys than in girls. This syndrome occurs most often in children between 3 and 7 years old. In 95% of patients, total recovery is the rule. Chronic glomerulonephritis develops in 3% of patients, and 2% have a second episode. This clinical syndrome can be associated with Henoch-Schönlein purpura (rash, arthritis of knees and ankles, and melena), Goodpasture syndrome (pulmonary hemorrhage), and hemolytic-uremic syndrome (see following discussion). For imaging, US is sufficient and (in the proper clinical setting) diagnostic. Increased echogenicity of the renal cortex in association with mild renal enlargement is common. The echogenicity of the kidney with acute nephritic syndrome is similar to that of the liver or spleen.

Nephrotic Syndrome

Nephrotic syndrome is defined as hypoproteinemia, proteinuria, and hypercholesterolemia and is predominantly a disease of young children (2 to 6 years). Most commonly, microscopic evaluation reveals that the underlying pathophysiology is the result of minimal change disease, which is treated with corticosteroids. Associated entities are numerous.

Imaging by US usually is useful to rule out anatomic anomalies and to show increased echogenicity of the renal cortex (Box 6-9). Pleural effusions are also frequently seen on chest radiographs.

Hemolytic-Uremic Syndrome

Hemolytic-uremic syndrome is the most common cause of acute renal failure in infants. It occurs occasionally in older children and adults. A microangiopathy is the proposed mechanism. Clinically, diarrhea, vomiting, or respiratory distress is followed by acute renal failure, hemolytic anemia, hypertension, and GI hemorrhage. The kidneys are affected in most (90%) instances. The acute renal failure lasts up to 4 weeks, then gradually improves. Imaging by US may show increased echogenicity of the renal cortex and/or bowel wall thickening. The latter finding can be confirmed on barium contrast studies of the GI tract. On Doppler US imaging, the vasculitic cause may be reflected in an increased resistive index. The majority of patients recover completely, with Doppler signal patterns returning to normal.

> **Box 6-9. "Medical Renal Disease": Increased Renal Parenchymal Echogenicity on Ultrasound**
>
> Nephrotic syndrome (minimal change disease; 85%)
> Glycogen storage disease (type I; von Gierke disease)
> Hemolytic-uremic syndrome
> Polycystic disease (autosomal recessive or autosomal dominant polycistic kidney disease)
> Glomerulonephritis, pyelonephritis
> Lymphoma/leukemia

GENITOURINARY TRAUMA

Kidneys

Blunt abdominal trauma, which is common in the pediatric age group, often involves the kidneys. Approximately 0.1% of pediatric hospital admissions are the result of renal injury. The kidneys are more prone to trauma in children than in adults because of their proportionally large size, less perirenal fat, and less developed surrounding (protective) musculature. In addition, children's kidneys may be more delicate because of the fetal lobulation, which may supply "cleavage" planes. Most injuries to the kidneys manifest as hematuria or flank pain. Twenty percent of all patients with renal injury also have associated organ trauma.

CT is the imaging technique of choice in blunt abdominal trauma. Helical CT is the best imaging technique for renal contusion or laceration. Extravasation of arterial or venous contrast agents can be detected in the nephrogenic phase. Delayed scanning may be useful if there is renal laceration or perinephric fluid suggesting a hematoma or urinoma.

US is not very specific or sensitive about renal trauma because it does not give functional information.

Radionuclide evaluation is very organ specific but time consuming, although it can be sensitive in the setting of renal trauma. Use of angiography in the renal trauma setting has largely been abandoned.

Therefore CT is the imaging modality of choice in renal trauma. Peritoneal lavage is invasive and is not generally performed in patients younger than 16 years, except in rare cases in which CT is difficult to perform; also, lavage has a higher false-positive result rate than CT.

The renal injuries are classified on CT (Fig. 6-42) as follows:
Group 1: minor (50%)—contusions, contained lacerations.

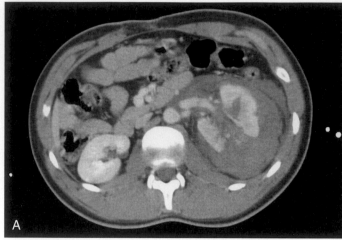

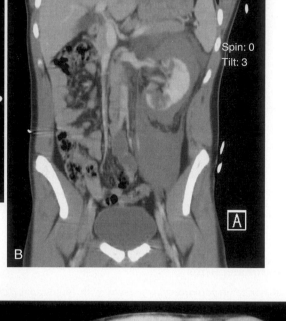

FIGURE 6-42. Renal trauma. Axial (A) and coronal (B) contrast-enhanced CT scans show a renal laceration extending into the collecting system with perirenal extravasation *(arrow)*.

Group 2: major (25%)—extension of injury into the pelvicalyceal system.

Group 3: critical (25%)—fragmentation of the kidney, with or without vascular pedicle injury.

Group 1 and 2 injuries are treated conservatively, and CT reliably identifies these cases. In 10% of traumatized kidneys, an underlying abnormality such as Wilms tumor, UPJ obstruction, or horseshoe kidney may be present.

Ureter

Injury to the pediatric ureter is uncommon. Most often, a UPJ avulsion or tear occurs in association with renal trauma.

▬ BLADDER

Rupture of the bladder is often associated with blunt pelvic fractures and may be intraperitoneal (20%) or extraperitoneal (80%), rarely both. CT accurately defines both soft tissue and osseous injuries (Fig. 6-43).

Urethra

Urethral injuries occur almost always in boys. They consist of tears, most commonly of the pendulous and posterior urethra, and are usually identifiable on a retrograde urethral contrast study. If a complete tear has occurred at the level of the pelvic floor, CT can be diagnostic when it shows elevation of the bladder floor within the pelvis.

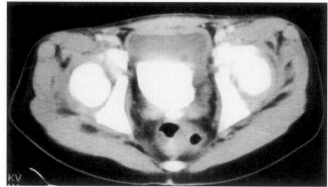

FIGURE 6-43. CT scan of trauma involving the bladder neck.

Genitalia

Female Genitalia
See Table 6-4.

Uterus
The neonatal uterus is quite large in relation to the bladder because of the presence of maternal estrogens. In the first month of life, the length ranges from 2.3 to 4.6 cm; in the subsequent months, a length regression totaling about 1 cm occurs (prepubertal uterine length ± 3 cm). The range of abnormalities of the uterus in infants and young children is very limited; most of them usually do not manifest

TABLE 6-4. Common Female Pediatric Abdominal and Pelvic Masses (By Age)

	Neonate (Less than 1 Month)	Child Younger than 2 Years	Child Older than 2 Years
Genitourinary (50%)	Hydronephrosis	Wilms tumor	
	Ovarian cyst	Hydronephrosis	
	Hydro(metro)colpos	Cystic disease	
Retroperitoneal (20%)	Neuroblastoma	Neuroblastoma	
	Adrenal hemorrhage	Teratoma	
Gastrointestinal (20%)	Duplications	Intussusception	Visceromegaly
		Appendix	Leukemia/lymphoma

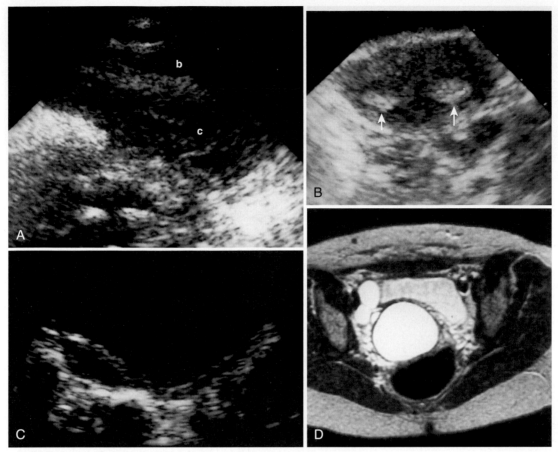

FIGURE 6-44. Uterus. **A,** Sagittal US scan of a normal infantile uterus (c, cervix; b, bladder). **B,** Transverse US scan identifies secretory endometrium in a bicornuate uterus *(arrows)*. **C,** US scan showing premenarchal "spadelike" uterus. **D,** MR image of a unilaterally obstructed bicornuate uterus.

until menarche. The infantile cervix (triangular on sagittal US scans) is often larger than the uterus. At 5 years of age, the uterus starts to become bigger than the cervix—a process that continues until puberty, when hormonal secretory changes result in the normal adult imaging relationship (Fig. 6-44). A hypoplastic uterus is occasionally identified. Congenital absence of the uterus and the upper two thirds of the vagina is diagnostic of the Mayer-Rokitansky-Küster-Hauser syndrome. Anatomic variants such as duplex uterus, retroverted uterus, and cloacal exstrophy may be identified by US, but MRI plays a more important role in these cases.

Hydro(metro)colpos

Hydro(metro)colpos is defined as a fluid-filled uterus and vagina. The causes of the obstruction range from (segmental) vaginal atresia (1 in 4000 live births) to imperforate hymen or vaginal diaphragm.

Hydro(metro)colpos may be accompanied by imperforate anus, dysraphic abnormalities of the vertebrae (12%), and urinary tract abnormalities such as solitary kidney and renal ectopia.

Most cases of hydro(metro)colpos caused by imperforate hymen are not discovered until menarche, when they may manifest as abdominal or pelvic masses. Infantile hydro(metro)colpos manifests as an abdominal mass; US is the screening modality of choice (Fig. 6-45).

Ovaries

The adnexa consists of ovaries, fallopian tubes, and supporting ligaments. In girls younger than 2 years, it is difficult to see the ovaries with US. In this age group, ovarian volume (0.5 × width × thickness × length) is less than 0.7 cm³, but ovarian volume increases to 1 to 3.5 cm³ in girls 2 to 12 years of age. The normal range for volume of postmenarchal girls is around 4 to 6 cm³. US is the diagnostic modality of choice, but it necessitates a full bladder to

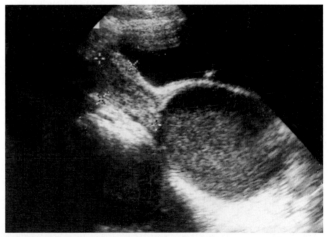

FIGURE 6-45. Hydrocolpos. Sagittal US scan demonstrates a fluid-fluid level in a markedly dilated vaginal vault and a normal uterus *(markers)*.

serve as a window to fully evaluate the retrovesical structures. In girls younger than 2 years, the normal ovarian appearance is that of a solid, ovoid structure with a mildly heterogeneous texture. In girls between 2 and 12 years, microcysts become apparent. With puberty, the number and size of physiologic (less than 0.9 cm) ovarian cysts increase. A corpus luteum cyst should be less than 3 cm in diameter. Neonatal ovarian cysts are fairly common and are probably caused by maternal hormonal overstimulation. Ovarian cysts may be quite mobile in the peritoneal cavity and may be located anywhere from the upper quadrants to the actual labia (Fig. 6-46).

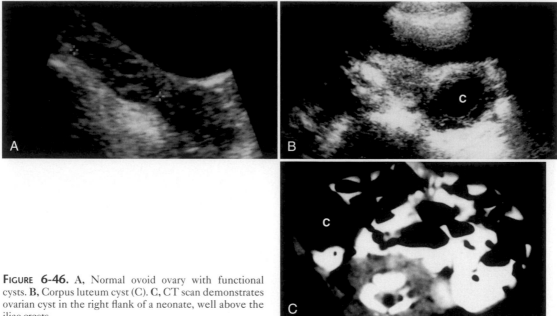

FIGURE 6-46. A, Normal ovoid ovary with functional cysts. **B,** Corpus luteum cyst (C). **C,** CT scan demonstrates ovarian cyst in the right flank of a neonate, well above the iliac crests.

When a normal mature follicle fails to involute and continues to enlarge, a functional ovarian cyst results. Because normal physiologic cysts are less than 3 cm, any (follicular or corpus luteum) cyst between 4 and 10 cm deserves serial imaging over two or three menstrual cycles. Failure of the cysts to involute may necessitate aspiration to relieve symptoms, exclude malignancy, or prevent torsion.

Polycystic Ovary Disease

Polycystic ovary disease (Stein-Leventhal syndrome) is not uncommon and is associated with amenorrhea, infertility, and hirsutism. Clinically, decreased levels of follicular-stimulating hormone and luteinizing hormone are present. On US, the imaging findings consist of bilateral ovarian enlargement (greater than 14 cm^3) with multiple small cysts.

Hemorrhagic Cysts

Hemorrhagic cysts can present difficult differential diagnostic problems in the teenage patient. They can be confused with endometriosis, ectopic pregnancy, or tubo-ovarian abscess (TOA). Internal debris in an ovarian cyst may suggest minimal hemorrhage; an echogenic cyst results from extensive hemorrhage (Fig. 6-47A). Presence of fluid in the cul-de-sac is often concomitant.

Ovarian Torsion

Ovarian torsion is uncommon in girls younger than 2 years except in the neonate, in whom it may be associated with ovarian tumors or cysts. Imaging findings are not unlike the clinical presentation and are nonspecific. There is arterial, venous, and lymphatic stasis, resulting in congestion and/or necrosis. Duplex Doppler US and color-flow Doppler US have had mixed success in distinguishing among hemorrhagic cysts, tumor, and TOA. The most reliable set of imaging findings is a larger-than-expected size of the ovary associated with fluid in the cul-de-sac and small cysts around the periphery of the ovary. Untreated, ovarian torsion leads to infarction, withering, and occasional calcification of the affected ovary (Fig. 6-47B).

Ectopic Pregnancy

Ectopic pregnancy is, like intrauterine pregnancy, a not unusual occurrence in teenage girls. Almost all ectopic pregnancies are located in the fallopian tubes and manifest by the seventh postmenstrual week on transabdominal US, earlier on transvaginal US. An extrauterine fetal pole is seen about 10% to 15% of the time. More often, imaging findings in an ectopic pregnancy consist of a nonspecific, echogenic, complex, adnexal mass, often with fluid in the cul-de-sac. Duplex Doppler imaging is quite specific in demonstrating ectopic fetal cardiac activity.

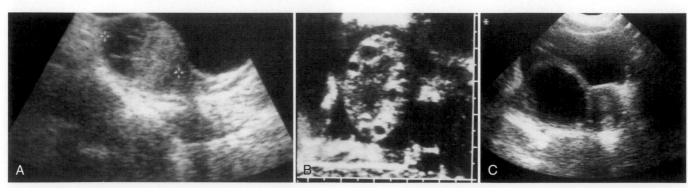

FIGURE 6-47. A, US scan of hemorrhagic cyst of the ovary. **B,** Ovarian torsion. Note peripheral cysts and surrounding cul-de-sac fluid. **C,** Tubo-ovarian abscess (TOA) in the right adnexa.

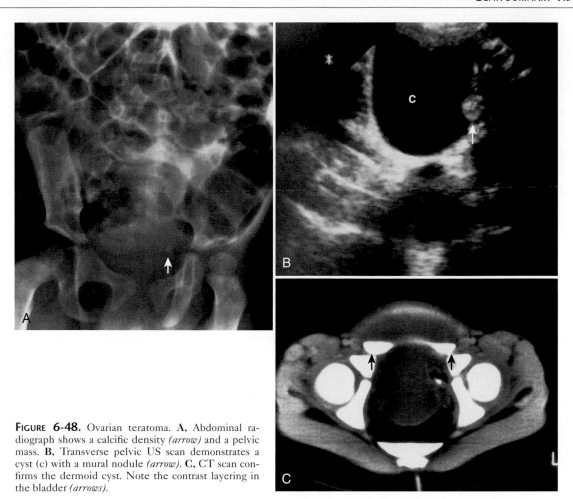

FIGURE 6-48. Ovarian teratoma. **A,** Abdominal radiograph shows a calcific density *(arrow)* and a pelvic mass. **B,** Transverse pelvic US scan demonstrates a cyst (c) with a mural nodule *(arrow)*. **C,** CT scan confirms the dermoid cyst. Note the contrast layering in the bladder *(arrows)*.

Tubo-ovarian Abscess

TOA is a sequela of pelvic inflammatory disease, often caused by *Neisseria gonorrhoeae* or *Chlamydia*. Pelvic inflammatory disease is caused by an ascending infection that originates in the cervix. The diagnosis is made clinically from the presence of symptoms of pain, vaginal discharge, and fever. US may detect a pyosalpinx, a TOA, or fluid or abscess in cul-de-sac. CT may be required in complicated cases (Fig. 6-47C).

Cloacal Malformation

Uncommonly (1 in 40,000 females), the rectum, vagina, and ureters may converge in the pelvis into a common outflow channel, the *cloaca* (Latin for "sewer"). This occurs if there is persistence of the cloacal membrane, which then interferes with normal closure of the anterior abdominal wall. Normal external genitalia are the rule. The anus is absent, because the rectum communicates with the often-septated vagina (cloaca). For diagnosis of cloacal malformation, the single perineal opening that is present is catheterized, and the anatomy is elucidated by injection of contrast material into the cloaca, which is then viewed in a lateral projection. Associated renal and spinal anomalies are common and can be screened for by US.

Ovarian Tumors

Benign ovarian teratomas (dermoid cysts) account for two thirds of pediatric ovarian tumors. The ovarian teratoma is the second most common after sacral teratoma. These tumors derive from totipotential cells, which then differentiate into ectodermal, mesodermal, and endodermal elements. This differentiation may go haywire, resulting in teratomas. The average age of the child at presentation is 6 to 11 years; the average diameter of these tumors is 10 cm, and they can be bilateral in 10% to 20% of patients. The most common presenting symptom is a mass, and 50% of children with ovarian tumors complain of pain. Abdominal radiographs show calcification in 50% of cases (Fig. 6-48). US demonstrates that two thirds of ovarian tumors are complex masses with both echogenic and cystic components. A mural nodule is characteristic and occurs in two thirds of cases. Fat-fluid levels may also be noted. CT and MRI may show calcifications of teeth or bone, hair, debris, or fat and may also demonstrate the mural nodule.

Malignant ovarian tumors, although rare, account for 35% of ovarian tumors in children. These malignant lesions can be of (1) the germ cell variety (85%; immature teratomas and dysgerminoma); (2) the stromal cell variety (10%; granulosa cell tumor, Sertoli-Leydig cell tumor); or (3) the epithelial cell variety (5%; cystadenocarcinoma). They usually come to clinical presentation in the postpubertal age group, are often large (more than 10 cm in diameter), and are mostly solid, although they may contain cystic areas caused by necrosis. Abdominal or pelvic pain is common. US is the initial imaging modality to determine the origin, size, and characteristics of the mass. Staging is better accomplished with CT or MRI.

Metastatic involvement of the ovaries is rare; lymphoma/leukemia and neuroblastoma have been reported.

Male Genitalia

Penile Urethra

The penile urethra and its abnormalities are usually evaluated on VCUG; they include a posterior urethral valve, strictures, and an anterior urethral valve (see Figs. 6-20 and 6-21). Strictures are postinflammatory or iatrogenic (after instrumentation) in origin.

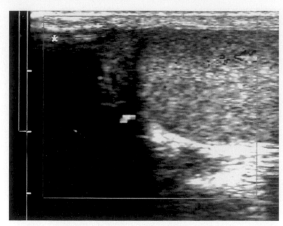

FIGURE 6-49. Normal testicular echogenicity and flow. See Plate 6 for color reproduction.

Scrotum

The scrotal contents consist of two testicles in 96% of all full-term male infants. Descent of testicles is related to birth weight, and only two thirds of premature infants have completed testicular descent at birth. Cryptorchidism (occurring in 10% of boys younger than 1 year) is a failure of descent, not a mechanical obstruction. Intra-abdominal location of undescended testes is uncommon; most (85%) lie within the inguinal canal. During the first year of life, 80% of cryptorchid testes in full-term neonates and 95% of cryptorchid testes in premature infants descend spontaneously to a normal scrotal position. The main concerns in cryptorchid testes are histologic changes, which can possibly lead to malignant transformation; they are shown not to occur before age 2 years. In boys older than 2 years, malignant degeneration in ectopic testes is 10 to 40 times more likely. Seminoma is the most common entity. To preserve fertility and prevent malignant change, some surgeons consider orchiopexy of the undescended testicle around age 2 years.

Total absence of one testis (1 in 5000) is four times as common as total testicular absence, and it usually occurs on the left side.

An imaging search for the undescended testicle usually involves US (90% specific and accurate) and MRI (more than 90% sensitive and specific).

US evaluation of the normal testis demonstrates an oval organ of uniform echogenicity (Fig. 6-49). The echogenic, linear mediastinum testis should be identified. Posteromedially, the epididymis is characterized as an echogenic structure adjacent to the testis. Measurements of the testes vary with age, ranging from 2 cm^3 in boys younger than 11 years, to 3 to 10 cm^3 in boys 12 to 14 years, to an average of 13 cm^3 in boys older than 14 years.

The imaging approach to scrotal pathology can be divided into two tiers: (1) painful scrotal mass, for which testicular nuclear scans reliably reveal torsion by demonstrating decreased flow to the affected testes, and color-flow Doppler US can reliably demonstrate epididymitis; and (2) painless scrotal mass, for which US is the imaging modality of choice to differentiate cystic from solid lesions.

Other infectious causes, such as mumps and coxsackievirus, are also common occurrences that can be associated with scrotal fluid, a reactive hydrocele. US findings vary and are often indistinguishable from those after scrotal or testicular trauma.

Scrotal Enlargement and Masses

Causes of a painless scrotal mass include hydrocele (with or without a hernia) and varicocele (dilatation of the pampiniform plexus of veins in the scrotum). Doppler US examination may show a venous flow pattern in the latter. Cysts or neoplasms of the spermatic cord may rarely occur. Testicular carcinoma is also rare, particularly in African-American and Asian boys.

Painful scrotal masses should be treated as torsion until proven otherwise. Torsion accounts for 20% of acute scrotal conditions. It is most common between the ages of 12 and 16 years, and the right side is affected more commonly than the left. The scrotum on physical examination is tender and swollen, and it does not transilluminate. Epididymitis, the main differential diagnostic consideration, is almost as common as testicular torsion and often is caused by *S. aureus*, *E. coli*, or *Chlamydia*.

The spermatic cord and testis should have demonstrable arterial flow on Doppler US imaging; the epididymis should not. Venous flow is difficult to appreciate in a testicle (Fig. 6-50).

Findings on color-flow Doppler US of the acute scrotum can be summarized as in Box 6-10. Overall US accuracy approaches 100%.

Because epididymitis and orchitis may be associated with urinary tract abnormalities, such as ectopic ureters, and can lead to abscess formation, further evaluation of the entire urinary tract with VCUG and US is needed.

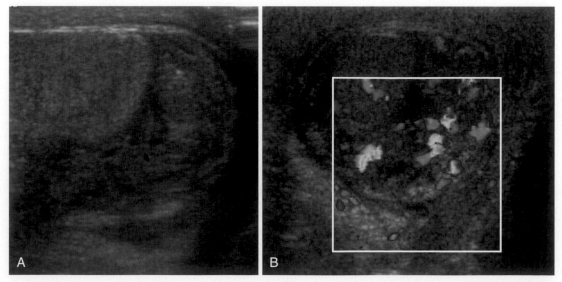

FIGURE 6-50. A, Color-flow Doppler US scan demonstrates increased flow (B) in the epididymis consistent with epididymitis. See Plate 7.

Neoplasms

About 80% of all testicular tumors in children are malignant. Clinically, such a tumor manifests as a painless, slowly enlarging testicular mass. About 25% have associated hydrocele. Two thirds of such tumors are of the germ cell variety; half of these are embryonal adenocarcinomas.

Embryonal adenocarcinoma (yolk-sac tumor or endodermal sinus tumor) is associated with high levels of seruma. Non–germ cell (Leydig cell) tumors manifest at around 4 years of age and are more common in African-American boys. Metastatic disease to the testis is seen in leukemia/lymphoma, neuroblastoma, and Ewing sarcoma. US examination is sensitive but not specific because it may show a variety of patterns, ranging from a diffuse decrease in echogenicity to an inhomogeneous parenchymal pattern.

■ ABDOMINAL MASSES (TABLE 6-5)

TABLE 6-5. Abdominal Masses

Type	Neonate	"Older Child"
Renal	Hydronephrosis Mesoblastic nephroma Cystic disease	Hydronephrosis Cystic disease Wilms tumor
Retroperitoneal	Adrenal hemorrhage Neuroblastoma	Neuroblastoma
Genital	Ovarian cyst or torsion Hydro(metro)colpos	Rhabdomyosarcoma of bladder or prostate Ovarian cyst, torsion, or mass Hematocolpos
Gastrointestinal	Malrotation/volvulus Meconium-related entities	Hypertrophic pyloric stenosis Inflammatory masses Duplication/cysts

■ SUGGESTED READINGS

TEXTS

Carty H, Shaw D, Brunelle F, et al (eds): Imaging Children, 1. London, Elsevier, 2005, pp 537-882 .

Dambro T, Stewart R, Carroll B: The scrotum. In Rumack C, Wilson S, Charboneau J (eds): Diagnostic Utrasound. St. Louis, Mosby, 1998, p 791.

Kirks DR (ed): Practical Pediatric Imaging, ed 3. Philadelphia, Lippincott-Raven, 1998, pp 1009-1171.

Kuhn JP, Slovis TL, In Haller JO (eds): Caffey's Pediatric X-Ray Diagnosis, ed 10, vol 1. Philadelphia, Elsevier, 2004, pp 186-264 1704-1987.

Skandalakis JE: In Gray SW (eds): Embryology for Surgeons, ed 2. Baltimore, Williams & Wilkins, 1994, pp 594-847.

Siegel MJ: Urinary tract. In Siegel MJ (ed): Pediatric Sonography, 3rd ed. Philadelphia, Lippincott/Williams & Wilkins, 2002, pp 385-473.

Siegel MJ: Female pelvis. In Siegel MJ (ed): Pediatric Sonography, 3rd ed. Philadelphia, Lippincott/Williams & Wilkins, 2002, pp 530-577.

Siegel MJ: Male genital tract. In Siegel MJ (ed): Pediatric Sonography, 3rd ed. Philadelphia, Lippincott/Williams & Wilkins, 2002, pp 579-624.

Taybi H, Lachman RS: Radiology of Syndromes. Metabolic Disorders, and Skeletal Dysplasias, ed 4. St Louis, Mosby-Year Book, 1996.

ARTICLES

Practice Parameter: The diagnosis, treatment, and evaluation of the initial urinary tract infection in febrile infants and young children. American Academy of Pediatrics, Committee on Quality Improvement, Subcommitee on Urinary Tract Infection. Pediatrics 1999;103:845.

Blickman JG: Pediatric urinary tract infection: Imaging techniques with special reference to voiding cystourethrography [doctoral thesis]. Rotterdam, 1991, Pasmans, The Hague, Netherlands.

Frush DP, Kliewer MA, Madden JF: Testicular microlithiasis and tumor risk in a population referred for scrotal US. AJR Am J Roentgenol 200;175:1703.

Karmazin B, Steinberg R, Korwreich L, et al: Clinical and sonographic criteria of the acute scrotum in children. Pediatr Radiol 2005;35:302.

Lonergan GJ, Martinez-Leon MI, Agrons GA, et al: Nephrogenic rest, nephroblastomatosis and associated lesions of the kidney. Radiographics 1998;18:947.

Lowe LH, Isuani BH, Heller RM, et al: Pediatric renal masses: Wilms' tumor and beyond. Radiographics 2000;20:1585.

McHugh K, Pritchard J: Problems in the imaging of three common paediatric solid tumours. Eur J Radiol 2001;37:72.

Patriquin H, Robitaille P: Renal calcium deposition in children: Sonographic demonstration of Anderson-Carr progression. AJR Am J Roentgenol 1986; 146: 1253.

Riccabona M, Simbrunner J, Ring E, et al: Feasability of MR urography in neonates and infants with anomalies of the upper urinary tract. Eur Radiol 2002; 12:1442.

Stalker HP, Kaufman RA, Stedje K: The significance of hematuria in children after blunt abdominal trauma. AJR Am J Roentgenol 1990;154:569.

Taylor GA: Assessing the impact of imaging information on clinical management and decision making in pediatric blunt trauma. Pediatr Radiol 1998;28:63.

Woodward PJ, Sohaey R, O'Donoghue MJ, et al: From the archives of the AFIP: Tumors and tumorlike lesions of the testis: Radiologic-pathologic correlation. Radiographics 2002;22:189.

CHAPTER 7

Skeletal System

Johan G. (Hans) Blickman and Geert Vanderschueren

■ IMAGING TECHNIQUES

Radiography

Conventional radiographs depict the bony density of the skeletal system quite adequately and remain the mainstay in the evaluation of musculoskeletal disease. Adequate evaluation by means of conventional radiographs must include imaging in at least two perpendicular directions. Oblique projections are useful in certain instances, whereas comparison views need be obtained only if there is confusion between a suspected abnormality and a possible normal variant.

Tomography

Computed tomography (CT), as well as conventional tomography in limited instances, is indicated in certain anatomic regions (e.g., the sternoclavicular joint for CT, the ankle for conventional tomography) to better delineate the extent of a bony lesion (e.g., stress or comminuted fractures, metastatic and primary bone lesions) and in preoperative and postoperative imaging. The reformatting and three-dimensional reconstruction capability and the superior visualization of trauma, the casted skeleton, and complex osseous structures are the most useful attributes of CT imaging. Spiral CT has allowed for faster throughput of patients and superior reconstruction capabilities—that is, better images.

The combination of CT with positron emission tomography (PET) either with image fusion algorithms or as a stand-alone in-line combination provides co-registered morphologic and functional data that holds great promise, particularly in malignant osseous disease.

Magnetic Resonance Imaging

Magnetic resonance imaging (MRI) has established itself as an excellent modality for directly imaging the bone marrow, joints, cartilaginous structures, and soft tissues. The extent and architecture of a tumor, the degree of vascular compromise, and intraosseous medullary involvement of bone lesions are best depicted by this modality. Positioning, surface coils, and slice thickness (thin slices give better resolution) are obviously important. Proton density sequences are less useful; T1-weighted sequences best assess marrow and fat, and edema is best depicted on short T1 inversion recovery (STIR) or T2-weighted sequences. Whole-body MR imaging has been shown to be of use in metastatic disease detection and follow-up as well as in cases of suspected child abuse (trauma X).

Ultrasonography

Ultrasonography (US) interacts with the skeletal system primarily in the evaluation of the neonatal hip but also the elbow and knee. With its Doppler capability, US is also used in the evaluation of soft tissue abnormalities, vascular anatomy, and potential complications of osteomyelitis. Best results are obtained with the use of linear transducers. This modality is used with more frequency outside the United States, being employed before MR imaging (see later).

Radionuclide Scintigraphy

Radionuclide scintigraphy remains the primary screening modality in the detection of osteomyelitis, metastatic bone lesions, and any disorder that may affect different portions of the skeleton (e.g., nonaccidental trauma in children older than 2 years). Agents used are technetium Tc 99m methylene diphosphonate (MDP) and, increasingly, indium In 111–labeled white blood cells and gallium Ga 67 citrate, although PET scanning with fluorine 18–labeled deoxyglucose (fluorodeoxyglucose; FDG) has become an efficient modality to localize bony lesion of a metastatic or infectious (i.e., glucose "eating") nature.

Arthrography

Arthrography of the double- or single-contrast variety—that is, the imaging of joints—has been replaced by MRI in most situations. CT arthrography plays a role in the detection of rotator cuff disease and labral disease in adults. Because sports injuries increase in incidence in the pediatric age group, and for osteochondral lesions of the shoulder, MRI would be preferred, not only because of the relative invasiveness of CT arthrography (needle puncture required) but also because of the vastly improved access to MRI.

■ NORMAL DEVELOPMENT AND VARIANTS

Bone is actually a constant balanced process of bone formation and resorption. Bone develops by intramembranous mesenchymal ossification (clavicle, skull, mandible/maxilla) or by enchondral or indirect conversion of cartilage to bone, and sometimes both (extremities, vertebral column).

This complex process is quite evident on imaging studies of the growing skeleton. Appreciation of the temporal sequences of these processes, as well as the effect of a variety of factors on them, is the main thrust of this chapter.

Normal Development

Skeletal structures are made up of four parts: the physis, or growth plate, and the *epiphysis*, *metaphysis*, and *diaphysis*. Each long bone (humerus, tibia) has a physis and thus metaphyses and epiphyses on either end. Each short tubular bone (metatarsal, metacarpal) has a physis, metaphysis, and epiphysis on one end only, they are located at the site of the greater joint motion.

In the fetus, primary ossification centers appear during the eighth and ninth weeks in the centers of the embryonal mesenchymal segments that become bone. This enchondral bone formation causes elongation and ossification of each bone. A secondary ossification center appears in the epiphysis after birth, and the appearance of the subsequent ossification process can range from solid to irregular and uneven when seen on radiographs or CT.

Remodeling (tubulation) of the shaft occurs concurrently with the increase in length and width of the bone and may be altered by any pathology that impedes that process.

An *apophysis* is defined as an ossification center at the end of, or on a protrusion from, a bone where a tendon inserts. It is usually located perpendicular to the bone, does not contribute to linear growth of the bone, and does not form an articular surface.

The secondary ossification center that appears earliest often fuses last. The relative contributions to bone length in the upper extremity reveal that the distal radius and proximal humerus grow the fastest and the elbow the slowest. In the lower extremity, this is particularly evident around the knee; the distal femur and the proximal tibia grow the fastest; the fibula is slowest. Overall, skeletal maturation generally occurs from proximal to distal.

Accessory Ossicles

Accessory ossicles are defined as accessory ossification centers; they are not always bilateral, and they may be the cause of pain. Conversely, a traumatic origin is also suggested, and many show uptake on scintigraphy.

An example is a bipartite patella. The division between parts of the patella is located in its superolateral portion, appears between 10 and 12 years of age, may persist into adult life, and is bilateral in about 40% of cases. Other common accessory ossicles are the accessory navicular and the os trigonum. These also appear around 10 to 12 years of age, are more commonly bilateral, and eventually fuse with their adjacent bones. False ossification centers (*pseudoepiphyses*) are seen in the proximal aspects of metacarpals or metatarsals II through V and in the distal aspect of the first metacarpal or metatarsal. Histologically a physis is not identified, so pseudoepiphysis is thus thought to be a radiographic finding only. These entities may originate from osteogenic tissue in continuity with the shaft. More commonly seen in cleidocranial dysostosis and hypothyroidism, they contribute little or nothing to linear growth (Fig. 7-1).

Sesamoid bones, named from their similarity in shape to sesame seeds, lie within the insertion of tendons. They articulate with the volar surface of the adjacent bony structure. These bones save on the wear and tear of joints, tendons, and ligaments because they ameliorate the tension on the tendons. The largest sesamoid in the body, the patella, as well as other sesamoids, may be bipartite or tripartite, an appearance that may occur bilaterally in 50% of patients. Other than the patella, sesamoid bones around the knee are the fabella (sesamoid in the lateral head of the gastrocnemius muscle) and the cyamella (located in the head of the popliteal muscle). Other sesamoids are most common in flexor tendons around the first and second rays of the feet and hands. They may ossify irregularly.

Upper Extrlemities

In the upper extremities, the proximal humeral ossification center usually ossifies between 38 and 42 weeks' gestational age. Therefore failure to identify this ossification in a neonate is no help; however, if the center *is* present, the infant has reached term. The proximal humeral ossification center has two parts, and the secondary proximal humeral growth center becomes radiographically visible around 1 year of age.

The multiple secondary ossification centers of the elbow can create confusion and may be difficult to differentiate from fractures in a trauma setting. The multiple secondary ossification centers, listed in order of the mnemonic CRITOE, are *c*apitellum, *r*adial head, *i*nternal or medial epicondyle, *t*rochlea, *o*lecranon, and *e*xternal or lateral epicondyle. Ossification of these centers occurs sequentially in boys at approximately 1, 3, 5, 7, and 9 years of age, respectively; in girls, each ossification occurs 6 to 9 months earlier (Fig. 7-2). In a trauma setting, a bony structure at or near any of these sites at an earlier stage than expected may represent a (avulsion) fracture. In such an instance, comparison views are often useful.

The distal radial epiphysis usually appears at around 2 years of age, the distal ulnar epiphysis at about 6 years of age.

The apophysis of the acromion and the coracoid processes of the scapula are evident within 6 months of birth and fuse during adolescence. Their well-ossified edges usually differentiate them from avulsion fractures. The last epiphysis to close is the medial clavicular epiphysis at the sternal notch, which is always closed after age 20 years (Fig. 7-3).

Lower Extremities

In almost all children, the earliest epiphysis to ossify is the distal femur, at birth. The head of the femur shows an ossification center at about 4 months of life. It may be irregular, and before fusing with the metaphyses, it may flatten somewhat. The centers for the proximal fibula and the patella often do not ossify until 5 years of age. The most striking epiphysis/physis is that of the proximal tibia on a lateral view. The anterior tibial tubercle "teardrop" reflects the differential growths of the main proximal tibial ossification center and the tubercle; it may be quite irregular in appearance (Fig. 7-4). Radiographic confirmation of the normal tubercle, however irregular, as opposed to Osgood-Schlatter disease, requires identification of the (infra) patellar tendon in its entire sharp course along the fat pad of Hoffa.

Secondary ossification centers can be confused occasionally with fractures, especially at the lesser trochanter, ischium, and base of the fifth metatarsal. To make matters even more difficult, scintigraphy is of little value because these centers generally

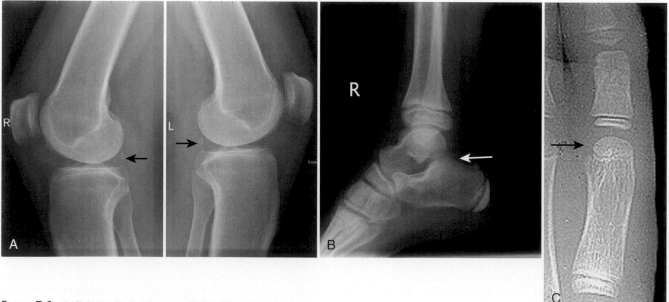

FIGURE 7-1. **A,** Fabella. **B,** Os trigonum. **C,** Pseudoepiphyses *(arrows)*.

show radionuclide uptake owing to normal bone growth. A diagnosis of an undisplaced fracture at these locations is made on the basis of clinical findings (presence of pain and/or soft tissue swelling). Thankfully, displacement frequently occurs in association with fracture. In addition, the apophysis of the fifth metatarsal is parallel to the long axis of the fifth metatarsal. A

fracture of the base of the fifth metatarsal is usually perpendicular to the long axis of the bone (Fig. 7-5).

The hamstrings are attached to the ischial apophysis; thus avulsion may occur in gymnasts or hurdlers. The lesser trochanter is the site of attachment of the iliopsoas tendon. Blood or pus can track down this muscle and affect the bony appearance. The anterior inferior iliac spine may be pulled off by excessive force on the rectus femoris (see Fig. 7-3B) or the sartorius muscle.

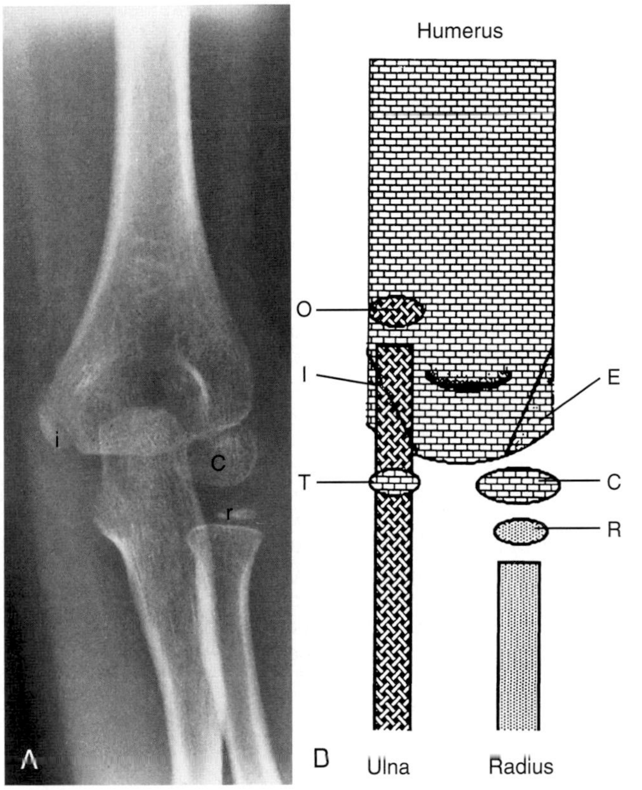

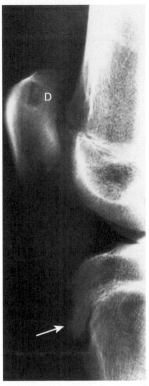

FIGURE 7-2. **A,** Anteroposterior radiograph of the elbow of a 5-year-old girl; C, capitellum; r, radius; i, medial epicondyle. **B,** CRITOE (capitellum, radial head, internal or medial epicondyle, trochlea, olecranon, and external or lateral epicondyle) mnemonic.

FIGURE 7-4. Lateral radiograph of the knee demonstrates a dorsal defect of the patella (D). Note the normal "teardrop" shape of the anterior tibial tubercle *(arrow)*.

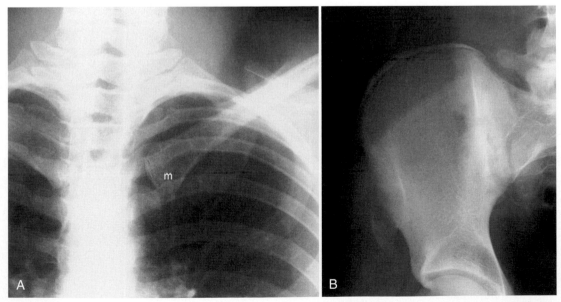

FIGURE 7-3. **A,** AP radiograph of the clavicle shows the last epiphysis to close (after age 20 years): the medial epiphysis (m). **B,** AP radiograph of the pelvis shows the last apophysis to close (around 24 years of age): the iliac crest. Note the avulsion fracture at the anterior inferior iliac spine.

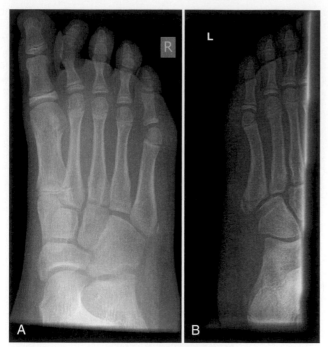

Figure 7-5. **A,** Normal apophysis at base of fifth metatarsal. **B,** Fracture.

Normal Variants

"Normal" Periosteal New Bone

The "normal" periosteal new bone of the newborn is seen in about 50% of all infants younger than 6 months. A result of relatively rapid growth during this time (Fig. 7-6), it is characterized by a thin, smooth layer of new bone paralleling the diaphysis of the humerus and radius as well as the femora. The bone itself is often dense and appears sclerotic; this appearance is due to the combined factors of cortical thickening, a normal medullary canal, and dense spongiosa bone. This finding disappears in the first weeks to months of life. The differential diagnosis of this normal variant includes osteomyelitis, Caffey disease, hypervitaminosis A, metastatic leukemia, or metastatic neuroblastoma,

although the medullary canal often is not normal in the last two instances (owing to the presence of pathologic marrow invasion). In premature infants treated with prostaglandins and those suffering from a TORCH (*t*oxoplasmosis, *o*ther [congenital syphilis and viruses], *r*ubella, *c*ytomegalovirus, and *h*erpes simplex virus) infection, this finding may also occur.

"Physiologic" Sclerosis

In children younger than 6 years, "physiologic" sclerosis is often present at the zone of provisional calcification (ZPC) of each metaphysis, particularly at the "fast" bone ends. This band is often difficult to distinguish from one caused by heavy metal (lead) intoxication or syphilis. "Lead" bands, because of inhibition of osteoclasts at the ZPC, consist of broader dense bands that are also noted in the slow-growing metaphyses such as the proximal fibulae. This feature helps distinguish them from the physiologic sclerosis and syphilis that primarily affect metabolically "fast" metaphyses (radius, tibia) (Fig. 7-6B).

Epiphyses

"*Ivory*" *epiphyses* are sclerotic-appearing epiphyseal variants seen most commonly in the distal phalanges and occasionally in the middle ones. The ratio of occurrence is 1 in 300 children. If they manifest elsewhere, epiphyseal dysplasia is suggested (Fig. 7-7A).

Cone-shaped epiphyses can be normal in 5% to 10% of children and are more common in such osteochondrodysplasias as achondroplasia, Ellis–van Creveld syndrome, cleidocranial dysostosis, and hereditary renal disease, which slow skeletal growth.

Fissures of the ossification centers, especially of the hallux (big toe), must not be mistaken for fractures (Fig. 7-7B).

Fissures and increased density are always noted in the calcaneal apophysis, which appears in children around 7 years of age. It is the result of the irregular coalescence of multiple ossification centers, which fuse in the middle teenage years. The incorporated apophysis then assumes the same density as the remainder of the calcaneus.

Supracondylar Process of the Humerus

A supracondylar process of the humerus is seen in approximately 1% of patients. It consists of an anteriorly projecting bony spur about 5 cm above the medial epicondyle. It is normally found in cats and other lower mammalian species. This process, which

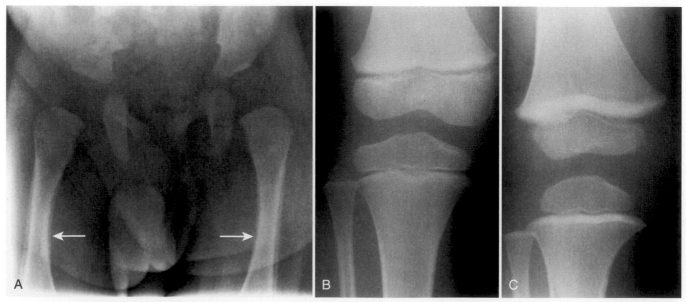

Figure 7-6. **A,** Normal newborn periosteal new bone formation. **B,** Normal "physiologic" sclerosis. **C,** "Lead" bands. Note the dense fibular metaphysis. There is also irregular ossification of the medial distal femoral epiphysis, a normal variant.

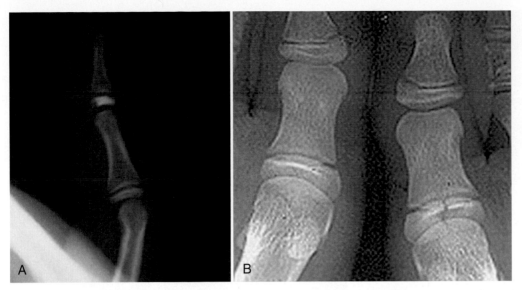

FIGURE 7-7. **A,** An "ivory" epiphysis. **B,** A "split" epiphysis.

rarely causes median nerve and/or brachial artery compression, may be palpable and may fracture.

"Air Vacuum" Phenomenon

In an immobilized patient, particularly when moderate to strong traction is applied to the shoulder, hip, knees, or ankles, an "air vacuum" phenomenon may occur. Negative *intra-articular* pressure allows mainly nitrogen gas to dissolve out of neighboring tissues into the joint space. The inability to elicit this crescent of air has been used to indicate the presence of joint effusions. This air vacuum sign is not very specific, however (Fig. 7-8A).

"Lucent" Anatomic Areas

"Lucent" anatomic areas consist of several "pseudocysts" that are due to composite shadows produced by the trabecular pattern (and thus normal), including the greater tuberosity of the

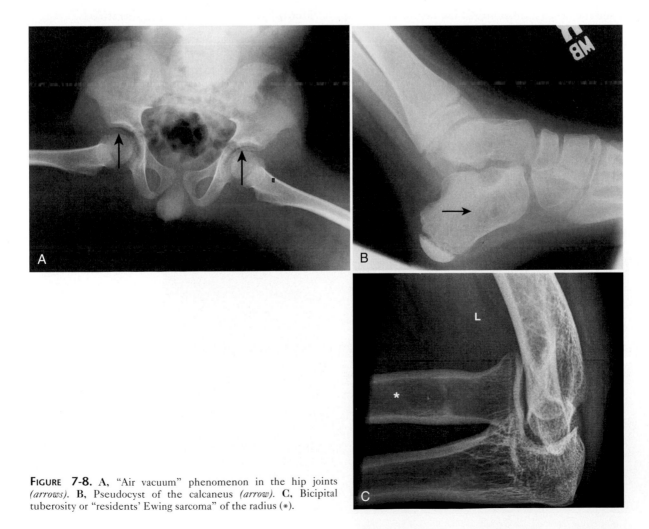

FIGURE 7-8. **A,** "Air vacuum" phenomenon in the hip joints *(arrows).* **B,** Pseudocyst of the calcaneus *(arrow).* **C,** Bicipital tuberosity or "residents' Ewing sarcoma" of the radius (∗).

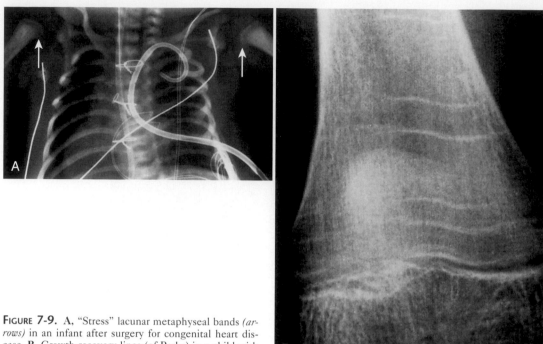

FIGURE 7-9. A, "Stress" lacunar metaphyseal bands *(arrows)* in an infant after surgery for congenital heart disease. B, Growth recovery lines (of Parks) in a child with cystic fibrosis and repeated bouts of pulmonary infection.

humerus and the bicipital tuberosity of the radius, as well as in the body of the calcaneus. These "cysts" are caused by an area of relatively sparse trabecula in comparison with the normal trabeculae around it (Fig. 7-8B and C).

The metaphysis may develop a lucent metaphyseal band as a result of "stress," such as prematurity, cyanotic congenital heart disease (CHD), or early scurvy. It is thought that blood flow and its resultant calcification function are slowed as blood flow is "diverted" to other parts of the body. When this stress is relieved, bone growth resumes, as evidenced by the growth "recovery" (or "arrest") line of Park (Fig. 7-9). Such lines fade into normal mineralization over months to years, from medial to lateral.

Metaphyseal Cortical Irregularities

A step-off, a spur, and a beak are common findings around the knee and wrist that must be differentiated from the classic findings of the "bucket handle" fracture characteristic of child abuse as well as from malignant bone lesions (e.g., Ewing sarcoma) (Fig. 7-10). These irregularities are frequently seen as cortical indistinctness, particularly on the dorsal and medial aspects of the distal femur and on the medial aspect of the distal fibula; they may also be seen proximally and distally in the humerus as well as in the distal radius. Each probably represents a projection and/or angulation of the cortex in the metaphysis and will disappear as the child grows.

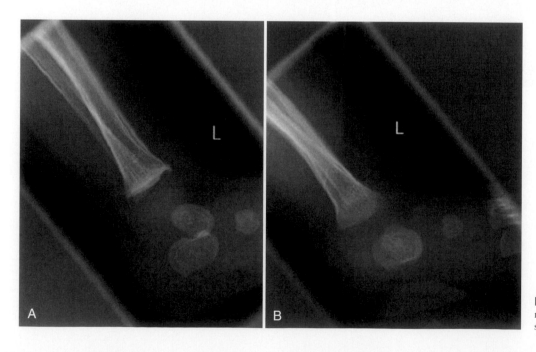

FIGURE 7-10. A, Metaphyseal irregularity. B, Bucket-handle tear in suspected child abuse (trauma X).

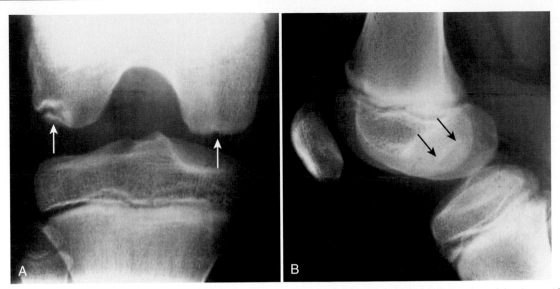

FIGURE 7-11. Irregular ossification. Tunnel view (**A**) demonstrates pseudo–osteochondritis dissecans of both femoral condyles *(arrows)* in a posterior, non–weight-bearing location *(arrows)* (**B**).

Irregular Ossification

Ossification is not a smooth, uninterrupted process. The radiographic result of irregular ossification is often seen in the lateral epicondyle of the distal humerus, as well as in the trochlea, and also at the medial and (less so) lateral edges of the distal femur.

Similar ossification irregularities of the more central portion of the distal femoral epiphysis can best be appreciated on the tunnel projection because they are located posteriorly. These findings must be differentiated from osteochondritis dissecans (Fig. 7-11).

Dorsal Defect of the Patella

A *dorsal defect of the patella* is an anomaly of ossification that is almost always located on the superolateral aspect of its dorsal surface. It manifests as a well-defined, round lucency with intact overlying articular cartilage (see Fig. 7-4). The differential diagnosis includes osteomyelitis and chondroblastoma as well as Langerhans cell histiocytosis (LCH) and osteomyelitis.

Fibrous Cortical Defect

Benign fibrous cortical defects (nonossifying fibromas) are most commonly seen in the distal femur and proximal tibia, appearing in children between 2 and 6 years of age. Occurring rarely before age 2 years and at tendinous insertions (of the adductor most commonly), they may be related to avulsive cortical forces during the learning process of walking and weight-bearing. These defects tend to disappear with age, but they may become quite large and may be complicated by fracture. They are distinctly uncommon in the upper extremities (Fig. 7-12).

▬ CONGENITAL ABNORMALITIES

Skeletal Dysplasias

Skeletal dysplasias are defined as congenital disturbances of bone growth, structure, and modeling. Shortening of the limbs or spine below the third percentile for a normal newborn constitutes congenital dwarfism.

Short stature can be symmetric or asymmetric. Symmetric short stature includes short-limb, short-trunk, and proportionate dwarfism.

Short-limb dwarfism is subdivided into rhizomelic, mesomelic, and acromelic categories. In *rhizomelia*, the proximal appendicular skeleton (the humeri and femora) is most severely shortened.

Mesomelia affects the middle skeletal segments (radius-ulna; tibia-fibula). In acromelia, the distal portions of the appendicular skeleton (metacarpals-phalanges; metatarsals-phalanges) are most severely involved.

Short-trunk dwarfism can be evident in a neonate as fatal achondrogenesis. In a surviving infant it manifests as metaphyseal chondrodysplasia, and in developing children as mucopolysaccharidosis, mucolipidosis, or spondyloepiphyseal dysplasia.

Proportionate short stature can vary from normal to being a sequela of systemic conditions, cleidocranial dysplasia, or osteopetrosis.

Asymmetric short stature includes osteogenesis imperfecta, multiple cartilaginous exostoses, and diaphyseal aclasis.

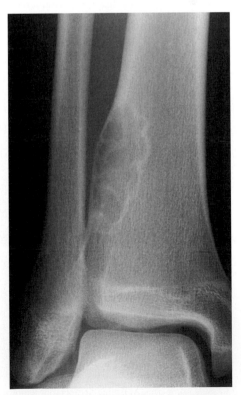

FIGURE 7-12. Typical appearance of a fibrous cortical defect.

The approach to diagnosis should start with a careful physical examination.

The skeletal images should minimally include:

- Anteroposterior (AP) and lateral views of the skull
- AP and lateral views of the entire spine
- AP view of the thorax; can include AP thoracic spine
- AP view of the pelvis/hips
- AP view of one entire upper limb, including hand
- AP view of one entire lower limb

Only after these views have been obtained can a systematic approach be undertaken to diagnosis and the assessment of prognosis.

Short-Limb Dwarfism

Rhizomelic Dwarfism

Noted at birth, *thanatophoric* (Gr. "death-bearing") dwarfism is a fatal condition in which the clinical and radiologic features differ from those of achondroplasia only in severity, especially in the ribs. The limb shortening predominantly affects the proximal segments (humeri, femora) of the extremities. In a surviving short-limbed dwarf, achondroplasia is the most common cause. Autosomal dominant (AD) inheritance is noted in both. The clinical features consist of shortening and bowing of the extremities with profound lumbar lordosis as well as an enlarged cranium with frontal bossing, a sunken nasal root, and prognathism. Knee pain is a common complaint. Key imaging findings are located in the spine and pelvis. In the spine they consist of narrow interpedicular (from *inter-pediculate*, "between lice") distances, posterior vertebral body scalloping, decreased vertebral body height (flattening), and short pedicles—all resulting in a narrow spinal canal and a thoracolumbar kyphosis. The ribs are short and broad. Characteristic findings in the pelvis include hypoplastic "square" iliac bones; the "champagne glass" pelvic inlet caused by small sacroiliac notches; and wide triradiate cartilages (Fig. 7-13). The bowed femora resemble old-fashioned telephone receivers.

A milder form of rhizomelic dwarfism, called *hypochondroplasia*, manifests in late childhood and demonstrates more subtle findings of achondroplasia. Clinically, the characteristic facies of achondroplasia are often not seen; radiographically, the features of achondroplasia are present in a milder form.

Mesomelic Shortening

Mesomelic shortening affects the middle segments (radius, ulna, tibia, and fibula) of the extremities. This often fatal form consists of *camptomelic* ("bent bones") dwarfism, which probably has an autosomal recessive (AR) mode of inheritance. Clinically, there is striking symmetric anterolateral bowing of the lower extremities with pretibial dimples. This disorder is further characterized by an enlarged cranium, micrognathia, cleft palate, and low-set ears. Diagnostic radiographic findings are tibial bowing, hypoplastic scapular wings (not spines), and absence of the thoracic pedicles. The tibial bowing can also be detected on antenatal US.

The vertebral bodies are normal. In addition, dislocated hips, kyphoscoliosis, and 11 pairs of ribs are often seen. Other severe forms of mesomelic dysplasia, characterized as dyschondrosteoses, are Cornelia de Lange syndrome and the Nievergelt and Langer types of limb shortening. AD entities occurring in girls are characterized by bilateral Madelung deformity—growth retardation of the medial portion of the distal radial growth plate, with resultant shortening and ulnar deviation of the radius causing ulnar deformity and occasional synostosis (Fig. 7-14). This deformity may also occur after trauma to or infection of the radius, as well as occasionally with multiple cartilaginous exostoses, enchondromatosis, and Turner syndrome, and in the mucopolysaccharidoses. It is more commonly bilateral and asymmetric than unilateral.

Acromelic Shortening

Acromelic shortening affects the distal segments of the extremities as well as the metacarpals, metatarsals, and phalanges. This entity is best exemplified by asphyxiating thoracic dystrophy (Jeune syndrome), a form of short-limb dwarfism that is usually fatal and inherited as an AR trait. Clinically, affected infants present with respiratory distress (short ribs resulting in a narrow tubular chest), with shortening of the tubular bones in the hands and feet, and polydactyly in up to one third of patients. Prenatal polyhydramnios is common, and frequent pulmonary infections, renal failure, and hypertension develop after birth. Radiographic findings feature the long and narrow chest as well as flattened acetabular angles and osseous spurs projecting interiorly from the medial and lateral aspects of the acetabula (trident acetabulum) (Fig. 7-15). Similar findings in surviving acromelic infants

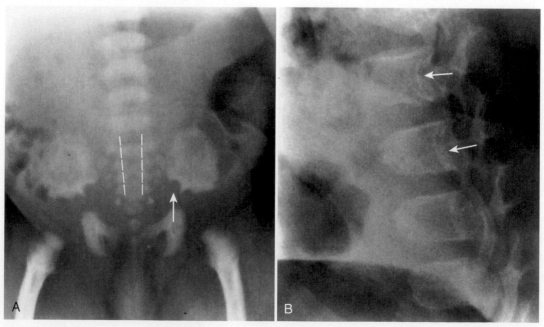

Figure 7-13. Achondroplasia. **A,** Frontal radiograph demonstrates tapering interpedicular distances (*dotted lines*), small sacroiliac notches (*arrows*), and wide acetabula. **B,** Lateral radiograph of the lumbar spine shows posterior scalloping (*arrows*).

are known as *chondroectodermal dysplasia* (Ellis–van Creveld syndrome, a triad of dwarfism, ectodermal dysplasia, and polydactyly). This condition has an AR mode of inheritance and manifests clinically as hypoplastic brittle nails, thin, sparse hair (including eyebrows, and eyelashes), and polydactyly on the ulnar aspects of the hands. There is associated CHD, most commonly an atrial or ventricular septal defect, in two thirds of patients. This syndrome is particularly common in the Amish community. Additional radiographic findings are wormian bones; the short bones, small thorax, and atrial or ventricular septal can be noted on prenatal US.

Another acromelic dwarf variant in surviving infants is referred to as *pyknodysostosis*. It is characterized by generalized osteosclerosis, short stature, short, broad hands, and bones that fracture

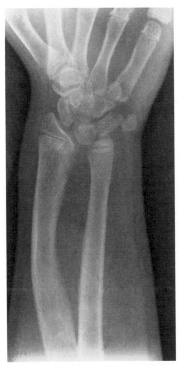

FIGURE 7-14. Madelung deformity. Shortening and ulnar deviation of the radius cause mild ulnar deformity (bowing). Carpal bones have wedged into the resulting V of the radius and ulna.

frequently. It is inherited as an AR trait. Clinically, there may be delayed closure of the anterior fontanelle in an enlarged cranium, bulging eyes, and a parrot-like nose as well as a receding chin. Radiography shows striking generalized osteosclerosis with multiple fractures of varying age. There may be multiple wormian bones and hypoplastic facial bones. Short phalanges of fingers and toes with hypoplastic terminal phalanges are common (Fig. 7-16). French artist Toulouse-Lautrec is said to have been affected by this variant.

Asymmetric Short Stature

Asymmetric short limbs may be seen in a form of multiple epiphyseal dysplasia called *chondrodysplasia punctata* (stippled epiphyses), which manifests at birth. There are two forms, an AR rhizomelic (symmetric and fatal) form and an AD (nonrhizomelic, asymmetric, and milder, nonlethal) form, the latter known as the Conradi-Hünermann variety. Mental retardation and facial features resembling those of achondroplasia are the clinical hallmarks, along with contractures of the extremities, cataracts, and long, delicate fingers. Transient calcifications in the skeletal and respiratory cartilage are the imaging hallmarks. Stippled epiphyses may also be seen in the gangliosidoses and in cretinism, fetal warfarin syndrome, and trisomy 18 (Fig. 7-17).

Nonspecific Short-Limb Dwarfism

Nonspecific short-limb dwarfism is best illustrated by osteogenesis imperfecta (OI), an inherited disorder of connective tissue (specifically, faulty collagen formation). Currently, gene probes have elucidated mutations in genes that regulate collagen formation and result in defective conversion of reticulum fibers to adult collagen fibers. This condition was classically divided into an AR lethal form (congenital, 10%) and an AD form (*tarda* ["late"], 90%) with a normal life expectancy. The former was characterized by thickened tubular bones resulting from multiple healing fractures, whereas the latter was characterized by thin tubular bones. Of the four clinical criteria—blue sclerae, fragile bones, otosclerosis, and poor teeth—the presence of two confirms the diagnosis.

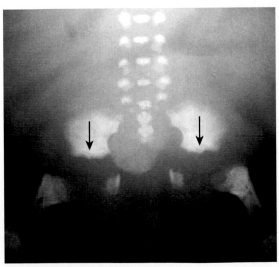

FIGURE 7-15. Trident acetabulum (Ellis–van Creveld syndrome and Jeune syndrome [asphyxiating thoracic dystrophy]) *(arrows)*.

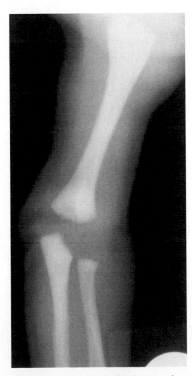

FIGURE 7-16. Pyknodysostosis: generalized osteosclerosis with multiple fractures.

Currently, four types of OI are recognized, as follows (Fig. 7-18):

Type I: Clinically, OI type I manifests in late teenage years as blue sclerae and occasional deafness (otosclerosis); it is AD-inherited with variable penetrance, and the most common form. This, previously known as the "tarda" form, is characterized by thin, brittle bones that fracture repeatedly. The fractures heal with exuberant callus formation, resultant skeletal bowing, and epiphyseal enlargement. In this progressive affliction beginning in infancy or early childhood, the rate of limb fractures decreases by the early teenage years. Other clinical hallmarks are blue sclerae, a small triangular face, and a bulging skull. Deafness due to otosclerosis may develop uncommonly. Radiographically, a progressive kyphoscoliosis (40%) is noted, wormian bones are present, and multiple (healing) fractures are noted in gracile, osteopenic bones. Medullary rods may be needed to splint these bones.

Type II: OI type II is the lethal, previously known as "congenital," form that can be recognized on prenatal US from findings of multiple fractures, demineralized calvaria, and a femur length more than 3 standard deviations (SD) below the mean for gestational age. Most infants with this form are born prematurely, and many are stillborn; in addition, blue sclerae are always present. Type II has AR inheritance. There are three subgroups, A, B, and C, which are distinguished most easily on the basis of broad, beaded, and stippled ribs, respectively; all of these rib findings are thought to be sequelae of fracture healing in utero.

Type III: OI type III features blue-gray sclerae, deafness, and progressive deformity of the limbs. Two thirds of affected infants present at birth with fractures that have a great deal of callus formation. OI type III is known as the severe deforming type.

Type IV: OI type IV is characterized by normal sclerae, by absence of wormian bones but presence of variable skeletal involvement consisting of osteoporosis and occasional fractures, and by the presence of discolored teeth.

OI has an equal gender incidence and no race predilection. Intramedullary rods correct bowing deformities and strengthen the bone to avoid new fractures.

The differential diagnosis of the imaging findings includes nonaccidental trauma, congenital insensitivity to pain, hypophosphatasia, and juvenile osteoporosis.

The most common limb-shortening syndromes are summarized in Box 7-1. Bowed bones occur in camptomelic dwarfs and in patients with OI, and occasionally in thanatophoric dwarfs.

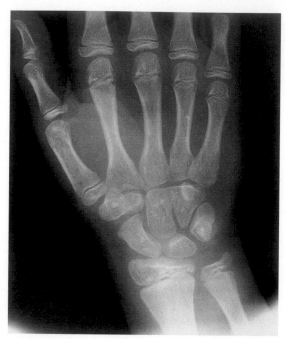

FIGURE 7-17. Stippled epiphyses—also seen in cretinism, fetal warfarin syndrome, and trisomy 18—in a child with asymmetric short stature.

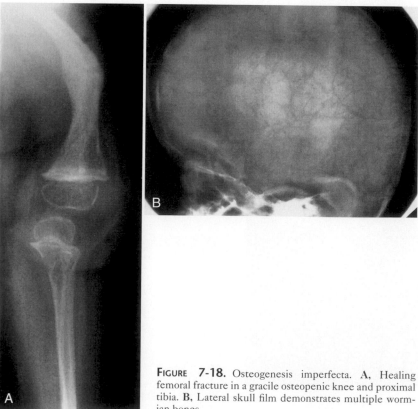

FIGURE 7-18. Osteogenesis imperfecta. **A,** Healing femoral fracture in a gracile osteopenic knee and proximal tibia. **B,** Lateral skull film demonstrates multiple wormian bones.

In summary, key points to assess whether dwarfism may be present according to imaging criteria include the pelvic and vertebral body shape; interpedicular distance; rib anatomy; and the prenatal US finding of polyhydramnios, short or bowed limbs, fracture or a thin calvaria.

Short-Trunk Dwarfism

Short-trunk dwarfism is the major manifestation of metaphyseal chondrodysplasias. The most severe, achondrogenesis, manifests as severe *micromelia* (shortening of proximal and distal limb portions), a large head, and neonatal death. In surviving infants, there are four types with decreasing levels of severity. Affected infants have severe micromelia, a large head, and bowed limbs. Decreased limb length can be diagnostic on prenatal US. On conventional radiographs, in types Jansen and Smid, both with AD inheritance, irregular metaphyses and widened growth plates are seen. The AR inheritance types, McKusick and the Shwachman-Diamond syndrome (associated with pancreatic exocrine insufficiency), are characterized by epiphyseal flattening and an irregular ZPC, as well as metaphyseal irregularity. Rarer forms of short-trunk dwarfism are Kniest dysplasia and spondylometaphyseal dysplasia (Kozlowski type), both with AD inheritance. Radiographic findings include platyspondyly, which is frequently associated with coronal clefts and anterior wedging. These characteristic vertebral anomalies are often associated with kyphosis, lordosis, or scoliosis. The metaphyses are irregular, and ossification of the epiphyses may be delayed.

Developing later in childhood, the mucopolysaccharidoses have skeletal findings that have been termed *dysostosis multiplex*. The abnormality of mucopolysaccharide or glycoprotein metabolism (incomplete degradation and resultant abnormal storage) manifests radiographically as osteopenia and as an enlarged cranium with a thick calvaria, poorly developed sinuses, and a J-shaped sella (difficult to appreciate today because the performance of skull films has all but ceased); anteroinferiorly beaked, oval vertebral bodies at the thoracolumbar junction (Fig. 7-19); dysplastic capital femoral epiphyses; and short, wide metacarpals and phalanges (hands).

The second through fifth rays of the hand tend to taper proximally, possibly resulting in a clawlike hand deformity. Clinically, knowledge of the patient's age, intelligence level, and the presence of urinary acid mucopolysaccharides is paramount for accurate diagnosis. Hurler syndrome (mucopolysaccharidosis I, AR), the most common, serves as a variant prototype both clinically and radiographically. A milder form, very similar to Hurler syndrome, is Hunter syndrome (mucopolysaccharidosis II, X-linked). The latter is characterized by a characteristic "gargoyle" face with a broad, flat nasal bridge, wide-spaced eyes, puffy cheeks, thick lips surrounding an open mouth, and a prominent tongue. Hepatosplenomegaly, abdominal hernias, and stiff joints are seen in addition to psychomotor retardation. Mucopolysaccharidosis III (Sanfilippo syndrome, AR) represents an even milder form of dysostosis multiplex. Morquio disease (mucopolysaccharidosis IV, AR) is characterized by short stature (less than 4 feet tall), lax joints, and a short neck, with normal intelligence.

Often, these children die before 10 years of age, and they are deaf and have CHD (murmurs of varying causes).

Another group of storage diseases is due to excess accumulation of glycolipids (mucolipidoses) or sphingolipids (sphingolipidoses) in the tissues. Basically, the mucolipidoses (types I, II, III) and sphingolipidoses are clinically and radiographically identical to the mucopolysaccharidoses, but they can be separated on clinical grounds because, in contradistinction to those with mucopolysaccharidoses, children with mucolipidoses or sphingolipidoses do not excrete mucopolysaccharides in their urine.

Proportionate Dwarfism

Proportionate dwarfism is seen in patients with short stature. However, skeletal dysplasias are not the most common cause. Affected children are more likely to have pituitary, renal, nutritional, or chromosomal abnormalities that contribute to or result in short stature. Proportional short stature can also be normal: 2% of all children measure below the third percentile on growth charts.

Box 7-1. Common Types of Short-Limb Dwarfism

SYMMETRIC LIMB SHORTENING

Rhizomelic Shortening (AD)
Thanatophoric dwarfism*
Achondroplasia
Hypochondroplasia

Mesomelic Shortening (AR)
Camptomelic dwarfism*
Dyschondrosteosis:
  Cornelia de Lange syndrome
  Langer and Nievergelt variants

Acromelic Shortening (AR)
Asphyxiating thoracic dystrophy*
Chondroectodermal dysplasia
Pyknodysostosis

ASYMMETRIC LIMB SHORTENING
Chondrodysplasia punctata

Nonspecific Shortening (AR/AD)
Osteogenesis imperfecta (types I-IV; AR/AD**)

---
*Fatal
**Previously classified as congenita and tarda forms.
  AD, Autosomal dominant inheritance; AR, autosomal recessive inheritance.

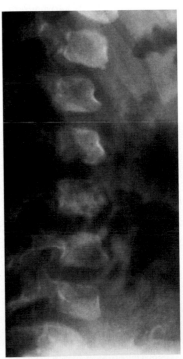

FIGURE 7-19. Dysostosis multiplex (mucopolysaccharidoses). Characteristic anteroinferiorly beaked oval vertebral bodies.

Asymmetric Dwarfism

The most common entities causing asymmetric dwarfism are osteogenesis imperfecta (discussed previously), multiple enchondromatosis, and diaphyseal aclasis (multiple exostoses).

Multiple Enchondromatosis

Multiple enchondromatosis, a nonhereditary disorder, is characterized by cartilaginous masses that infiltrate the metaphyses of long and short tubular bones as well as the flat bones. *Enchondral* bones are not affected. There are six types, and usually the three most common types involve the following conditions: If the multiple enchondromas are purely unilateral, or if they are unevenly distributed throughout the metaphyses of the long bones, sparing the cranium and spine, the type is Ollier disease. If the enchondromas are associated with multiple cutaneous hemangiomas, the type is Maffucci syndrome. If the enchondromas are symmetrically distributed throughout the body with involvement of the cranium and hands and feet, the type is known as generalized enchondromatosis. The former two (Ollier and Maffucci syndrome) are more common in boys (2:1). Less common variants are metachondromatosis, affecting the short tubular bones of the hands and feet; spondyloenchondroplasia, in which the enchondromas are associated with platyspondyly; and a variant consisting of enchondromas with irregular vertebral lesions called vertebral enchondromas.

Radiographically, multiple lucent metaphyseal lesions often containing punctate ("popcorn") calcifications are characteristic. Eventually these lesions may result in angular limb deformities (Fig. 7-20). Chondrosarcomas can reportedly occur in both Maffucci syndrome and Ollier disease, usually in adults; 5% of patients with chondrosarcomas have Ollier disease. Sudden increase in size of such lesions and symptoms such as pain may indicate malignant transformation. MRI is the imaging modality of choice for depiction of the extension and morphology of the lesion. The differential diagnosis includes polyostotic fibrous dysplasia and diaphyseal aclasis.

Multiple Hereditary Cartilaginous Exostoses

Multiple hereditary cartilaginous exostoses (osteochondromas, AD) are one of the most common bone dysplasias. The disorder is characterized by multiple cartilaginous exostoses arising from the metaphyses of, in particular, the tubular bones (distal femur, proximal tibia) and ribs (80%) and the pelvis and scapulae (10%) (bones preformed in cartilage or enchondral ossification) (Fig. 7-21). If the resultant pain or deformity created by these lesions causes discomfort to the patient, the osteochondromas may be surgically resected. They may cause pain and neurovascular compromise as a result of direct compression upon adjacent neurovascular structures. Sarcomatous degeneration occurs in less than 5% of patients. Multiple hereditary exostoses are more common in males, and about 50% of affected patients have affected parents. CT may best image a cartilaginous cap that is thin and sharp. A thick cap (more than 2.3 cm) raises the possibility of malignant degeneration. MRI is more specific than CT in identifying and measuring the cartilaginous cap.

Focal Bony Deficiencies

Focal congenital malformations of the extremities are thought to be caused by a variety of insults: drugs (thalidomide), vascular occlusion (radial aplasia), intrauterine adhesions (amniotic band syndrome), and genetic disorders (trisomy 13 or 18). The majority, however, are of unknown cause.

Hypoplasia or Aplasia

Hypoplasia and aplasia constitute more common congenital skeletal malformations than short stature. Unilateral absence of the fibula is most common, more common than bilateral absence. Clinically, there is pitting of the skin over the apex of a bowed lower leg. The next most common malformations, listed in decreasing order of frequency, are absence of the radius, femur, ulna, and humerus. Radial deviation of the hand is usually seen accompanying radial ray absence. This may be observed in Holt-Oram syndrome (associated with atrial septal defect), the VACTERL (*v*ertebral abnormalities, *a*nal atresia, *c*ardiac abnormalities, *t*racheoesophageal fistula and/or *e*sophageal atresia, *r*enal agenesis and dysplasia, and *l*imb defects) association, Fanconi anemia, and trisomies 13 and 18. The femur may be hypoplastic to absent, a spectrum of femoral abnormalities grouped together as proximal femoral focal deficiency (Fig. 7-22). Most cases (90%) are unilateral; the deficiency is more common in boys and on the right, and it may be associated with aplasia or hypoplasia elsewhere in the same limb. These anomalies may also occur as part of the caudal regression syndrome (maternal diabetes).

Hyperplasia

Hyperplasia may include (hemi)hypertrophy and an excess number of structures (e.g., polydactyly). Overgrowth of one half of the body can be segmental or total. Associated anomalies include renal polycystic disease, Wilms tumor, adrenal and hepatic neoplasms, focal nodular hyperplasia, and hepatoblastoma. Other syndromes in which polydactyly is seen are asphyxiating thoracic dystrophy, acrocephalosyndactyly (Apert syndrome), Ellis–van Creveld syndrome (short ribs, polydactyly syndrome), Holt–Oram syndrome, and trisomy 13.

Synostoses, which most commonly affect the carpal or tarsal bones, are failures of cartilaginous segmentation. Of these, tarsal coalition (fusion) is the most common synostoses as well as the most common cause of foot pain in an adolescent; although most cases are congenital (failure of segmentation), the disorder can be the result of trauma, surgery, arthritis, or infection. A tarsal coalition often results in a spastic flatfoot (pes planus) deformity. A coalition may be bony, fibrous, or cartilaginous. The calcaneonavicular coalition is the most common form of tarsal coalition (60% of patients with tarsal coalition), followed by talocalcaneal coalition (30%). The talonavicular coalition, the least common (approximately 10%), is bilateral in 25% of affected patients. CT is the imaging modality of choice for detection and characterization of the (bony) bridging tissue (Fig. 7-23).

Congenital Amputations

Constricting amniotic bands may result in stumps (amputation) or focal soft tissue constrictions of limbs (Streeter bands), fused digits, or clubfoot deformity (Fig. 7-24). These disorders are grouped

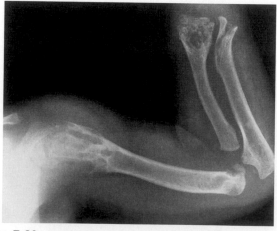

FIGURE 7-20. Enchondromatosis. Characteristic metaphyseal lesions with "popcorn" calcifications that have resulted in radial ulnar deformities and contour abnormalities of the proximal humerus.

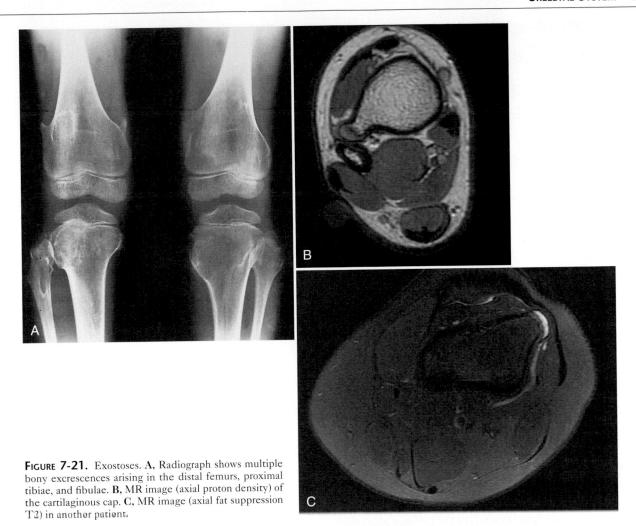

FIGURE 7-21. Exostoses. **A,** Radiograph shows multiple bony excrescences arising in the distal femurs, proximal tibiae, and fibulae. **B,** MR image (axial proton density) of the cartilaginous cap. **C,** MR image (axial fat suppression T2) in another patient.

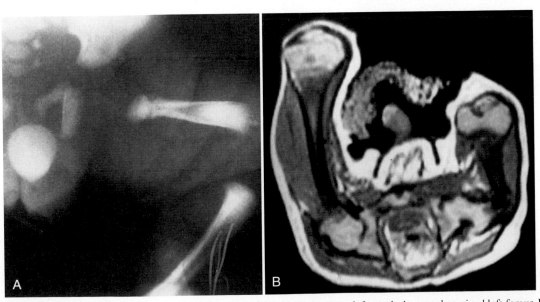

FIGURE 7-22. Proximal femoral focal deficiency. **A,** Conventional radiograph demonstrates a deformed, shortened proximal left femur. **B,** MR image of the same, with striking angular deformity of the shortened left femur.

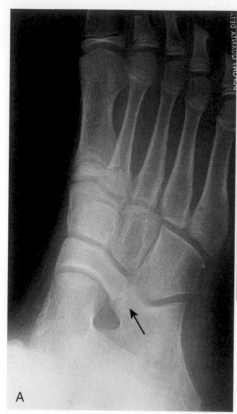

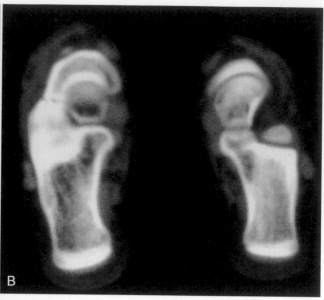

FIGURE 7-23. Right tarsal (calcaneonavicular) coalition. **A,** Radiograph *(arrow).* **B,** CT scan illustrating bony bridge.

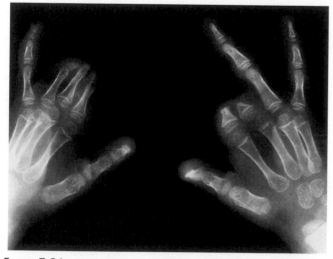

FIGURE 7-24. Amniotic bands in ADAM (amniotic deformity, adhesion, mutilation) complex. There are amputations of multiple phalanges of both hands.

together as the ADAM (*a*mniotic *d*eformity, *a*dhesion, *m*utilation) complex. Disruption of the amniotic membrane from the chorion is thought to lead to adhesions that may trap parts of the developing fetus. Alternatively, vascular constriction and/or deficient blood supply causing "tissue necrosis" may be the underlying cause.

Dysplasias Due to Defects of Ossification

Cleidocranial Dysostosis

An AD disorder of mesenchymal skeletal development (30% are spontaneous mutations), cleidocranial dysostosis is characterized by a triad of cranial, clavicular, and pelvic abnormalities. Clinically,

an affected patient is presented with a soft cranium and delayed closure of the fontanelles resulting in a brachycephalic skull with a small face; eventually, drooping shoulders, short stature, and an abnormal gait develop. On radiography, wormian bones are common in widely patent sutures; there are hypoplastic facial bones and widely placed orbits with delayed closure of the sutures. Clavicles are completely absent in 10% to 15% of patients; they are partially absent in most, with the lateral aspect affected most often. There is delayed ossification of the symphysis pubis, an abnormality that creates the appearance of widening of the symphysis pubis (Fig. 7-25). Affected patients have normal maturation and can expect a normal life span.

Sclerosing Bone Dysplasias

Increased bone density and abnormalities of tubulation are the characteristic radiographic findings in sclerosing bone dysplasias. There are two groups, osteosclerosis, caused by increased mineralization, and hyperostosis, caused by active bony overgrowth.

Osteosclerosis

In osteopetrosis, osteoblast dysfunction (carbonic anhydrase II deficiency) causes a failure of resorption of cartilage and bone matrix (primary spongiosa). The result is dense bones caused by marrow underdevelopment (marble bones). This disorder can be of a congenital infantile (Albers-Schönberg disease) or adult (tarda) type. In the former (AR), there is an increase in the density of all the bones with club-shaped metaphyses ("Erlenmeyer flask") and "bone-within-bone" appearance of the vertebral bodies. The base of the calvaria is thickened, with obliteration of the mastoids and paranasal sinuses, and this can lead to deafness or optic atrophy. Hepatosplenomegaly and anemia are present at birth, and recurrent infections are common. There may be longitudinal striations in the distal long bone shafts and rachitic-like changes at the ends of the bones.

The tarda variant is usually noted incidentally in childhood or adolescence and has AD inheritance. Transverse lucent bands in the phalanges, arcuate bands in the iliac bones, and "bone-within-bone" appearance of vertebral bodies are manifestations of the temporal fluctuations of this disorder. Bone pain and a propensity for fractures or infection are the presenting symptoms if the disease becomes clinically evident (Fig. 7-26).

Pyknodysostosis, which has been discussed previously, is characterized by generalized sclerosis with overmodeled (narrow) shafts. Clinically, there is delayed closure of the fontanelle and failure to thrive. The bones of the hands and feet are short, with hypoplastic tufts. A thickened sclerotic skull base, a persistent anterior fontanelle, wormian bones, and hypoplasia of the sinuses are characteristic radiographic findings.

In osteopoikilosis, multiple small rounded foci of osteosclerosis may be present in the carpus, tarsus, pelvis, and scapulae in a periarticular distribution. The disorder, which is asymptomatic,

is an AD dysplasia that can be regarded as an incidental finding in the epiphyses and metaphyses. It does not progress with age (see Fig. 7-17).

Osteopathia striata (Voorhoeve disease), characterized by fine linear striations in the metaphyses of long bones, may represent an intermediate stage in the development of an osteosclerosis. The findings, usually bilateral, may coexist with described osteopetrosis or osteopoikilosis or with melorheostosis (discussed later).

Hyperostosis

Caffey disease (infantile cortical hyperostosis) is of unknown etiology. It occurs during the first few months of life (average age of onset 9 weeks; seldom after 6 months), often in clusters of patients and locales. Clinically, the affected child is irritable, with an elevated temperature and soft tissue swelling around affected areas: most commonly the mandible, clavicle, and tubular bones. There is an elevated erythrocyte sedimentation rate. Prostaglandin E, a virus, and a familial tendency have been implicated. The disorder is a self-limited disease that affects boys and girls equally.

Imaging demonstrates periosteal new bone in relation to the following bones, listed in decreasing order of frequency: mandible, ribs, clavicle, and ulna (Fig. 7-27A). The findings usually resolve in 6 to 12 months.

Melorheostosis is an uncommon and painless disorder manifesting in children with asymmetry of the limbs. Boys and girls are equally affected. It is characterized radiographically by usually unilateral extracortical and endosteal hyperostotic "waves" resembling molten wax flowing down the side of a candle. The findings are usually limited to a single limb, the lower extremity more often than the upper (Fig. 7-27B).

Diaphyseal dysplasia (Camurati-Engelmann disease) is rare; of AD inheritance, it manifests as a waddling gait in a malnourished child. Radiographically there is endosteal and periosteal thickening of the diaphyses of the tubular bones. The bones affected most, listed in decreasing frequency, are tibia, femur, and humerus.

In the differential diagnosis of these sclerosing bone dysplasias, only melorheostosis and Caffey disease produce a radionuclide bone scan with a markedly increased uptake. Mild uptake may occasionally be seen in diaphyseal dysplasia. This differential diagnosis includes, in addition to the three previously described conditions, healing rickets, healing scurvy, trauma X, hypervitaminosis A, and long-term prostaglandin E administration.

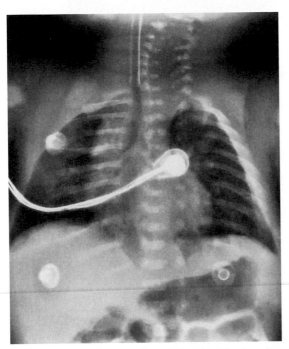

FIGURE 7-25. Cleidocranial dysostosis. Delayed ossification of the posterior neural arches, absence of the clavicles, and short ribs are demonstrated on a chest radiograph of a newborn.

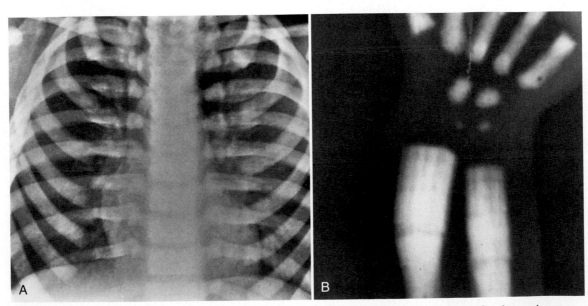

FIGURE 7-26. Osteopetrosis. **A,** Generalized osteosclerosis of all bony structures. **B,** Fine, longitudinal striations in flared metaphyses.

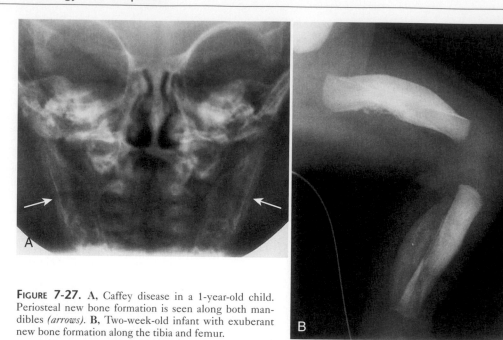

FIGURE 7-27. A, Caffey disease in a 1-year-old child. Periosteal new bone formation is seen along both mandibles *(arrows)*. **B,** Two-week-old infant with exuberant new bone formation along the tibia and femur.

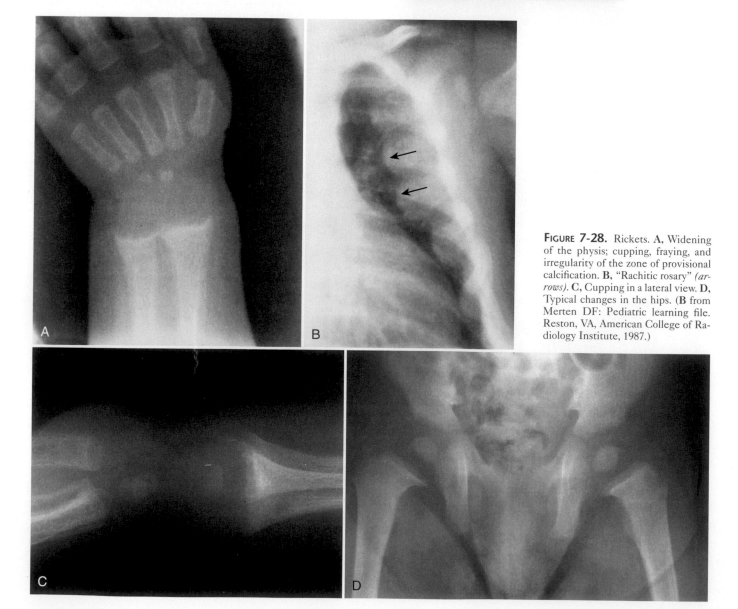

FIGURE 7-28. Rickets. **A,** Widening of the physis; cupping, fraying, and irregularity of the zone of provisional calcification. **B,** "Rachitic rosary" *(arrows)*. **C,** Cupping in a lateral view. **D,** Typical changes in the hips. **(B** from Merten DF: Pediatric learning file. Reston, VA, American College of Radiology Institute, 1987.)

▬ SYSTEMIC SKELETAL DISORDERS

Metabolic Disorders

Rickets

A relative or absolute deficiency in vitamin D or its derivatives causes failure of mineralization of the normal growing cartilage into bone. There are several causes of rickets: poor nutrition, due to deficiency of vitamin D in the diet or lack of sunlight (ultraviolet); malabsorption, resulting from hepatobiliary disease (anticonvulsant medication, neonatal hepatitis) or small bowel disorders (sprue, celiac disease); and a defect in synthesis, such as in renal glomerular failure, vitamin D–resistant rickets, or inherited renal tubular (phosphate loss) acidosis (RTA). Rarely, rickets also may be due to familial vitamin D resistance (X-linked hypophosphatemia). Rickets is almost always diagnosed in an individual younger than age 2 years; it may be seen radiographically before it is clinically evident in up to one third of patients. The classic radiographic appearances occur after 4 to 6 weeks of vitamin D deficiency, especially in the most rapidly growing ends of bones. The most rapidly growing areas of the skeleton are the ZPCs of the wrist, knees, and proximal humeri. Because of the calcium deficiency, it does not become mineralized, yet the ZPC itself continues to expand. Imaging findings thus include widening of the physis (growth plate), cupping, fraying, and irregularity of the distal metaphysis accompanied by generalized osteopenia (Fig. 7-28).

Bone age may be delayed. The classic "rachitic rosary" at the anterior rib ends and transverse radiolucent bands in the diaphyses (umbauzonen) is rarely seen today.

Hyperparathyroidism

Primary hyperparathyroidism is due to a parathyroid adenoma secreting increased levels of parathormone. In children this disorder is rare and commonly hereditary. *Tertiary* hyperparathyroidism occurs after the prolonged presence of secondary hyperparathyroidism. Escape of the parathyroid glands from the regulatory effects of serum calcium levels is the underlying mechanism. *Secondary* hyperparathyroidism ("renal rickets") is due to chronic hypocalcemia. The radiographic changes are seen most commonly in children with renal failure or chronic renal disease that is treated with peritoneal dialysis and in those suffering from intestinal malabsorption. Growth retardation may accompany renal osteodystrophy. Radiographic changes include generalized osteopenia with areas of subperiosteal resorption ("cut-back" zones), initially seen along the radial margins of the middle phalanges. The *distal* clavicles and inner aspects of the femoral necks are also frequently involved with more advanced disease (Fig. 7-29). Soft tissue calcification or chondrocalcinosis may occur, but this is rarely detected radiographically in the pediatric age group. Intraosseous localized fibrous tissue accumulations (osteoclastomas), known as "brown" tumors, may be diagnostic if seen in conjunction with the rachitic changes already described.

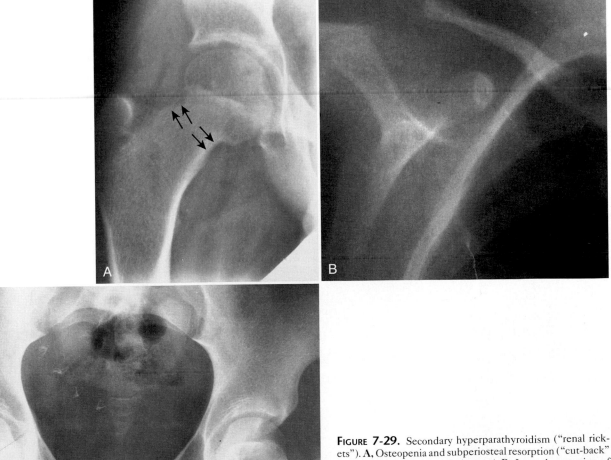

FIGURE 7-29. Secondary hyperparathyroidism ("renal rickets"). **A,** Osteopenia and subperiosteal resorption ("cut-back" zone) of the femoral neck *(arrows)*. **B,** Lateral resorption of the clavicle. **C,** Brown tumor (b) in the left superior pubic ramus of a patient who has undergone renal transplantation (note the right lower quadrant sutures) for chronic glomerulonephritis.

Renal Osteodystrophy

Renal osteodystrophy refers to changes that occur in children with chronic renal insufficiency, in which retention of phosphate leads to osteopenia and secondary hyperparathyroidism. The underlying causes can be thought of as broadly belonging to two groups: tubular disease, including congenital (renal tubular acidosis) and acquired (nephrotic syndrome) variants, and glomerular disease (chronic pyelonephritis, glomerulonephritis, polycystic disease). Both result in rachitic-like changes in the metabolically less active bones (femoral neck, pubic rami, scapulae) (Box 7-2). In renal osteodystrophy, if growth failure is severe, the radiographic alterations of hyperparathyroidism predominate. With skeletal growth, the changes of rickets appear.

The differential diagnosis of rickets includes hypophosphatasia, metaphyseal chondrodysplasia (Schmidt variant), and copper deficiency (premature neonates).

Hypothyroidism

Cretinism is the most common metabolic abnormality found in the routine laboratory testing of newborns. Thyroid hormone is necessary for bone growth and maturation as well as for development of the central nervous system. Hypothyroidism slows both skeletal growth and maturation. It is usually the result of congenital absence or hypoplasia of the thyroid gland. The inheritance of congenital hypothyroidism is usually sporadic, but it may occasionally have AR inheritance. It occurs three times more frequently in girls than in boys. Radiographically, the bone age is usually more than 2 SD below the mean. The epiphyseal ossification centers may be irregular and fragmented; there is delay in closure of the physes and cranial sutures, with wormian bones common.

Abnormalities commonly associated with hypothyroidism include Down syndrome, autoimmune endocrine abnormalities, and CHD.

Hyperthyroidism is extremely rare in neonates and rare in childhood. Advanced bone age is the hallmark. (Pre)adolescent girls may present with a toxic goiter called juvenile myxedema, in which skeletal maturation is usually normal.

Scurvy

Today scurvy occurs very rarely, mostly in infants fed boiled-milk formulas or in children older than 6 months. It is due to a vitamin C deficiency, which results in poor bone matrix (collagen) formation. Calcium deposition at the ZPC is not affected. Radiographic findings include generalized demineralization and a

lucent band subjacent to the ZPC (the "scurvy" line, or zone of Fränkel). Subperiosteal hemorrhage associated with metaphyseal pathologic fractures leads to exuberant periosteal new bone formation and prominent metaphyseal spurs (the "corner" or "angle" sign of scurvy, a "Pelkan spur"). The epiphysis is osteopenic with a relatively dense ZPC, resulting in a prominent ring: the Wimberger ring (Fig. 7-30).

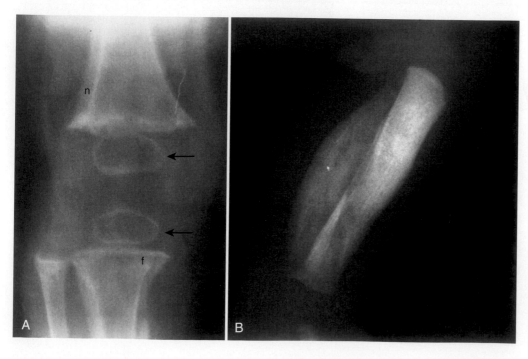

Figure 7-30. Scurvy. **A,** Osteopenia, periosteal new bone (n), and a relatively dense zone of provisional calcification, resulting in an epiphyseal Wimberger ring *(arrows)*. A zone of Fränkel (f) is shown in the proximal tibia. **B,** Calcified subperiosteal hemorrhage.

Hypervitaminosis A

The acute sequelae of a massive dose of vitamin A are clinical: nausea, vomiting, lethargy. The chronic form of excessive vitamin A intake results in radiographic findings consisting of periosteal new bone formation along the shafts of mostly the ulna and phalanges. Clinically, these patients are presented between 1 and 3 years of age with pruritus, often painful lumps in the soft tissue, and loss of appetite. With the cessation of vitamin A intake, symptoms and radiographic findings disappear. Differentiation of the radiographic findings from those of infantile cortical hyperostosis (Caffey disease) can be difficult, except for the fact that in the latter condition there is a predilection for hyperostosis of the mandible and clavicles.

Lead Poisoning

Acute lead poisoning occurs primarily after the ingestion (pica) of the lead found in paint chips or fumes (Fig. 7-31); the hematogenous lead interferes with the resorption of primary spongiosa by paralyzing the osteoclasts. The resultant dense bands, the so-called lead lines, are a *late* manifestation of long-term lead exposure and are best seen in the fastest-growing metaphyses in children between 3 and 6 years of age. It may be difficult to differentiate bands of lead poisoning from bands of "physiologic" sclerosis, in which case the principle of differential bone growth can be useful (see Fig. 7-6C). Dense metaphyses evident in the proximal fibular metaphyses and in the other slow-growing bones of the body (e.g., iliac wings) help differentiate lead bands from "physiologic" sclerosis, which is also noted most often in the first 6 months of life.

Anemias

Hemophilia

Classic hemophilia occurs as the result of the deficiency in the procoagulant portion of factor VIII, whereas Christmas disease is due to a deficiency of the partial thromboplastin portion of factor IX. The incidence of classic hemophilia is approximately 1 in 10,000 newborn male infants; it occurs five times as frequently as Christmas disease. Both are gender-linked, recessively inherited traits.

Hemophilia primarily affects joints, most often (95%) the large joints. Synovial hemorrhage leads to hemosiderin deposition and fibrosis, which results in synovial hypertrophy/overgrowth and

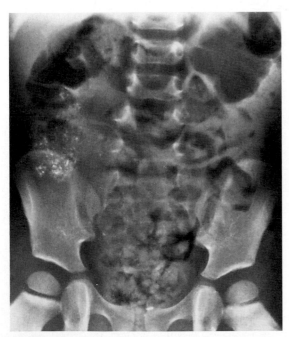

FIGURE 7-31. Acute heavy metal poisoning seen as radiodense "pica" in the ascending colon. Chronic "lead bands" are noted in all visualized metaphyses.

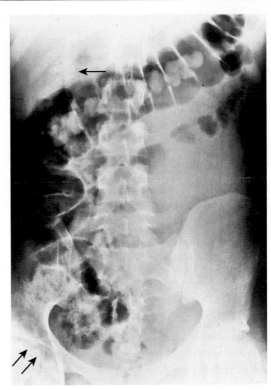

FIGURE 7-32. Hemophilia. Abdominal radiograph demonstrates gallstones *(single arrow)*, destructive arthritis of the right hip joint *(double arrows)*, and a soft tissue mass in the left lower quadrant, with bowel displacement (hemophilic pseudotumor).

inflammation that subsequently destroy the joint cartilage and subchondral bone.

The frequency of joint involvement, listing in descending order, is knee, elbow, ankle; the hip, wrist, and shoulder are less frequently involved. Imaging may show an effusion that may be seen on conventional radiographs or US as well as with other cross-sectional imaging modalities in the acute phase.

Chronic hemophilic arthropathy is characterized by thickening of the synovium, premature ossification of epiphyses, epiphyseal overgrowth, and resultant premature fusion of the growth plates; all of these changes are due to increased blood flow to this region. Avascular necrosis may also occur secondary to occlusion of epiphyseal vessels by the hemarthrosis. The cartilage destruction results in joint space narrowing, subchondral cyst formation, and eburnation of the articular cortex. In the knee, the classic findings are epiphyseal overgrowth and widening of the intercondylar notch (differential diagnosis includes juvenile rheumatoid arthritis [JRA] and tuberculous arthritis); there may be squaring of the inferior aspect of the patella. Pseudotumor formation occurs in about 1% of patients with severe hemophilia. The majority occur in the femur and pelvis, manifesting as painless, slowly expanding masses. There may be calcification within such a mass, as well as associated bone erosion and periosteal new bone formation. Conventional radiographs (Fig. 7-32) and CT are the primary diagnostic modalities. Marrow recruitment and resultant hyperplasia can be seen on MRI of the marrow (T1-weighted). Owing to compensatory red marrow hyperplasia, there is retardation of the normal conversion process of red marrow into yellow (high T1 signal) marrow.

Sickle Cell Disease

Hemoglobin S (HbS), the most common hemoglobin variant, results from substitution of valine for glutamic acid on the sixth position of the beta-chain. HbS as the predominant hemoglobin indicates homozygosity (HbSS, 1 in 650 African Americans); however, HbSA and other variants (e.g., HbS thalassemia) may result in sickle cell disease, which occurs in approximately 7% of African Americans.

The presence of HbF (fetal hemoglobin) prevents symptoms in the first 6 months of life. Swollen fingers (dactylitis) or toes (the hand-foot syndrome) may be the first clinical signs of HbSS disease, appearing between ages 6 months and 2 years in about one third of children with sickle cell disease.

Abdominal pain, bone infarction, and joint pain become more common presentations through childhood. Skeletal abnormalities in sickle cell disease are due to three factors: bone infarction, bone infection, and marrow hyperplasia.

On conventional radiographs, hand-foot syndrome is characterized by soft tissue swelling, periosteal new bone formation along the phalangeal shafts, and mild expansion. This disorder may be difficult to distinguish from osteomyelitis. The skull may show diploic space widening with vertical striations, causing the so-called hair-on-end pattern, although this finding is seen much less commonly in hand-foot syndrome than in thalassemia. Infarction is uncommon in the skull. In the spine, however, on the lateral view, the end plates demonstrate central cupping, causing the vertebral body to resemble the letter H (also known as "Lincoln Log" deformity) (Fig. 7-33). These findings are probably due to the infarction secondary to "rouleaux" (stack-of-coins) formation of red blood cells in the smaller vessels supplying the central portion of the end plates; the larger vessels supplying the epiphyseal rings or the vertebral bodies are not affected and thus remain patent. These changes may also be seen on the anteroposterior view of the vertebral body, the so-called fish-mouth appearance.

Infarction of the long bones, most commonly the femur, occurs at the junction of the metaphysis and diaphysis because the epiphyses and metaphyses are individually supplied by collateral circulation. Infarction of the marrow may heal with fibrosis, which can calcify, or may be complicated by osteomyelitis, most often caused by *Staphylococcus aureus*.

Salmonella organisms occur with greater frequency (20 times more often) in patients with sickle cell disease than in the general population. Scintigraphy has been used in the acute phase of suspected marrow infection, but because patients with sickle cell disease often have had previous infarctions, the findings on bone scintigraphy, that is, focal areas of decreased uptake, are less reliable. Combining bone and marrow imaging has been helpful in differentiating osteomyelitis from infarction immediately after the occurrence of an infarct. The combination of a large defect on marrow scan and a smaller defect on radionuclide bone scan is typical of osteonecrosis; in other words, there is a mismatch between bone scan and bone marrow imaging in a bone infarction but not (or less pronounced) in osteomyelitis. Avascular necrosis of the epiphyseal portion of the long bone usually occurs after closure of the growth plate. The hip is the most common site for this to occur; it is seen in approximately one third of patients with sickle cell disease, usually adults. MRI is the modality of choice to detect avascular necrosis in its earliest phase.

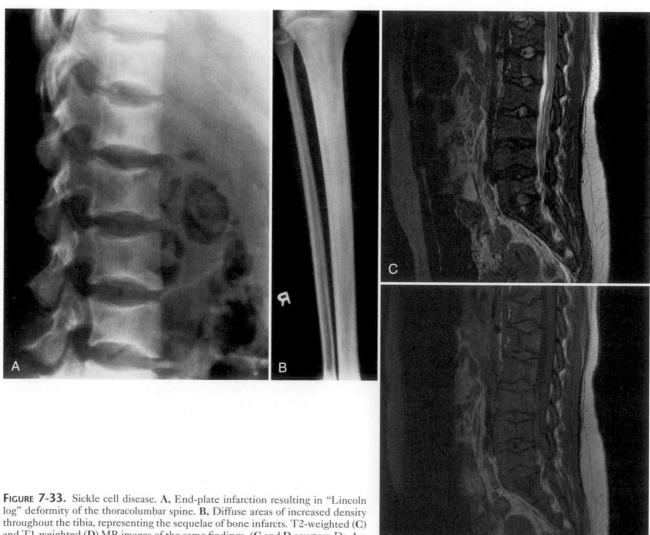

FIGURE 7-33. Sickle cell disease. **A,** End-plate infarction resulting in "Lincoln log" deformity of the thoracolumbar spine. **B,** Diffuse areas of increased density throughout the tibia, representing the sequelae of bone infarcts. T2-weighted (**C**) and T1-weighted (**D**) MR images of the same findings. (**C** and **D** courtesy Dr. Ara Kassarjian, Madrid, Spain.)

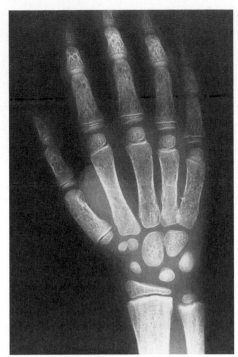

FIGURE 7-34. Thalassemia. Hand shows widened medullary cavities with coarse trabecular markings of the metacarpals and phalanges.

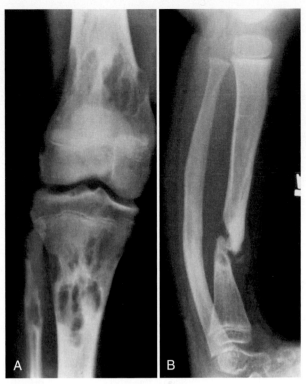

FIGURE 7-35. Neurofibromatosis. **A,** "Erosive" cortical defects consistent with multiple neurofibromas impinging on the distal femur, proximal tibia, and fibula. **B,** Congenital pseudarthrosis of the distal tibia and bowing deformity of the fibula.

Thalassemia

Cooley anemia is the major (homozygous) form of this severe childhood anemia (often leading to death by age 12 years); thalassemia minor is a milder (heterozygous) form. Both occur more frequently in patients of Eastern Mediterranean descent (from Gr. *thalassa*, "the sea"). The polypeptide chain involved determines further characterization of the variants. The alpha-chain variant occurs in the fetus (HbF), the beta-chain variant after the newborn period. The homozygous form is called thalassemia major, the heterozygous form thalassemia minor. Radiographic changes are mainly the result of marrow hyperplasia. In particular, the hands and feet show widened medullary cavities with coarse trabecular patterns and squaring of the bones (Fig. 7-34). During adolescence, these peripheral findings involute and sclerose as a result of the conversion of hematopoietic marrow to fat. In the calvaria, diploic widening with hair-on-end appearance (radiodense cortical striations) may be seen, and there may be progressive obliteration of the paranasal sinuses ("rodent facies"). In the axial skeleton there is osteopenia, especially of the vertebral bodies, and expansion of the shafts and ribs. Undertubulation in the long bones may lead to an Erlenmeyer flask deformity. Extramedullary hematopoiesis may also be seen paraspinally, best identified on CT or MRI (see Fig. 2-64). Spinal cord compression caused by the extramedullary hematopoietic tissue may occur.

The differential diagnosis of metaphyseal widening (Erlenmeyer flask deformity) includes the anemias, marrow storage disease (e.g., Gaucher disease), mucopolysaccharidoses, and osteopetrosis as well as metaphyseal dysplasias (classically, Pyle disease).

Neurofibromatosis

The gene for neurofibrosis (NF), an AD trait with variable penetrance and an almost 50% mutation rate, has been mapped to 17q21 (NF type 1; NF-1) and 22q12 (NF type 2; NF-2). Neurofibromatosis is a hereditary hamartomatous disorder with potential for involvement of any organ system of the body.

Musculoskeletal involvement occurs in about 80% of patients with NF. von Recklinghausen first described it in 1882 as one

of the most devastating, destructive, and debilitating diseases known to humans. Its incidence is 1 in 3000 live births. The classic clinical triad consists of café au lait (coffee-brown) spots, mental deficiency, and skeletal deformities. If neurofibromas of the peripheral nerves, Lisch nodules in the iris, and café-au-lait spots are present at any age, the NF diagnosis is established. Half of patients with NF have a family history, and about half suffer from scoliosis that is indistinguishable from idiopathic scoliosis. The presence of more than five café-au-lait spots, each 0.5 cm or larger in diameter, is considered the hallmark of NF. Characteristic skeletal radiographic findings in NF include "erosive" cortical defects, which are probably related to adjacent nerve enlargement caused by NF, and the "empty orbit" sign.

A bony defect in the (left) lambdoid suture is also often present. The most commonly associated skeletal lesion is a congenital pseudarthrosis, most often of the tibia. This occurs when a long bone such as the tibia is fractured in a patient with NF, with subsequent incomplete fracture healing resulting in non-union (tibia) and an associated bowing deformity (fibula) (as seen in Fig. 7-35). Kyphoscoliosis occurs in more than 20% of patients with NF-1, often in association with posterior scalloping and dumb-bell neurofibromas causing widened neural foramina.

This "erosion" of adjacent bony structures, particularly in the spine, is best seen on conventional radiographs, although MRI may be necessary to differentiate meningoceles from neurofibromas.

Tuberous Sclerosis

AD inheritance, Bourneville disease presents with the triad of mental retardation, seizures, and adenoma sebaceum. It has neither gender nor ethnic or geographic predilection. Cystlike or osteoblastic lesions are noted in the phalanges in up to 60% of affected patients, probably representing subungual fibromas. Localized multifocal areas of bony sclerosis are characteristically

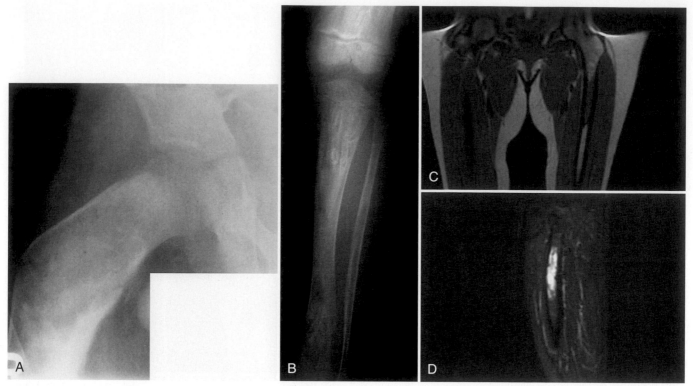

FIGURE 7-36. Fibrous dysplasia (FD). **A,** Radiograph of the proximal femur shows a mildly expansile "ground-glass" lesion with a pathologic fracture ("shepherd's crook" deformity). **B,** Radiograph of tibia illustrating typical FD. **C,** Sagittal short T1 inversion recovery (STIR) MR image. **D,** Coronal T1 MR image of a femoral lesion.

seen in the posterior elements of the spine and pelvis. The central nervous system lesions of this disease are described in Chapter 8 (see Figs. 8-93 and 8-94).

Fibrous Dysplasia

Fibrous dysplasia (FD), a nonhereditary, common disorder of unknown cause, involves replacement of bone by fibrous tissue because of failure of osteoblasts to undergo their usual differentiation. It occurs in a monostotic (70%) and polyostotic form. Both, although mainly the polyostotic form, may be associated with endocrine dysfunction and precocious puberty in a girl.

About one third of patients have the *polyostotic* form. About one third to one fifth have cutaneous café-au-lait spots of the "coast of Maine" variety. Males and females are affected about equally. The association of precocious puberty in girls, café-au-lait spots, and polyostotic (typically unilateral) FD is known as the McCune-Albright syndrome. It occurs in about one third of girls with FD. Polyostotic FD is also associated with bilateral, asymmetric limb involvement, and it may spare the axial skeleton.

In monostotic FD, occurring in the second and third decades, the severity and extent of bone involvement are more severe than in polyostotic FD. Both forms may manifest as an alkaline phosphatase elevation.

Radiography demonstrates expansile lytic lesions occupying the medullary canal. They may thin the cortex and involve the diaphysis, but they may extend into the metaphysis (Fig. 7-36). A "ground-glass" appearance may result from a preponderance of abnormal (dysplastic) trabeculae in areas of bone marrow replaced by fibrous tissue. The proximal femur (35%), tibia (20%), and facial bones and ribs (15%) are the most common sites of involvement. Bowing deformities such as the "shepherd's crook" deformity of the proximal femur occur in one third of patients, probably as a result of biomechanical forces. Involvement of the facial bones may lead to asymmetric sclerotic thickening, called *leontiasis osseae* ("resembling a lion's face"). Skull lesions, which occur in 20% of patients, are characterized by radiolucent or sclerotic lesions. CT is most useful in the facial region, as well as elsewhere in the skeleton, to define extent of involvement; radionuclide bone scanning shows the distribution of lesions most reliably in the polyostotic form by usually producing intense uptake. MRI is adjunctive.

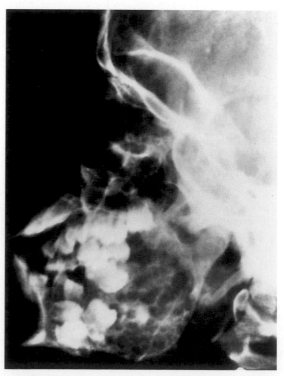

FIGURE 7-37. Cherubism. Extensive multilocular lesions of the mandible in a patient presenting with swelling of the jaw.

Cherubism is a rare disorder manifesting as bilateral swelling in the jaw with expansile, multilobular bony lesions. It may simulate FD, but it is a familial disorder most often occurring in children younger than 4 years (Fig. 7-37).

Langerhans Cell Histiocytosis

LCH is a disease complex of unknown cause (a defect in immunoregulation?) that is characterized by proliferation of a distinct histiocyte called a Langerhans cell; the LCH designation includes the often fatal Letterer-Siwe disease, the slowly progressive Hand-Schüller-Christian disease, and eosinophilic granuloma (EG). In LCH there is considerable overlap between these groups, yet up to 50% of patients are not clearly "groupable." EG is a self-limiting disease in most cases. Age at diagnosis (younger than 2 years) and severity of liver, lungs, or bone marrow involvement are important prognostic factors. Prevalence is higher in Caucasians with a 2:1 male preponderance.

Letterer-Siwe Disease

Letter-Siwe disease represents less than 10% of cases of LCH. It is the acute disseminated form of LCH seen in infants younger than 6 months. The disorder manifests as hepatosplenomegaly, lymphadenopathy, purpura, and anemia. Skeletal lesions are rare, and the prognosis is poor.

Hand-Schüller-Christian Disease

Accounting for 10% to 20% of cases of LCH, Hand-Schüller-Christian disease is a more slowly progressive form of disseminated LCH that manifests in children between 3 and 6 years of age. The children are often presented with polydipsia, polyuria (diabetes insipidus), and bone pain. Lymphadenopathy, hepatosplenomegaly, and exophthalmos also are common presentations. The classic triad consisting of exophthalmos, diabetes insipidus, and lytic cranial bony lesions occurs in 10% to 15% of cases. Skeletal lesions are present in 85% of children with this disease. Prognosis is related to the extent of organ involvement, and mortality is about 10%.

Eosinophilic Granuloma

In EG, which accounts for 75% of cases of LCH, the Langerhans cell proliferation is limited to bone. It is a disease affecting children and young adults between 6 and 10 years of age. EG is a painful lesion, often accompanied by fever and most often monostotic. Skeletal involvement is common, but the overall prognosis is excellent.

This skeletal involvement (Fig. 7-38A to C) is most common in the (anterior) skull (25%), ribs (14%), femur (14%), and pelvis (10%), followed by the spine, mandible, and humerus (each about 8%). Thus about 70% of EGs affect the flat bones, and about 30% the long bones. The lesions in the skull and shoulder

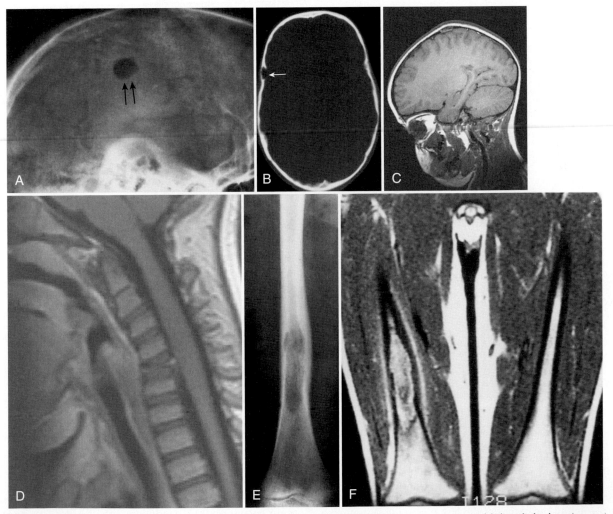

FIGURE 7-38. Langerhans cell histiocytosis. Lateral skull radiograph (**A**) and CT scan (**B**) show a lytic lesion with beveled edges *(arrows)*. **C,** MR image of the same finding. **D,** MR image illustrates vertebra plana of C5. **E,** Destructive central lesion of the distal femoral diaphysis is well defined and slightly expansile. A periosteal reaction can be seen. **F,** MR imaging better delineates the marrow extent and degree of expansion of the lesion, as well as extent of the soft tissue involvement.

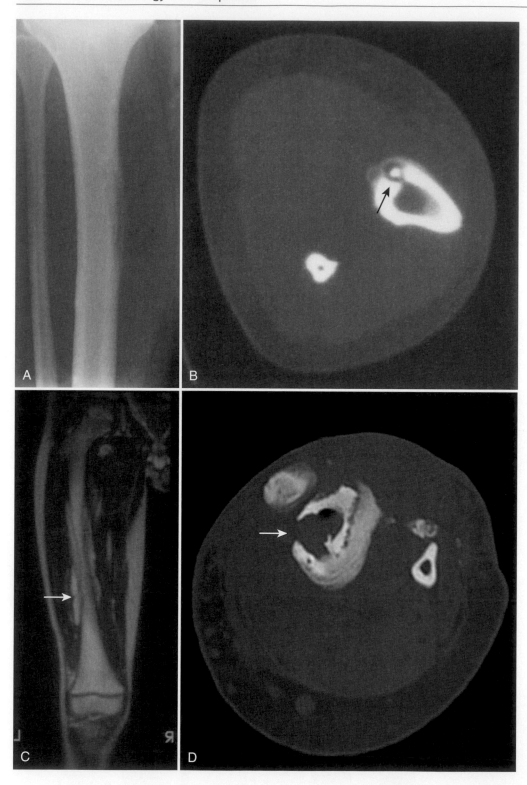

FIGURE 7-39. Acute osteomyelitis. **A,** Subperiosteal resorption and periosteal elevation demonstrated in the tibia. **B,** CT scan demonstrates a sequestrum *(arrow)*. MR scan **(C)** and CT image **(D)** show a cloaca *(arrow)*.

girdle are characteristically punched out and destructive, with well-defined but not sclerotic, although often beveled, margins. In the vertebral column, an almost pathognomonic finding is a uniformly flattened "vertebra plana." Affected vertebral bodies may return to normal or to at least half-normal height over the years. Long bones demonstrate lytic lesions. CT and MRI exquisitely define the extent of the lesion into the surrounding tissues (Fig. 7-38D). Bone scintigraphy is less reliable because not all lesions (about 60%) take up the radioisotope; the uptake depends on active skeletal response. The differential diagnosis includes metastatic disease, osteomyelitis, lymphoma, and Ewing sarcoma.

■ INFECTION

Bones and joints can become infected from (1) the bloodstream (most common), (2) a contiguous site of infection, or (3) direct penetration of infected foreign material into the bone. Hematogenous osteomyelitis is primarily a disease of infants and children. Its origin is hematogenous seeding, and it may arise from transient, asymptomatic bacteremia. Spread from adjacent structures or puncture wounds is a less frequent infectious route. There are three classic forms of osteomyelitis: acute, subacute, and chronic.

Acute Osteomyelitis

Acute hematogenous osteomyelitis primarily affects the metaphyses. Blood-borne organisms flourish in the large, slow-flowing venous sinusoids (terminal capillary loops) within the intramedullary portion of the metaphysis, aided by a decrease in the phagocytic ability of macrophages. Spread of the organism may occur through transphyseal vessels to the physis, epiphysis, and joints. However, because transphyseal vessels disappear after 12 to 18 months of age, transphyseal spread becomes unlikely after that time. The inflammatory response, exudate, and increased intraosseous pressure cause stasis of blood flow and thrombosis and then may result in bone necrosis and bone resorption as the inflammatory process traverses the haversian and Volkmann canals, lifts up the periosteum, and finally penetrates the periosteal membrane, causing soft tissue extension of the infectious process.

A *sequestrum* is a piece of necrotic bone embedded in the inflammatory process, whereas periosteal new bone formation around dead bone constitutes the *involucrum*, which may contain an exit tract to the skin, a *cloaca* (Latin for "sewer"). Today, because of proper and timely antibiotic therapy, an involucrum or sequestrum is seldom seen. More than three fourths of cases of osteomyelitis involve the long bones, with the faster-growing and largest metaphyses usually affected first (wrist, humerus, knee). Flat bones (ilium, vertebrae, and calcaneus, etc.) are involved in 25% of cases. One third of all cases of osteomyelitis occur in the first 2 years of life, and osteomyelitis is more common in boys than girls (2:1). The most common organism in this age group is *S. aureus* (85%), followed by group B β-hemolytic *Streptococcus*. In older children with sickle cell disease, *Salmonella* is most common. The erythrocyte sedimentation rate is always elevated, but the white blood cell count and blood cultures are positive for infection in only 50% of cases.

Conventional radiographic findings should never be used to exclude acute osteomyelitis in a patient who has had symptoms less than 10 days. Deep soft tissue swelling may be seen within days after onset of infection. Destructive bone changes do not occur until 7 to 10 days after the onset of infection. These consist first of subperiosteal resorption ("scalloping"), creating radiolucencies within cortical bone that then may progress to irregular destruction with periosteal new bone formation (Fig. 7-39). Subperiosteal resorption is caused by resorption of the bone cortex and, subsequently, the bone trabeculae of the endosteal and intramedullary bone. It is due in part to pressure erosion caused by the attendant soft tissue swelling. As the periosteal membrane is perforated and disrupted by the infectious process, and as the increased pressure is relieved through the haversian and Volkmann canals of the cortex and the exudate exits to the subperiosteal space, an abscess may form in the neighboring soft tissues. During the first 2 to 3 days of symptoms, radionuclide imaging may be particularly useful in showing this well-defined focus of increased radioactivity on the dynamic perfusion, as well as early blood pool and delayed images corresponding to the area of hyperemia. Greater than 90% sensitivity and specificity for increased blood flow can be expected, especially with three- or four-phase bone scans, although experience in pediatric bone scanning is mandatory because the main issue with scintigraphy is poor spatial resolution. When needed, gallium 67 citrate or indium In 111–labeled leukocyte scanning may raise the specificity for infection to 80%.

Multiple foci of osteomyelitis are seen in children with sickle cell disease, diabetes, or chronic granulomatous disease of childhood. Cross-sectional imaging modalities such as US may confirm periosteal elevation in the first few days; MRI—and to a lesser degree CT—can detect marrow (with use of high T2-weighting, fat suppression, and short T1 inversion recovery [STIR] techniques), cortex, and soft tissue alterations caused by edema and destruction (Figs. 7-39 and 7-40). The sequestrum and/or cloaca is well shown by both CT and MRI. Whole-body MRI has been shown to be useful in detecting multiple sites of infection.

Subacute Osteomyelitis

Subacute osteomyelitis is more insidious in presentation (2 weeks of symptoms) and more classic on conventional radiographs: single or laminated periosteal new bone formation or a

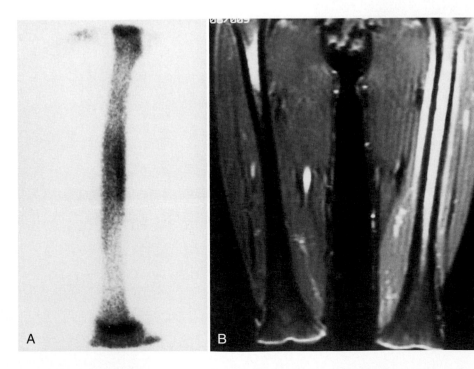

FIGURE 7-40. Acute osteomyelitis. **A,** Radionuclide scan demonstrates an area of increased uptake in the left femoral diaphysis. **B,** MR images better illustrate extent of marrow involvement *(right)* and soft tissue edema *(left)* of the left femur.

lucent circumscribed lesion (a Brodie abscess) in the metaphyses of long bones, predominantly abutting the growth plate with well-defined dense margins, is most commonly seen in the tibia and femur (Fig. 7-41). CT and MRI delineate the extent of these findings exquisitely, but they are not really necessary or diagnostic. Differentiation of subacute osteomyelitis from an osteoid osteoma (less than 2 cm in diameter) or a stress fracture may be difficult. Metastatic neuroblastoma and Ewing sarcoma may also be included in the differential diagnosis.

Chronic Osteomyelitis

Chronic osteomyelitis, defined as continuous infection of a low-grade type or of a recurrent type, is characterized predominantly by bony sclerosis, periosteal new bone formation, and the presence of sequestra and/or draining sinuses. It is uncommon in children. CT or MRI defines the extent better than conventional radiographs. If the new bone formation is considerable, the imaging findings are known as Garré sclerosing osteomyelitis, which is due to multiple small foci of repeated infarction at the infection site that result in new bone formation. This entity may occasionally be difficult to distinguish from osteoid osteoma, Ewing tumor, and FD (Fig. 7-42).

Unique Forms of Inflammation

Juvenile Rheumatoid Arthritis

Infection of the joints, or arthritis, is the most important chronic disease of children. There are two types: (1) adult type (rheumatoid factor [RF] positive) and (2) a pauciarticular form (RF negative), which is known as Still disease if it coexists with splenomegaly and lymphadenopathy. Iridocyclitis may or may not coexist with JRA. The disorder manifests in children between 3 and 5 years of age, predominantly girls, as pain and swelling of joints.

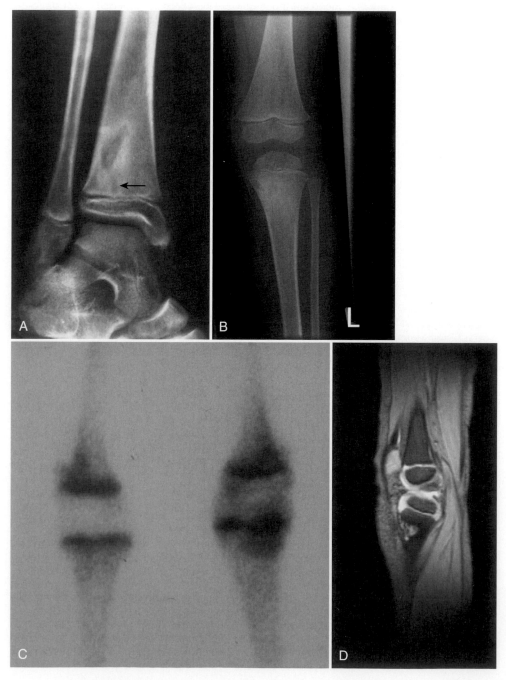

FIGURE 7-41. Subacute osteomyelitis. **A,** Brodie abscess extending to the growth plate *(arrow)* of the distal tibia. The same findings in the proximal tibia of another patient are shown in a radiograph (**B**), radionuclide scan (**C**), and MR image (**D**).

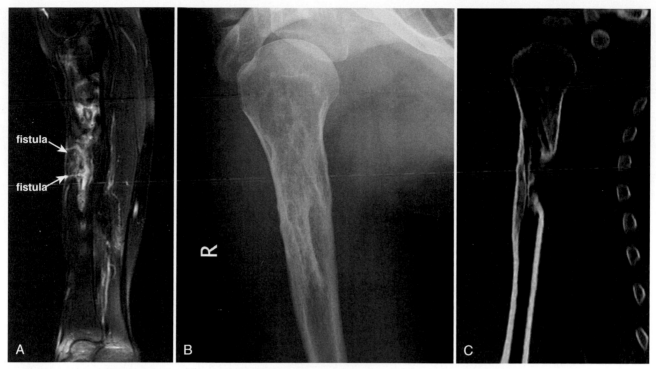

FIGURE 7-42. Chronic osteomyelitis. **A,** Fistulae after 3 months of infection. **B,** Radiograph showing chronic remodeling changes. **C,** CT scan of chronic skeletal changes.

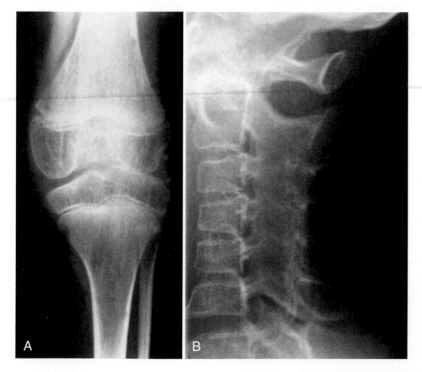

FIGURE 7-43. Juvenile rheumatoid arthritis. **A,** Epiphyseal overgrowth and widening of the intercondylar notch. **B,** Bony fusion of the cervical apophyseal joints.

Sites of involvement in chronic polyarthritis are hands (50%), wrist (70%), and feet and knees (90%). Cervical spine involvement is seen in 2% of both variants. Radiographic findings are identical to those in adult rheumatoid arthritis but lack the symmetric involvement. They include soft tissue swelling; accelerated bony maturation with early closure of the physes and epiphyseal overgrowth; periosteal new bone formation with growth recovery lines; and bony erosions (Fig. 7-43). Joint space narrowing, widening of the intercondylar notch, and effusions,

as well as ankylosis of the apophyseal joints (cervical spine, sacroiliac joints), may supervene. Skeletal scintigraphy is useful to monitor distribution and progression of the disease. MRI is superior for joint imaging, especially for cartilage assessment and the detection of response to hemosiderin therapy.

The rheumatoid variants, such as psoriatic arthritis, arthritis of inflammatory bowel disease, and Reiter syndrome, are rare in children but may be considered in the differential diagnosis of JRA.

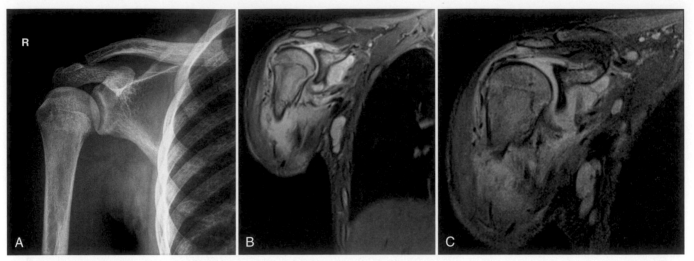

FIGURE 7-44. **A,** Plain film in a 17-year-old patient with known β-thalassemia who presented to the emergency department with right shoulder pain. Note the abnormal bone marrow pattern in the diaphysis and in the ribs, with normal alignment of the humeral head and glenohumeral joint. **B,** Coronal image using intravenous contrast agent, T1 weighting, and fat suppression; **C,** axial short T1 inversion recovery (STIR) image. Both show marked joint effusion with hypertrophic enhancing synovium, indicating septic arthritis. The subperiosteal extension is the key finding, because it requires surgical treatment. (Courtesy Mario Maas, MD, PhD, Amsterdam Medical Center, The Netherlands.)

Septic Arthritis

Septic arthritis is frequently encountered in the neonate, often in the intensive care unit. It is due to secondary joint involvement in osteomyelitis by an infecting organism that crosses the growth plate via vascular channels. It is most often seen in the shoulder or hips, followed by the knee, elbow, and ankle. Polyarticular involvement is common, with the hip the most common site (60%). *S. aureus* is the most likely organism in children younger than 2 years; after that age, group B *Streptococcus* or coliform bacteria are the most common organisms. Imaging findings, often absent in the first few days, include joint effusion, periarticular osteopenia, and apparent joint dislocation or fracture through the growth plate (type 1 epiphysiolysis). Characteristically, this fracture through the growth plate is seen in the hip because increased

joint pressure compresses the vascular supply to the femoral head, which also puts the patients at risk for avascular necrosis. Joint space narrowing occurs within days; bone destruction and subsequent remodeling are rare late sequelae. The differential diagnosis of a widened joint space includes JRA, hemarthrosis (hemophilia), and toxic synovitis (Fig. 7-44).

Toxic (transient) synovitis (irritable hip) consists of pain and a limp and/or spasm. It affects children younger than 10 years, and it has a male preponderance. Although there is joint fluid, a causative organism is seldom if ever found. A recent viral illness is often noted.

Radiographic findings in the hips are usually normal. Any effusion (e.g., inflammatory, hemarthrosis, or JRA) may increase the teardrop–femoral head distance. A difference of more than 1 mm

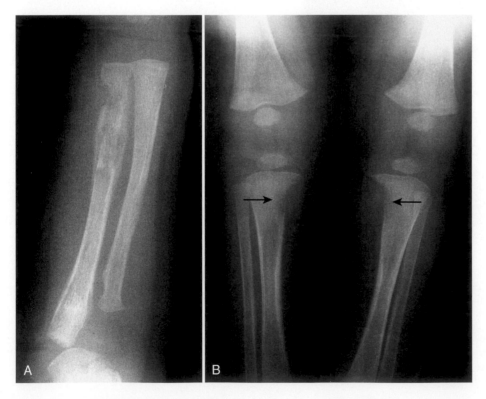

FIGURE 7-45. Syphilis. **A,** Destructive metadiaphysitis in an infant's ulna. **B,** Wimberger sign in proximal tibiae: destruction of the medial metaphyses *(arrows).*

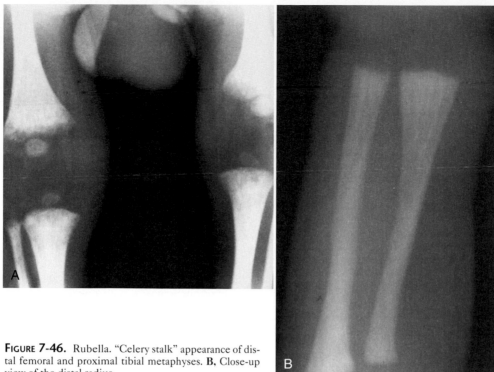

FIGURE 7-46. Rubella. "Celery stalk" appearance of distal femoral and proximal tibial metaphyses. **B,** Close-up view of the distal radius.

from side to side is considered significant for the presence of an effusion. US, which is much more sensitive for detection of joint effusions is the imaging modality of choice. Radionuclide scanning may show increased periarticular activity or, if vascular compression has occurred, a photopenic femoral head area. Neither imaging modality is specific for synovitis. MRI may be adjunctive.

Congenital Syphilis

As a result of transplacental spread of *Treponema pallidum* in the second or third trimester, an infected infant may present with a rash, anemia, hepatosplenomegaly, ascites, and nephrotic syndrome. Because the skeletal manifestations (eventually present in 80% of patients) of syphilis may take up to 2 months to appear, radiographic diagnosis may be delayed. Bilateral symmetric involvement of the long bones is characteristic. A metaphyseal lucent band ("metaphysitis") is directly subjacent to a dense band in the subphyseal region. Focal areas of lytic destruction may occur in the diaphyses (Fig. 7-45). The bilateral metaphyseal destruction in the upper medial tibia is seen in 50% of patients, known as the (other) Wimberger sign (see under "Scurvy"). This destructive lesion may also be seen in bacterial osteomyelitis and hyperparathyroidism. There may be pathologic fractures and abundant periosteal new bone formation, in both the metaphyses *and* the diaphyses. In the cranium and flat bones, lytic lesions may occur. With specific therapy, most lesions heal. Thickening of the anterior tibial cortex during healing leads to the so-called saber shin deformity.

Congenital Rubella

Maternal rubella infection during the first half of pregnancy results in intrauterine growth retardation, cataracts, deafness, hepatosplenomegaly, and cardiovascular lesions as well as skeletal changes in about half of infants. Conventional radiographs demonstrate irregular metaphyses characterized by the classic "celery stalk" appearance, particularly around the knee (Fig. 7-46). All of the TORCH entities (*t*oxoplasmosis, *o*ther [congenital syphilis and viruses], *r*ubella, *c*ytomegalovirus, and *h*erpes simplex virus)

TABLE 7-1. Differential Diagnosis of Radiographic Findings in the Skeleton*

Metaphyseal lucency ("lines")	**Leukemia**
	Infection: syphilis, TORCH (*t*oxoplasmosis, *o*ther [congenital syphilis and viruses], *r*ubella, *c*ytomegalovirus, and *h*erpes simplex virus) **syndrome**
	Neuroblastoma
	Endocrine (rickets, hypophosphatasia)
	Scurvy
"Celery stalking"	Rubella
	Syphilis
	Toxoplasmosis
	Cytomegalovirus
Widened joint space	Transient synovitis
	Septic arthritis
	Juvenile rheumatoid arthritis
	Hemarthrosis (trauma, hemophilia)

***Boldface type** indicates lines.

should be included in the differential possibilities. Periosteal new bone formation is rare in these entities except for syphilis. Most changes are trophic and heal by 3 to 6 months of life. Skeletal maturation is often delayed (Table 7-1).

Ankylosing Spondylitis

The onset of spondylitis is usually in early adulthood; so-called juvenile ankylosing spondylitis may also occur in children, more commonly in boys, especially those older than 8 years of age. Chronic inflammatory changes of the spine and sacroiliac joints resulting in ascending ankylosis and spine deformity are of unknown cause and are partly genetic (positive HLA B27 response in 95% of patients). In the pediatric age group, blurring and sclerosis with eventual fusion of the sacroiliac joint is the most common radiographic finding, but syndesmophytes are rare.

■ AGGRESSIVE LESIONS

Osteosarcoma

Osteosarcoma is the most common primary malignant neoplasm of bone that occurs in older children and young adults (10 to 25 years of age). It accounts for 60% of malignant bone lesions in the first two decades of life. The neoplasm affects males more than females (1.4:1) and is usually located in the metaphysis of a long bone (80%), especially around the knee (65%). There are three subgroups of osteosarcoma: osteoid producers (50%), predominantly cartilaginous (chondroblastic; 25%), and predominantly fibroblastic (an abundance of spindle cells; 25%). The difference in cell types affects the radiographic appearance. Pain and swelling of the affected area are the common clinical findings, not seldom the result of pathologic fracture.

Conventional radiographic findings include a mixed lytic and sclerotic, aggressive, and eccentric metaphyseal lesion that penetrates the cortex and is accompanied by "sunburst" periosteal new bone formation that may be flocculent.

A Codman triangle may be present. Multicentric or metachronous (skip) lesions may occur in up to 10% of cases. MRI exquisitely defines the extent of bone marrow and soft tissue involvement both before and after therapy (Fig. 7-47). Metastatic lesions are most commonly noted in the lung on CT and may ossify; they are found in 10% to 20% of patients at presentation. The role of radionuclide scintigraphy in assessment for osteosarcoma has diminished with the availability of CT and MRI and does not reliably detect skip lesions. Treatment consists of preoperative and/or postoperative chemotherapy, resection, and allograft replacement. Overall, the probability of 5-year survival is about 70% in the absence of metastatic disease.

The varieties of osteosarcoma are all rare in children. A parosteal osteosarcoma occurs in the third decade, more often in females; it manifests radiographically as a lobulated ossified mass, most often in the distal femur. Parosteal osteosarcoma has the best prognosis of all forms of osteosarcoma.

A telangiectatic osteosarcoma looks like an aneurysmal bone cyst, measuring more than 5 cm; it is purely lytic with fluid-fluid levels and very destructive, and it most often occurs in the metaphyses around the knee. The differential diagnosis of this form of osteosarcoma consists of aneurysmal bone cyst (ABC) and other sarcomas.

A periosteal osteosarcoma is a diaphyseal lesion that has chondroblastic characteristics yet has a better prognosis than a conventional osteosarcoma.

Except for the telangiectatic variety, the differential diagnosis of osteosarcoma includes myositis ossificans, chondrosarcoma, and giant cell tumor.

Ewing Sarcoma

Although Ewing sarcoma affects a somewhat younger age group than osteosarcoma, it is also more common in males (2:1). The tumor is rare in African Americans and Asians and in patients older than 30 years. It is the most common bone lesion in the first decade, is second only to osteosarcoma in the second decade, and rarely occurs before age 5 years. Peak incidence is at 5 to 15 years of age. In 30% to 40% of cases, the child presents with pain, fever, and leukocytosis, findings that mimic osteomyelitis. Because both the clinical picture and imaging appearance of Ewing sarcoma may mimic those of osteomyelitis, biopsy is required. Long bones (femur) are primarily affected, followed by the spine and ribs; 25% of cases occur in the pelvis.

On conventional radiographs, this diaphyseal lesion is characteristically permeative with poorly defined margins, often lytic. There may be periosteal new bone formation with an "onion-skin" appearance. CT and MRI clearly delineate the

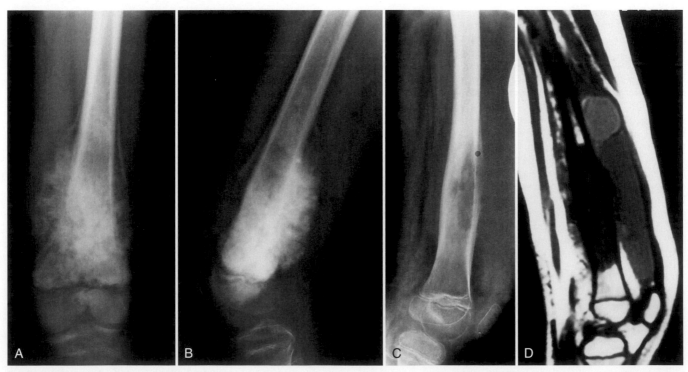

FIGURE 7-47. Osteosarcoma. **A** and **B,** Conventional radiographs of a classic bone-forming tumor of the distal femur, with "sunburst" periosteal new bone formation and elevation. **C,** Conventional radiograph of a lytic osteosarcoma of the distal femur. **D,** T1-weighted MR image exquisitely delineates the extent of marrow and soft tissue involvement.

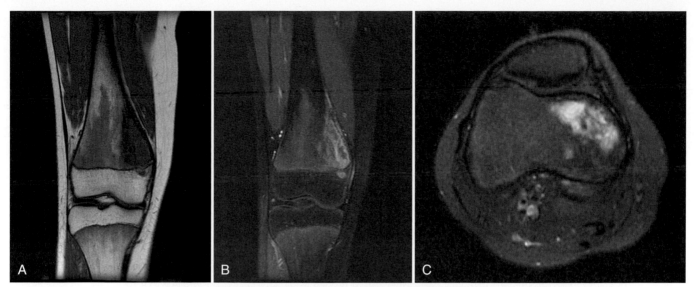

FIGURE 7-48. Ewing sarcoma. **A,** Coronal T1-weighted MR image in a patient who had thigh pain 2 weeks after soccer trauma. Conventional film findings were normal. **B,** Coronal T1-weighted MR image with fat suppression obtained after administration of contrast agent. **C,** Axial T2-weighted MR image using fat suppression.

often very large soft tissue component of Ewing sarcoma, especially in the flat bones of the pelvis and thoracic cage (Fig. 7-48). Bone scintigraphy is useful for the early detection of bone metastases, which are common in Ewing sarcoma. Metastatic lesions are seen in the lungs, skeletal system, and lymph nodes and are present in 15% to 25% of children at presentation. Treatment primarily consists of radiotherapy and chemotherapy, sometimes in combination with resection. Five-year survival approaches 50%.

The differential diagnosis of Ewing sarcoma includes EG, non-Hodgkin lymphoma, osteosarcoma, osteomyelitis, and metastatic neuroblastoma.

Primitive Neuroectodermal Tumor of Childhood

Clinically similar to Ewing sarcoma, primitive neuroectodermal tumor (PNET) of childhood consists of small round cell tumors that are likely neural in origin. A highly malignant tumor, PNET is located most often in the thoracopulmonary region and has been called an Askin tumor. Often the tumor is associated with a pleural effusion and a rapidly enlarging soft tissue mass (see Fig. 2-24). CT defines its extent well. If there is no metastatic disease or locoregional invasion of cardiomediastinal or pulmonary structures at the time of diagnosis, the probability of 5-year survival is approximately 50%.

Chondrosarcoma

Chondrosarcoma is rare in children (less than 5% of cases) and may occur centrally (medullary) or peripherally (cortical or juxtacortical). The medullary version occurs exclusively in adults. The peripheral lesions arise in osteochondromas (exostoses) and tend to occur in the third through fifth decades. These peripheral lesions are more than 5 cm in diameter; they have a cartilaginous cap greater than 1 cm and are of a low-grade malignancy. Overall, this tumor of cartilaginous origin is characterized by slow growth and progression, and it may manifest as a very large lesion. The central lesion is often metaphyseal in location, occurring in the femur, ribs, and humerus, as well as in the pelvis; however, the peripheral lesion is more often diaphyseal in location. A chondrosarcoma that has arisen in a (preexisting) benign cartilaginous lesion, such as multiple enchondromatosis or osteochondromatosis, or after radiation therapy is more commonly located in the

flat bones (scapula, pelvis). Chondrosarcomas clinically manifest as pain and interval growth and/or swelling of the lesion. Conventional radiographs may show the typical "popcorn" or "cumulus cloud" type of calcification; the calcification is best seen, and its extent best delineated, on CT or MRI (Fig. 7-49). MRI does show the extent of bone and soft tissue involvement but may not identify the calcific component of the tumor. These lesions are often radioresistant, and treatment consists of wide excision.

Metastatic Lesions

Box 7-3 outlines the differential diagnosis of metastatic bone lesions.

Leukemia

Leukemia constitutes the most common childhood cancer. Eighty percent of cases are the acute lymphoblastic type. The peak age incidence is 2 to 5 years. Bone and joint pain is a common clinical finding, and there may be tenderness and swelling of the extremities. More than half of patients with leukemia have skeletal findings classically consisting of osteopenia (metaphyseal lucent bands), focal osteolytic lesions, and, in 35%, periosteal new bone formation in association with generalized demineralization (Fig. 7-50). The periosteal new bone formation is due to subperiosteal infiltration of leukemic cells and is more often seen in the terminal phalanges. MRI exquisitely delineates the low-signal cellular infiltrate of leukemia/lymphoma (or metastatic neuroblastoma), which contrasts with the high signal of the fatty marrow on T1-weighted images. Because leukemia, lymphoma, and neuroblastoma may be indistinguishable on imaging, the definitive diagnosis of leukemia is made with bone marrow aspiration. A *chloroma* is an extramedullary manifestation of leukemia in which leukemic cell aggregates are noted in the soft tissues (e.g., retropharyngeal space).

Lymphoma

Lymphoma in children only rarely affects the skeleton (and then only secondarily as metastatic disease).

Non-Hodgkin Lymphoma

Only rarely are bone lesions the only manifestation of non-Hodgkin lymphoma. When they are, however, their appearance may mimic leukemia, neuroblastoma, and EG as well as

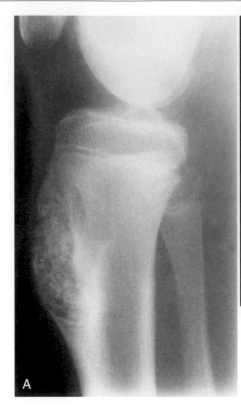

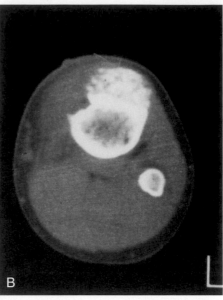

FIGURE 7-49. Chondrosarcoma. **A,** Lateral radiograph of proximal tibia shows an expansile lesion with "popcorn" calcification in the region of the tibial tubercle. **B,** CT scan confirms extent of lesion and "popcorn" calcification.

Ewing sarcoma. Permeative lesions are usually seen, vertebra plana may occur, and periosteal new bone formation, if present, is minimal.

Hodgkin Lymphoma

Radiographic findings in Hodgkin lymphoma do not differ significantly from those in non-Hodgkin lymphoma, although vertebral involvement, as in adults, usually manifests as an ivory vertebra.

Rhabdomyosarcoma

Rhabdomyosarcoma is the most common soft tissue sarcoma in children. One third of these lesions occur in the head and neck,

Box 7-3. Differential Diagnosis of Lytic (Metastatic) Bone Lesions

Lymphoma/leukemia
Neuroblastoma
Rhabdomyosarcoma
Wilms tumor
Retinoblastoma
Medulloblastoma
Ewing sarcoma or multicentric (metachronous) osteosarcoma

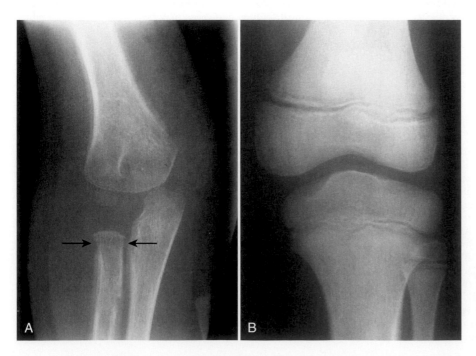

FIGURE 7-50. Acute lymphocytic leukemia. **A,** Anteroposterior radiograph of the elbow in a 6-month-old infant demonstrates the metaphyseal lucent band as part of the "moth-eaten" appearance of the proximal radius *(arrows)*. There is periosteal new bone formation of all visualized bones. **B,** Metaphyseal lucent bands in a 6-year-old child.

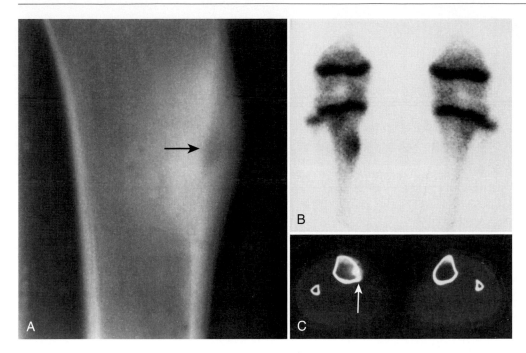

FIGURE **7-51.** Osteoid osteoma. **A,** Conventional tomography demonstrates cortical thickening and a lucent nidus *(arrow).* **B,** Radionuclide bone scan confirms increased uptake. **C,** Axial CT scan delineates the nidus as well in the right proximal tibia *(arrow).*

one third in the genitourinary tract, and one third in the bony skeleton. There are two types: the *embryonal* type, which is the more common, and the *alveolar* type, which contains slightly more mature muscle cells and more often involves the extremities. Cytologic classification seems to have more bearing on prognosis: anaplastic, monomorphous round cell, and mixed types have been described. Conventional radiographs may show an indistinct soft tissue mass with adjacent bone erosion, best seen on CT or MRI. Metastatic disease occurs primarily to the lung and regional lymph nodes (15%).

▬ BENIGN AND CYSTIC LESIONS
Osteoid Osteoma

Osteoid osteoma is a common bone-forming lesion that occurs in children older than 3 years (most commonly between 10 and 20 years) and twice as often in boys as in girls. The classic clinical presentation consists of pain, which is characteristically worse at night and is relieved by aspirin in 75% of patients. The majority of these lesions are seen in the femoral neck and tibia, as well as in the posterior elements of the vertebral column. The nidus may be cortical, periosteal, or intramedullary, and it is usually less than 1.5 cm in diameter. It is usually lucent but may calcify, and it is surrounded by an exuberant zone of reactive sclerosis. This dense sclerosis may obscure the nidus, which is then best demonstrated on CT; MRI is less useful. Radionuclide scintigraphy shows a well-circumscribed area of intense uptake (Fig. 7-51). The differential diagnosis includes healing stress fracture and chronic osteomyelitis. Surgical curettage is the treatment of choice, with confirmative imaging of the excised specimen a necessity. Thermo-ablation with radiofrequency probes in mainly peripheral nonspinal osteoid osteomas with fluoroscopic guidance is also gaining acceptance. Thermo-ablation is performed mainly with guidance from "standard" CT or CT fluoroscopy.

Much less common (<1% of all primary bone tumors) but with the same age and gender incidence and microscopic and radiographic appearance as osteoid osteoma is the *giant osteoid osteoma,* or *osteoblastoma.* There is less reactive sclerosis and more expansion of the lesion, and the nidus is more than 1.5 cm in diameter. More than half of such lesions occur in the posterior elements of the spine, and ABCs may be secondarily associated. Curettage with grafting is curative.

Chondroblastoma (Codman Tumor)

Chondroblastoma is an uncommon lesion usually seen in teenagers, with affected boys outnumbering affected girls (1.7:1). The proximal humerus and proximal tibia, as well as the distal femur, are commonly involved; 50% of lesions are located around the knee. Conventional radiographs show a well-defined, lytic, rounded lesion located in an epiphysis, a sesamoid bone, or an apophysis (Fig. 7-52). There may be cartilaginous calcification within half the lesions, which is often best seen on CT. The differential diagnosis includes osteomyelitis (classically tuberculosis), LCH, and FD. Curettage is curative.

Other differential diagnostic possibilities for this tumor are giant cell tumor (affects an older age group), avascular necrosis, and clear cell chondrosarcoma.

Benign Fibrous Cortical Defect (Nonossifying Fibroma)

The benign, asymptomatic lesions of benign fibrous cortical defect and nonossifying fibroma derive from fibrous tissue and are eccentrically metaphyseal or diaphyseal in location in the major long bones, often posteromedially. These lesions affect boys more often than girls (1.6:1). The differentiation between these two lesions is based primarily on age and size of lesion, but pathologically they are identical. Fibrous cortical defects occur in young children. They are usually round to ovoid, less than 2 cm in size, with a well-defined, sclerotic margin located in the cortex. They disappear (resorb) during teenage years (see Fig. 7-12). More than 80% occur in the lower extremities, and 25% are polyostotic. Nonossifying fibromas, which occur in older children, are more than 2 cm in diameter; they are most often seen in the distal tibia and may manifest as pathologic fracture. They do not grow or spread, and they regress spontaneously with age.

Multiple nonossifying fibromas may be found in association with NF (see Fig. 7-35A). The differential diagnosis of nonossifying fibroma includes ABC, chondromyxoid fibroma, and brown tumor.

Chondromyxoid Fibroma

Chondromyxoid fibroma, the least common benign cartilaginous tumor, is most often seen in the metaphyseal region of long bones,

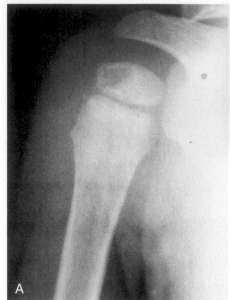

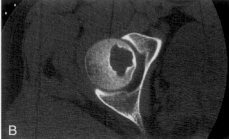

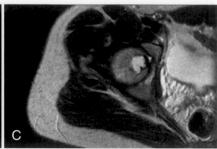

Figure 7-52. Chondroblastoma. **A,** Frontal radiograph of the proximal humerus illustrates a well-demarcated, lytic, round epiphyseal lesion. **B,** CT scan demonstrates a lesion in the femoral head. **C,** Axial T$_2$-weighted MR image of the same lesion.

with approximately one half in the proximal tibia. It occurs in the teenage years with a predilection for boys (1.6:1). There is no soft tissue involvement. The scalloped, oval, and lytic eccentric lesions with chondroid flecks of calcification (5%) are defined best on CT (Fig. 7-53). MRI also delineates the extent of the lesion and its chondromyxoid contents well. Malignant transformation of chondromyxoid fibroma has been described.

Desmoplastic Fibroma

Desmoplastic fibroma, a rare lesion, is a member of the family of fibromatosis lesions. Occurring in the distal femur and proximal tibia and more than 5 cm in diameter, desmoplastic fibroma constitutes purely lytic monostotic lesions without matrix or soft

tissue extension. The lesion manifests as pain and swelling in the second decade of life, occurring with equal frequency in men and women. CT or MRI is necessary for delineation and characterization (Fig. 7-54). It may locally recur; therefore wide (cryo)resection and curettage are necessary.

Hemangioma

Hemangiomas are the most common benign tumors in infancy and childhood, usually occurring in the skin and subcutaneous tissues. The two main forms are capillary hemangiomas and cavernous hemangiomas. Capillary hemangiomas consist of masses of capillaries that, in contrast to cavernous hemangiomas, have a connection to the systemic circulation. Cavernous hemangiomas

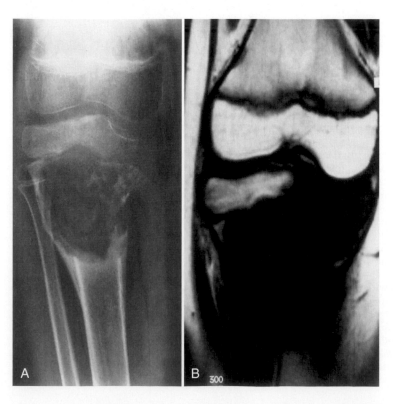

Figure 7-53. Chondromyxoid fibroma. **A,** Expansile metaphyseal lesion with chondroid flecks and scalloping, and cortical thinning and disruption. A pathologic fracture is suspected (asymmetric height loss of the proximal tibial metaphysis and diaphysis). **B,** MR image demonstrates the epiphyseal extension of the lesion.

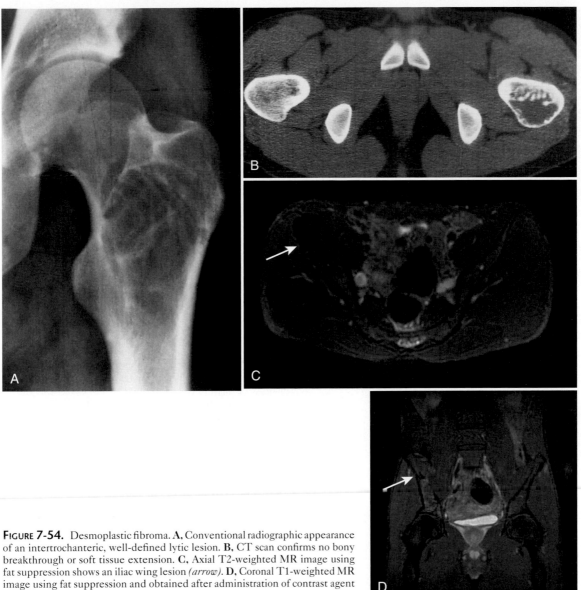

FIGURE 7-54. Desmoplastic fibroma. **A,** Conventional radiographic appearance of an intertrochanteric, well-defined lytic lesion. **B,** CT scan confirms no bony breakthrough or soft tissue extension. **C,** Axial T2-weighted MR image using fat suppression shows an iliac wing lesion *(arrow)*. **D,** Coronal T1-weighted MR image using fat suppression and obtained after administration of contrast agent shows the same lesion.

may be visible on radiographs because of calcified phleboliths. If these calcified phleboliths coexist with enchondromas, the condition is called the Maffucci syndrome. Capillary hemangiomas range from the juvenile form (strawberry nevus in 1 out of 200 live births) to deep skeletal involvement, which is most common in the lower extremity. Diffuse involvement in hemangiomatosis characteristically involves one extremity, which often enlarges because of the hyperemia; this condition is known as Klippel-Trenaunay syndrome.

Intraosseous hemangiomas are rare and more commonly found in the spine (75%) and in skull and facial bones. The typical radiographic finding is prominent bony trabeculation in vertebral bodies represented by vertical prominent dense trabeculation with mild expansion. There is no sex predilection.

Giant Cell Tumor (Osteoclastoma)

Giant cell tumors are very rarely seen before closure of the growth plate. Only 5% to 10% of giant cell tumors occur in patients younger than 15 years, and 85% occur after age 20 years. Radiographically, they often resemble ABCs and appear eccentric, with

cortical disruption in 25% of cases. They seldom cause symptoms. There is an equal sex incidence and are rare in African Americans.

Osteoclastic overactivity results in essentially fibrous lesions that histologically resemble brown tumors. Approximately 15% of tumors exhibit metastasis, primarily to the legs. Treatment consists of curettage and packing with methylmethacrylate cement. The recurrence rate is 10% to 15%. A pathologic fracture occurs in up to one third of patients with giant cell tumor.

Solitary, Unicameral, or Simple Bone Cysts

Solitary, unicameral, or simple bone cysts are relatively common bone lesions that are usually (80%) found in the proximal metaphysis of the humerus and femur. They contain clear, yellow fluid. These lesions are most common in patients between 2 and 20 years old, with boys outnumbering girls by a 3:1 ratio. Radiographically (Fig. 7-55) they appear as well-demarcated, central lucent lesions that may be mildly expansile or contain septa, and they are occasionally complicated by pathologic fracture. Like fibrous cortical defects, they gradually disappear and are seldom seen in adulthood. A "fallen fragment," resulting

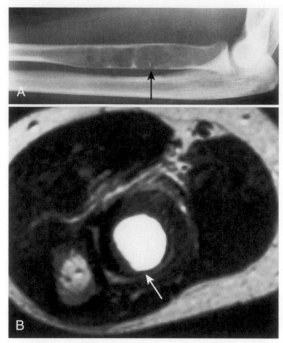

FIGURE 7-55. Unicameral bone cyst. **A,** Mildly expansile lytic lesion of the proximal radius with a "fallen fragment" *(arrow)*. **B,** MR image confirms the cystic nature and the fluid-fluid level *(arrow)*.

from a pathologic fracture, may be noted in 15% to 20% of such bone cysts. If it is a totally "free" fragment, it will be located in the most dependent portion of the lesion. It may also be mimicked by overlapping bone fragments after a pathologic fracture. CT findings are comparable to findings on conventional radiographs; MRI demonstrates the cyst contents as uniformly high T2 signal. There is no soft tissue extension except for edema after a pathologic fracture. If for mechanical reasons treatment is necessary, it consists of curettage and packing with bone chips. Intracavitary steroid or methylmethacrylate injection has also had success, but with such therapy there is a 20% recurrence rate of the cyst. The differential diagnosis includes ABC, LCH, and FD.

Aneurysmal Bone Cysts

Although once considered a giant cell variant, ABCs are cavernous, blood-filled spaces that are most often seen in the metaphyses of tubular bones and in the posterior elements of the vertebral column. ABC is the only bone tumor named after its radiographic appearance, and it is slightly more common in girls than in boys. Eighty percent occur in patients younger than 20 years. Located eccentrically, ABCs are expansile and considered posttraumatic or reactive lesions; a preexisting osseous lesion (nonossifying fibroma, single bone cyst, or osteoblastoma) is associated in 30% to 50% of cases. Expansion of the cortex may cause focal cortical disruption, resulting in associated reactive periosteal new bone formation that mimics an aggressive lesion. CT and MRI may show fluid-fluid levels in one third of cases; this finding is highly suggestive but not diagnostic of ABC, differential diagnosis of which includes telangiectatic osteosarcoma, aggressive lesions, and osteosarcoma (Fig. 7-56). Treatment for ABCs consists of resection or curettage, and there is a 50% recurrence rate.

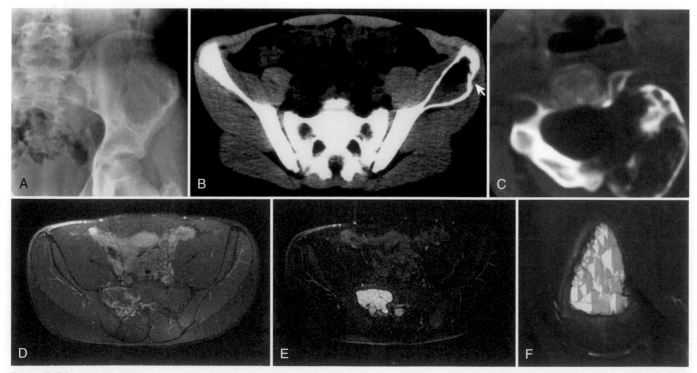

FIGURE 7-56. Aneurysmal bone cyst (ABC). **A,** Frontal radiograph of pelvis demonstrates a lucent, well-demarcated left iliac lesion with minimal internal architecture. **B,** Axial CT scan shows both a fluid-fluid level within the expansile left iliac lesion and the pathologic fracture *(arrow)*. **C,** Axial CT scan illustrates an ABC of the posterior elements of C5. **D,** Axial T1-weighted MR image with fat suppression obtained after administration of contrast agent shows a sacral lesion. **E,** Axial T2-weighted MR image using fat suppression showing the same lesion. **F,** Classic "fluid-fluid" levels in a distal femoral lesion.

■ TRAUMA

Injuries

The pattern of fractures in the pediatric population depends on the age of the child, the stage of the child's development, and the knowledge that dislocations and ligamentous injuries are uncommon in children. Pediatric fractures generally occur as a result of abnormal stress on normal bone, and less often secondary to normal stress on abnormal (pathologic) bone. Rapid repair and remodeling are the rule in children with more than 2 years of growth remaining; only rotational injuries to bone do not follow this rule, especially if the physis is involved.

There are also age-related differences in the composition of the bones and soft tissues. In the soft tissues, the relatively stronger and thicker periosteum and the stronger but slightly more lax ligaments are relatively resistant and/or resilient to external forces applied. In addition, the haversian canals constitute more of the cortical bone in children than in adults, making children's bones more pliable. This difference explains why children have more incomplete fractures than adults—the forces can be more easily absorbed. On the other hand, the weakest point in the pediatric bony skeleton is the physis or growth plate. Finally, the type of fracture is often influenced by the kind of activity in which the child of a certain age is engaged; for example, toddler's fractures seldom occur after age 2 years, shoulder dislocations and/or clavicular fractures are more characteristic of birth trauma, and a femoral or humeral shaft fracture seldom occurs accidentally in an infant.

The extent of fracture healing is also an important adjunct in the correct evaluation of pediatric fractures. There are three stages: the inflammatory stage, with an acute hematoma; the callus formation stage, with immature bony bridging; and the reparative stage, when mature bone replaces the fibrocartilage and immature bone bridges the fracture site. The callus formation stage can be radiographically identified by 10 to 14 days after the fracture; at 6 weeks, well-organized bone is usually present. The amount of callus formation depends on the fracture site and amount of displacement, as well as the extent of immobilization during the healing phase. These same factors also directly affect the amount of remodeling that can be achieved in the healing process. The younger the child, the greater the potential for remodeling. Internal fixation is rarely necessary because nonunion seldom occurs.

This means that the most important complications of pediatric fractures are due to growth disturbances that may occur when the fracture involves the growth plate. Resultant bony bridging of the growth plate is exquisitely delineated on MRI (Fig. 7-57).

As stated, different fracture mechanisms are identified in children according to age. In infants and toddlers, incomplete fractures may be of the bowing (plastic) type, with no obvious break in the cortex; of the greenstick type, defined as a fracture on the convex side of the cortex but not on the concave side; and of the buckle type, possibly occurring on the opposite side of the greenstick fracture. This buckling is also known as a *torus* (*protuberance*, or "little hill") fracture (Fig. 7-58). Stress fractures can be the result either of abnormal stress to normal bone (march fractures) or of normal stress placed on abnormal bone (rickets, OI). Radionuclide scintigraphy is most sensitive early on for detection of stress fractures; lucent lines surrounded by sclerosis can be noted radiographically after about 1 week.

Fractures involving the growth plate reflect the relative weakness of the growth plate cartilage and the greater laxity and strength of the ligaments, as well as the tight attachment of the periosteum. In order from the epiphysis to the metaphysis, there are four zones in the growth plate: the germinal zone, the proliferating zone, the hypertrophic zone, and the ZPC. Because of the relative abundance of collagen matrix in the germinal and proliferating zones, as well as the calcium deposition in the ZPC, the hypertrophic zone is the relatively weakest zone. It is here that fractures occur.

The Salter-Harris classification of epiphyseal complex fractures recognizes at least five types, as follows (Fig. 7-59):

Type I: The fracture passes through the growth plate only; more common in children younger than 5 years.

Type II: The fracture line exits through the metaphysis; accounts for approximately 70% of all fractures involving the growth plate; most commonly seen in the distal radius and tibia.

Type III: Accounts for 10%; the fracture line extends through the epiphysis; it is thus intra-articular and is most often seen affecting the ankle and knee and the medial epicondyle of the distal humerus.

Type IV: Accounts for 10%; occurs when the fracture extends through both the metaphysis and the epiphysis; is seen most often in the lateral epicondyle of the distal humerus.

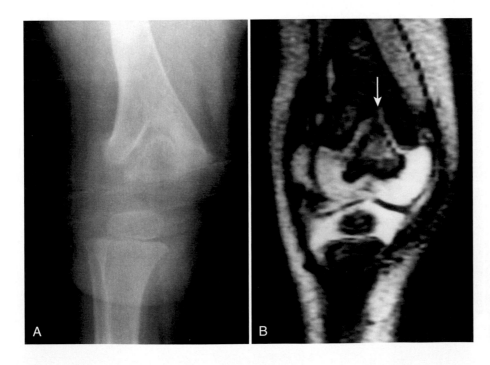

FIGURE 7-57. Posttraumatic bony bridge (and secondary focal growth deformity). **A,** Frontal radiograph. **B,** MR image illustrates the bony bridge well *(arrow).*

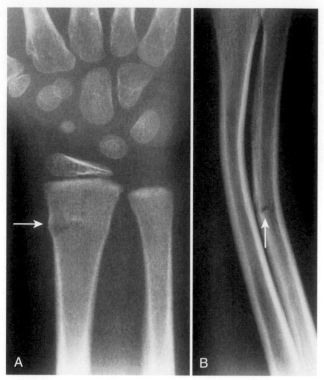

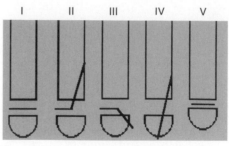

FIGURE 7-59. Schematic diagram of the Salter-Harris classification of epiphyseal complex fractures. *Left* to *right,* types I through V; see text for explanation.

FIGURE 7-58. A, Torus fracture resembling a "little hill" *(arrow).* **B,** Bowing fracture of the radius and "greenstick" fracture of the ulna *(arrow).*

Type V: Rare (1%); involves a crush of the growth plate and may lead to premature fusion.

Salter-Harris type I and II fractures have an excellent result if properly treated, as will type III if properly reduced. Type IV and V fractures may result in growth deformity, and they often need open reduction and/or internal fixation (Fig. 7-60).

Common Fractures/Dislocations in the Upper Extremity

Two thirds of fractures of the clavicle occur in children younger than 10 years. The part of the clavicle most commonly fractured is the middle third, followed by the lateral third. These fractures heal completely most of the time. Acromioclavicular separations are rare.

The surgical neck of the humerus is the second most common site of injury. On the AP view the radiographic appearance of the growth plate at two (differential) levels which is a normal variant, should not be mistaken for a fracture (Fig. 7-61). Midshaft fractures are unusual, but they put the radial nerve and brachial artery at risk for injury. These fractures also heal well, without the need for internal fixation. The pseudosubluxation of the glenohumeral joint seen in association with midshaft humeral fractures may persist for several weeks but eventually resolves spontaneously.

The elbow is one of the more common sites of injury and the most difficult area in which to interpret the imaging findings. In addition to understanding the normal ossification sequence (see Fig. 7-2), one should note that an effusion most likely indicates a fracture even if it is not found after a diligent search. The quintessential finding on the lateral view is known as the "fat pad" sign. Normally, fat is "visible" in the shallow anterior coracoid fossa, whereas the fat in the deep posterior olecranon fossa is not normally noted (Fig. 7-62A and D-1). An effusion (traumatic, secondary to blood dyscrasia or infection) elevates these fat pads, deforming and elevating the anterior fat pad as well as the posterior fat pad, resulting in the latter's "visualization." In a trauma setting, a nondisplaced distal humeral (supracondylar) fracture is most commonly the culprit in younger children, whereas an occult radial head fracture is more likely in older children (Fig. 7-62A). More than half of the fractures around the elbow are of the supracondylar variety.

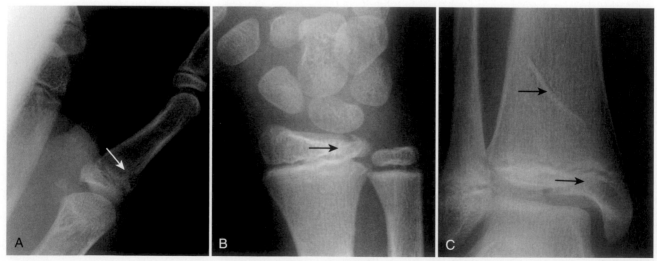

FIGURE 7-60. Salter-Harris fractures of the epiphyseal complex. **A,** Type II, fracture through the metaphysis *(arrow).* **B,** Type III, fracture through the epiphysis *(arrow).* **C,** Type IV, fracture through the metaphysis and epiphysis *(arrows).*

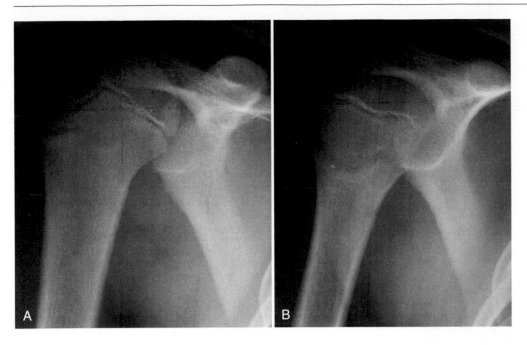

FIGURE 7-61. Normal proximal humeral growth plate in external rotation (**A**) and internal rotation (**B**).

To assess the extent of dislocation and determine subsequent avenues of treatment, several lines may be drawn in the lateral view of the elbow: the *anterior humeral line* is a line drawn down the anterior aspect of the shaft of the humerus. It should pass through the middle of the ossification center of the capitellum. This line aids in assessing the amount of dorsal or ventral angulation. The *radiocapitellar line* through the center of the radius

should do the same, to allow detection of radial head dislocation. The extent of dislocation, within a spectrum ranging from mild avulsion to fractures with posterior dislocation of the ulna, determines the need for open or closed reduction (Fig. 7-62D-3).

Avulsion fracture of the medial epicondyle is seen in up to 15% of elbow injuries in children. This fracture—known as a "Little Leaguer's" elbow because it occurs when the flexor carpi ulnaris

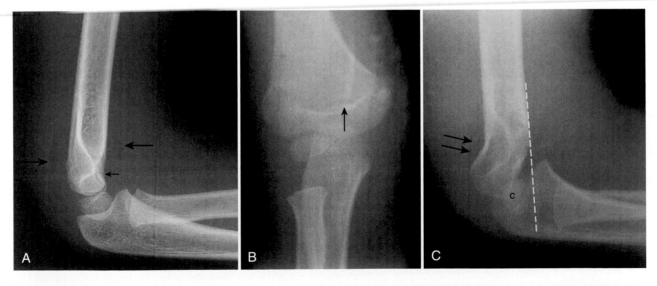

FIGURE 7-62. Elbow trauma. **A,** Fat pad sign *(arrows)* indicates an elbow effusion in a patient with a nondisplaced distal humeral fracture *(small arrow)*. **B,** Anterior view demonstrates the fracture line *(arrow)*. **C,** Lateral view shows the extent of dislocation. Note the location of the capitellum (c) posterior to the anterior humeral line *(dashed line)*. A fat pad sign is also present *(arrows)*. **D,** Schematic representation of (1) normal joint, (2) effusions *(arrows)*, and (3) anterior humeral line and radiocapitellar line.

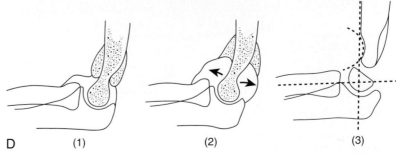

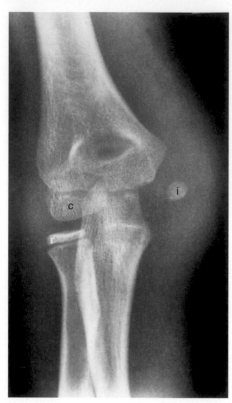

FIGURE 7-63. "Little Leaguer's elbow." Avulsion fracture of the medial epicondyle (i) with marked soft tissue swelling. c, capitellum.

tendon pulls off the medial condyle—classically is the result of snapping the wrist and/or elbow when throwing a curve ball at too early an (skeletal) age. Significant soft tissue swelling is usually associated with this fracture (Fig. 7-63). The fragment, often still attached to the tendon, may be trapped within the elbow joint, causing pain and/or locking. Internal fixation by pinning the fragment is the treatment of choice.

Traumatic dislocation of the elbow joint is virtually always in a posterior direction. Avulsion of the medial epicondyle is often associated.

In infants, the "nursemaid's" elbow is the result of pulling (extension) of the arm by an adult. The radial head slips out of its figure-of-eight annular ligament. This dislocation is usually readily reduced by supination of the forearm. When positioning the child for a radiograph, the radiographer frequently accomplishes the reduction; this is the reason that radiographs are frequently

noncontributory to diagnosis, except for an occasional avulsion fracture. Carpal injuries are very rare before the teenage years, and rare in fact until adulthood.

Common Fractures/Dislocations in the Lower Extremity

In children, fractures/dislocations in the lower extremity mostly occur in the hip and the ankle, followed by the knee.

Slipped capital femoral epiphysis (SCFE) in children is a Salter-Harris type I fracture of the proximal femoral growth plate. It is relatively common in adolescents who are obese, and is more likely in boys and in African Americans. It may be a hereditary condition and is more common on the left side. Both mechanical and endocrine factors have been implicated as causes. SCFE has also been associated with hypothyroidism, rickets, osteomyelitis, and developmental dysplasia of the hip (DDH).

The fracture occurs between the proliferative and hypertrophic zones of the metaphysis, as opposed to a classic Salter-Harris type I fracture. Because of normal muscular forces, the femoral neck moves anteriorly and slightly superolaterally, so that the epiphysis is rotated posteriorly and inferomedially (retroversion).

Conventional radiographs can show (1) a subtle difference in joint and femoral head symmetry, with the frontal view revealing loss of height of the affected epiphysis; (2) widening of the affected growth plate (AP view); and (3) the lateral femoral neck (Klein) line traversing the lateral aspect of the ipsilateral epiphysis (AP view). An additional aid is the finding that on the frog-leg lateral view, the widened growth plate is better delineated (as a result of the posterior and inferior displacement of the epiphysis). Both views are useful, although pain may make it difficult to obtain the frog-leg lateral view (Fig. 7-64). Contralateral SCFE occurs in 10% to 15% of patients.

In summary:

AP view: femoral head asymmetry (loss of height), widening of the growth plate, abnormal lateral femoral neck (Klein) line.

Lateral view: widened growth plate, posterior and inferior slippage.

Treatment of SCFE consists of internal pin fixation of the epiphysis, usually in situ. If there has been an acute slip, the pinning may be accomplished after closed reduction. Late sequelae include avascular necrosis (10%) and chondrolysis, especially in teenage girls and African Americans, and especially if the subchondral cortex is penetrated by the fixation pin. Controversy exists about prophylactic contralateral pin fixation.

Fractures around the knee in children are not common, but those of the Salter-Harris types II (70%) and III (15%) do occur. The knee is the most common site for a Salter type V fracture, especially the proximal tibial physis. Fractures of the patella are uncommon; they are transverse or stellate in configuration and

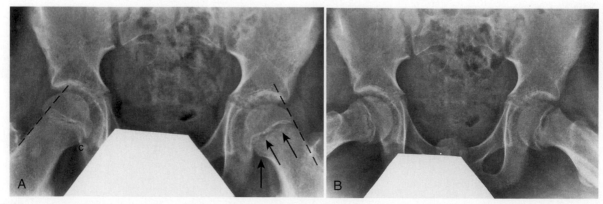

FIGURE 7-64. Slipped capital femoral epiphysis (SCFE). **A,** Anteroposterior radiograph reveals a widened physis *(double arrows)* and decreased height of the epiphysis on the left. Also Klein's line does not intersect epiphysis on affected side *(dotted line)*. In addition, there is loss *(arrow)* of the Capener triangle (c) (normal double density of the medial metaphysis superimposed on the posterior acetabular rim on right). **B,** Frog-leg (Lauenstein) lateral view confirms the inferomedial position of the SCFE.

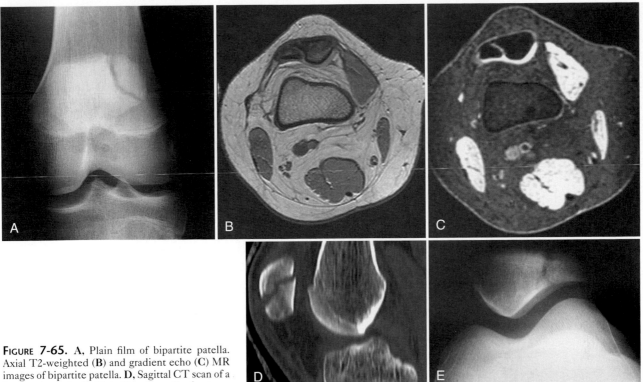

FIGURE 7-65. A, Plain film of bipartite patella. Axial T2-weighted (**B**) and gradient echo (**C**) MR images of bipartite patella. **D,** Sagittal CT scan of a fractured patella. **E,** Plain film of patellar fracture.

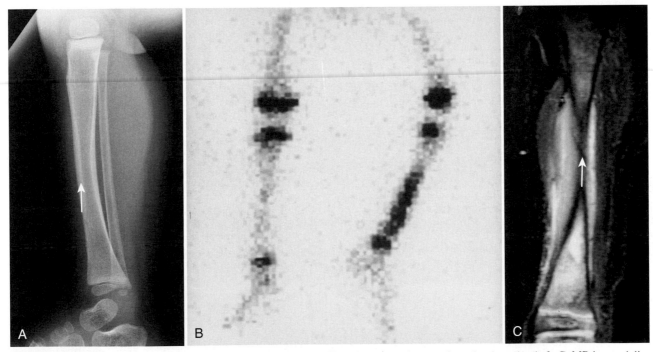

FIGURE 7-66. Toddler's fracture. **A,** Spiral fracture *(arrow)* of the tibia. **B,** Bone scan shows increased uptake along the shaft. **C,** MR image delineates the fracture *(arrow)* surrounded by bone and soft tissue.

often associated with dislocation. A bipartite patella should not be confused with a fracture (Fig. 7-65).

Toddler's Fracture

A spiral fracture of the tibia in a child who is starting to walk (between ages 1 and 2 years) is called a toddler's fracture. It consists of an undisplaced fracture of the middle to distal tibial shaft. Oblique radiographs may be necessary for confirmation.

Radionuclide bone scanning reveals increased uptake along the entire tibial shaft. A child who has a toddler's fracture usually has a limp and is afebrile (Fig. 7-66).

Osteochondroses

Osteochondroses most often become apparent in the first decade of life, during growth spurts.

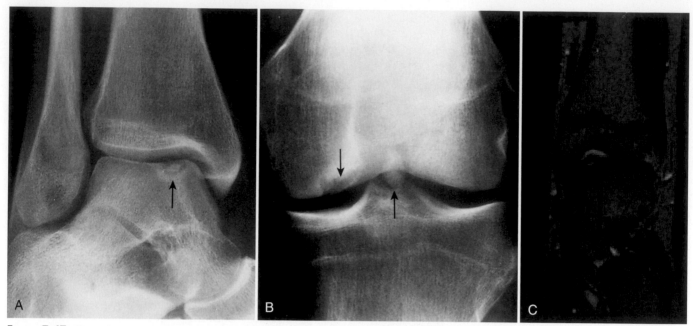

FIGURE 7-67. Osteochondritis dissecans. **A,** "Lytic" talar dome lesion with a sclerotic margin and a sclerotic nidus *(arrow).* **B,** Loose bony fragment in the joint space *("up" arrow)*; the donor site for the fragment *("down" arrow).* **C,** MR image illustrates cartilaginous continuity.

Osteochondrosis Dissecans

Often misnamed as osteochond*ritis* dissecans, osteochondrosis dissecans predominantly affects teenagers and young adults and most likely has a traumatic origin (impaction). It affects males more than females (3:1), and the condition most commonly occurs in the lateral aspect of the medial condyle of the femur, followed by the talus and the elbow. The patella is rarely involved. The lesion is bilateral in 25% of cases. Conventional radiographs are often diagnostic (Fig. 7-67). A linear lucency may be the earliest finding in the subchondral bone; more commonly, the fragment of articular cartilage with or without some underlying bone may be freely floating in the joint space, thus causing pain and/or locking. Whether the covering cartilage is intact can be assessed on arthrography as well as on MRI. If the cartilage covering is intact, intervention is not deemed necessary.

Legg-Calvé-Perthes Disease

Idiopathic avascular necrosis of the femoral head is the most common cause of hip pain in the young child (4 to 8 years of age), and it may cause a limp or knee pain. Bilateral but not symmetric involvement is seen in less than 20% of patients, and a familial history is present in 10%. There may be delayed skeletal maturation of more than 2 SD. The condition affects boys more

than girls (5:1). The cause is deemed ischemic, but the exact cause (trauma?) is unclear. Classic radiographic findings initially consist of subchondral fractures, the extent of which may be best appreciated on the frog-leg lateral view. These (micro)fractures then may progress to fragmentation and flattening of the femoral head. Attendant joint space widening may be seen (Fig. 7-68). The epiphysis may be smaller than the contralateral one. The medial increase in the joint space, often the initial finding, may be due to swelling of the ligamentum teres, hypertrophy of the articular cartilage (nourished by synovial fluid), and/or continued growth of unossified cartilage. In about 75% of patients there is slight lateral displacement of the femoral head. Progression is variable over time, with metaphyseal "cysts" and shortening and widening of the femoral neck being most often observed.

MRI may demonstrate avascular necrosis, although conventional radiographic findings are still normal. MRI is thus a much better suited modality than CT for treatment planning. Bilateral avascular necrosis of the femoral heads may be seen in multiple epiphyseal dysplasia, Gaucher disease, and sickle cell disease; unilateral SCFE, as well as chronic dislocation of the hip, should also be considered. The patient's age and pertinent clinical findings are essential components in the consideration of this differential diagnosis.

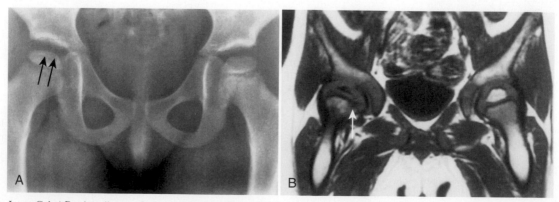

FIGURE 7-68. Legg-Calvé-Perthes disease. **A,** Conventional radiograph demonstrates increased sclerosis of the right femoral epiphysis with a subchondral lucent line *(arrows).* **B,** MR image shows signal void in the right femoral epiphysis and synovial hypertrophy *(arrow).*

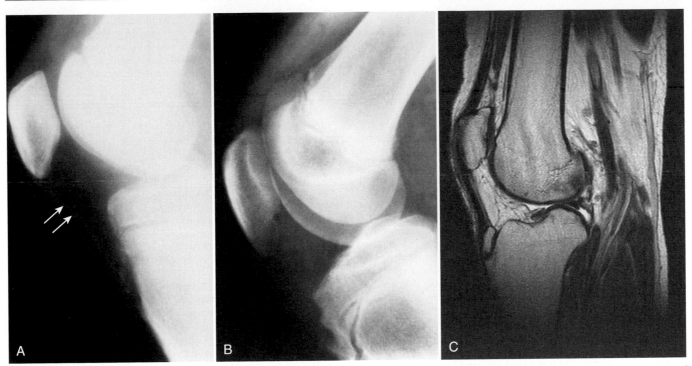

FIGURE 7-69. Osgood-Schlatter disease. **A,** Normal infrapatellar tendon *(arrows)* and normally "fragmented" anterior tibial tubercle. **B,** Obliteration of the infrapatellar tendon–Hoffa's fat pad interface, associated with irregular osseous hypertrophy of the proximal tibial apophysis. **C,** Sagittal T2-weighted MR image shows sequelae of an old Osgood-Schlatter disease in an adult, with a nonfused apophysis.

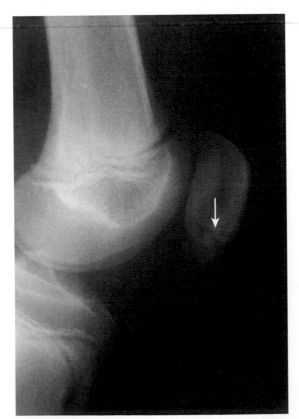

FIGURE 7-70. Sinding-Larsen-Johansson disease. Avulsive (traumatic) changes *(arrow)* on the inferior aspect of the patella, with a thickened patellar tendon.

Osgood-Schlatter Disease

Osgood-Schlatter disease is clinically characterized in a teenager by tenderness over the tibial tubercle. Overuse and repeated trauma to the infrapatellar tendon insertion site may lead to tearing of the infrapatellar tendon fibers without evidence of inflammation, avascular necrosis, or osteochondritis. The disease is seen in more boys than girls (3:1), and 30% of patients have bilateral involvement. Conventional radiographs support the diagnosis if there is obliteration of the posterior aspect of the infrapatellar tendon bordering Hoffa's infrapatellar fat pad as a result of soft tissue edema (Fig. 7-69). Fragmentation and/ or soft tissue swelling of the anterior tibial tubercle alone are not sufficient for the radiographic diagnosis. Thus, in the presence of pain, the radiographic diagnosis of Osgood-Schlatter disease is as previously described; the clinical diagnosis remains symptom based. Rest, physiotherapy, and anti-inflammatory medications are usually the treatment of choice. The differential possibilities are infection, chondrosarcoma (rare), and stress fractures.

Sinding-Larsen-Johansson Disease

Sinding-Larsen-Johansson disease is exemplified by changes similar to those in Osgood-Schlatter disease at the lower margin of the patella (Fig. 7-70). A similar avulsive mechanism is involved, usually in active children, and therapy is identical to that for Osgood-Schlatter disease.

Köhler Disease

More common in boys, irregular ossification of the tarsal navicular, also known as Köhler disease, is a relatively rare unilateral entity. In 80% of patients, it represents a normal variant. It is self-limited, and in 2 to 4 years the navicular becomes totally normal.

Freiberg Infraction

Most commonly affecting the head of the second metatarsal unilaterally, Freiberg infraction is usually seen in teenagers who present with pain and swelling of the foot. Radiographically, it features flattening of the metatarsal head, subchondral cysts, and widening of the joint space. Early degenerative changes of the joint are late sequelae.

Blount Disease

Blount disease is a developmental deformity of the proximal tibial epiphysis (osteochondrosis deformans tibiae) that may be traumatic in origin and/or a sequela of physiologic bowing (tibia vara). The early-onset (infantile) form develops between the ages of 1 and 3 years, when the child begins ambulating. It is therefore often (80%) bilateral and symmetric, affecting boys and girls equally, and is more common in African Americans. Disordered ossification of the medial portion of the proximal tibial growth plate results in tibia vara. The characteristic radiographic features are sloping and medial fragmentation of the epiphyseal center, widening and irregularity of the growth plate, and beaking of the metaphysis. The bony bridging of the growth plate that may occur may be well seen on MRI (Fig. 7-71). Physiologic bowing of the legs, OI, trauma, infection, and rickets are the main differential diagnostic possibilities.

In children between 7 and 14 years of age, sclerosis and narrowing of the medial tibial growth plate along with widening of the lateral aspect of the growth plate is sometimes seen. This has been called late-onset (adolescent) Blount disease, and it results from similar premature fusion of the medial portion of the proximal tibial growth plate and varus deformity. It is almost exclusively unilateral.

Nonaccidental Trauma (Trauma X, Child Abuse)

The diagnosis of child abuse (also known as trauma X, nonaccidental injury) is predicated on combining the knowledge of the mechanics of injury, the location of injury, the sequential findings of skeletal healing, and an appreciation of the development of the child. In a sense, one must compare and contrast normally expected children's activity and injury against what is presented on the radiographs.

Child abuse traverses all social lines. It occurs in rich and poor households, among people of all races, both educated and illiterate. It is estimated that 1.5 million children per year in the United States are abused or neglected in some way, and that approximately 1000 children die annually as a result of trauma X. Boys and girls are affected equally, and almost all are younger than 2 years. Imaging plays an important role in physical abuse because in about two thirds of cases the findings, although subtle, are positive for this diagnosis.

Although physical trauma does occur in other types of abuse (e.g., sexual, psychologic), in only about 20% of such cases does skeletal trauma, which may be evident on imaging, occur. If the imaging findings are suspicious, it is the radiologist's legal obligation to report these findings as compatible with child abuse. Usually, reporting the findings to the referring (pediatric) clinician, either in the report or via telephone, is sufficient. The latter means is preferable.

In the case of a child younger than 2 to 3 years, it is often difficult to obtain a satisfactory history from the child; thus a skeletal survey is the screening modality of choice. In children younger than 2 years this survey is done radiographically after suspicion has been raised.

The skeletal survey for suspected nonaccidental trauma consists of the same views obtained in the evaluation for syndromes, with oblique views of the ribs, and both lower extremities in two directions added. AP views of the hands and feet complete the survey. A "babygram" or a single film is not satisfactory. Imaging systems with a spatial resolution of more than 10 line pairs per millimeter are recommended, although digital radiography probably ensures this quality.

In the child older than 5 years, a skeletal series can be cumbersome, with many films exposing the child to a lot of radiation. In these circumstances, a radionuclide bone scan is considered the optimal initial study, with subsequent radiographs of the areas that are suspicious. CT and MRI, particularly in the neuraxis, play complementary imaging roles (see Figs. 8-28 to 8-34).

In children between 2 and 5 years old, each case should be imaged individually according to the information needed.

Following are characteristic imaging findings in nonaccidental trauma (Fig. 7-72):
1. Metaphyseal corner fractures, the so-called bucket handle fractures, are most common in the distal femur, distal humerus, wrist, and ankle (Fig. 7-72A).

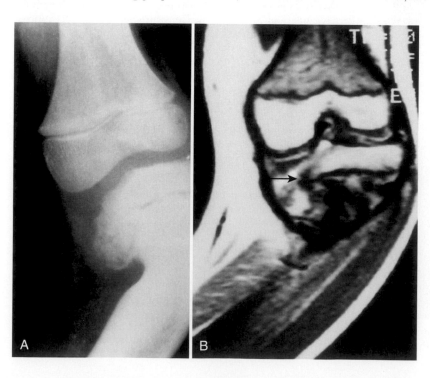

FIGURE 7-71. Blount disease. **A,** Sloping and medial fragmentation of the proximal tibial epiphysis. **B,** MR image depicts bony bridge of the growth plate *(arrow).*

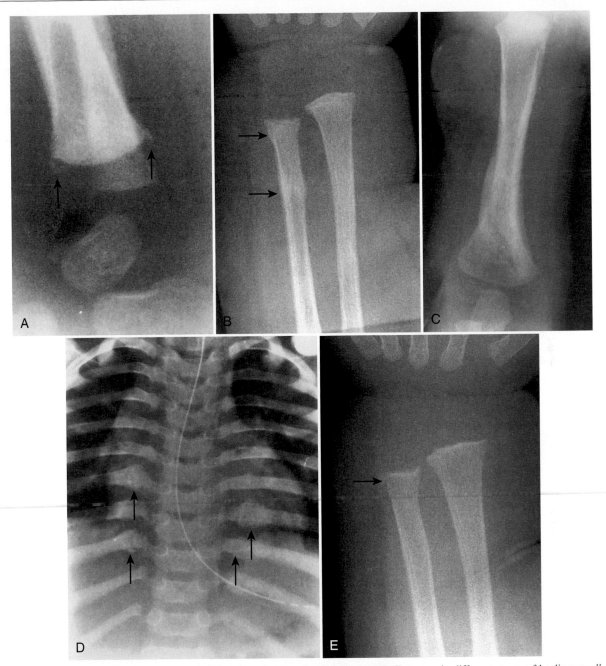

FIGURE 7-72. Nonaccidental trauma (trauma X). **A,** Metaphyseal corner fracture *(arrows).* **B,** Fractures in different stages of healing; *small arrow* indicates old injury; *large arrow* indicates recent injury. **C,** Healing spiral humeral fracture. **D,** Bilateral posterior rib fractures *(arrows).* **E,** Fracture in an unusual site (ulna).

2. Fractures in different stages of healing (Fig. 7-72B).
3. Spiral fractures in infants and toddlers, particularly in the femur, humerus, and tibia (Fig. 7-72C).
4. Fractures caused by unusual mechanisms (i.e., posterior ribs, spinous processes, or of metacarpals and metatarsals) (Fig. 7-72D).
5. Fractures in unusual locations, multiple skull fractures, or fractures of the scapular spine or thoracic spinous process (Fig. 7-72E).

Multiple fractures, especially in different stages of healing, as well as those occurring in "unusual" locations, can contain abundant callus as a result of repeated injury, poor immobilization, and hemorrhage. In long bones of young children, the "bucket handle" or "corner" fracture is considered pathognomonic of child abuse. Periosteal avulsion with microfractures of the growing bone at its metaphyseal insertion is considered the causative mechanism; it is most likely caused by the forces generated in the act of shaking the child. Posterior rib fractures and avulsion fracture of the spinous processes are highly suggestive of abuse, particularly in children younger than 5 years. The same holds true for spiral fractures of long bones in children younger than 1 year. Metacarpal and metatarsal fractures, fractures of the lateral end of the clavicle, and sternal fractures are similarly rare and should be viewed with suspicion. Cranial CT classically reveals a parieto-occipital subdural hematoma, often associated with parenchymal injury ("shaken-baby" syndrome). Visceral trauma may also accompany skeletal trauma; abdominal CT is thus the imaging modality for demonstrating hepatic or splenic tears, duodenal hematomas, and pancreatic injury. The differential diagnosis of the skeletal findings includes true accidental trauma, birth trauma, and variants of ossification (e.g., acromion, physiologic periosteal new bone formation, OI, congenital syphilis, leukemia, multifocal osteomyelitis [including meningococcemia]; however, scurvy, Caffey disease, hypervitaminosis A, copper deficiency (Menkes syndrome), and prostaglandin therapy in infants should also be considered.

Birth Trauma

The passage of the fetus down the birth canal can be traumatic. Trauma may occur in approximately 5 of every 1000 live births. The most common skeletal manifestation is a clavicular fracture, but humeral or femoral fractures as a result of breech delivery, as well as shoulder or hip dislocation caused by complications of position, occur as well. Soft tissue deformity of the cranium is a frequent occurrence after the birthing process. The generalized form of cranial deformity is due to subcutaneous edema and possible hematomas; this edema, called caput succedaneum, resorbs within a couple of weeks. A localized form of soft tissue trauma is seen in a cephalohematoma, a subperiosteal hematoma that does not cross suture lines because of its containment by the periosteum. It may ossify, resulting in asymmetry of the skull that may persist for months. Conversely, subgaleal hematomas do cross suture lines but are rarely present. In all of these soft tissue anomalies, associated skull fractures are quite rare, although molding of the skull tables may resemble a depressed fracture (see Figs. 8-28 and 8-29).

▬ MISCELLANEOUS CONDITIONS
Developmental Dysplasia of the Hip (Congenital Dislocation of the Hip)

To develop normally, the femoral head and the acetabulum depend on being in intimate contact. Lack of these normal stress forces may lead to deficient development of the acetabulum, femoral head cartilage, or entire proximal femur. The hip is formed by 11 weeks' gestation. Most dislocations are thought to occur postnatally. Risk for DDH may be caused by intrauterine forces, the most common being breech presentation, but bony dysplasias and oligohydramnios can also contribute. Generally, ligamentous laxity is the major contributing factor. This laxity is increased because of endogenous estrogens/relaxin, particularly in the female infant. This partially explains the female-to-male incidence ratio (9:1). Infants with a first-degree female family history are also at risk. More than 60% have no identifiable risk factors.

Overall, the incidence of DDH is 1 in 200 live births; it is rare in African Americans and Asians. It may be bilateral in up to 30% of patients. Ossification of the femoral head is usually seen by 2 months of age in girls and by 3 months of age in boys. Asymmetric ossification of the femoral head may be an indication of subluxation, but it may also be a normal variant. Conventional radiographs of the pelvis make use of several lines that assist in assessing whether the femoral heads are normally seated.

On the AP pelvis view, the horizontal line of Hilgenreiner connects the superior portions of the triradiate cartilage. A perpendicular line of Perkins is then drawn from the lateral

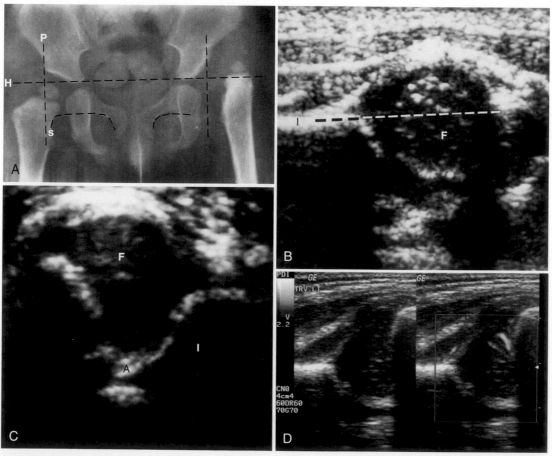

FIGURE 7-73. Developmental dysplasia of the hip (DDH). **A,** Conventional radiograph depicting the lines of Hilgenreiner (H), Perkins (P), and Shenton (s), and a left hip dislocation. **B,** Normal US scan findings. "Lollipop" coronal view, with the iliac wing (I) bisecting *(dotted line)* the femoral head (F). **C,** "Seagull" or "rising sun transverse" US scan; A, acetabulum; F, femoral head; I, ischium. **D,** Coronal left hip US scan showing normal alignment and normal vascular supply (color-flow Doppler US). See Plate 8 for color reproduction.

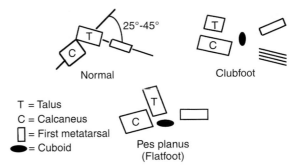

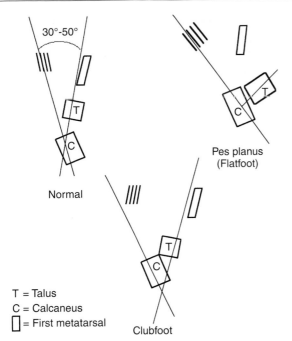

FIGURE 7-74. Schematic diagram of the foot as seen on anteroposterior view: normal, clubfoot, and pes planus (flatfoot).

FIGURE 7-75. Schematic diagram of the foot as seen on lateral view: normal, clubfoot, and pes planus (flatfoot).

margin of the ossified rim of the acetabular roof. The femoral head should normally project into the inferior medial quadrant created by these lines. The acetabular angle can then be computed as well. It normally measures between 15 and 30 degrees, the larger of these values pertaining to the younger neonate (average 27 degrees). Values above 30 degrees or an asymmetry of more than 7.5 degrees suggests dysplasia. The curved line along the undersurface of the lesser trochanter and the superior portion of the obturator foramen, the line of Shenton, is not very useful in infants (Fig. 7-73A). The lines and measurements should be performed on the AP view because the frog-leg lateral view often reduces the dislocation, creating a false-negative result.

Although universal clinical screening of the hip has been deemed worthwhile, radiographic findings are falsely negative at a high rate in infants younger than 6 weeks. This is why US has gained great popularity. It has become the primary imaging technique to screen the infant hip for stability, visualize the hip cartilage, and assess the acetabular morphology. It is best performed at 4 to 6 weeks in infants in whom clinical findings are equivocal or in a high-risk infant for whom physical findings are negative. Monitoring satisfactory relocation with a Pavlik harness is also easily achieved with US.

CT images through the acetabulum are useful for postreduction evaluation of femoral head position, especially postoperatively. MRI is helpful in further assessment of the joint space cartilage.

Although US is operator dependent, it is 100% sensitive and highly specific for evaluating the position of the femoral head and the anatomy of the hip joint. Neonates may have up to 6 mm of physiologic laxity during the first week of life, so care must be taken not to overdiagnose this entity.

The normal US appearance of the hip in the coronal plane with the hip flexed should resemble a "lollipop," whereas the configuration on the transverse view in the flexed hip should resemble a "seagull," or "rising sun" (Fig. 7-73B and C). The alpha angle measures acetabular depth. It is the complementary angle of the acetabular angle measured on the conventional anteroposterior hip radiograph. Normal values are 55 to 65 degrees. Stress views can then dynamically assess the stability of the joint, and

application of color-flow Doppler US may elucidate the vascular perfusion of the femoral epiphysis (Fig. 7-73D). Correlation of these maneuvers with results of the Barlow (adduct to dislocate) and Ortolani (abduct to relocate) tests is disappointing.

Clubfoot

Clubfoot (talipes equinovarus), slightly more common unilaterally, affects males more commonly and occurs in 1 in 500 live births. It may be familial. The cause is unknown, although it is often associated with cerebral palsy or myelo(meningo)celes. Medical or surgical intervention depends on severity.

Basic assessment of the anatomy of the feet, depicted schematically in Figures 7-74 and 7-75, is best assessed on weight-bearing radiographs.

The talus is the bone of reference. If the lateral radiograph finding is normal but the posteroanterior view demonstrates forefoot varus, one may identify the most common structural foot deformity of infancy: metatarsus adductus. Metatarsus adductus is more common in females, and the incidence is 1 in 100 births.

Down Syndrome

Skeletal manifestations of trisomy 21 include 11 pairs of ribs, DDH in 40% of patients, short stature, and atlantoaxial instability. There may be two manubrial ossification centers (hypersegmentation of the sternum), flared iliac wings, and short tubular fingers. The differential diagnosis of atlantoaxial instability includes JRA, rheumatoid variants (Reiter syndrome), and Morquio syndrome.

Turner Syndrome

Abnormalities of the skeleton found in Turner syndrome include short stature, foot deformities (tarsal coalition), decreased bone mineralization, and short fourth metacarpals and metatarsals. The last abnormality may also occur in pseudopseudohypoparathyroidism.

▬ SUGGESTED READINGS

TEXTS

Carty H, Shaw D, Brunelle F, Kendall B (eds): Imaging Children, vol 1. London, Elsevier/Churchill Livingstone, 2005, pp 45-537.
Keats TE, Anderson MW: An Atlas of Normal Roentgen Variants that May Simulate Disease, ed 8. St. Louis, Mosby/Elsevier, 2007.
Kirks DR (ed): Practical Pediatric Imaging, Philadelphia, Lippincott-Raven, 1997, pp 327-510.
Kleinman PK: Diagnostic Imaging of Child Abuse, ed 2. St. Louis, Mosby, 1998.
Kuhn JP, Slovis TL, Holler JD (eds): Caffey's Pediatric Diagnostic Imaging, ed 10, vol 2. Philadelphia, Mosby, 2004, pp 1443-1966, pp 1998-2502.
Taybi H, Lachman RS: Radiology of Syndromes, Metabolic Disorders, and Skeletal Dysplasias, ed 4. St Louis, Mosby-Yearbook, 1996.

ARTICLES

Babcock DS, Hernandez RJ, Kushner DC, et al: Developmental dysplasia of the hip: American College of Radiology. ACR Appropriateness Criteria. Radiology 2000;215:819.

Blickman JG, Wilkinson RH, Graef AW: The radiologic lead band revisited. AJR Am J Roentgenol 1986;146:245.

Borsa JJ, Peterson HA, Ehman RL: MR imaging of physeal bars. Radiology 1996;199:683 .

Burrows PE, Mulliken JB, Fellow KE, et al: Childhood hemangiomas and vascular malformations: Angiographic differentiation. AJR Am J Roentgenol 1983;141:483.

Caffey J: Infantile cortical hyperostosis. J Pediatr 1946;29:541.

Colaita N, Orazii C, Danza SN, et al: Premature epiphyseal fusion and extramedullary hematopoiesis in thalassemia. Skeletal Radiol 1987;16:533.

Eggli KE, King SH, Boal DK, et al: Low dose CT of developmental dysplasia of the hip after reduction: Diagnostic accuracy and dosimetry. AJR Am J Roentgenol 1994;163:1441.

Gylys-Morin VM: MR imaging of pediatric musculoskeletal inflammatory and infectious disorders. Magn Reson Clin North Am 1998;6:537.

Harcke HT, Grissom LE: Performing dynamic sonography of the infant hip. AJR Am J Roentgenol 1990;155:837.

Konez O, Burrows PE: Magnetic resonance of vascular anomalies. Magn Reson Clin North Am 2002;10:363.

Lamer S, Dorgeret S, Khaironni A, et al: Femoral head vascularization in Legg-Perthes disease. Pediatr Radiol 2002;32:580.

Park EA: The imprinting of nutritional disturbances on the growing bone. Pediatrics 1964;33(Suppl):815.

Rogers LF, Malave S, White H, et al: Plastic bowing, torus and greenstick supracondylar fractures of the humerus. Radiology 1978;128:145.

Rohrschneider WK, Fuchs G, Tröger J: US evaluation of the anterior recess in the normal hip: A prospective study in 166 asymptomatic children. Pediatr Radiol 1996;26:629.

Zawin JK, Hoffer FA, Rand FF, et al: Joint effusion in children with an irritable hip: US diagnosis and aspiration. Radiology 1993;187:459.

CHAPTER 8

Brain Imaging

Patrick D. Barnes

The central nervous system (CNS) consists of the skull, brain, spine, and spinal cord. The head and neck region contains the face, eye and orbit, nasal cavity and paranasal sinuses, ear and temporal bone, oral cavity, jaw, and neck. Modalities used for the imaging of the pediatric CNS and head and neck region include plain film/computerized radiography (PF/CR), ultrasonography (US), computed tomography (CT), magnetic resonance imaging (MRI), radionuclide imaging (RI), catheter angiography, and myelography. Imaging modalities may be classified as structural or functional. Structural imaging modalities provide spatial resolution primarily on the basis of anatomic or morphologic data (e.g., CT). Functional imaging modalities (including molecular imaging) provide spatial resolution on the basis of physiologic, metabolic, or biologic data or markers (e.g., positron emission tomography [PET]). Some modalities may actually be regarded as providing both structural and functional information (e.g., MRI, PET-CT). The technical and procedural descriptions of angiography, myelography, and other invasive and interventional modalities are detailed in other texts. In this presentation, guidelines for their utilization are presented by region and modality.

▪ BRAIN IMAGING GUIDELINES

Skull Plain Films and Computerized Radiography

Skull PF/CR is most often obtained for trauma (e.g., fracture) or craniofacial anomalies (e.g., craniosynostosis), or to evaluate a lump or bump. It may also clarify cranial findings suggested by CT or MRI. PF and CR are x-ray–based techniques that are being increasingly displaced, or replaced, by the other modalities, especially CT; they are best used in a limited and selective manner to minimize radiation exposure.

Ultrasonography

US is readily accessible, portable, fast, and multiplanar, and provides real-time images. It is less expensive than other cross-sectional imaging modalities and relatively noninvasive (non-ionizing radiation). It requires no contrast agent and infrequently needs patient sedation. The resolving power of US is based on variations in acoustic reflectance of tissues. Its diagnostic effectiveness, however, depends primarily on the skill and experience of the operator and interpreter. Also, US requires a window or path unimpeded by bone or air.

Probably the most important uses of US are (1) fetal and neonatal screening; (2) screening of the infant who cannot be examined in the radiology department (e.g., because of prematurity [neonate], use of extracorporeal membrane oxygenation [ECMO], or need for intraoperative imaging); (3) when important adjunctive information is quickly needed (e.g., cystic versus solid, vascularity, vascular flow, or increased intracranial pressure); and (4) for real-time guidance and monitoring of invasive diagnostic or therapeutic surgical and interventional procedures. Brain US is principally used as a screening procedure to evaluate and follow up on premature infants with intracranial hemorrhage or periventricular leukomalacia. Other common indications are screening for the sequelae of hypoxia-ischemia in the term infant and searching for hemorrhage or infarction in infants undergoing ECMO. Doppler US is often used to specifically evaluate intracranial arterial and venous abnormalities in these infants. Any lesion (particularly a cystic one) identified by US should be evaluated by Doppler US

to determine its vascularity (e.g., galenic vascular malformation). Although intracerebral mass lesions (cystic or solid) may be detected by real-time US, CT or MRI is often necessary to characterize and determine the extent of disease.

Computed Tomography

Although it uses ionizing radiation, current-generation CT effectively collimates and restricts the exposure to the immediate volume of interest. This applies to the more advanced multidetector/multislice CT (MDCT) technology, which provides ultrafast, high-resolution imaging with direct acquisition in the axial plane and retrospective isotropic multiplanar reformatted or three-dimensional (3D) reconstructions using a variety of soft tissue, bone, vascular, and other high-resolution spatial or temporal algorithms. MDCT is now the preferred method for CT imaging of the pediatric CNS and head and neck region. In fact, MDCT is becoming the standard for the emergency evaluation of trauma. The reasons are its speed and its obviation of the necessity for, and potential risk of, repositioning for direct coronal imaging. As a result, the need for sedation or anesthesia has been dramatically reduced. Also, as previously mentioned, MDCT employs algorithms that are specific to patient age, size, and region in order to minimize radiation exposure. Projection scout images in the frontal or lateral plane are used to plan image acquisition and may provide information similar to that provided by PF/CR but with less spatial resolution. CT requires sedation in infants and young children more often than US but less often than MRI. CT occasionally needs intravenous (IV) contrast enhancement, and sometimes opacification of the cerebrospinal fluid (CSF) with contrast material.

High-resolution bone and soft tissue algorithms are important for demonstrating fine anatomy (e.g., skull base). The bone algorithm is also important for delineating the sutures as an indicator of normal versus deficient brain growth, increased intracranial pressure, and dysplastic versus metabolic bone conditions. Advances in computer display technology include image fusion (e.g., MRI/single-photon emission CT [SPECT], CT/PET), two-dimensional reformatting, 3D volumetric and reconstruction methods, segmentation, and surface rendering techniques. These high-resolution display techniques are used for CT angiography (CTA) and venography (CTV) and in the planning and image guidance of stereotactic neurosurgery and head and neck surgery, radiotherapy, radiosurgery, craniofacial reconstructive surgery; to aid in the surgical stabilization of craniocervical anomalies and scoliosis; and to provide real-time or stereotactic image guidance for interventional and neurosurgical procedures. The surface 3D reconstructions can also assist in differentiating accessory sutures and fissures from fractures.

Contraindications to CT in childhood are unusual, particularly with the proper application of radiation protection, dose reduction, and dosage monitoring in compliance with the "as low as reasonably achievable" (ALARA) principle, the appropriate use of non-ionic contrast agents, the proper administration of sedation or anesthesia, and the use of vital monitoring and support technology when indicated.

The role of CT has been redefined in the context of accessible and reliable US and MRI. US is the procedure of choice for primary imaging or screening of the brain, neck, and spinal neuraxis in the fetus, neonate, and young infant. When US does not satisfy the clinical inquiry or an acoustic window is not available, CT becomes the primary postnatal modality for brain imaging in children, especially in acute or emergency presentations. Its use is especially important for acute trauma, acute neurologic deficit, encephalopathy, increased intracranial pressure, macrocephaly, headache, unexplained or complicated acute episodic disorder (e.g., seizure, apnea), visual symptoms or signs, suspected CNS infection, shunted hydrocephalus with suspected shunt malfunction, and suspected postoperative complication. In these situations, CT is used primarily to screen for acute or subacute hemorrhage, edema, herniation, fractures, hypoxic-ischemic injury, focal infarction, hydrocephalus, tumor mass, or abnormal collection (e.g., pneumocephalus, abscess, empyema). It may be particularly important to rule out an intracranial mass or collection as a potential source for herniation in a child who must undergo lumbar puncture for diagnostic collection of CSF (e.g., in suspected infection). Another primary indication for CT is the evaluation of bony or airspace abnormalities of the head and neck region, including the skull base, cranial vault, orbit, paranasal sinuses, facial bones, and the temporal bone, especially for trauma and infection (see later). Additionally, CT is the definitive procedure for detection and confirmation of calcification. Secondary indications for CT are often primary indications for MRI (see later); although preferred to CT, MRI is sometimes not readily available or feasible. In these situations, CT is clearly less desirable than MRI.

When CT is used, IV enhancement for blood pool effect (e.g., CTA), blood-brain barrier disruption, or abnormal vascular permeability is additionally recommended for the evaluation of suspected or known vascular malformation, infarction, neoplasm, abscess, or empyema. Enhanced CT may help evaluate a mass or hemorrhage of unknown etiology and identify the membrane of a chronic subdural collection. By identifying the cortical veins, enhanced CT may distinguish prominent low-density subarachnoid collections (benign extracerebral collections or benign external hydrocephalus of infancy) from low-density subdural collections (e.g., chronic subdural hematomas or hygromas). It also may help differentiate infarction from neoplasm or abscess, serve as an indicator of disease activity, for example, in degenerative or inflammatory disease and vasculitis, or provide a high-yield guide for stereotactic or open biopsy (e.g., tumor core). Ventricular or subarachnoid CSF contrast opacification may further assist in evaluating or confirming CSF compartment lesions or communication (e.g., arachnoid cyst, ventricular encystment, CSF leak) or may be used for myelographic evaluation in patients unable to undergo MRI or in whom diagnostic-quality MRI cannot be obtained (e.g., because of an electronic implant or metallic instrumentation). As a rule, and with the possible exception of suppurative infection, MRI is the preferred alternative to CT using IV or CSF contrast administration in the circumstances just enumerated.

CTA and CTV provide vascular spatial and temporal resolution equal or superior to that of MRI; the contrast agent may be administered by rapid hand injection in infants or by power injection in older children. Such dynamic techniques are particularly expedient in the evaluation of acute traumatic vascular injuries (e.g., carotid dissection or transection), hemorrhage due to vascular anomalies (e.g., aneurysm, vascular malformation), for acute vascular occlusive disease (e.g., carotid or vertebrobasilar occlusion, dural sinus or venous thrombosis), including CT perfusion imaging, and for vascular mapping for surgical or radiotherapy planning (e.g., arteriovenous malformation [AVM]).

Radionuclide Imaging

PET has the unique ability to provide specific metabolic tracers (e.g., oxygen utilization and glucose metabolism). The wider availability and relative simplicity of SPECT allows more practical functional assessment of the pediatric CNS. Clinical and investigative applications of SPECT and PET at this time include the assessment of brain development and maturation, focus localization in refractory childhood epilepsy, assessment of tumor progression versus treatment effects in childhood CNS neoplasia, the evaluation of occlusive cerebrovascular disease for surgical revascularization (e.g., moyamoya disease), the diagnosis of brain death, the use of brain activation techniques in the elucidation of childhood cognitive disorders, and the assessment of CSF kinetics (e.g., in hydrocephalus, CSF leaks).

Magnetic Resonance Imaging

MRI is one of the less invasive or relatively noninvasive imaging technologies. Furthermore, the MRI signal is exponentially derived from multiple parameters. MRI also employs many more basic imaging techniques than other modalities. Advancing MRI capabilities have further improved its sensitivity, specificity, and efficiency. They include the fluid attenuation inversion recovery (FLAIR) technique, fat-suppression short T1 inversion recovery (STIR) imaging, gradient recalled echo (GRE) sequence, magnetization transfer imaging (MTI), and vascular gadolinium enhancement for increased structural resolution. IV gadolinium is administered to provide enhancement for blood pool effects, blood-brain barrier disruption, and abnormal vascular permeability. It is recommended for the evaluation of suspected or known vascular malformation, infarction, neoplasm, abscess, or empyema. Fast and ultrafast MRI techniques (fast spin echo, fast gradient echo, echo planar imaging [EPI]) have also been developed to reduce imaging times, improve structural resolution, and provide functional resolution. Important applications include MR vascular imaging (MR angiography [MRA] and MR venography [MRV]) and perfusion MRI (PMRI), diffusion-weighted and diffusion tensor MRI (DWI and DTI), CSF flow and brain/cord motion imaging, brain activation techniques (functional MRI [fMRI]), and MR spectroscopy (MRS). Fast and ultrafast imaging techniques are also being used for fetal imaging, morphometrics, treatment planning, and "real-time" MRI-guided surgical and interventional procedures.

The role of MRI in imaging of the pediatric CNS and head and neck region is defined by its superior sensitivity and specificity in a number of areas in comparison with US and CT. MRI has also redefined the roles of invasive procedures like myelography, ventriculography, cisternography, and angiography. MRI provides multiplanar imaging with equivalent resolution in all planes without repositioning of the patient. Bone does not interfere with soft tissue resolution, although metallic objects often produce signal void or field distortion artifacts. Some ferromagnetic or electronic devices (e.g., pacemakers) pose a hazard, and MRI is usually contraindicated in the presence of such devices. MRI is not as fast as US or CT, and sedation or anesthesia is required in most infants and younger children, because image quality is easily compromised by motion. MRI may not be as readily accessible to the pediatric patient as US or CT, particularly in emergencies or for intensive care cases, although magnet-compatible vital monitoring and support technology are now widely available for these patients.

The FLAIR sequence attenuates the signal from flowing water (i.e., CSF) and increases the conspicuity of nonfluid water-containing lesions lying in close approximation to the CSF-filled subarachnoid and ventricular spaces. The STIR technique suppresses fat signal to provide improved conspicuity of water-containing lesions in regions where fat dominates (e.g., orbit, head and neck, spine). The GRE sequence is used to enhance magnetic susceptibility (T2*) effects to detect iron, calcium, or hemorrhage. The MTI method suppresses background tissues and increases conspicuity for vascular flow enhancement (e.g., MRA) and gadolinium enhancement (e.g., tumor seeding). Diffusion MRI (DWI/DTI), as provided by EPI or line-scan spin echo imaging techniques, generates images based on differences in the rate of diffusion of water molecules and is especially sensitive to intracellular changes. This is particularly true for primary or secondary derangements of cellular energy metabolism. The classic examples are hypoxia and ischemia; other examples are hypoglycemia, other metabolic disorders (e.g., mitochondrial), viral encephalitis, and status epilepticus. The rate of diffusion, or apparent diffusion coefficient (ADC), is higher for free or pure water (e.g., CSF) than for macromolecular bound water (e.g., gray matter and white matter). Fractional anisotropy, as provided by DTI, addresses the differences in directionality of ADC (e.g., along white matter fiber tracts). The ADC and fractional anisotropy vary according to the microstructural or physiologic state of a tissue, including the level of maturation. Current clinical applications include the assessment of brain maturation, the evaluation of ischemia, and the characterization of tumors. A particularly important application of DWI is in the early detection of diffuse and focal ischemic injury. The ADC of water is reduced within minutes of an ischemic insult and is progressive within the first hour. High intensity is demonstrated on DWI (low intensity on ADC maps) at a time when conventional MRI findings are negative and likely reflects cytotoxic edema. Further investigation is under way regarding the roles of DWI, PMRI, and MRS in the early diagnosis and treatment of potentially reversible ischemic injury. An emerging application of DTI is the assessment of microstructural injury in the neonate as a predictor of neurodevelopmental outcome. Such early indicators may become the basis for interventional trials that may improve outcomes (e.g., in at-risk premature infants). The line-scan technique may be a more useful method for imaging of the spine and spinal cord.

PMRI is currently being used to evaluate cerebral perfusion dynamics through the application of a dynamic gadolinium-enhanced T2*-weighted MRI technique. This new technique is undergoing further development to qualitate and quantitate normal and abnormal cerebrovascular dynamics of the developing brain by analyzing hemodynamic parameters, including relative cerebral blood volume, relative cerebral blood flow, and mean transit time, all as complementary to conventional MRI, MRA, and gadolinium-enhanced MRA. Current applications of this and noncontrast-enhanced methods of PMRI—for example, arterial spin labeling (ASL), flow-sensitive alternating inversion recovery (FAIR), and blood oxygen level–dependent (BOLD)—include the evaluation of ischemic cerebrovascular disease (e.g., hypoxia-ischemia, moyamoya, sickle cell disease), the differentiation of tumor progression from treatment effects, and fMRI. One of the most active areas of research is fMRI for the localization of brain activity. *Functional MRI* is the term often applied to brain activation imaging in which local or regional changes in cerebral blood flow are displayed that accompany stimulation or activation of sensory (e.g., visual, auditory), motor, or cognitive centers. fMRI is providing important information about cognitive and behavioral disorders. Also, it may serve as a guide for safer and more effective tumor resection, AVM resection, and seizure ablation.

MR spectroscopy offers a noninvasive in vivo approach to biochemical analysis. Furthermore, this modality provides additional quantitative information regarding cellular metabolites, because signal intensity is linearly related to steady-state metabolite concentration. MRS can detect cellular biochemical changes prior to the detection of morphologic changes by MRI or other imaging modalities. MRS may therefore provide further insight into both follow-up assessment and prognosis. With advances in instrumentation and methodology and utilization of the high inherent sensitivity of hydrogen-1, single-voxel and multivoxel proton MRS is now carried out with relatively short acquisitions to detect low-concentration metabolites in healthy and diseased tissues. Phosphorus 31 (P-31) spectroscopy has also been developed for pediatric use. Currently, MRS has been used primarily in the assessment of brain development and maturation, perinatal brain injury, childhood CNS neoplasia versus treatment effects, and metabolic and neurodegenerative disorders.

Motion-sensitive MRI techniques not only are used to evaluate vascular flow (e.g., MRA) and perfusion but also may be used to demonstrate the effect of pulsatile cardiovascular flow on other fluid tissues (e.g., CSF) and on nonfluid tissues such as the brain and spinal cord. With the utilization of cardiac or pulse gating, these MRI techniques may be used for preoperative and postoperative evaluation of abnormalities of CSF dynamics (e.g., hydrocephalus, hydrosyringomyelia) as well as abnormalities of brain motion (e.g., Chiari malformation) and spinal cord motion (e.g., tethered cord syndrome).

Brain MRI is the imaging modality of choice in a number of clinical situations. These include developmental delay (e.g., static encephalopathy vs. neurodegenerative disease); unexplained seizures (especially focal), unexplained neuroendocrine disorder, or unexplained hydrocephalus; the pretreatment evaluation of neoplastic processes and the follow-up of tumor response and treatment effects; suspected infectious, postinfectious, and other inflammatory or noninflammatory encephalitides (e.g., encephalitis, postinfectious demyelination, vasculitis); migrational and other submacroscopic dysgeneses (e.g., cortical dysplasia); neurocutaneous syndromes (e.g., neurofibromatosis 1 [NF-1], tuberous sclerosis); intractable or refractory epilepsy; and vascular diseases, hemorrhage, and the sequelae of trauma. A basic, but comprehensive, screening whole-brain MRI protocol, for example, includes the following images:

- Sagittal T1-weighted imaging
- Axial T2-weighted imaging
- Axial FLAIR imaging
- Axial GRE imaging
- Angled coronal STIR imaging
- Axial DWI

Depending on the clinical indication or the results of this basic protocol, other sequences may be prospectively added to the protocol or retrospectively obtained, including use of gadolinium enhancement, MRA/MRV, MRS, PMRI, and higher-resolution regional examination. Real-time radiologist monitoring of these procedures, especially in children requiring sedation, anesthesia, or intensive care or in emergencies, facilitates the process.

MRI frequently offers greater diagnostic specificity than CT or US for delineating vascular and hemorrhagic processes. Advantages include the clear depiction of vascular structures and abnormalities based on proton flow parameters and software enhancements not requiring the injection of contrast agents (e.g., MRA/MRV). MRI with angiography or venography can be used to differentiate arterial from venous occlusive disease. Using magnetic susceptibility sequences, MRI also provides more specific identification and staging of hemorrhage and clot formation according to the evolution of hemoglobin breakdown using T1-weighted, T2-weighted, and GRE sequences. MRI is often reserved for more definitive evaluation of hemorrhage and as an indicator or guide for angiography in a number of special situations. MRI may be used to evaluate an atypical or unexplained intracranial hemorrhage by distinguishing hemorrhagic infarction from hematoma and by distinguishing among the types of vascular malformations (e.g., cavernous malformation vs. AVM). MRA may obviate the need, in some cases of vascular malformation, for conventional angiography during follow-up after surgery, interventional treatment, or radiosurgery.

In the evaluation of intracranial vascular anomalies (e.g., vascular malformation, aneurysm), MRI may identify otherwise unsuspected prior hemorrhage (i.e., hemosiderin). When CT demonstrates a nonspecific focal high density (calcification vs. hemorrhage), MRI may provide further specificity, for example, by distinguishing an occult vascular malformation (e.g., cavernous malformation) from a neoplasm (e.g., glioma). It may further assist US or CT in differentiating benign infantile extracerebral subarachnoid collections from subdural hematomas.

■ NORMAL DEVELOPMENT

Morphologic CNS development during the embryonic and fetal stages may be subdivided into two basic phases, formation and maturation. More recently, genetic and molecular principles of CNS development have been elucidated. Early formation involves

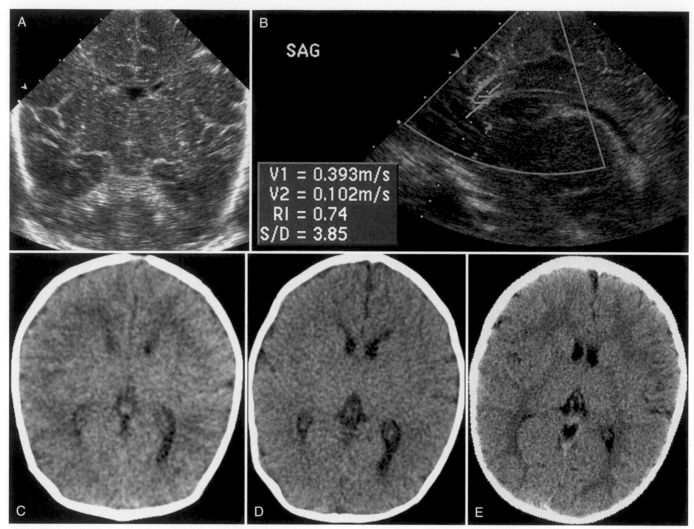

FIGURE 8-1. Normal infant and child brain. **A** and **B,** Coronal US scan (**A**) and sagittal US plus Doppler scan (**B**) with resistive indices (RI) in a term infant. **C** to **E,** CT scans of a term neonate (**C**), a 2-month-old infant (**D**), and a 2-year-old child (**E**) show progress of maturation, including myelination.

neural tube development (0-10 weeks) from the neuroectoderm as induced by the notochord. This development includes dorsal and ventral neural tube closure to form the brain, face, and spinal cord. Later formation involves neuronal, glial, and mesenchymal development (2-6 months) during the stages of proliferation, differentiation, histogenesis, migration, and cortical organization. The result is the formation of the gray and white matter structures, the glia, and the vascular, meningeal, CSF, and supportive musculoskeletal (i.e., skull and spinal column) structures.

Subsequently the CNS primarily undergoes maturational changes, including myelination, cortical maturation, and further connectivity (i.e., synaptogenesis, neuroplasticity). A fundamental understanding of normal development and its variants is necessary for the accurate interpretation of imaging of the CNS in the child. More detailed descriptions of CNS embryology and development are covered in other texts. Knowledge of the normal skull and brain, and their variations of normal, according to stage of development and maturation, is important for proper image interpretation using PF/CR, US, CT, and MRI (Fig. 8-1). This subject is also covered in greater detail elsewhere.

■ CONGENITAL AND DEVELOPMENTAL ABNORMALITIES

Congenital and developmental abnormalities of the CNS have been classified by van der Knaap and Valk according to the timing

(i.e., weeks of gestational age—WGA) of the disorder, rather than the etiology, as the major determinant of the type of malformation (Table 8-1). CNS malformations are also a major cause of childhood hydrocephalus (Table 8-2).

Disorders of Dorsal Induction

Dorsal induction is the process whereby the notochord induces the adjacent ectoderm to form the neural plate. Neural folds develop from the plate to form the primitive neural tube (i.e., primary neurulation), which gives rise to the brain and spinal cord. Malformations associated with disorders of dorsal induction have their origin within the embryonic period (0-4 WGA) and include anencephaly, cephaloceles, Chiari malformations, dermal sinus, spinal dysraphism, and hydrosyringomyelia. The last three malformations are discussed in Chapter 9.

Anencephaly

Anencephaly is due to failure of early cephalic neural tube closure and results in complete absence of the cranium and brain above the brainstem. It is fatal, is associated with elevated alpha-fetoprotein concentrations, and is readily detected by fetal US.

Cephalocele

Cephaloceles are extensions of intracranial tissues through a skull defect. They are classified, according to content and location,

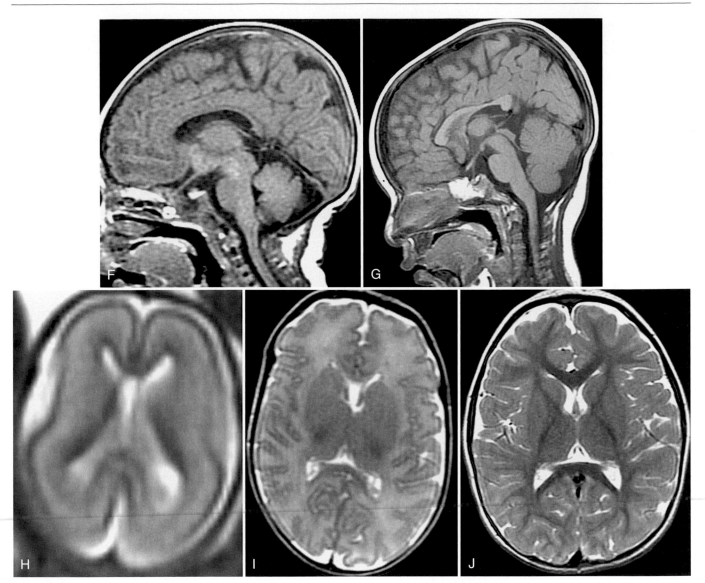

FIGURE 8-1.—CONT'D F and G, Sagittal T1-weighted MR images of a term neonate (**F**) and a 1-year-old infant (**G**) show progress in brain growth, myelination of the corpus callosum, and pituitary maturation. **H** to **J**, T2-weighted MR images of a 20-week fetus (**H**), a term neonate (**I**), and a 2-year-old child (**J**) show progress in maturation, i.e., decreasing water content along with increasing myelination and cortication.

as meningoceles (meninges only), encephaloceles (brain tissue), and encephalocystomeningoceles (meninges, brain, and ventricles). Cephaloceles may extend through either the calvarium or the skull base. Occipital cephaloceles are most common in western European and North American cultures (Fig. 8-2). They may occur with the Dandy-Walker spectrum of malformations or the Meckel-Gruber syndrome. Occipital cephaloceles often contain dysplastic occipital lobe or cerebellar tissue, and anomalies of the venous sinuses are common. MRI (e.g., in the lateral decubitus position) is best for delineating the contents of cephaloceles as well as venous or dural sinus anomalies or involvement, associated CNS anomalies, and hydrocephalus. Cervico-occipital cephalocele is a component of the Chiari III malformation.

Frontoethmoid cephaloceles are most common in Southeast Asian populations. They are subcategorized as nasoethmoidal, nasofrontal, naso-orbital, and interfrontal. Frontoethmoidal encephaloceles may manifest as hypertelorism or as a glabellar mass. Associated anomalies include corpus callosal hypogenesis, holoprosencephaly, migrational disorder, and hydrocephalus. Failure of closure at the foramen cecum or persistence of the dural projection at that level may result in nasofrontal cephalocele,

dermoid-epidermoid, or nasal "glioma" (i.e., isolated ectopic and dysplastic brain tissue; Fig 8-3). Sphenoidal cephaloceles occur through defects of the sella turcica and sphenoid body (Fig. 8-4). There is potential herniation of the pituitary stalk, third ventricle, and optic apparatus into the sphenoid, ethmoid, or nasopharynx. Associated anomalies include corpus callosum hypogenesis, hypertelorism, and midline facial clefts. Sphenoid wing cephaloceles are usually associated with NF-1.

Parietal cephaloceles occur at the vertex near the posterior fontanelle and are often atretic (Fig. 8-5). The straight sinus is often replaced by an anomalous falcine vein that extends to the defect. Also, emissary veins or the superior sagittal sinus may traverse the defect. Possible associated anomalies are the Dandy-Walker spectrum, callosal hypogenesis, holoprosencephaly, and Chiari II malformation.

Chiari Malformations

The *Chiari I malformation* is defined as an extension of the cerebellar tonsils below the foramen magnum (e.g., > 3-5 mm). It may be associated with hydrocephalus, craniocervical junction anomalies, basilar invagination, scoliosis, or hydrosyringomyelia, or with intracranial hypotension (e.g., spinal CSF leak). Other

TABLE 8-1. Classification of Central Nervous System Malformations by Gestational Timing

I. Disorders of dorsal neural tube development	3-4 weeks	Anencephaly Cephaloceles Dermal sinus Chiari malformations Spinal dysraphism Hydrosyringomyelia
II. Disorders of ventral neural tube development	5-10 weeks	Holoprosencephalies Agenesis of the septum pellucidum Optic and olfactory hypoplasia/aplasia Pituitary-hypothalamic hypoplasia/aplasia Cerebellar hypoplasia/aplasia Dandy-Walker spectrum Craniosynostosis
III. Disorders of migration and cortical organization	2-5 months	Schizencephaly Neuronal heterotopia Agyria/pachygyria Lissencephaly Polymicrogyria Agenesis of the corpus callosum
IV. Disorders of neuronal, glial, and mesenchymal proliferation, differentiation, and histogenesis	2-6 months	Micrencephaly Megalencephaly Hemimegalencephaly Aqueductal anomalies Colpocephaly Cortical dysplasias Neurocutaneous syndromes Vascular anomalies Malformative tumors Arachnoid cysts
V. Encephaloclastic processes	>5-6 months	Hydranencephaly Porencephaly Multicystic encephalopathy Encephalomalacia Leukomalacia Hemiatrophy Hydrocephalus Hemorrhage Infarction
VI. Disorders of maturation	7 mo-2 yr	Hypomyelination Delayed myelination Dysmyelination Demyelination Cortical dysmaturity

TABLE 8-2. Childhood Hydrocephalus

Developmental	Chiari II malformation Aqueductal anomalies Congenital cysts Encephalocele Hydranencephaly Craniosynostosis Skull base anomalies Foraminal atresia Immature arachnoid villi Vein of Galen malformation
Acquired	Posthemorrhage Postinfection Posterior fossa tumors Tumors about the third ventricle Cerebral hemispheric tumors

intracranial anomalies are rarely present. Hydrosyringomyelia is commonly associated with Chiari I malformation in childhood (see Chapter 9).

Chiari II malformations are complex congenital anomalies affecting the craniospinal neuraxis (Fig. 8-6). This primary hindbrain anomaly is characterized by a variable spectrum including caudal displacement of a dysplastic cerebellum and brainstem from a small posterior fossa into an enlarged foramen magnum and upper cervical canal. It is almost always associated with myelomeningocele (see Chapter 9). There are a small fourth ventricle, an elongated medulla, and a cervicomedullary "kink." Hydrocephalus commonly occurs at birth or following surgery for the myelomeningocele. Associated anomalies include callosal hypogenesis, colpocephaly, stenogyria, fenestrated falx with gyral interdigitation, large massa intermedia, tectal "beaking," aqueductal anomalies (e.g., stenosis), heterotopias, persistent or accentuated Lückenschädel (i.e., lacunar) skull, and petrous temporal scalloping. New or progressive neurologic impairment following surgery often requires imaging to evaluate for hydrocephalus, shunt malfunction, encysted or entrapped fourth ventricle, craniocervical compromise (e.g., stenosis), hydrosyringomyelia, or spinal cord "retethering" at the surgical site. A *Chiari III malformation* is a rare disorder in which a cervico-occipital cephalocele contains cerebellum and sometimes brainstem (see Fig. 8-2).

Disorders of Ventral Induction

During ventral induction (4-10 WGA) the cephalic neural tube expands to form the brain, and the notochordal mesoderm induces the overlying ectoderm to form the facial structures.

FIGURE 8-2. A, Fetal sagittal T2-weighted MR image showing a cervico-occipital cephalocele (*posterior arrow*), Chiari III malformation (*anterior arrow*), and microcephaly. **B,** Neonatal sagittal T1-weighted MR image shows an occipital cephalocele (*posterior arrows*) with a kinked brainstem (*anterior arrow*).

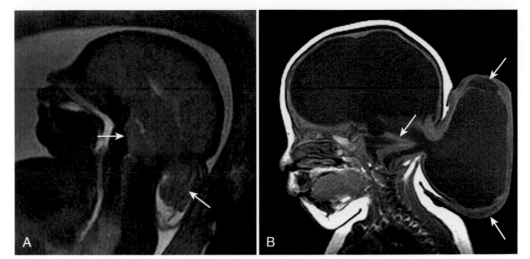

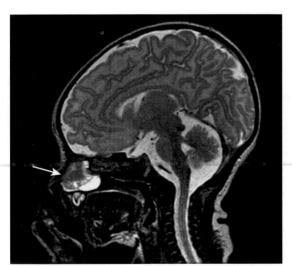

FIGURE 8-3. Nasoethmoidal cephalocele—nasal "glioma" (*arrow*) on a sagittal T2-weighted MR image.

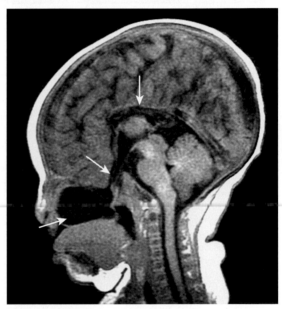

FIGURE 8-4. Sphenoidal cephalocele (*lower arrows*) and hypogenesis corpus callosum (*upper arrow*) on a sagittal T1-weighted MR image.

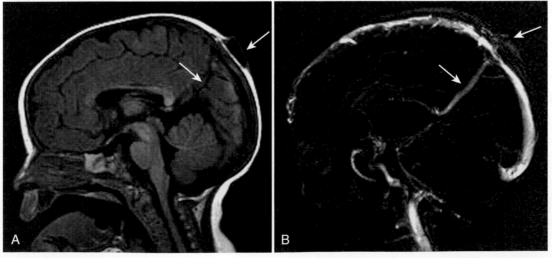

FIGURE 8-5. Parietal cephalocele (*upper arrow*) and transfalcine vein (*lower arrow*) on a sagittal T1-weighted MR image (**A**) and an MR venogram (**B**).

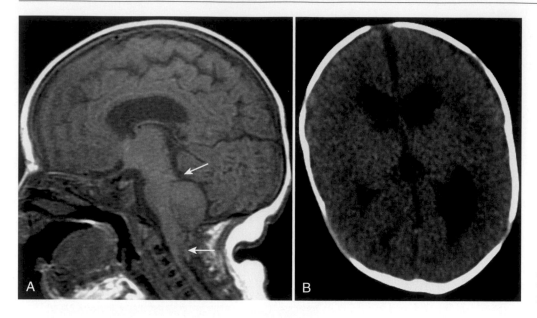

FIGURE 8-6. **A,** Chiari II malformation (*arrows*) on a sagittal T1-weighted MR image. **B,** Ventriculomegaly on CT.

Diverticulation results in formation of the prosencephalon (forebrain), the mesencephalon (midbrain), and the rhombencephalon (hindbrain). Disorders in this category include the holoprosencephalies, absence of the septum pellucidum, craniosynostosis, and the Dandy-Walker spectrum of malformations.

Holoprosencephaly

The holoprosencephalies (HPEs) are a spectrum of disorders resulting from lack of normal cleavage of the telencephalon into two cerebral hemispheres and lack of separation of the telencephalon from the diencephalon (Fig. 8-7). Associated facial anomalies include cyclopia, ethmocephaly, cebocephaly, and hypotelorism. Alobar HPE, the most severe form, is often fatal (Fig. 8-7A). It is composed of microcephaly, a common hemisphere, a monoventricle with dorsal cyst, thalamic fusion, absence of the falx and septum pellucidum, corpus callosum agenesis, and absence of olfactory apparatus. There is an azygous (single) anterior cerebral artery with absence of the superior sagittal sinus, straight sinus, and internal cerebral veins. Semilobar HPE is an intermediate form (Fig. 8-7B). Facial features are less common and less severe. It consists of microcephaly, partial posterior cleaving of the cerebral hemispheres, absence of the septum pellucidum and of anterior portions of the corpus callosum, partial separation of the thalami, partially formed temporal horns, and a posterior falx and interhemispheric fissure. Lobar HPE is the third classic form (usually no facial anomalies) along with the middle interhemispheric subtype (Fig. 8-7C and D). There is failure of cleavage of the cerebral hemispheres frontally or parietally. The septum pellucidum is absent, and the corpus callosum may be incomplete or dysplastic.

Absence of the Septum Pellucidum

Absence of the septum pellucidum is characterized by complete or partial absence of the leaflets of the septum pellucidum (Fig. 8-8). Septo-optic dysplasia (de Morsier syndrome) includes hypoplasia of the optic nerves. Schizencephaly or heterotopias are present in half the cases. Pituitary-hypothalamic dysfunction occurs in most (e.g., growth hormone or thyroid-stimulating hormone deficiencies), including ectopia of the posterior pituitary bright spot. In some patients there is complete absence of the septum pellucidum and hypoplasia of the cerebral white matter without other anomalies. Absence of the septum pellucidum may also occur with Chiari II malformation, holoprosencephaly, callosal agenesis, and severe hydrocephalus.

Posterior Fossa Cystic Malformations

Posterior fossa cystic malformations are subdivided along a continuum that includes the Dandy-Walker malformation, Dandy-Walker variant, mega cisterna magna, and Blake's pouch or arachnoid cyst. The classic *Dandy-Walker malformation* is characterized by complete or partial vermian agenesis (especially of the inferior vermis), a large retrocerebellar cyst communicating with the fourth ventricle, an enlarged posterior fossa, elevation of the torcular above the lambda, and absence of the falx cerebelli (Fig. 8-9). Associated CNS and systemic anomalies are common, including corpus callosum hypogenesis, polymicrogyria, heterotopias, cephalocele, and holoprosencephaly. Macrocephaly and hydrocephalus are common. Evaluation of aqueductal patency is important before surgery for ventricular or cyst shunting.

In *Dandy-Walker variant*, the cerebellar vermis is hypogenetic (i.e., inferior vermis), the posterior fossa is usually of normal size, and there is separation of the fourth ventricle from a smaller retrocerebellar space (Fig. 8-10A). If the cerebellar vermis is completely formed and an enlarged retrocerebellar CSF space is present, the anomaly is usually designated *mega cisterna magna* (Fig. 8-10B). If the retrocerebellar CSF collection exerts mass effect on a completely formed cerebellum, then *Blake's pouch or arachnoid cyst* may be diagnosed, especially if there is hydrocephalus (Fig. 8-11). Other CNS or systemic anomalies are uncommon in Dandy-Walker variant, mega cisterna magna, and Blake's pouch or arachnoid cyst. The cystic posterior fossa anomalies are to be distinguished from cerebellar hypoplasia (formed but small cerebellum without cyst), pontocerebellar hypoplasia (formed but small pons and cerebellum), Joubert syndrome (superior or total vermian hypogenesis), rhombencephalosynapsis (absence of vermis with fused hemispheres), and cerebellar atrophy or degeneration (small cerebellum with prominent fissures).

Craniosynostosis

Craniosynostosis (premature fusion of the sutures) may be primary or secondary. Primary synostosis is probably related to an anomaly of skull base development. Secondary synostosis may be due to external compression of the calvarium, metabolic abnormalities, or failure of brain growth. Primary craniosynostosis may also be syndromic. Examples are Apert, Crouzon, and Pfeiffer syndromes (see Chapter 10). Sutural synostosis may be identified on PF/CR or CT as bony bridging of the affected suture. 3DCT is the best procedure for surgical planning. Sagittal synostosis produces elongation of the skull (dolichocephaly)

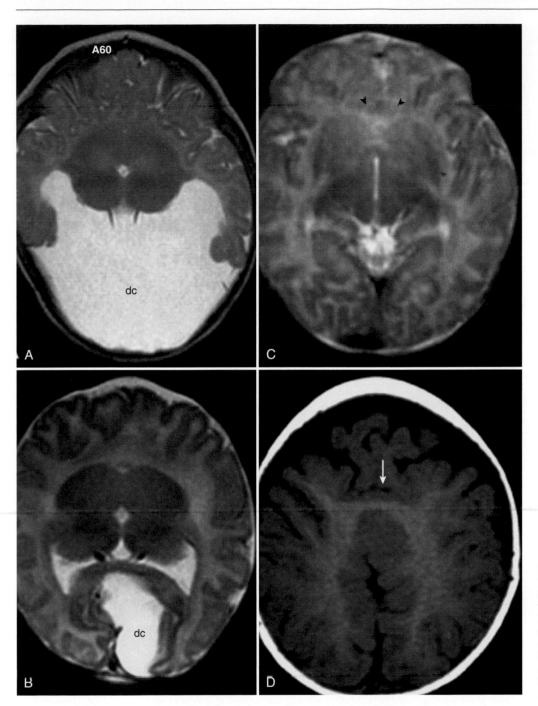

FIGURE 8-7. The spectrum of holoprosencephaly (HPE) on MR images. **A,** Alobar HPE on an axial T2-weighted image; dc, dorsal cyst. **B,** Semilobar HPE on an axial T2-weighted image. **C,** Lobar HPE on an axial T2-weighted image. **D,** Middle interhemispheric subtype of HPE on an axial T1-weighted image; *arrowheads* (**C**) and *arrow* (**D**) indicate midline fusion.

(Fig. 8-12A and B). Coronal synostosis results in anterior plagiocephaly (unilateral) or brachycephaly (bilateral) with elevation of the ipsilateral orbit yielding a "harlequin eye" appearance (Fig. 8-12C and D). Metopic synostosis produces trigonocephaly. Lambdoidal synostosis results in posterior plagiocephaly (unilateral) or brachycephaly (bilateral). The latter is to be distinguished from the more common deformational plagiocephaly or brachycephaly resulting from intrauterine or postnatal molding. Fusion of the sagittal, coronal, and lambdoid sutures produces a cloverleaf skull (kleeblattschädel), which may be seen in thanatophoric dwarfism.

Disorders of Neuronal Proliferation and Differentiation

Micrencephaly, megalencephaly, aqueductal abnormalities, and arachnoid cysts are discussed here. Other anomalies often included in the category "disorders of neuronal proliferation and

differentiation" are colpocephaly, neurocutaneous syndromes, vascular anomalies, and malformative tumors; the last three are discussed in later sections.

Micrencephaly
Micrencephaly (smaller than normal brain mass) is a primary form of microcephaly (small head) that is often genetic. The brain is small but may be morphologically normal on imaging. This is contrasted with microcephaly related to other malformations (e.g., lissencephaly) or to acquired conditions (e.g., post-infection). In these cases, the brain is morphologically abnormal (see Fig. 8-2).

Megalencephaly
Megalencephaly (larger than normal brain mass) may be bilateral or unilateral. The bilateral form is most commonly familial but also occurs in other conditions, such as cerebral gigantism, the phakomatoses, and Beckwith-Weidemann syndrome. Unilateral

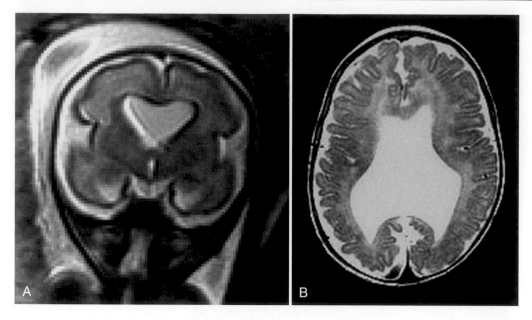

FIGURE 8-8. Absence of the septum pellucidum on a fetal coronal T2-weighted MR image (**A**) and a postnatal axial T2-weighted MR image (**B**).

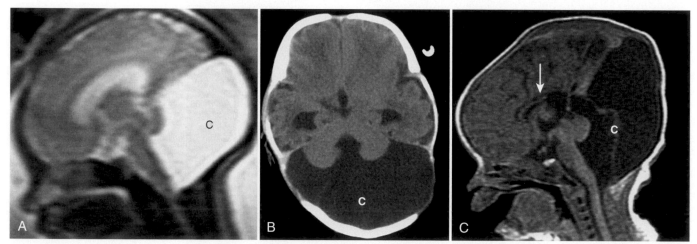

FIGURE 8-9. Dandy-Walker cyst (c) on a fetal sagittal T2-weighted MR image (**A**), a neonatal axial CT scan (**B**), and a sagittal T1-weighted MR image, which also shows hypogenesis of the corpus callosum (*arrow*).

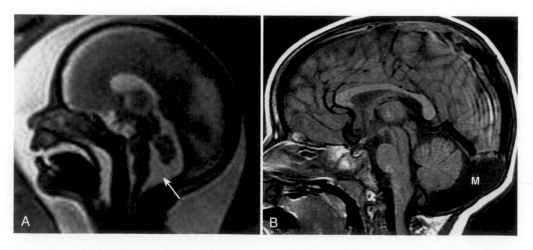

FIGURE 8-10. A, Dandy-Walker variant (*arrow*) on a fetal sagittal T2-weighted MR image. **B,** Mega cisterna magna (M) on a sagittal T1-weighted MR image.

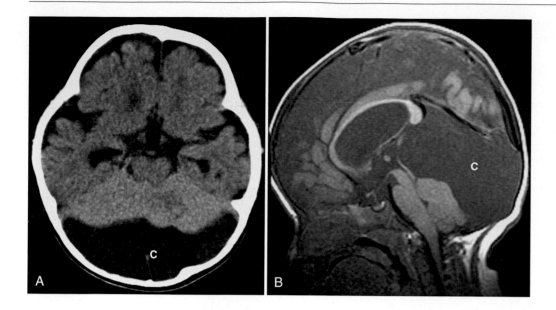

FIGURE 8-11. Retrocerebellar arachnoid cyst (c) and hydrocephalus on a CT scan (**A**) and a sagittal T1-weighted MR image (**B**).

megalencephaly is a hamartomatous cerebral overgrowth that may be isolated or may occur with ipsilateral hemihypertrophy of the body, linear sebaceous nevus syndrome, NF-1, and hypomelanosis of Ito. Intractable seizures, developmental delay, or hemiparesis is common. On imaging there is unilateral cortical thickening with polymicrogyria, pachygyria, or agyria (Fig. 8-13). Enlargement of the lateral ventricle and abnormal white matter densities/intensities are common. A more localized cortical form of this disorder may be seen as one of the focal cortical dysplasias that characteristically manifests as seizures (Fig. 8-14). This form may have a similar appearance to an isolated "tuber" (see tuberous sclerosis) and must be differentiated from other focal cortical lesions that manifest as seizures (see neoplasms).

Aqueductal Abnormalities

Aqueductal narrowing may be primary and maldevelopmental or secondary (acquired). It is a common cause of hydrocephalus (see Table 8-2) and may be isolated or associated with other developmental or acquired conditions. Developmental narrowing may occur in the form of stenosis, gliosis, forking (i.e., fenestration), or a membrane. Hemorrhage, infection, or tumors may lead to acquired aqueductal stenosis. Imaging often shows hydrocephalus with lateral and third ventricular enlargement and a normal-sized or small fourth ventricle (Fig. 8-15). There may be tectal dysplasia with thickening or beaking. This is to be distinguished from tectal glioma (see neoplasm discussion).

Arachnoid Cyst

Arachnoid cysts, which are CSF-containing lesions within an arachnoid membrane, may be primary and malformative. There may be hypogenesis or dysplasia of adjacent brain structures. Arachnoid cysts may expand the cleft of schizencephaly.

Secondary, or acquired, arachnoid cysts are CSF loculations produced by arachnoidal scarring, for example, as a result of inflammation or hemorrhage. Occasionally they are associated with neoplastic invasion of the subarachnoid space (e.g., pilocytic astrocytoma). Common sites include the middle cranial fossa and sylvian fissure, suprasellar, quadrigeminal plate cistern, and posterior fossa. They may be solitary or multiple. Occasionally, they may occur intraventricularly, periventricularly, or along the cerebral convexities. On CT and MRI, arachnoid cysts have CSF density and intensity characteristics, respectively (see Fig. 8-11; Figs. 8-16 and 8-17). The cyst wall may not be visualized, but septations may be present. Calcification or enhancement with contrast agent is not expected unless the cyst is associated with

an inflammatory or neoplastic process. Vascular displacement and bony remodeling are often seen. Hydrocephalus may occur, especially with midline cysts (e.g., retrocerebellar, suprasellar). Arachnoid cysts may occasionally be complicated by intracystic, subarachnoid, or subdural hemorrhage (or hygroma).

Disorders of Neuronal Migration and Cortical Organization

Disorders of neuronal migration and cortical organization include lissencephaly, pachygyria, polymicrogyria, heterotopia, schizencephaly, and hypogenesis of the corpus callosum. More localized defects may manifest as congenital hemiparesis or focal seizures, including medically refractory epilepsy that may be amenable to surgery. More extensive defects are often associated with more global neurodevelopmental delay.

Lissencephaly

Lissencephaly may be considered a spectrum of diffuse cortical malformations resulting from faulty migration and including agyria (absence of sulci and gyri), pachygyria (coarse, broad, flat gyri with shallow intervening sulci), or a combination (agyria-pachygyria). Type I (classical lissencephaly; LIS I gene) results from undermigration, which leads to a four-layer cortex with a "smooth" surface, microcephaly, and severe developmental delay. In this group are the Miller-Dieker, X-linked, and isolated forms. Lissencephaly may also result from toxins (e.g., alcohol) or congenital infection (e.g., cytomegalovirus with associated periventricular calcifications). Agyria, pachygyria, or a mixed pattern may be seen (Fig. 8-18) along with abnormal myelination, band heterotopia ("double cortex"), deficient gray matter–white matter interdigitation, abnormal sylvian fissures (incomplete opercularization), ventriculomegaly, or colpocephaly.

Type II (cobblestone) lissencephaly results from overmigration, which leads to an irregular cortex (cobblestone dysplasia, polygyria, or polymicrogyria) with hypomyelination and hindbrain plus ocular anomalies. It occurs with the merosin-positive congenital muscular dystrophies and includes Walker-Warburg syndrome, Fukuyama syndrome, and cerebro-ocular muscular syndrome (Haltia-Santavuori or muscle-eye-brain disease). The prototypical Walker-Warburg syndrome is characterized by a variable combination of cobblestone lissencephaly, hypomyelination, vermian hypogenesis, kinked brainstem, cerebellar polymicrogyria or cysts, cephalocele, callosal hypogenesis, hydrocephalus, and ocular abnormalities (e.g., retinal, optic dysplasia) (Fig. 8-19).

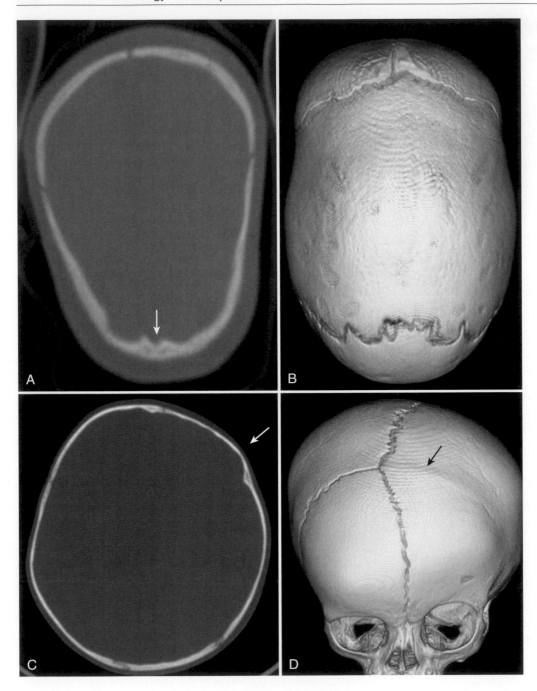

FIGURE 8-12. Craniosynostosis (*arrows*): sagittal type on axial CT (**A**) and top view 3DCT (**B**); coronal type on axial CT (**C**) and front view 3DCT (**D**).

Polymicrogyria

Polymicrogyria (PMG; also known as microgyria) results from a late migrational or post-migrational disorder in which the cortex has an irregular, serrated, or pebble-like appearance. PMG is the major component of a number of focal and diffuse forms of cortical dysgenesis or dysplasia and often occurs with other disorders of migration, differentiation, and proliferation. Early gestational cytomegalovirus (CMV) infection may result in diffuse PMG (Fig. 8-20). The underlying cortex is serrated or thickened and of gray matter intensity on all MRI sequences. PMG lines the complete cleft of a schizencephalic defect and the partial cleft of some forms of focal cortical dysgenesis/dysplasia (Fig. 8-21). Associated white matter hyperintensity on T2-weighted sequences reflects undermyelination. Often there is reduced white matter volume and decreased gray matter–white matter interdigitation.

It may be difficult to distinguish PMG from pachygyria in some cases. Occasionally anomalous veins or arachnoidal cysts are associated with the cleft.

Schizencephaly

A migrational anomaly, schizencephaly manifests as a transmantle cleft. It may occur at any site and may be unilateral or bilateral, and symmetric or asymmetric. The cerebral cleft is classically a CSF-containing hemispheric defect that communicates with the lateral ventricle and the subarachnoid space. It is lined by PMG and covered by an ependyma-to-pia membrane. The cleft may be narrow (i.e., closed-lip) or wide (open-lip). Occasionally an incomplete, or partial, cortical cleft is present that does not communicate with the ventricle. Schizencephaly is frequently associated with absence of the septum pellucidum, including septo-optic dysplasia (de Morsier syndrome). On MRI, the cleft is identified

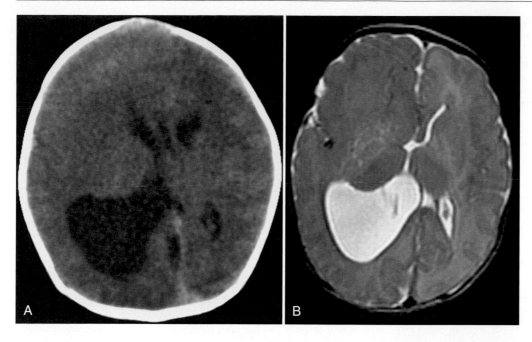

FIGURE 8-13. Hemimegalencephaly and cortical dysplasia on CT scan (**A**) and axial T2-weighted MR image (**B**).

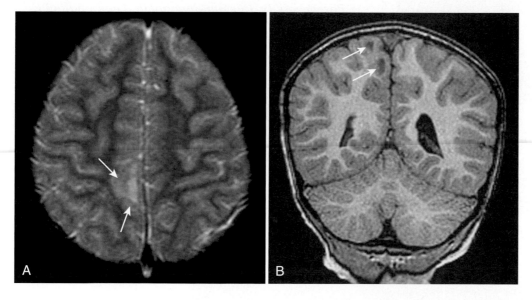

FIGURE 8-14. Focal cortical dysplasia (*arrows*) on axial T2-weighted (**A**) and coronal T1-weighted (**B**) MR images.

as a CSF-intensity defect lined by thickened or irregular gray matter intensities and associated with cortical and ventricular dimples (see Fig. 8-21). This appearance differentiates it from porencephaly, which is encephaloclastic (e.g., post-infarction or post-hemorrhagic) and is a glial-lined defect that extends through both gray and white matter.

Neuronal Heterotopia
Neuronal heterotopias arise as a result of arrested radial neuronal migration from the subependymal germinal matrix zone to the cortical plate. They may be nodular or laminar and single, multiple, or diffuse. They may occur in a cortical, subcortical, periventricular, or transmantle distribution. Neuronal heterotopia may manifest as an isolated anomaly (e.g., nodular type) or may occur in association with other migrational disorders (e.g., laminar or band type in lissencephaly). Isolated heterotopias typically manifest as seizures that may be refractory. Periventricular nodular heterotopia may be associated with the filamin-1 gene

mutation. On MRI, neuronal heterotopias are usually of gray matter intensity on all sequences (Fig. 8-22).

Hypogenesis of the Corpus Callosum
The development of the corpus callosum (CC; at 8-20 weeks' gestation) normally proceeds from the genu bidirectionally—that is, posteriorly to the body and the splenium, and anteriorly to the rostrum (see Fig. 8-1). With agenesis, the entire CC is absent. With partial agenesis, the posterior body, splenium, and rostrum are commonly absent. Absence of only the anterior CC may indicate a destructive process. An exception is holoprosencephaly, in which only the splenium and posterior body may be present. CC hypogenesis may be isolated or associated with other anomalies, including the Chiari malformations, the Dandy-Walker malformation spectrum, the HPEs, median cleft face syndromes, encephaloceles, and Aicardi syndrome (female, CC hypogenesis, interhemispheric cyst, lacunar chorioretinopathy, mental retardation, and infantile spasms).

Sagittal MRI best shows the extent of the CC hypogenesis (see Figs. 8-4 and 8-9; Figs. 8-23 and 8-24). The cingulate gyri remain everted, and the cingulate sulcus does not form. As a result, the parasagittal gyri appear to radiate about the roof of the third ventricle. Additionally, the axons, which would normally cross through the CC, are diverted and extend along the medial surface of the lateral ventricles (Probst bundles). The third ventricle is frequently "high-riding." The bodies of the lateral ventricles typically assume a parallel configuration on axial images, and colpocephaly is commonly present. There may be an associated interhemispheric cleft, arachnoid cyst (Fig. 8-24A and B), neuroepithelial cyst, or pericallosal lipoma (Fig. 8-24C and D).

Encephaloclastic Disorders: Secondarily Acquired Injury of Formed Structures

The expression of an intrauterine insult depends on its severity and timing. First-trimester and early second-trimester insults usually result in malformations, whereas later insults more often

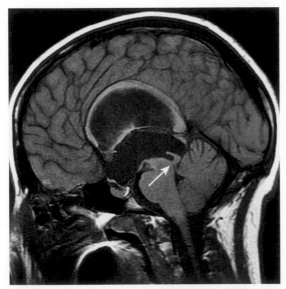

FIGURE 8-15. Aqueductal stenosis (*arrow*) and hydrocephalus on sagittal T1-weighted MR image.

produce injury to formed structures (i.e., destructive or disruptive). The latter are classified as *encephaloclastic*. Also, these later injuries are more commonly associated with a reactive astroglial response (i.e., gliosis). Some transgestational insults may have both malformative and encephaloclastic features (e.g., CMV infection). The encephaloclastic category includes hydranencephaly, porencephaly, encephalomalacia, leukomalacia, hemiatrophy, hydrocephalus, hemorrhage, and infarction.

Hydranencephaly

Hydranencephaly is a condition in which most of the cerebrum in the distribution of the internal carotid arteries is replaced by thin-walled, CSF-filled cavities. There is relative preservation of structures in the vertebrobasilar arterial territories (occipital lobes, inferior temporal lobes, thalami, brainstem, and cerebellum). This pattern implicates bilateral internal carotid arterial occlusions as the cause. Hydranencephaly has also been observed with intrauterine infection (e.g., toxoplasmosis and CMV). The presence of the falx and the separation of paired structures at the midline differentiate hydranencephaly from alobar HPE (Fig. 8-25). However, it may be difficult to distinguish hydranencephaly from severe hydrocephalus associated with marked attenuation of the cerebral mantle. Treatment with CSF shunting is important in both cases in an attempt to preserve tissue and prevent massive macrocephaly.

Porencephaly, Encephalomalacia, Leukomalacia, and Hemiatrophy

The response of the brain to focal, multifocal, or diffuse injury (e.g., ischemia, hemorrhage, infection) changes during gestation. The result of an earlier insult may be one or more thin-walled, CSF-containing cavities known as a porencephaly or multicystic encephalomalacia (Fig. 8-26). The glial-lined cysts often have no septations or associated gliosis. Porencephaly may have a ventricular communication and may be associated with hydrocephalus. Encephalomalacia, leukomalacia, and hemiatrophy, which are due to later insults, may be multicystic, macrocystic, microcystic, or noncystic. Gliosis and septations are commonly present.

Disorders of Maturation

Neuronal and glial proliferation and axonal myelination continue in a predictable pattern during maturation of the developing brain. The process of myelination begins during the fifth month

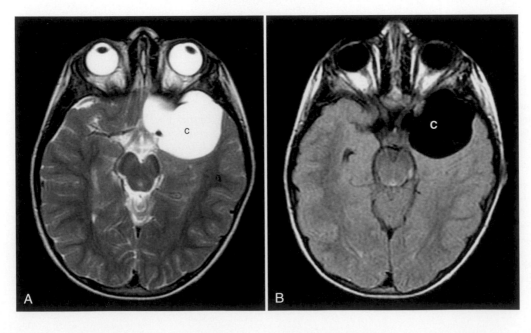

FIGURE 8-16. Middle cranial fossa/ sylvian arachnoid cyst (c) on axial T2-weighted (**A**) and FLAIR (**B**) MR images.

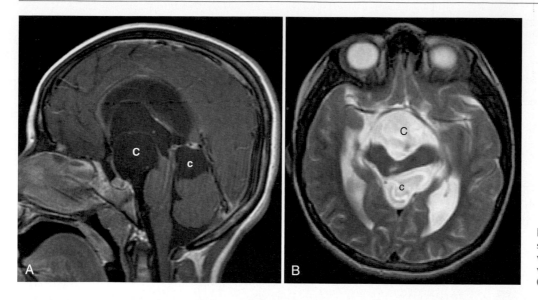

FIGURE 8-17. Suprasellar (**C**) and supracerebellar (**c**) arachnoid cysts with hydrocephalus on sagittal T1-weighted (**A**) and axial T2-weighted (**B**) MR images.

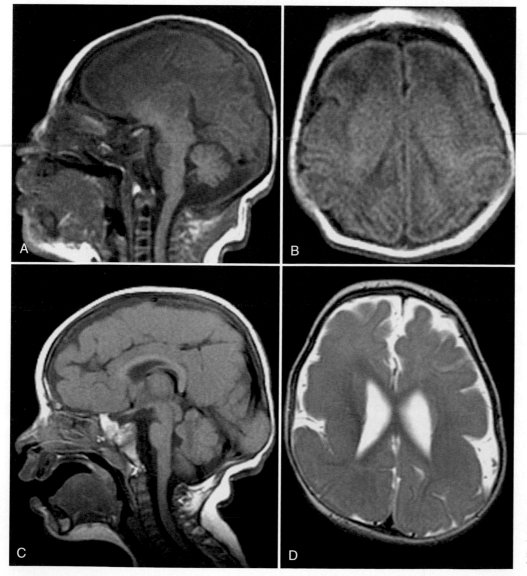

FIGURE 8-18. Agyria (lissencephaly) on sagittal (**A**) and axial (**B**) T1-weighted MR images. Pachygyria on sagittal T1-weighted (**C**) and axial T2-weighted (**D**) MR images.

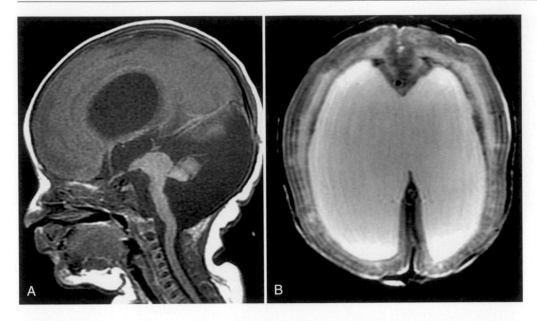

FIGURE 8-19. Cobblestone lissencephaly (Walker-Warburg syndrome) on sagittal T1-weighted (**A**) and axial T2-weighted (**B**) MR images.

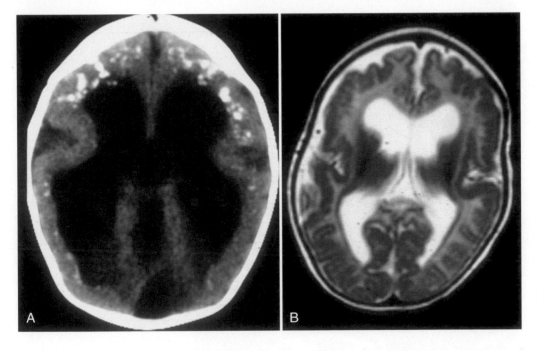

FIGURE 8-20. A, Cytomegalovirus infection with calcification on CT scan. **B,** Diffuse polymicrogyria on axial T2-weighted MR image.

of fetal life and continues into adulthood. However, these changes are most dramatic during the first 2 to 3 years of postconceptional life. MRI provides the best assessment of maturation, including evaluation of myelination based on T1 and T2 relaxation (see Fig. 8-1). The watery, unmyelinated white matter of the immature brain is hypointense on T1-weighted imaging (T1-hypointense) and hyperintense on T2-weighted imaging (T2-hyperintense). Myelinated areas appear T1-hyperintense and T2-hypointense, approaching an adult pattern after 18 to 24 months of postnatal age. At the same time, cortical maturation occurs and is manifest as progressive secondary and tertiary gyral and sulcal development along with frontal, temporal, and parietal opercularization about sylvian fissures to cover the insula (see Fig. 8-1).

The ability to diagnose a delay in maturation depends on recognition of the normal pattern at any given age. In general, normal myelination proceeds in a caudal to cephalad direction, which parallels sensory and motor development. CNS myelination first begins within the spinal cord and brainstem and progresses rapidly into the cerebellum, the midbrain, the posterior thalami, the posterior limb of the internal capsule, and deep white matter tracts of the corona radiata and centrum semiovale, leading to the paracentral cortical motor strips by 40 to 44 weeks' gestation. The optic tracts and radiations begin to myelinate early, usually appearing anteriorly within the first 2 to 3 months and extending to involve the calcarine cortex by 4 to 6 months. Myelination of the corpus callosum first begins within the splenium at 2 to 3 months and progresses anteriorly to the genu and rostrum by 6 to 8 months. Myelination of the centrum semiovale extends from a central focus, first posteriorly and finally anteriorly to the frontal cortex.

A number of conditions may result in underdevelopment and undermyelination, including malformative disorders (e.g., genetic), hypoxia-ischemia, infection, trauma, and metabolic diseases. The pattern of abnormal maturation is commonly nonspecific as to the etiology. Distinguishing cortical immaturity from dysmaturity, or delayed myelination from hypomyelination, demyelination,

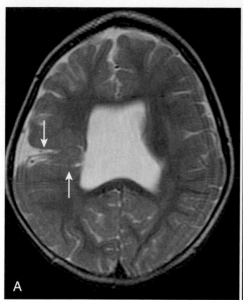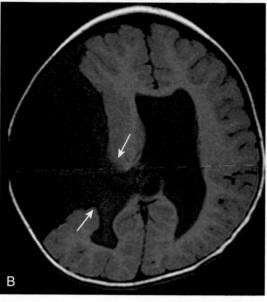

FIGURE **8-21.** Schizencephaly (*arrows*) with polymicrogyria and absence of the septum pellucidum on axial MR images. **A,** Closed-lip schizencephaly on a T2-weighted image. **B,** Open-lip schizencephaly on a T1-weighted image.

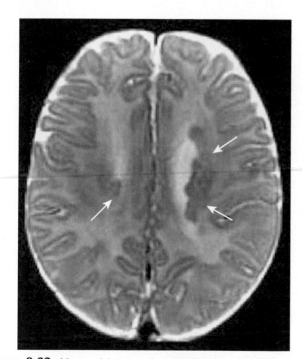

FIGURE **8-22.** Neuronal heterotopia (*arrows*) on an axial T2-weighted MR image.

or dysmyelination, is often difficult. Therefore, it may be impossible from a single examination to distinguish an encephaloclastic and static process (e.g., postischemic) from a progressive and degenerative one (e.g., leukodystrophy). This issue may be clarified only by the clinical evaluation and follow-up MRI.

TRAUMA

The immaturity of the skull and brain during infancy is associated with patterns of traumatic injury that are special to this group. With further maturation, the manifestations of trauma in the older child and adolescent are similar to those in the adult. It is often not possible to distinguish accidental from nonaccidental injury (i.e., child abuse) on the basis of imaging findings.

Parturitional and Neonatal Injury

Neonatal extracranial hemorrhage may be associated with labor and delivery, including instrumentation (forceps, vacuum), coagulopathy, or both. These are the caput succedaneum, subgaleal hemorrhage, and cephalohematoma. Caput succedaneum is usually a self-limited subcutaneous hemorrhage. Subgaleal hemorrhage occurs beneath the galea aponeurotica of the occipitofrontalis muscle; the hemorrhage may be very large and extensive within this space and a potential cause of anemia or circulatory compromise (Fig. 8-27). A cephalohematoma is a subperiosteal hemorrhage. The bleeding is usually confined and may occasionally be associated with skull fractures. Over time, the lesion may calcify and may manifest as skull mass, but it usually disappears over a period of months to years.

Neonatal skull fractures are deformational in origin (e.g., impact) and may be linear, buckled, or depressed (Fig. 8-28). Linear fractures most frequently occur in the parietal region and may be associated with cephalohematoma. It may be difficult to distinguish a linear fracture from any of a number of normal skull variants (e.g., fissures, accessory sutures). Depressed fractures occur readily because of the immaturity of the cranial vault (i.e., "ping-pong" fracture). They are best evaluated with CT, especially for planning of surgical intervention. Occasionally, a congenital skull deformation, resulting from intrauterine forces (e.g., amniotic bands), may mimic a depressed fracture (see Fig. 8-28).

The intracranial trauma associated with the birth process (i.e., parturitional and/or coagulopathy) often results in small subarachnoid or subdural hemorrhages, especially along the tentorium and posterior falx (Fig. 8-29) about the dural venous sinuses. Such trauma may be difficult to distinguish from venous sinus thrombosis. Posterior fossa subdural hemorrhage may be associated with tentorial laceration, occipital osteodiastasis, or dural venous sinus injury. If it is massive, there may be brainstem compression or hydrocephalus. Neonatal supratentorial subarachnoid and subdural hemorrhages may be associated with injury to the falx or a superficial cerebral vein. An accompanying fracture may be present. There may be injury to the inferior sagittal sinus with interhemispheric hemorrhage, or tearing of a cortical vein with a convexity hemorrhage. Traumatic intracerebral or intraventricular hemorrhage is unusual, particularly in the absence of extracerebral hemorrhage. Brain injury may be directly or indirectly associated with parturitional trauma.

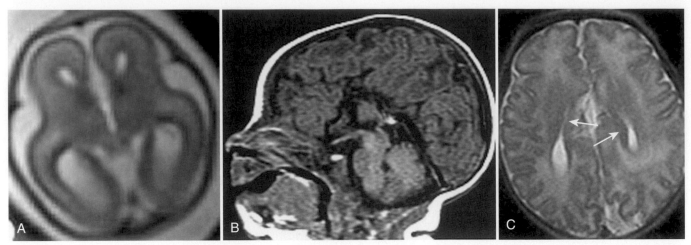

FIGURE 8-23. Agenesis corpus callosum on MR images: **A,** Fetal axial T2-weighted image. **B,** Neonatal sagittal T1-weighted image. **C,** Axial T2-weighted image showing Probst bundles (*arrows*).

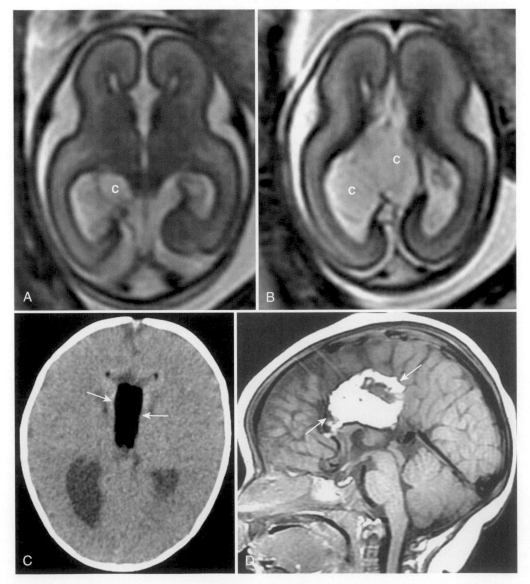

FIGURE 8-24. Agenesis corpus callosum with cyst (c) on fetal axial (**A,B**) T2-weighted MR images. Agenesis corpus callosum with lipoma (*arrows*) on axial CT scan (**C**) and sagittal T1-weighted image (**D**) in another neonate.

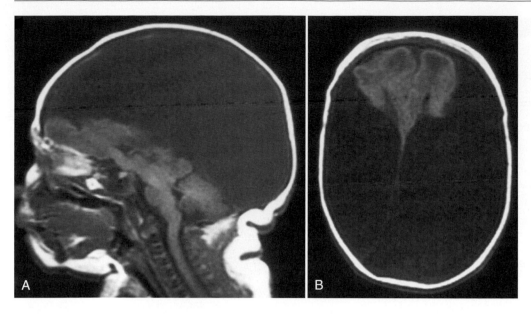

FIGURE 8-25. Hydranencephaly on sagittal (**A**) and axial (**B**) T1-weighted MR images.

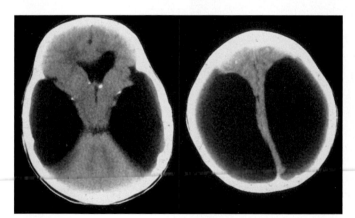

FIGURE 8-26. Congenital toxoplasmosis. CT scans show hydrocephalus, porencephaly, and calcifications.

Injury to the Infant, Child, and Adolescent

Skull Fractures

The dynamics of head trauma in childhood depend on the level of maturity and relate biomechanically to a spectrum from deformation to acceleration-deceleration regarding the relationships of brain tissues, vasculature, CSF, meninges, and skull. Trauma is often associated with deformation (i.e., impact), which may or may not produce a skull fracture. The brain of the infant is surrounded by large amounts of CSF that separate it from the cranial vault and base. Therefore, movement of the brain within the cranium may be considerable. Skull fracture may occur at the site of cranial inbending or as a secondary outbending. Suture diastasis may also be the result of such forces. Skull fractures, including simple fissure fractures and diastatic and/or depressed fractures, are relatively common in pediatric head trauma (see Fig. 8-28). However, skull fracture does not always indicate intracranial injury, nor does the absence of fracture exclude such injury. Multiple comminuted linear fractures may occur in infants without evidence of depression or sutural diastasis. Linear fractures may be straight or irregular. They may also be diastatic without being depressed. Healing of linear fracture in an infant or young child usually occurs over

3 to 6 months; it may require up to a year in older children and teenagers. Dural tears are present in approximately one third of children with depressed or diastatic fractures. There may be concomitant brain damage or an associated subdural or extradural hematoma. Surgical repair depends on the severity of deformity. Failed fracture healing or increasing diastasis—that is, growing fracture—suggests the presence of a leptomeningeal cyst. Often there are associated subgaleal and subdural collections along with underlying encephalomalacia. Occasionally, brain tissue may herniate into the defect or there may be a pseudoaneurysm.

Intracranial Hemorrhage

Hemorrhage is a common finding in acute intracranial injury in children. Extraparenchymal hemorrhages may be categorized by their subarachnoid, subdural, or epidural location. Any or all of the compartments may be involved. Subarachnoid hemorrhage is a common finding with head injury and often accompanies parenchymal trauma. CT demonstrates subarachnoid hemorrhage as an area of high density extending into the sulci or layering along the tentorium (see Fig. 8-29).

Subdural hematomas usually result from a "tear" in the bridging veins. These veins are particularly vulnerable to injury in the infant owing to the relatively soft consistency of the immature brain and the prominent extracerebral subarachnoid spaces. They may be unilateral or bilateral. Imaging often reveals a crescentic collection (Fig. 8-30). In the acute phase, the hemorrhages are hyperdense on CT. Hyperacute hemorrhage (i.e., unclotted) may be isodense to low-density. Isolated or associated traumatic arachnoid tear may produce acute subdural hygromas which may be of CSF density on CT and may follow CSF intensity on MRI. After 7 to 10 days, the subdural hemorrhages usually appear isodense or of low density on CT. It is not possible, in a mixed-density collection, to distinguish a hyperacute-acute hemorrhage from a chronic collection associated with acute rehemorrhage (Figs. 8-30 and 8-31). MRI may provide better precision regarding the timing (Table 8-3).

On occasion it may be difficult to distinguish chronic subdural hematoma from benign extracerebral collection (BEC) in an infant with macrocephaly, particularly on CT (see Fig. 8-30). The differentiation, however, has significant implications because subdural hematoma is often of a traumatic origin and BEC is a self-limited, often familial, condition resulting from immaturity of the arachnoid granulations (decreased CSF absorption rate).

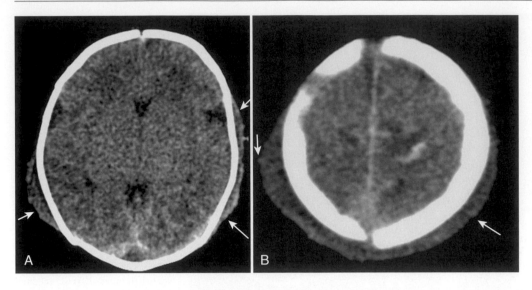

FIGURE 8-27. A and B, Subgaleal collections (*arrows*) on neonatal CT scans.

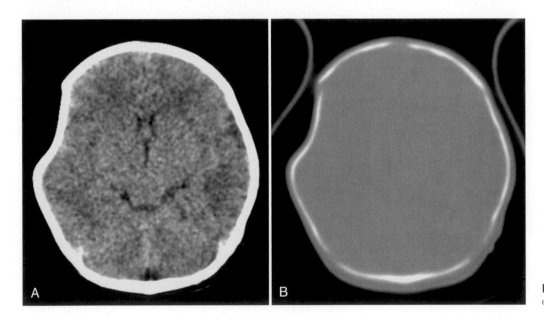

FIGURE 8-28. A and B, CT scans of cranial depression in a newborn.

The two conditions may coexist on a spontaneous, accidental, or nonaccidental basis (see Fig. 8-30). BEC is usually associated with mild prominence of the ventricular system and extracerebral CSF spaces, especially over the frontal lobes. It typically resolves by 2 years of age. The gyri are not compressed, the fluid follows CSF on all MRI sequences, and the cortical vessels traverse the collections. Chronic subdural hematomas are usually of non-CSF intensity, may compress the gyri, and displace the cortical vessels toward the brain surface.

Subarachnoid hemorrhage is a common finding with head injury and often accompanies parenchymal trauma. CT demonstrates subarachnoid hemorrhage as an area of high density extending into the sulci or layering along the tentorium. Epidural hematoma may be of arterial origin (e.g., middle meningeal artery) or venous origin. Therefore, the presentation may be acute (e.g., arterial) or subacute (e.g., venous). CT usually shows a lentiform, high-density collection that is often confined by the sutures. Low-density appearance or fluid-fluid levels may indicate active hemorrhage (Fig. 8-32). An accompanying fracture is often present. The intensities of the lesion on MRI depend on the age of the hemorrhage at the time of imaging (Table 8-3).

Brain Injury

The range of brain injury includes acute to subacute injuries (e.g., contusion, shear injury, intracerebral hemorrhage, edema, hypoxia-ischemia) and chronic injuries (e.g., atrophy, encephalomalacia, mineralization). Contusions may be hemorrhagic or nonhemorrhagic, typically occur in cortical gray matter along brain surfaces next to hard tissues (e.g., bone, dura), and may appear near or opposite the point of impact (i.e., coup or contrecoup, respectively). Shear injury occurs deeper in the brain within the subcortical and periventricular white matter at gray matter–white matter junctions, is more often nonhemorrhagic than hemorrhagic, and may appear as gross tears or as more subtle axonal injury. This injury has been previously referred to as "diffuse axonal injury" but is more properly termed *multifocal or traumatic axonal injury*, because diffuse axonal injury is more characteristic of hypoxic-ischemic damage.

Edema or swelling may be traumatic, hyperemic, hypoxic-ischemic, or related to other factors (e.g., seizures, metabolic). Traumatic edema is related to direct traumatic effects such as contusion, shear, and vascular injuries (e.g., associated with dissection or herniation). Malignant brain swelling in children with

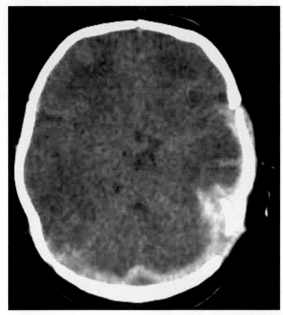

FIGURE 8-29. CT scan showing birth-related high-density hemorrhage along the tentorium and falx in a neonate.

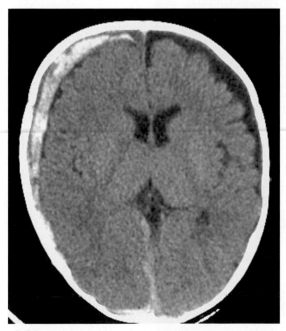

FIGURE 8-30. CT scan demonstrating high-density right subdural hematoma superimposed upon low-density benign extracerebral collections in a premature infant.

head trauma may also occur because of cerebrovascular congestion (i.e., hyperemia) as a vasoreactive or an autoregulatory phenomenon (see Fig. 8-31). Global hypoxia (e.g., apnea, respiratory failure) or ischemia (e.g., cardiovascular failure) is likely a major cause of, or contributor to, brain edema in the child with head trauma. Other contributors to edema or swelling include such complicating factors as seizures (e.g., status epilepticus), fluid-electrolyte imbalance, and other systemic or metabolic derangements (e.g., hypoglycemia). The type (e.g., cytotoxic, vasogenic) and pattern of edema conforms to the nature and distribution of the causative insult. Traumatic edema is often focal or multifocal (e.g., in areas of contusion, shear, or hemorrhage). Hyperemic edema is often diffuse and may appear early as accentuated gray matter–white

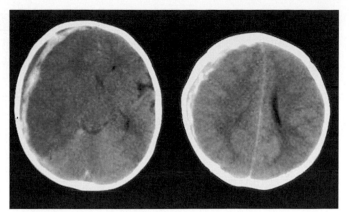

FIGURE 8-31. CT scans of acute-hyperacute right subdural hematoma and cerebral edema in an infant.

matter differentiation. Hypoxic-ischemic injury may have a diffuse appearance acutely with decreased gray-white differentiation throughout the cerebrum (e.g., "white cerebellum" sign; Fig. 8-33) and then evolve to a more specific pattern—for example, border zone or watershed, basal ganglia/thalamic, cerebral white matter necrosis, and reversal sign (reversed gray-white differentiation; Fig. 8-33). The subacute to chronic sequelae of traumatic brain injury include hydrocephalus, atrophy, encephalomalacia, gliosis, mineralization, and chronic extracerebral collections.

Vascular Trauma

Vascular trauma may result in dissection or pseudoaneurysms. The vascular injury may be the result of penetrating or nonpenetrating trauma or may be spontaneous (i.e., no history of significant trauma). Dissection of the internal carotid artery typically involves the cervical or supraclinoid segments. Dissection of the vertebrobasilar system most commonly involves the distal cervical segments of the vertebral artery at the C1 to C2 level. Intracranial or multiple dissections are rare. Dissection often results in distal embolic infarction. Pseudoaneurysms may be associated with hemorrhage. Dissection is demonstrated on MRA, CTA, or angiography as vascular narrowing or occlusion with or without a pseudoaneurysm (Fig. 8-34). A beaded vascular appearance may indicate an underlying arteriopathy (e.g., fibromuscular dysplasia).

Nonaccidental Injury

Intracranial injury is reportedly the leading cause of death and disability in nonaccidental injury (NAI)—that is, inflicted injury or child abuse (also called trauma X). The spectrum of lesions encountered as a result of NAI is similar to those produced by accidental injury (see Figs. 8-28 to 8-34). Fractures, subdural and subarachnoid hemorrhage, cortical contusion, axonal shear injury, and cerebral edema may all result from NAI or accidental trauma. NAI may be suspected when the extent of injury is excessive for the given history or when injuries of varying ages are present. This statement includes injury by strangulation or suffocation. CNS lesions previously reported to be suspicious for NAI are the interhemispheric subdural hematoma, retinal hemorrhages, and subdural hematoma, particularly when associated with characteristic skeletal fractures demonstrated by bone survey. However, such findings may also be seen with accidental trauma and certain medical conditions. "Mimics" of NAI (e.g., dural and retinal hemorrhages) include accidental trauma (e.g., short falls), hypoxia-ischemia (e.g., dysphagic choking), coagulopathies, vascular diseases (e.g., venous thrombosis), infectious or postinfectious conditions (e.g., after vaccination), metabolic disorders, neoplastic diseases, certain therapies, and some congenital and dysplastic disorders (e.g., vitamin C, D, and K deficiencies, osteogenesis imperfecta). CT and MRI both assist with the evaluation of pattern of injury and timing issues. A timely and thorough clinical,

TABLE 8-3. Magnetic Resonance Imaging of Intracranial Hemorrhage and Thrombosis

Stage of Disease	Features and Timing	T1-Weighted Imaging	T2-Weighted Imaging	Biochemical Form(s)
Hyperacute	Edema <24 hours	Isointense-low I	High I	OxyHb
Acute	Edema 1-3 days	Isointense-low I	Low I	DeoxyHb
Early subacute	Edema 3-7 days	High I	Low I	MetHb, intracellular
Late subacute	No edema 1-2 weeks	High I	High I	MetHb, extracellular
Early chronic	No edema >2 weeks	High I	High I	Transferrin
Chronic	Cavity	Isointense-low I	Low I	Ferritin, hemosiderin

Hb, hemoglobin; I, signal intensity.

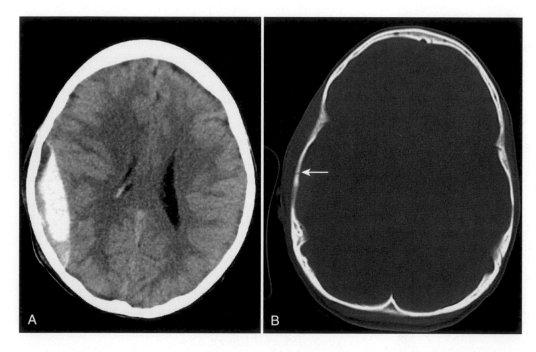

FIGURE 8-32. **A** and **B,** CT scans of linear right temporoparietal skull fracture (*arrow*) with hyperacute epidural hematoma.

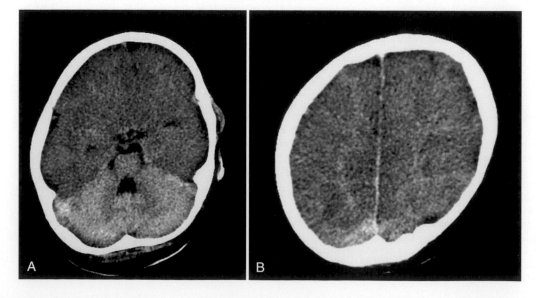

FIGURE 8-33. CT scans of hypoxia-ischemia injury. **A,** The "white cerebellum sign." **B,** The "reversal sign."

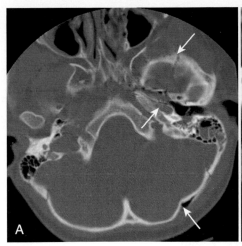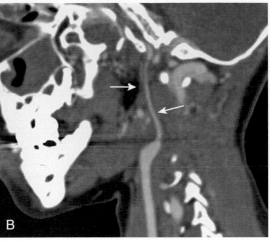

FIGURE 8-34. A, CT scan shows skull base fracture (*arrows*) from the occipital bone through the mastoid, petrous, and carotid canal. **B,** Sagittal reformatted CT angiogram shows internal carotid arterial dissection with narrowing (*arrows*).

radiologic, and biomechanical evaluation of childhood CNS trauma and alleged NAI, in addition to the social service assessment, may make the difference between appropriate child protection and an improper breakup of the family or a wrongful indictment and conviction.

■ INTRACRANIAL INFECTIONS AND INFLAMMATORY DISEASE

Congenital and Neonatal Infections

The most common congenital and neonatal infections involving the CNS are those related to the TORCH agents—that is, toxoplasmosis (TXP), other (e.g., syphilis), rubella, CMV, herpes simplex 2 (HSV-2), human immunodeficiency virus type 1 (HIV-1)—and bacterial infections. TXP, rubella, CMV, and HIV are transmitted to the fetus through the placenta. HSV-2 and bacterial infections are often acquired via the birth canal during parturition. The manifestations of congenital and neonatal infections depend more on the timing than on the agent. Infections in the first trimester and early second trimester (e.g., CMV) commonly result in malformations. Later infections (e.g., TXP) are often associated with encephaloclastic lesions, hydrocephalus, undermyelination, calcification, and gliosis. Transgestational infections (e.g., CMV) may result in combined malformative and destructive lesions. Rarer congenital infections (e.g., congenital lymphocytic choriomeningitis viral syndrome) may mimic the findings of CMV or TXP infection.

Cytomegalovirus

CMV is the most common of the TORCH infections. Clinical manifestations include microcephaly, hearing loss, seizures, chorioretinitis, developmental delay, hepatosplenomegaly, and petechiae. Depending on the timing of the infection, the result is varying degrees of cortical dysgenesis (e.g., lissencephaly, heterotopia, polymicrogyria; see Fig. 8-20), ventriculomegaly, gliosis, delayed myelination, cysts, calcifications, or cerebellar hypoplasia. The calcifications are typically periventricular and are best shown by CT (see Fig. 8-20).

Toxoplasmosis

TXP is an intracellular infection with a parasite (*Toxoplasma gondii*) that usually occurs by maternal ingestion of oocytes from undercooked pork or beef and transplacental spread to the fetus. The second most common TORCH infection, it manifests as seizures, mental retardation, and chorioretinitis. Calcifications are common and more random in distribution, including periventricular, cortical, and basal ganglia. Hydrocephalus often results from the granulomatous meningeal or ependymal reaction, including aqueductal stenosis (see Fig. 8-26). Cortical dysgenesis/

dysplasia is infrequent. Occasionally, there is porencephaly or hydranencephaly.

Rubella

Congenital rubella viral infection has decreased in prevalence as the result of maternal screening and immunization. Infections occurring early in pregnancy are more likely to produce disease, including microcephaly, infarctions, chorioretinitis, cataracts, glaucoma, sensorineural hearing loss, and cardiac disease. Imaging often shows calcifications in the basal ganglia and cortex, infarctions, and undermyelination.

Herpes Simplex Virus Type 2

Neonatal HSV-2 infection (sexually acquired form) usually results from maternal genital transmission during parturition. Characteristic manifestations include neonatal cutaneous, ocular, and mucous membrane lesions or jaundice, fever, and respiratory distress. Meningoencephalitis may result in seizures or lethargy. Imaging shows that the involvement tends to be diffuse, multifocal, or asymmetric; the findings include edema, petechial hemorrhages, and enhancement with contrast agent (Fig. 8-35). Restricted diffusion may be seen early. The sequelae include gliosis, undermyelination, and multicystic encephalomalacia.

Syphilis

Fetal syphilis infection (with the spirochete *Treponema pallidum*) is most commonly associated with maternal secondary syphilis. Clinical signs are condylomata, lymphadenopathy, meningitis, periostitis, and osteochondritis. Basal meningitis with perivascular extension occurs and may be associated with hydrocephalus, but parenchymal lesions are uncommon. The meningovascular involvement rarely results in aneurysm and intracranial hemorrhage.

Human Immunodeficiency Virus Type 1

HIV-1 infection is often a congenitally acquired disease. It may also occur through transfusions with infected blood products. The virus is both lymphotropic and neurotropic. Symptoms are variable and usually delayed for a few months after the initial infection. The acquired immunodeficiency syndrome (AIDS) is the most severe form. CNS disease usually results from HIV infection alone (e.g., leukoencephalopathy). Less often there may be associated opportunistic infections (e.g., TXP, CMV, *Mycobacterium avium-intracellulare*, and papovavirus) or neoplasia (e.g., lymphoma). Thromboses and embolization with infarction may result from an aneurysmal arteriopathy of the circle of Willis. Hemorrhage may rarely occur, especially if there is thrombocytopenia. Progressive encephalopathy is common, along with movement disorder, ataxia, developmental delay, and microcephaly. Imaging

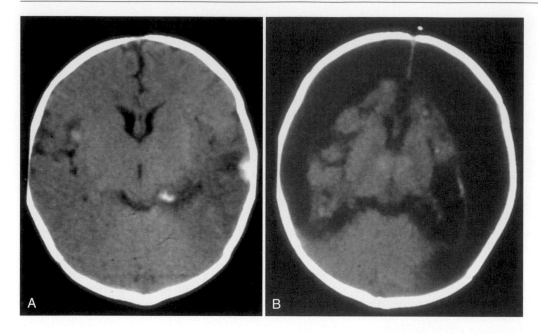

FIGURE 8-35. Herpes simplex virus type 2 encephalitis on CT. **A,** Acute phase including hemorrhages. **B,** Chronic phase with atrophy and calcifications.

shows atrophy, symmetric undermyelination/demyelination, and calcification (e.g., basal ganglia, frontal lobe, cerebellum). Lymphadenopathy and parotid lymphoepithelial cysts are also characteristic. Superimposed infection or tumor occurs less commonly in the childhood form and may produce one or more focal lesions. A ring-enhancing lesion may suggest TXP. A T2-hypointense lesion with marked ring or solid enhancement suggests lymphoma. Areas of asymmetric demyelination may indicate progressive multifocal leukoencephalopathy (PML).

Neonatal Meningitis

Neonatal meningitis is most commonly due to infection with group B streptococcus (GBS), *Escherichia coli*, or *Listeria monocytogenes*. Other bacterial causes include *Staphylococcus*, *Proteus*, and *Pseudomonas*. Newborn meningitis may be related to maternal urogenital infection, premature membrane rupture, or nosocomial conditions. The immaturity of the CNS and immune system predisposes the neonate to severe injury. The clinical onset (e.g., of GBS) may be early postnatal or may be delayed for a few months. Hematogenous infection often produces purulent ventriculitis and arachnoiditis. Venous or arterial occlusions (vasculitis, thrombosis) often result in hemorrhagic or ischemic infarctions. Hydrocephalus is also common. Imaging may show edema, ischemic or hemorrhagic infarction, and ependymal or leptomeningeal enhancement. With ventriculitis, US may show abnormal intraventricular and periventricular echoes plus ventricular wall thickening. In chronic infection, there may be hydrocephalus, ventricular encystment, atrophy, calcification, cavitations, or encephalomalacia. Rim-enhancing necrotic cavitation or abscess may rarely occur (e.g., with *Citrobacter* infection; Fig. 8-36).

Suppurative Infections

Osteomyelitis

Osteomyelitis of the skull is rare in childhood and may be primary (tuberculosis, fungal, syphilis) or secondary (e.g., bacterial from sinusitis, mastoiditis, cellulitis, sepsis, trauma, or surgery). PF/CR or CT may show lytic destruction or soft-tissue swelling. CT or MRI may show associated intracranial suppuration or venous thrombosis (Fig. 8-37). Sclerosis may appear with chronic infection. Radionuclide imaging may be helpful in selected cases.

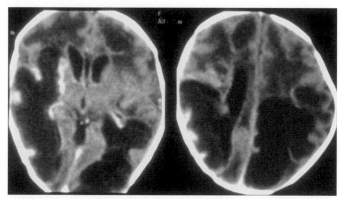

FIGURE 8-36. *Citrobacter* meningitis. CT scans show enhancing abscesses, ventriculitis, and hydrocephalus.

Meningitis

Meningitis may be either bacterial (purulent, suppurative, or septic meningitis) or viral (aseptic meningitis) in origin. Brain involvement results in cerebritis or meningoencephalitis. Meningitis from *Haemophilus influenzae* type B infection in older infants and young children has been reduced in prevalence by immunization. In older children, meningitis is often due to *Streptococcus pneumoniae* or *Neisseria meningitides*. Infections (e.g., *Staphylococcus aureus* or *Staphylococcus epidermidis*) may also be associated with ventricular shunt malfunction or dermal sinus. Meningitis in older children may be hematogenous or due to direct spread from adjacent mastoiditis or sinusitis, CSF leak, congenital or acquired defects, trauma, or surgery. Fever, meningismus, headache, seizures, and photophobia may be present. Vasculitis or thrombosis may produce arterial or venous infarction. Subdural effusions are often small and bilateral but may be asymmetric or unilateral. Surgical intervention may be considered for large or purulent collections.

Recurrent meningitis may suggest a parameningeal focus (e.g., mastoiditis, sinusitis) or abnormal communication (e.g., traumatic fistula, dermal sinus, cephalocele, inner ear anomaly, or primitive neurenteric connection). Noninfectious causes of meningitis in childhood include leukemia and disseminated CNS neoplasia (e.g., medulloblastoma). Imaging findings for meningitis are often negative in the acute stage. Other findings in purulent meningitis include subarachnoid or ventricular enlargement, subdural effusion, ependymal or leptomeningeal enhancement, and single or multiple focal infarctions (Fig. 8-38). Hemorrhagic infarction may result from cortical venous or dural sinus thrombosis. The sequelae may include atrophy, encephalomalacia, or hydrocephalus.

Cerebritis, Abscess, and Empyema

Suppurative infections are usually bacterial and may be blood-borne (e.g., systemic infection or a remote source) or occur from direct inoculation (e.g., trauma), contiguous infection (e.g., sinusitis), or septic thrombophlebitis of bridging veins (see Fig. 8-37). At-risk children include those with uncorrected or palliated cyanotic heart disease, pulmonary arteriovenous malformations, chronic pulmonary conditions (e.g., cystic fibrosis), and immune-compromised states (oncologic treatment, transplantation). Infecting agents include *S. aureus*, streptococci, gram-negative bacilli, anaerobes, and, rarely, *Nocardia, Mycobacterium tuberculosis*,

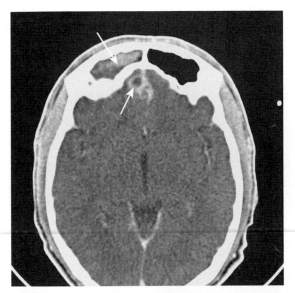

FIGURE 8-37. Frontal sinusitis (*upper arrow*) with subdural empyema and cerebral abscess (*lower arrow*) on enhanced CT scan.

or fungi. If such infections are untreated, the result may be cerebritis, abscess, or empyema.

In cerebritis, there is inflammation, which progresses to tissue necrosis and edema. Without treatment, the inflammation may evolve to abscess (single or multiple) with collagenous encapsulation over 1 to 2 weeks. Antibiotic therapy alone may be ineffective, and surgical drainage or excision may be warranted. In early cerebritis, edema (hypodensity, T2/FLAIR hyperintensity) and irregular enhancement may be present. With evolution, the necrosis and abscess are more defined. The abscess rim becomes T1-hyperintense and then T2-hypointense. The center typically shows restricted diffusion. Intense rim enhancement progresses with chronicity.

Epidural abscess and subdural empyema occur more often in teenagers than in younger children, and more often with sinusitis than with mastoiditis (see Fig. 8-37). The overlying collection may be small or may have a mass effect (Fig. 8-39). Associated brain edema, cerebritis, infarction, or abscess may occur. Imaging demonstrates crescentic or lentiform extracerebral collections with peripheral enhancement and restricted diffusion.

The Encephalitides

Encephalitis, meningoencephalitis, leukoencephalitis, cerebellitis, and encephalomyelitis may be the result of a primary viral infection or an immunologic reaction to prior infection or vaccination (i.e., acute disseminated encephalomyelitis [ADEM]). Viral infection may occur sporadically (e.g., HSV-1, HIV, Ebstein-Barr virus [EBV], *Mycoplasma*) or in epidemics (e.g., spread by ticks, mosquitoes). The major involvement may be meningeal (i.e., aseptic meningitis, due to mumps or coxsackievirus), gray matter (e.g., HSV-1, arboviruses, rabies, Rasmussen encephalitis), or white matter (e.g., eastern and western equine virus, HIV, ADEM, PML, subacute sclerosing panencephalitis [SSPE]). Reye syndrome is an uncommon parainfectious encephalopathy associated with viral illness, salicylate intake, hepatotoxicity, and cerebral edema. Although the clinical and imaging findings in the encephalitides are often nonspecific, some processes may have characteristic features. The differentiation of primary viral encephalitis (usually gray matter involvement) from ADEM (predominant white matter involvement) is important, because the former may require antiviral therapy and the latter may respond only to corticosteroids.

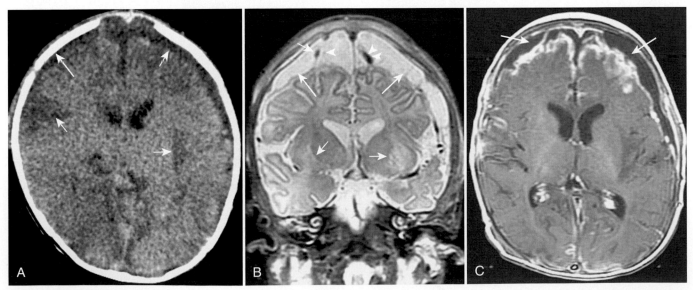

FIGURE 8-38. Pneumococcal meningitis. CT scan (**A**) and coronal T2-weighted (**B**) and gadolinium-enhanced T1-weighted (**C**) MR images demonstrate enhancing subdural collections (**A** to **C**, *top long and short arrows*), venous thromboses (**B**, *top short arrows and arrowheads*), and infarctions (**A** and **B**, *bottom short arrows*).

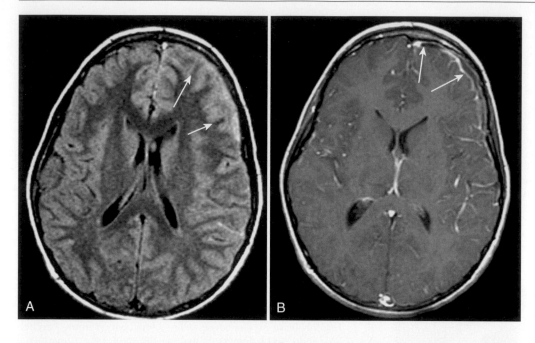

FIGURE 8-39. Left frontal cerebritis on axial FLAIR MRI (*arrows* in **A**) associated with left frontal subdural empyema on axial gadolinium-enhanced T1-MRI (*arrows* in **B**).

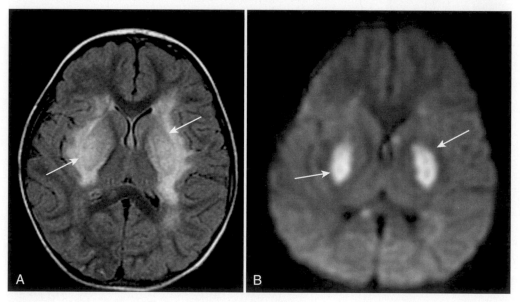

FIGURE 8-40. Viral encephalitis with bilateral subinsular/basal ganglia involvement (*arrows*) on MRI. **A**, Axial FLAIR image. **B**, Diffusion-weighted image shows reduced diffusion.

Herpes Simplex Virus Type 1

HSV-1 is probably the most common cause of sporadic encephalitis in childhood and is usually associated with orofacial herpes. CNS disease most often results from reactivation of a latent infection involving the gasserian ganglion and trigeminal nerve branches. The necrotic or hemorrhagic meningoencephalitis involves one or both temporal lobes, often spreads to the subfrontal region and insula, but spares the basal ganglia. Imaging findings may be negative early or there may be CT hypodensity, T2 hyperintensity, leptomeningeal or cortical enhancement, and petechial hemorrhage. Reduced or restricted diffusion may also be seen. Other types of encephalitis may involve the cerebral cortex or basal ganglia (e.g., EBV, *Mycoplasma*, Japanese; Fig. 8-40), the brainstem, or the cerebellum (Fig. 8-41).

Acute Disseminated Encephalomyelitis

ADEM is a postinfectious or parainfectious inflammatory condition of the brain or spinal cord that primarily involves white matter (i.e., demyelination). It probably represents an immunologic response to a viral infection. Seizures, lethargy, or neurologic deficit often arise several days following a viral infection or immunization (e.g., measles, mumps, chickenpox, rubella, or pertussis). Complete recovery is common, and corticosteroid therapy may help. Occasionally there may be residual or recurrent disease. In such cases, it may difficult to distinguish ADEM from vasculitis or multiple sclerosis, particularly if there is optic pathway involvement. Multifocal or diffuse CT hypodensity or T2/FLAIR hyperintensity is seen in the cerebral white matter, brainstem, or cerebellum (Fig. 8-42; see Fig. 8-41). Basal ganglia and thalamic involvement may also be present. Enhancement with a contrast agent is variable, but may be very prominent. ADEM must be distinguished from other infectious and postinfectious leukoencephalopathies (as mentioned previously) as well as from metabolic disorders (e.g., leukodystrophies), toxic reactions (e.g., methotrexate, cyclosporin), and reversible conditions (e.g., hypertensive, posterior reversible leukoencephalopathy).

Cerebellitis

Cerebellitis is very common in childhood, may be viral or postviral (e.g., ADEM), and must be distinguished from neoplasm (see Fig. 8-41). Persistent ataxia is a common presentation. CT findings may be negative or unilateral or bilateral hypodensities may be seen. MRI findings are more often abnormal, with T2/FLAIR hyperintensities. Enhancement with contrast agents is variable. With severe swelling there may be upward or downward herniation and/or hydrocephalus.

Rasmussen Encephalitis

Rasmussen encephalitis is a chronic focal encephalitis that may be viral, postviral, or autoimmune in origin. Intractable focal seizures (epilepsy partialis continua) are characteristic. Imaging shows early edema followed by progressive regional or hemispheric atrophy (including crossed cerebellar diaschisis). Hemispherectomy may be necessary for seizure control.

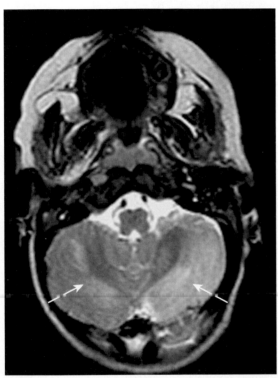

FIGURE 8-41. Cerebellitis with diffuse bilateral areas of high intensity (*arrows*) on axial T2-weighted MR image.

Progressive Multifocal Leukoencephalopathy and Subacute Sclerosing Panencephalitis

PML is an opportunistic papovaviral leukoencephalitis occurring primarily in cell-mediated immunocompromised states (e.g., AIDS, congenital immunodeficiency, immunosuppressive therapy). It is rare in childhood. Regional cerebral demyelination is usually seen and may involve the corpus callosum. Brainstem or cerebellar forms may also be seen. The abnormality is hypodense on CT scans (CT-hypodense) and T2-hyperintense. Mass effect and enhancement are uncommon.

SSPE is probably the result of reactivation of a latent measles infection. Mental status and behavioral changes are often accompanied by seizures and irritability. Imaging shows nonspecific atrophy and patchy white matter hypodensity or T2 hyperintensity without enhancement or mass effect.

Subacute and Chronic Infections

Tuberculosis

Tuberculosis (TB) remains a frequent cause of fatal childhood meningitis worldwide. It results from the miliary spread of *Mycobacterium tuberculosis*. Basilar granulomatous meningitis probably results from rupture of parenchymal tuberculomas (caseating granulomas) into the subarachnoid space (Fig. 8-43). Marked enhancement of the basal leptomeninges is characteristic. Hydrocephalus is usually present. Lenticulostriate/thalamoperforate arterial involvement often results in basal ganglia and thalamic infarction (CT-hypodense, T2-hyperintense, presence or absence of enhancement). Parenchymal tuberculomas appear as enhancing nodular or ring lesions and may occasionally calcify. Other less common, or rare, *Mycoplasma* or mycobacterial CNS infections include *Mycoplasma pneumoniae* meningoencephalitis and leprosy (Hansen disease).

Fungal Infections

Fungal infections of the CNS may result from pathogenic fungi (e.g., *Blastomyces, Histoplasma, Coccidioides, Nocardia*) in immunocompetent patients or from saprophytic fungi (e.g., *Cryptococcus, Actinomyces, Aspergillus, Candida, Mucormycosis*) in immunocompromised individuals. CNS fungal infections may produce a granulomatous basal meningitis similar to that seen in TB, including meningeal and cranial nerve enhancement. Enhancing abscesses or granulomas may also be present as well as white matter lesions. Aspergillosis or mucormycosis may cause a vasculitis resulting in infarction or hemorrhage (Fig. 8-44). Sarcoidosis is very rare in childhood and may mimic TB or fungal infection.

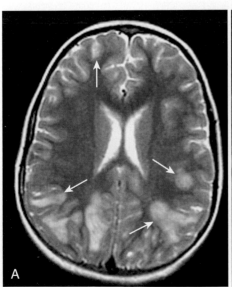
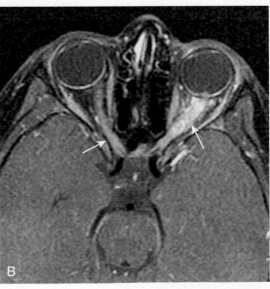

FIGURE 8-42. Acute disseminated encephalomyelitis on MRI. **A,** Multiple white matter lesions (*arrows*) on axial T2-weighted image. **B,** Asymmetric optic nerve enhancement (*arrows*) on gadolinium-enhanced T1-weighted image.

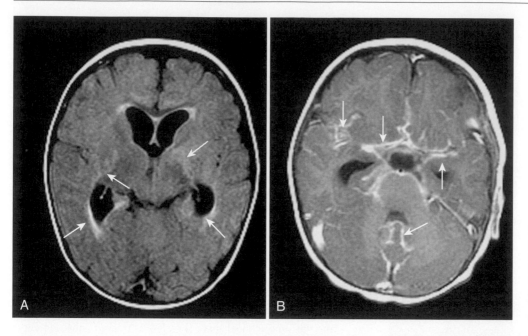

FIGURE 8-43. Tuberculous meningitis on MRI. **A,** Axial FLAIR image shows basal ganglia infarctions (*short arrows*) and hydrocephalus with periventricular edema (*long arrows*). **B,** Gadolinium-enhanced T1-weighted image shows basilar cistern enhancement (*arrows*).

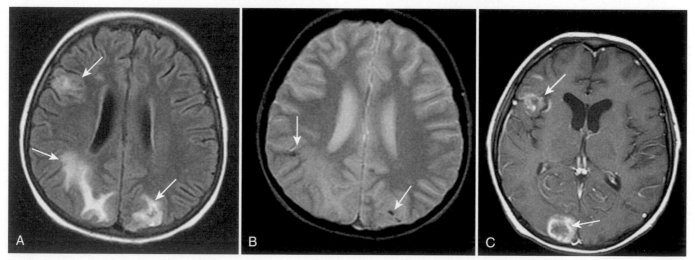

FIGURE 8-44. Aspergillosis on MRI. **A,** Edema (*arrows*) on axial FLAIR image. **B,** Hemorrhage (*arrows*) on GRE image. **C,** Abscess (*arrows*) on gadolinium-enhanced T1-weighted image.

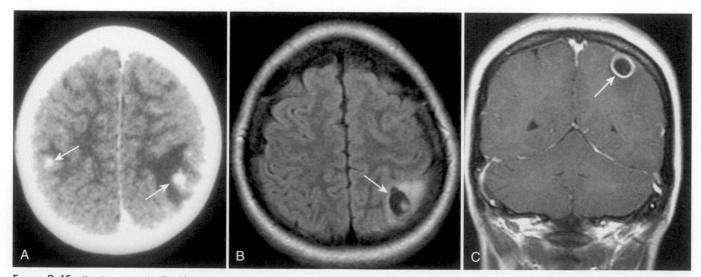

FIGURE 8-45. Cysticercosis. **A,** Calcification (*arrows*) on CT scan. Axial FLAIR (**B**) and coronal gadolinium-enhanced T1-weighted (**C**) MR images show ring-enhancing cyst with larva (*arrows*) and edema.

Parasitic Infections

Toxoplasmosis (discussed earlier) and cysticercosis are the most common parasitic infections of the CNS. Cysticercosis results from ingestion of material contaminated with pork tapeworm eggs. Seizures are common, and hydrocephalus and vasculitis may also occur. Patterns of involvement include parenchymal, leptomeningeal, intraventricular, and racemose. Parenchymal lesions are the most common form and usually involve gray matter–white matter junctions (Fig. 8-45). The lesions containing live cysticerci are cystic and contain the nodular scolex. The dying, or dead, larval lesions are often associated with edema and peripheral enhancement. The nonviable lesions frequently calcify over a long period. Leptomeningeal cysticercosis is often an enhancing basal granulomatous meningitis that may produce vasculitis with infarction. Intraventricular cysts may be identified from the nodular density or intensity of the contained scolex and may result in hydrocephalus. Racemose cysts lack larvae and most commonly occur in the basal cisterns and sylvian fissures.

Spirochete Infections

Spirochete infections of the CNS other than syphilis (discussed earlier) include Lyme disease and leptospirosis. The tick-transmitted Lyme disease (due to *Borrelia burgdorferi*) usually involves the CNS in the second stage. There may be predominant white matter involvement (CT hypodensity; T2 hyperintensity; presence or absence of ring enhancement) of the cerebrum and cerebellum along with brainstem, basal ganglia, or thalamic lesions. The findings may mimic those in ADEM. CNS disease rarely occurs in the second phase of leptospirosis (i.e., meningoencephalitis).

Vascular Sequelae of Infection

The vascular sequelae of systemic or CNS infection include vasculitis with arterial or venous thrombosis and ischemic or hemorrhagic infarction, mycotic aneurysm with hemorrhage, and hemorrhage related to associated coagulopathy. Vasculitis involving small arteries (arteritis) or small veins (phlebitis) is a common sequela of some meningitides (e.g., TB, fungal, or severe bacterial infections) and encephalitides (e.g., rubella, herpes). Basal ganglia and thalamic infarction is seen with basal meningitis (see Figs. 8-38 and 8-43). Hemorrhagic cortical or subcortical infarction occurs with cortical venous thromboses associated with meningitis or encephalitis (see Fig. 8-38). Smaller vessel occlusions associated with encephalitis (e.g., HSV, aspergillosis) may produce petechial hemorrhagic infarctions (see Figs. 8-35 and 8-44).

Involvement of medium-sized and larger vessels with thrombosis may be associated with CNS or systemic infections or the postinfectious immune-mediated encephalitides; this may include internal carotid or vertebrobasilar arterial or branch arterial occlusions with major arterial territorial infarctions, as has been reported following varicella zoster infection (chickenpox). Superficial or deep dural venous sinus thrombosis may be associated with CNS or systemic infections, particularly when complicated by fluid/electrolyte imbalance (e.g., dehydration). The result may be cortical and subcortical hemorrhagic infarction, deeper periventricular infarction, or intraventricular hemorrhage.

Mycotic aneurysms may be associated with bacterial or fungal infections. The aneurysms are usually fusiform and may be multiple. Risk factors include bacterial endocarditis, heart disease, intravenous drug use, and immunosuppression. Rupture with hemorrhage is often the presenting event.

■ NEUROVASCULAR DISEASES

Neurovascular disease includes abnormalities of hemodynamics (e.g., hypoxia-ischemia), hematology (e.g., coagulopathy), and vasculature (e.g., angiopathies, malformations), which characteristically manifest as acute neurologic events. Occasionally, the acute deficits may be episodic (e.g., migraine, seizures). A recently discovered but fixed deficit (e.g., hemiplegia) may be the first indication of a remote prenatal or perinatal neurovascular injury. Imaging assists in the clinical evaluation and differentiation of hypoxia-ischemia, hemorrhage, and occlusive vascular disease (Boxes 8-1 and 8-2; Tables 8-3 and 8-4).

Hypoxic-Ischemic Brain Injury

Brain injury may result from decreased oxygenation (e.g., airway obstruction, respiratory failure) or decreased blood flow (i.e., circulatory failure). Hypoxic-ischemic (HI) injury in the fetus is most often related to abnormal hemodynamics (i.e., hypoperfusion). Postnatal HI injury may be hypoxic, ischemic, or combined. HI injury is an important cause of neurodevelopmental decline (e.g., cerebral palsy). HI encephalopathy due to prenatal, peripartum, or postnatal insults may cause seizures, developmental delay, movement disorders, or spasticity. Dysautoregulation, reperfusion, hypercarbia, and acidosis, along with chemical mediators and inflammatory responses, also contribute to the clinical and imaging findings.

The pattern of HI injury depends on the severity and duration of the insult, or insults (e.g., profound, partial prolonged, combined) as well as the timing of the insult (e.g., gestational age [GA]). The maturational state of the brain and its vulnerability vary with GA. Areas of high metabolic activity (i.e., cellular turnover, active myelination) and regions with high concentrations of excitatory neurotransmitters are especially vulnerable. US during the acute phase may show nonspecific hyperechogenicity (Fig. 8-46A). Decreased resistive indices on Doppler US may be more suggestive of HI injury. In the acute phase, CT often shows nonspecific hypodensity and decreased gray matter–white matter differentiation (Fig. 8-46B). Such nonspecific findings may be seen with HI injury, infection, or metabolic disorders. Early-onset encephalopathy (<24 hours after birth) may suggest HI injury, whereas later onset may indicate infection (e.g., GBS, HSV-2)

Box 8-1. Imaging Patterns of Diffuse or Global Hypoxic-Ischemic Encephalopathy (HIE)*

HEMORRHAGE
Germinal matrix—intraventricular hemorrhage
Choroid plexus—intraventricular hemorrhage
Subarachnoid hemorrhage
Hemorrhagic infarctions

PARTIAL PROLONGED HIE
Preterm: Periventricular leukomalacia
Term/post-term: Cortical/subcortical injury (border-zone, watershed, parasagittal)
Intermediate: combined or transitional pattern
Ulegyria
Cystic encephalomalacia

PROFOUND HIE
Thalamic and basal ganglia injury
Brainstem injury
Hippocampal injury
Cerebral white matter injury
Paracentral injury
Global injury (prolonged profound)

COMBINED PROFOUND AND PARTIAL PROLONGED HIE
Total asphyxia

*Depends on gestational age, chronological age, and duration and severity of the insult.

or metabolic disorders (e.g., hypoglycemia, hyperbilirubinemia, inborn errors of metabolism). In the acute and subacute phases, MRI often shows a more definitive morphologic HI injury pattern (T1 hyperintensity, T2 hypointensity), including restricted diffusion and lactate elevation on MRS, and provides timing and outcome parameters. The long-term result of HI injury is a static encephalopathy (e.g., cerebral palsy). MRI best demonstrates injury in the chronic phase, including atrophy, periventricular leukomalacia, cystic encephalomalacia, and gliosis or mineralization in a characteristic distribution (see later).

Profound HI injury reflects a state of anoxia or circulatory arrest. The injury is shown best by MRI (Fig. 8-47). Although there may be some variation from preterm to term, profound HI primarily involves the basal ganglia (i.e., posterior putamina), thalami (i.e., ventrolateral), posterior limbs of the internal capsule, corona radiata, perirolandic cerebrum, and, occasionally, the cerebellar vermis, midbrain, and hippocampi. The profound HI injury pattern is to be distinguished from other causes of basal ganglia injury, including infection (e.g., neonatal meningitis with basal ganglia infarctions) and metabolic disorders (e.g., kernicterus, aminoacidopathy, organic acidopathy, sulfite oxidase deficiency).

Partial prolonged HI injury reflects a state of hypoxia or hypoperfusion in which there is relative shunting of blood flow from the cerebrum to the vital centers of the basal ganglia and brainstem. The result is cerebral injury along the major arterial border zone or "watershed" regions. In the preterm (e.g., 24-36 weeks' GA) fetus or neonate, the injury may be "multifocal" and predominantly involve the periventricular white matter (e.g., periventricular leukomalacia [PVL]), or there may more "diffuse" white matter injury. US displays early PVL as parietal or frontal periventricular hyperechogenicity. Similar findings, however, may be seen with infection, ischemia (e.g., maternal cocaine use), or metabolic disorders. Evolution to the cystic form of PVL occurs 2 to 6 weeks later (Fig. 8-48A). Hemorrhage may also occur. In chronic PVL, imaging often shows decreased white matter volume, lateral ventricular irregularity with variable enlargement, periventricular CT hypodensity or T2/FLAIR hyperintensity, and thinning of the corpus callosum (Fig. 8-48B). It may mimic colpocephaly. Partial prolonged HI injury in the term, full-term, or post-term fetus (or newborn) (e.g., 37-44 weeks' GA) primarily results in cortical and subcortical cerebral injury along the parasagittal border zones (Fig. 8-49). The base of each gyrus is particularly vulnerable to hypoperfusion. This is reflected in the chronic phase by the characteristic ulegyria pattern ("mushroom-shaped" gyri).

Combined profound and partial prolonged HI injury patterns may be encountered, including components that differ in timing. Very severe partial prolonged, or combined, HI insults may result in cystic encephalomalacia (Fig. 8-50). Injury patterns in the preterm or term child that may mimic HI injury (e.g., PVL or leukoencephalopathy pattern) include infection (e.g., chorioamnionitis, CMV), congenital heart disease, venous thrombosis, hypoglycemia, and other metabolic disorders (e.g., maple syrup urine disease, nonketotic hyperglycinemia, neonatal leukodystrophy).

In older children, HI insults may produce generalized cerebral edema with diffuse CT hypodensity and decreased gray matter–white matter differentiation. Hypodensity of the basal ganglia may be the earliest sign. Differential perfusion renders the brainstem, cerebellum, and tentorium hyperdense ("white cerebellum" sign—see Fig. 8-33A). Capillary and venous congestion renders the cerebral white matter hyperdense relative to the gray matter ("reversal sign"; see Fig. 8-33B) and is a poor prognostic sign. With primarily hypoxic/anoxic insults in infants and young children (e.g., near-drowning), the only imaging abnormality may be restricted diffusion of the cerebral white matter in the subacute phase. Similar findings may be seen with prolonged seizures. Atrophy frequently follows severe HI injury. There may be mineralization, gliosis, or cystic encephalomalacia.

Box 8-2. Occlusive Neurovascular Disease in Childhood

Idiopathic
Cardiac disease:
  Congenital
  Acquired
Vascular maldevelopment:
  Atresia
  Hypoplasia
Traumatic:
  Dissection
  Vascular distortion
  Air or fat emboli
Vasculopathy:
  Moyamoya disease
  Fibromuscular dysplasia
  Marfan syndrome
  Takayasu arteritis
  Kawasaki disease
  Vasculitis
  Polyarteritis nodosa
  Systemic lupus erythematosus
Vasospasm:
  Migraine
  Ergot poisoning
  Subarachnoid hemorrhage
Drugs:
  Cocaine
  Amphetamines
  L-asparaginase
  Oral contraceptives
Hypercoagulopathy:
  Protein S deficiency
  Protein C deficiency
  Antithrombin III deficiency
  Factor V (Leiden) and prothrombin mutations
  Antiphospholipid antibody (lupus, anticardiolipin)
  Heparin cofactor II deficiency
  Dehydration
  Nephrotic syndrome
  Oncologic disease
  Hemolytic-uremic syndrome
Hemoglobinopathy:
  Sickle cell disease
Infection:
  Meningoencephalitis
  Varicella
Metabolic disease:
  Homocystinuria
  Dyslipoproteinemia
  Fabry disease
  Mitochondrial cytopathies
  MTHFR deficiency
  Familial lipid disorders
Other:
  Radiation
  Emboli from involuting fetal vasculature
  Placental vascular anastomoses (twin gestation)
  Co-twin fetal death
  Fetofetal transfusion

Intracranial Hemorrhage

Intracranial hemorrhage may result from prematurity, trauma, HI injury, a coagulopathy (e.g., thrombocytopenia, disseminated intravascular coagulation, ECMO), or vaso-occlusive disease (e.g., venous thrombosis). Hemorrhage may occasionally be associated with infection (e.g., HSV-2). Vascular malformations and aneurysms producing intracranial hemorrhage are rare in the neonate and young infant and usually are not encountered until later childhood (see later).

Postischemic reperfusion is a proposed cause for the germinal matrix hemorrhage (GMH), intraventricular hemorrhage (IVH), and the resultant posthemorrhagic hydrocephalus associated with prematurity (<34 weeks' GA). GMH-IVH has been divided into four categories. Grade I is subependymal hemorrhage confined to the germinal matrix (caudothalamic groove). Grade II denotes intraventricular extension without ventricular dilatation. Grade III is subependymal and intraventricular hemorrhage with hydrocephalus. Grade IV refers to additional hemorrhagic periventricular infarction resulting from subependymal venous thrombosis (Fig. 8-51). Poor neurodevelopmental outcome in preterm brain injury generally correlates with the higher grades of GMH-IVH, parenchymal injury (e.g., PVL), and ventriculomegaly (e.g., PVL, posthemorrhagic hydrocephalus).

TABLE 8-4. Central Nervous System Vascular Anomalies of Childhood

Low-flow anomalies	Capillary malformations (telangiectasias)
	Capillary-venous malformations (e.g., Sturge-Weber)
	Venous malformations (developmental venous anomaly)
	Cavernous malformations
High-flow anomalies	Arteriovenous fistulae (dural, pial, intraparenchymal)
	Arteriovenous malformations (AVMs)
	Vein of Galen malformations (choroidal, mural, AVM subtypes)
	Hemangiomas (rare, multisystem hemangioendotheliomas)
Aneurysms	Traumatic (e.g., neonatal peritentorial)
	Mycotic (endocarditis, sepsis, human immunodeficiency virus)
	Familial
	Hypertension
	Collagen disorders
	Autosomal dominant polycystic kidney disease
	Neurofibromatosis
	Fibromuscular dysplasia
	Tuberous sclerosis
	Coarctation of the aorta
	Klippel-Trenaunay-Weber
	AVMs (Osler-Weber-Rendu)
	Radiation
	Moyamoya disease
	Metastatic atrial myxoma
	Craniopharyngioma post-surgery

GMH at term is unusual. Parenchymal hemorrhage in the term infant is most often subpial, in the choroid plexus, subependymal, or thalamic. Such hemorrhage may result from trauma (e.g., subpial), hypoxia-ischemia (e.g., in the choroid plexus, thalamic), coagulopathy, or venous thrombosis (e.g., subpial, subependymal, thalamic). There may be accompanying subarachnoid, subdural, or intraventricular hemorrhage. Hydrocephalus may be a sequela.

Occlusive Vascular Disease

These are single (focal) or multiple (multifocal) infarctions that result from arterial or venous occlusion. The arterial or venous distribution of the lesion(s) may help distinguish occlusive vascular injury from HI injury. Arterial occlusion may result from thrombosis, embolism, or stenosis. This often leads to ischemic infarction. Venous occlusion is usually the result of thrombosis and often produces hemorrhagic infarction.

Arterial Occlusive Disease

Encephalopathy including seizures may indicate acute cerebral infarction (i.e., "stroke") in the newborn. Prenatal stroke, however, may not manifest until later infancy, with early hand preference (i.e., contralateral "congenital hemiplegia") or focal seizures. Acute infarction in an older child, as in an adult, usually manifests as an acute neurologic deficit. Focal cortical ischemic lesions most often involve the middle cerebral artery territory and, less often, the posterior or anterior cerebral artery territory (Fig. 8-52). Multifocal territorial involvement may occasionally be seen, particularly with embolic infarction. The causes of arterial infarction in childhood are diverse (Box 8-2). In addition to heart disease, arteriopathies such as dissection as well as sickle cell, Kawasaki, and moyamoya diseases may result in pediatric stroke. Coagulopathies (e.g., antithrombin III, factor V, antiphospholipid antibody), drug use (e.g., cocaine), and metabolic disorders (e.g., mitochondrial encephalomyopathy with lactic acidosis, and stroke-like episodes [MELAS] syndrome, homocysteinuria) may also be responsible. Meningoencephalitis (e.g., pneumococcal, tuberculosis, varicella) may be complicated by stroke.

Characteristic imaging findings for acute arterial infarction include a wedge-shaped lesion involving the cortex with gyral swelling. Gyriform enhancement may be present in the subacute phase, and there may be petechial or frank hemorrhage (e.g., reperfusion). In the chronic phase there may be focal, or multifocal, atrophy with variable gliosis, porencephaly, or cystic encephalomalacia. MRI offers greater sensitivity for the early detection of infarction than US or CT, but conventional MRI findings may be negative in the early hours after the insult. PWI and DWI now offer earlier demonstration of ischemic lesions. MRA or CTA may show the site of vascular occlusion, especially

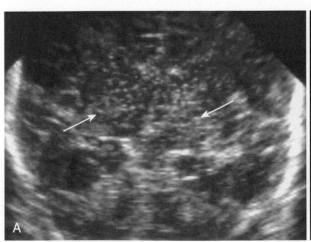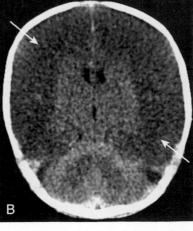

FIGURE 8-46. Acute hypoxia-ischemia with edema. **A,** US scan in a term newborn shows increased echoes of the basal ganglia and thalami (*arrows*). **B,** CT scan in another term newborn shows bilateral cerebral low densities (*arrows*) with decreased gray matter–white matter differentiation.

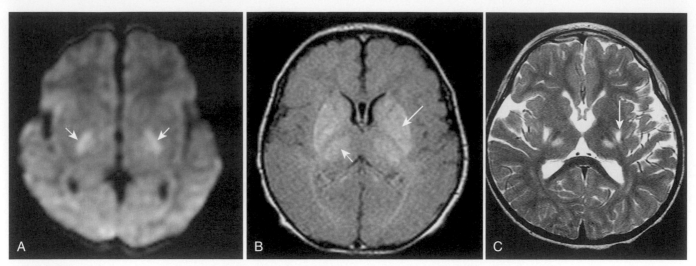

FIGURE 8-47. Profound hypoxia-ischemia on MRI. Acute phase with bilateral putaminal (*long arrow*) and thalamic (*short arrows*) necrosis on axial diffusion-weighted (**A**) and T1-weighted (**B**) images. **C,** Chronic phase with matching gliosis on axial T2-weighted image.

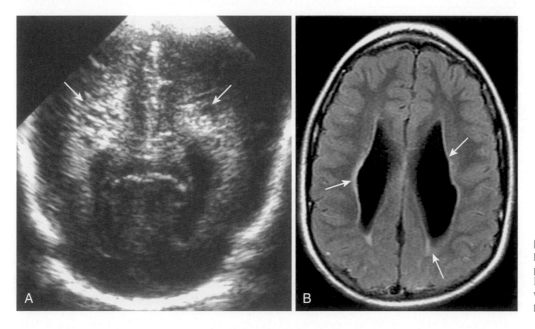

FIGURE 8-48. Periventricular leukomalacia. **A,** US scan of subacute phase with cysts (*arrows*). **B,** Axial FLAIR MR image of chronic phase with irregular ventriculomegaly and periventricular gliosis (*arrows*).

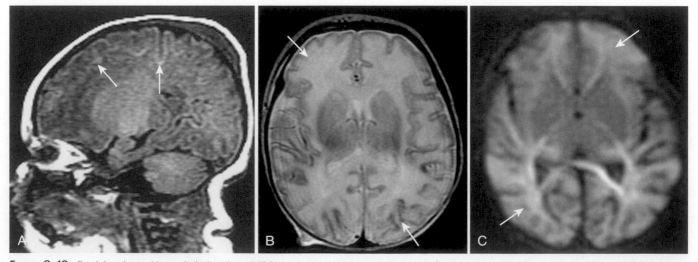

FIGURE 8-49. Partial prolonged hypoxia-ischemia on MRI. Acute phase with watershed injury (*arrows*) on sagittal T1-weighted (**A**), axial T2-weighted (**B**), and axial diffusion-weighted (**C**) images.

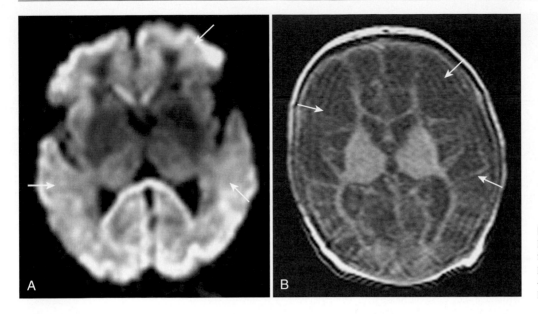

FIGURE 8-50. Cystic encephalomalacia on MRI. **A,** Axial diffusion-weighted image of acute phase showing edema (*arrows*). **B,** Axial T1-weighted image of chronic phase showing cysts (*arrows*).

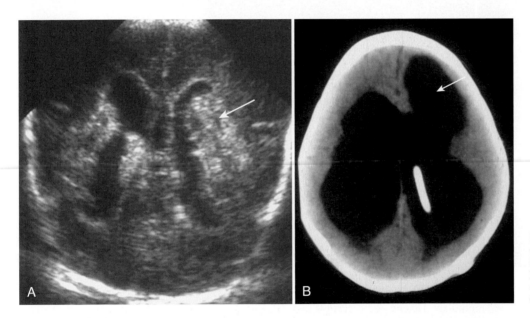

FIGURE 8-51. A, Grade IV intraventricular hemorrhage with hemorrhagic infarction (*arrows*) on coronal US scan. **B,** Post-hemorrhagic hydrocephalus with porencephaly (*arrows*) on axial CT scan with shunt catheter.

in large or medium-sized vessels. Smaller vessel lesions (e.g., vasculitis) often require catheter angiography for delineation.

Moyamoya disease is the prototype for pediatric stroke. It is characterized by progressive stenosis and occlusion of the internal carotid artery bifurcation along with the development of prominent basal, leptomeningeal, and transdural arterial collaterals. This disease is usually idiopathic but it may occur in association with neurofibromatosis, radiation therapy, sickle cell disease, or Down syndrome. In the childhood form, the disease is usually bilateral and the collateral vessels are prominent (Fig. 8-53). Ischemia occurs much more frequently than hemorrhage. There may be progressive developmental delay and focal neurologic deficits. Direct or indirect surgical transcranial revascularization between the superficial temporal artery and middle cerebral artery is the treatment of choice. Infarction or gliosis may be shown by CT or MRI and often occurs along the border zones. The basal collateral vessels may appear as flow voids or as enhancement on MRI. Vascular slow-flow areas of high intensity may be seen on FLAIR images. PMRI, perfusion SPECT, or xenon CT may be used for preoperative and postoperative hemodynamic evaluation. Catheter angiography is the procedure of choice for confirmation and preoperative planning.

Venous Occlusive Disease

Venous thrombosis is a common cause of infarction in childhood, including the perinatal period. There may be involvement of the dural venous sinuses or of the cortical, subependymal, or medullary veins. Etiologies include congenital heart disease, dehydration, infection, hypercoagulable states, toxins, chemotherapy (e.g., L-asparaginase) and oral contraceptives. Seizure or neurologic deficits are common, and hemorrhagic infarction is characteristic. Subarachnoid or subdural hemorrhage may also be seen, especially in infants, and the imaging findings may mimic those of NAI. Doppler US, contrast-enhanced CT, CTA, MRI with MRV and gadolinium enhancement, or catheter angiography may be needed to directly demonstrate dural venous sinus thrombosis

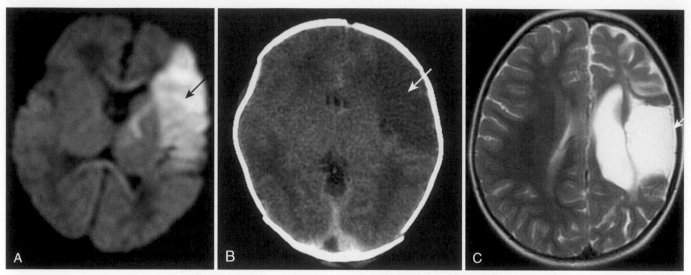

FIGURE 8-52. Middle cerebral arterial infarction (*arrows*). **A,** Axial diffusion-weighted MR image shows acute phase with edema. **B,** CT scan shows subacute phase. **C,** Axial T2-weighted MR image shows chronic phase with hemiatrophy.

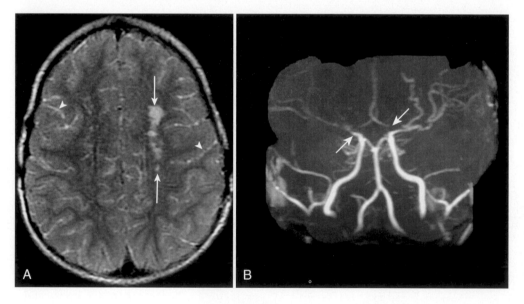

FIGURE 8-53. Moyamoya disease on MRI. **A,** Axial FLAIR image shows left anterior border-zone infarction (*arrows*) and vascular slow flow (*arrowheads*). **B,** Frontal MR angiogram shows bilateral arterial stenosis of the internal carotid bifurcation (*arrows*).

(Fig. 8-54). Cortical, subependymal, or medullary venous occlusion may not be directly demonstrated by these techniques, although hemorrhages or thromboses may be present in those distributions. The thrombosis may appear hyperdense on CT, of high intensity on T1-weighted MR images, of low intensity on T2-weighted images, or hypointense on GRE images and may mimic hemorrhage (Fig. 8-54). Intravenous enhancement about the thrombus may be seen on CT as an "empty delta" sign. Depending on the clinical context, treatment may be directed only to the specific cause (e.g., infection) or may also include anticoagulation or thrombolysis.

Vascular Anomalies

Clinically important vascular anomalies of the CNS in childhood include vascular malformations and aneurysms. Vascular malformations are categorized as AVM and arteriovenous fistula (AVF), cavernous malformations, developmental venous anomalies, and capillary telangiectasias. Aneurysms are rare in childhood and of diverse etiology.

AVMs are high-flow malformations in which there are abnormal connections between arteries and veins (no intervening capillaries). The lesions consist of enlarged arterial feeders, a vascular nidus, and draining veins. AVFs are high-flow malformations with one or more direct arteriovenous connections without a nidus. Common presentations include headache, seizure, and neurologic deficit and are often due to hemorrhage. Associated high-flow vasculopathy may produce aneurysms or venous stasis, increasing the risk of hemorrhage. Ischemic injury may result from the associated steal phenomenon. CT may detect high-density hemorrhage, blood pool, or calcification (Fig. 8-55). Contrast-enhanced CT or CTA may show the AVM. MRI using MRA, MRV, and gadolinium enhancement best shows the AVM, its hemorrhagic or ischemic components, and its anatomic relationships. Catheter angiography is required to precisely define the vascular components of the AVM. Treatment options include surgery, endovascular interventional procedures, conformal radiotherapy, or a combination.

The vein of Galen malformations (VGMs) are the prototypical AVM/AVF of infancy. VGMs are classified as choroidal, mural, and AVM types. The choroidal VGM manifests in the neonate as high-output congestive heart failure. Multiple deep AVFs connect with the persistent median prosencephalic vein, which drains into a persistent falcine sinus in the absence of the vein of Galen

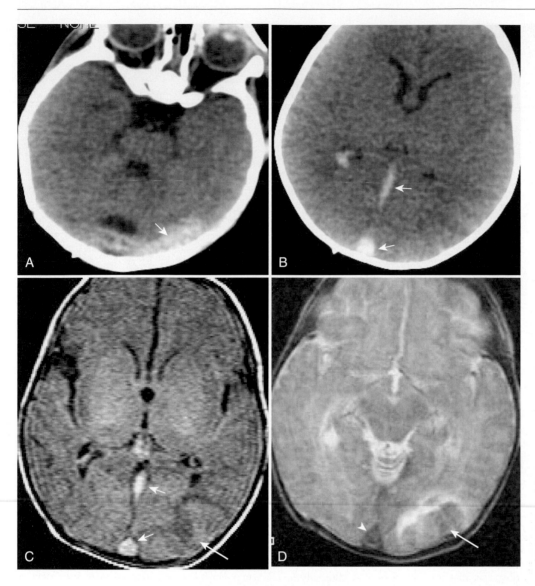

FIGURE 8-54. Venous thromboses (**A** to **C**, *short arrows*; **D**, *arrowhead*) with hemorrhages and infarctions (*long arrows*) on axial CT scans (**A** and **B**) as well as axial T1-weighted (**C**) and GRE (**D**) MR images in an infant with hypercoagulable state (mimicking nonaccidental injury).

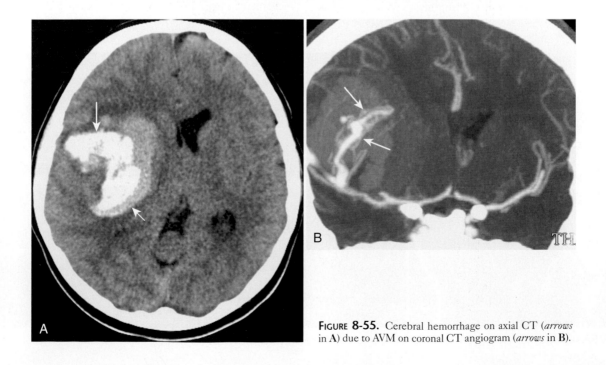

FIGURE 8-55. Cerebral hemorrhage on axial CT (*arrows* in **A**) due to AVM on coronal CT angiogram (*arrows* in **B**).

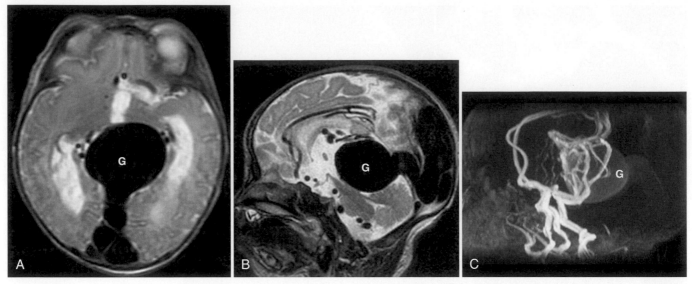

FIGURE 8-56. Vein of Galen (G) arteriovenous fistula (choroidal type) on axial (**A**) and sagittal T2-weighted (**B**) MR images as well as a lateral MR angiogram (**C**).

and straight sinus (Fig. 8-56). The mural VGM manifests later in infancy as hydrocephalus or seizures. One or more AVFs may be present within the wall of the median prosencephalic vein. Often there is outflow venous stenosis, which limits the AV shunting. The third type of VGM is composed of a deep AVM with venous drainage into a dilated vein of Galen. It often manifests as hemorrhage in older children and adults. US with Doppler imaging may provide the diagnosis in the fetus or neonate. CT, contrast-enhanced CT, and CTA may demonstrate the lesion, but MRI and catheter angiography are the best procedures for fully de-lineating the VGM and its complications, and for planning treat-ment and follow-up. Depending on the type and presentation, the options for therapy are similar to those described previously.

Cavernous malformations (CMs), also known as cavernomas or cavernous angiomas, are low-flow vascular malformations composed of endothelium-lined spaces without the components of AVM or AVF. They are probably the most common vascular

malformation of childhood. Similar lesions may occur following radiotherapy for CNS neoplasia. CMs may be asymptomatic or may manifest as hemorrhage, headache, or seizure. They may be single or multiple, and familial. Occasionally, a CM is associated with a developmental venous anomaly. Nonenhanced CT scans may show a hyperdense lesion with occasional calcification. On MRI, a T1- or T2-hyperintense focus with a T2-hypointense rim is often present (Fig. 8-57). Blood products of varying ages may be evident. These lesions are occult to CTA, MRA, and catheter angiography.

Developmental venous anomalies (DVAs), also called venous angiomas, are low-flow malformations in which one or more anomalous veins drain normal or dysplastic brain. No AVM or AVF components are present. Common sites are the frontal lobes and cerebellum. DVA may be associated with cortical dysplasias or migrational abnormalities. They are typically asymptomatic and incidental findings. DVA may rarely be associated with seizures or

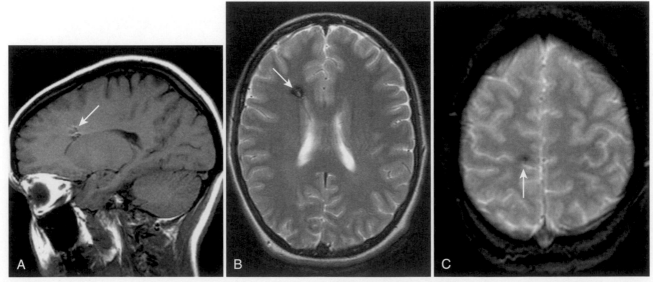

FIGURE 8-57. Familial multiple cavernous malformations (*arrow*) on sagittal T1-weighted (**A**), axial T2-weighted (**B**), and axial GRE (**C**) MR images.

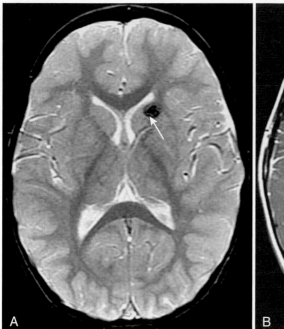
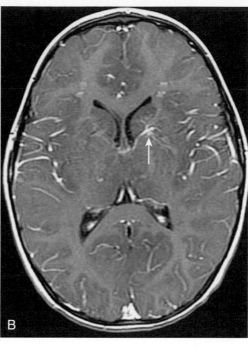

FIGURE 8-58. Cavernous malformation on axial GRE image (*arrow* in **A**) associated with developmental venous anomaly on axial gadolinium-enhanced T1 MR image (*arrow* in **B**).

hemorrhage, particularly when there is a concomitant cavernous malformation (Fig. 8-58). DVA is often demonstrated by imaging as a collection of dilated medullary veins that converge into a single vein that drains into the superficial or deep venous system. These lesions are frequently evident on CT only after contrast enhancement. MRI may show them as vascular flow voids or as gadolinium vascular enhancement. They are also demonstrated by catheter angiography.

Capillary telangiectasias are slow-flow capillary malformations. The lesions usually occur in the pons and are rarely symptomatic in children. They may be detected only on CT or MRI with contrast enhancement or if there is rare hemorrhage. They are usually occult to angiography.

Aneurysms are rare in childhood. They tend to be large (> 1 cm diameter), occur more often in males, and have a higher incidence within the vertebrobasilar system and at the internal carotid artery bifurcation. Aneurysms outside the circle of Willis are common and are usually mycotic or traumatic in origin. Increased risk of aneurysm is associated with certain conditions, such as coarctation of the aorta, polycystic kidney disease, neurofibromatosis, and a positive family history. The clinical presentation is often related to rupture with hemorrhage (e.g., headache) or is due to mass effect (e.g., third cranial palsy). Unenhanced CT often detects subarachnoid or intracerebral hemorrhage and may detect the aneurysm as a focal blood-pool of high density. On MRI, an aneurysm may appear as a focal flow void or as a focal hemorrhage or thrombosis. Catheter angiography is necessary for delineating site and morphology as well as for detecting additional aneurysms. CTA is also useful for surgical planning. MRA or CTA may be useful for aneurysm screening of at-risk patients. Treatment options include surgery and endovascular interventional techniques.

▬ CRANIAL AND INTRACRANIAL TUMORS OF CHILDHOOD

Classification

Tumors of the nervous system constitute the largest group of solid neoplasms in childhood. Neuroepithelial tumors contain cell types derived from the embryonic neuroepithelial tube (e.g., gliomas). Tumors of nonneuroepithelial tissues include those of neural crest or peripheral nervous system origin (e.g., neuroblastoma) as well as those of other cell types (e.g., germinoma and craniopharyngioma). Tumors are generally classified pathologically according to cell type and level of malignancy (World Health Organization [WHO] classification) (Box 8-3). Location and resectability, however, are often more important prognostic factors. Although primary CNS tumors may spread within the subarachnoid space (e.g., medulloblastoma), metastases beyond the CNS are uncommon. From a clinical and imaging perspective, CNS tumors may be categorized according to the major region of involvement, for example, in the posterior fossa, about the third ventricle, in the cerebral hemisphere, and parameningeal.

Although US or CT may detect neoplastic processes manifesting as large masses, MRI is preferred for complete evaluation, including treatment planning and the follow-up of tumor response and treatment effects. Important treatment effects after radiotherapy and chemotherapy include mineralization, ischemic vasculopathy, hemorrhagic vasculopathy, leukoencephalopathy, and second tumors. Functional imaging, including MRS, PMRI, SPECT, and PET, may be needed to distinguish treatment effects from tumor progression.

Posterior Fossa Tumors

Posterior fossa tumors occur more often in childhood than in adulthood. They often manifest as hydrocephalus, cerebellar signs (ataxia), brainstem signs (cranial nerve palsies), or meningeal signs (head tilt). Common lesions include embryonal tumors (i.e., medulloblastoma), cerebellar astrocytoma, brainstem glioma, and ependymoma. Less frequent tumor types are dermoid-epidermoid, teratoma, ganglioglioma, gangliocytoma of Lhermitte-Duclos, choroid plexus papilloma or carcinoma, sarcoma, acoustic neuroma, meningioma, and hemangioblastoma. Nonneoplastic lesions included in the differential diagnosis of posterior fossa "masses" are the Dandy-Walker-Blake spectrum of retrocerebellar cysts, arachnoid cyst, cavernous malformation, abscess, and hemorrhage. Skull base or petrous temporal parameningeal tumors that may invade the posterior fossa include sarcomas, histiocytosis, neuroblastoma, primitive neuroepithelial tumor (PNET), carcinoma, metastases, paraganglioma, and chordoma.

Box 8-3. Neuropathologic Classification of Central Nervous System Tumors*

I. Neuroepithelial tumors
  A. Astrocytic (e.g., astrocytoma, anaplastic, pilocytic, glioblastoma, subependymal Giant Cell Tumor)
  B. Oligodendroglial (e.g., oligodendroglioma, anaplastic)
  C. Ependymal (e.g., ependymoma, anaplastic)
  D. Mixed gliomas (e.g., oligoastrocytoma)
  E. Choroid plexus (e.g., papilloma, carcinoma)
  F. Uncertain origin (e.g., gliomatosis cerebri)
  G. Neuronal/mixedneuronal-glial(e.g.,ganglioglioma,dysembryoplastic neuroepithelial tumor, neurocytoma)
  H. Pineal (e.g., pineoblastoma, pineocytoma)
  I. Embryonal (e.g., primitive neuroepithelial tumor, medulloblastoma, atypical teratoid rhabdoid tumor)
II. Cranial and spinal nerve tumors
  A. Schwannoma
  B. Neurofibroma
  C. Malignant peripheral nerve sheath tumor
III. Meningeal tumors
  A. Meningothelial (e.g., meningioma)
  B. Mesenchymal, nonmeningothelial (e.g., sarcoma, rhabdoid)

  C. Primary melanocytic (e.g., melanosis)
  D. Uncertain histogenesis (e.g., hemangioblastoma)
IV. Lymphomas and hemopoietic neoplasms
V. Germ cell tumors
  A. Germinoma
  B. Embryonal carcinoma
  C. Yolk sac tumor
  D. Choriocarcinoma
  E. Teratoma
  F. Mixed
VI. Cysts and other tumor-like lesions (e.g., Rathke cyst, dermoid-epidermoid, colloid cyst, neuroglial cyst, hamartoma, heterotopia)
VII. Tumors of the sellar region
  A. Pituitary adenoma
  B. Pituitary carcinoma
  C. Craniopharyngioma
VIII. Localextensionsfromregionaltumors(e.g.,parameningeal neoplasms)
IX. Metastatic tumors (e.g., seeding)
X. Unclassified tumors

*Modified from Louis D, Ohgaki H, Wiestler O, et al: The 2007 WHO classification of tumours of the central nervous system. Acta Neuropathol 2007;114:97-109.

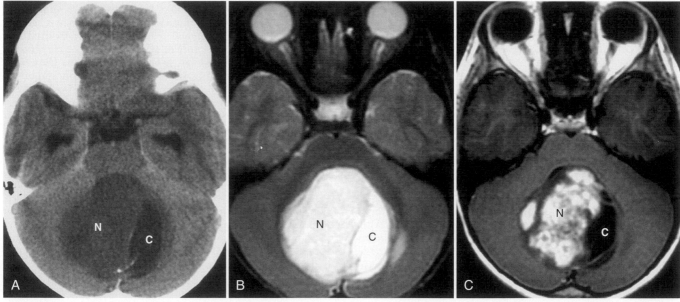

FIGURE 8-59. Cerebellar astrocytoma with nodular (N) and cystic (C) components on axial CT scan (**A**) as well as axial T2-weighted (**B**) and gadolinium-enhanced T1-weighted (**C**) MR images.

Cerebellar Astrocytoma

Cerebellar astrocytoma is one of the most common posterior fossa neoplasms of childhood. The pilocytic subtype far outnumbers the fibrillary and anaplastic forms. These tumors tend to be slow-growing, circumscribed, and differentiated. They have a good prognosis and usually require only surgical excision. Cerebellar astrocytomas usually arise within the vermis, hemisphere, or both (e.g., paramedian). They may be microcystic or macrocystic and may contain solid or laminar tumor. Associated displacement of the fourth ventricle or aqueduct results in hydrocephalus. On CT, the cystic portion is usually low density and the solid tumor is isodense (Fig. 8-59). Iodine enhancement of the solid component is common. Infrequently

the tumor appears more heterogeneous with variable enhancement. Unlike medulloblastoma or ependymoma, cerebellar astrocytomas rarely demonstrate tumor hyperdensity, hemorrhage, or calcification. On MRI, the macrocystic component usually displays intensity patterns characteristic of proteinaceous fluid (see Fig. 8-59). The microcystic component is commonly of low intensity on T1-weighted MRI and isointense to hyperintense on FLAIR and T2-weighted images. The nodular or laminar solid component is commonly isointense on T1-weighted images and isointense to hyperintense on T2-weighted images. Gadolinium enhancement of cerebellar astrocytoma on MRI is quite variable and similar to that described for iodine enhancement on CT.

Medulloblastoma

Medulloblastoma is a PNET in the embryonal category and, in many reported series, the most common posterior fossa tumor of childhood. A number of subtypes exist. *Atypical teratoid rhabdoid tumor* (ATRT), formerly mistaken for medulloblastoma, may be of choroid plexus origin, has the worst prognosis of tumors in the embryonal category, and may arise in the posterior fossa or cerebrum. For all the embryonal tumors, there is a tendency for seeding, although systemic metastasis is rare.

Medulloblastoma usually arises in the midline from the cerebellar vermis and grows into the fourth ventricle. It is often infiltrative, adheres to adjacent structures, and may directly involve the brainstem. It is the most common childhood tumor producing intracranial and intraspinal seeding, which may be present initially. Occasionally the tumor contains areas of necrosis, cysts, hemorrhage, or calcification, appearing similar to ependymoma (Fig. 8-60). In older children, medulloblastoma may arise from the cerebellar hemisphere (e.g., desmoplastic or nodular subtype). This hypercellular tumor is usually isodense to hyperdense on CT and T2-hypointense on MRI (see Fig. 8-60). Marked enhancement is characteristic. A mass with a more heterogenous

intensity and enhancement appearance in an infant or very young child should also prompt consideration of ATRT, ependymoma, and choroid plexus carcinoma. Seeding is best demonstrated on gadolinium-enhanced T1-weighted MRI as laminar or nodular enhancing lesions along pial or ependymal surfaces of the brain or spinal cord (see Fig. 8-60). Treatment of medulloblastoma requires a combination of surgery, chemotherapy, and craniospinal radiotherapy.

Ependymal Tumors

Ependymal tumors show considerable histologic diversity. Most ependymomas grow in or adjacent to the ventricular system, although extraventricular (e.g., cortical) lesions also occur. The tumors may be circumscribed and contain calcification, thrombosis or hemorrhage, necrosis, vascular proliferation, or other elements. Anaplastic forms also exist.

Ependymoblastoma is a variant of PNET. Ependymomas often arise within or about the fourth ventricle and produce hydrocephalus. Such a tumor may be small, midline, and confined to the fourth ventricle. Often, however, the tumor is large and eccentric, obliterating posterior fossa landmarks. Commonly

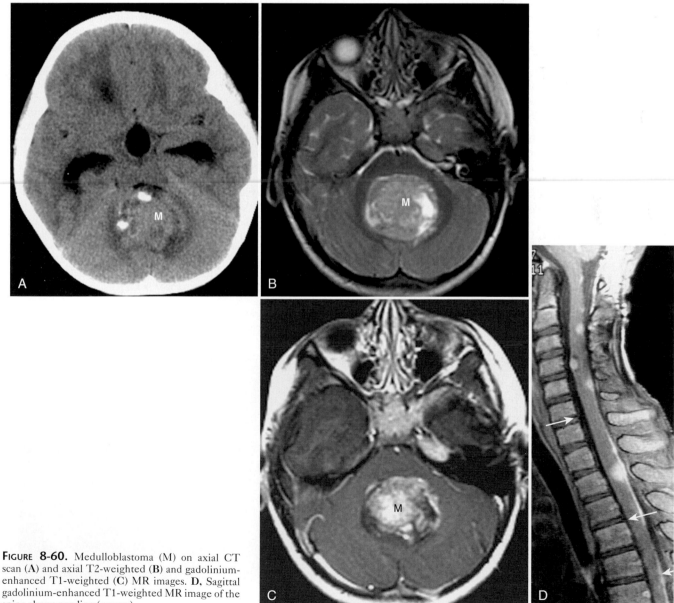

FIGURE 8-60. Medulloblastoma (M) on axial CT scan (**A**) and axial T2-weighted (**B**) and gadolinium-enhanced T1-weighted (**C**) MR images. **D**, Sagittal gadolinium-enhanced T1-weighted MR image of the spine shows seeding (*arrows*).

there is extension through the outlet foramina into the cisterna magna, the cisterns about the brainstem, and the foramen magnum and upper cervical canal about the spinal cord. Involvement of the cerebellum, brainstem, and vertebrobasilar arterial and cranial nerve structures is common. Seeding may rarely occur, especially with anaplastic ependymoma. Associated hemorrhage and hemosiderosis is rare in childhood. Density, intensity, and enhancement heterogeneity is characteristic of ependymomas and represents a mix of tumor, cysts, necrosis, edema, calcification, or hemorrhage (Fig. 8-61). ATRT, nontypical medulloblastoma, and choroid plexus carcinoma are in the differential diagnosis.

Brainstem Tumors

Brainstem tumors are most often gliomas of varying histologic types and grades of malignancy, including pilocytic or anaplastic astrocytoma, glioblastoma, mixed gliomas, and neuronal tumors (e.g., ganglioglioma). Anatomic subtypes include diffuse, focal, cystic, and cervicomedullary. Brainstem gliomas commonly arise in the pons, often diffusely infiltrate into the medulla and midbrain, require chemotherapy and radiotherapy, and have a very poor prognosis (Fig. 8-62). Symptomatic hydrocephalus is unusual early. There may be symmetric expansion with obliteration of the cisterns and fourth ventricle or asymmetric growth with exophytic extension and encasement of the basilar artery or adjacent cranial nerves. Cystic or necrotic changes may be seen with glioblastoma. Focal or cystic tectal, midbrain, thalamic, and cervicomedullary tumors are often lower grade and have a better prognosis. They may require only surgery or conformal radiotherapy. Tectal tumors occur as low-grade gliomas, hamartomas, or gliosis, and may be detected only on MRI (Fig. 8-63). They produce aqueductal stenosis and manifest as hydrocephalus. Cervicomedullary tumors may manifest as recurring emesis and are often only shown on MRI (Fig. 8-64). On imaging, brainstem tumors are often CT-isodense or hypodense, T1-isointense/hypointense, and T2/FLAIR-isointense to hyperintense. Enhancement is variable (e.g., diffuse, nodular, or ring). MRI helps distinguish these tumors from infarction, encephalitis, demyelination, and vascular malformation (e.g., cavernous malformation).

Other Tumors

Choroid plexus papilloma or carcinoma occasionally arises within the fourth ventricle or the angle (also see "Cerebral Tumors"). Mixed gliomas, neuronal, or mixed neuronal-glial tumors may also arise in the posterior fossa, including the dysplastic gangliocytoma (Lhermitte-Duclos). Tumors of cranial and spinal nerves occurring in childhood include schwannoma (neurilemmoma or neurinoma), neurofibroma, and malignant peripheral nerve sheath tumors. Solitary schwannomas (e.g., eighth nerve vestibular schwannoma or acoustic neuroma) are generally sporadic, whereas multiple schwannomas are characteristic of neurofibromatosis 2 (NF-2). Plexiform neurofibromas occur in NF-1. A number of malformative tumors occasionally arise in the posterior fossa, including dermoid/epidermoid, arachnoid cyst, and hamartomas. Epidermoids are of epidermal origin and usually arise in the cisterns about the angles. They are nonenhancing masses with CSF-like density or intensity that are hyperintense on FLAIR MRI and DWI. The latter feature assists in distinguishing them from arachnoid cysts. Dermoids contain epidermal and dermal elements and tend to arise midline in relation to the cerebellar vermis, brainstem, fourth ventricle, or cisterna magna. They exhibit fatlike densities and intensities as well as calcification. Hemangioblastoma rarely occurs in childhood in the absence of von Hippel–Lindau syndrome (see "Neurocutaneous Syndromes"). Lymphomas and hematopoietic neoplasms may also arise in the posterior fossa (see "Parameningeal Tumors"). Germ cell tumors, except teratoma, are extremely rare in the posterior fossa (see "Tumors About the Third Ventricle").

Tumors About the Third Ventricle

Tumors about the third ventricle may be subdivided as to suprasellar/anterior third ventricular tumors, pineal region/posterior third ventricular tumors, intraventricular tumors, and paraventricular tumors. Clinical manifestations often reflect hydrocephalus, neuroendocrine disorder (growth failure, hypopituitarism, precocious puberty, amenorrhea, galactorrhea, diabetes insipidus, diencephalic syndrome, syndrome of inappropriate antidiuretic hormone secretion), and optic pathway or other cranial nerve involvement. In childhood, common neoplasms in this region are optic and hypothalamic glioma, craniopharyngioma, and germ cell tumors. Less common tumors include pituitary adenoma, dermoid/epidermoid, choristoma, histiocytosis, pineal cell tumors (pinealoma, pineoblastoma), third ventricular glioma, ganglioglioma, ependymoma, meningioma, choroid plexus papilloma, paraganglioma, schwannoma, or neoplastic seeding. Nonneoplastic tumors include arachnoid cyst, sphenoidal encephalocele, colloid cyst, Rathke cyst, hamartoma (glial, neuronal, or mesenchymal, e.g., lipoma), ectopic posterior pituitary, aneurysm, galenic varix, cavernous angioma, granuloma, arachnoiditis, infundibulitis, hypophysitis, and sarcoidosis. Extracranial (parameningeal) processes of bone or sinus origin that may invade the midline brain structures include neuroblastoma, PNET, histiocytosis, esthesioneuroblastoma, sarcomas, chordoma, angiofibroma, carcinoma, mucocele, granulomatous processes (aspergillosis, etc.), and metastatic disease.

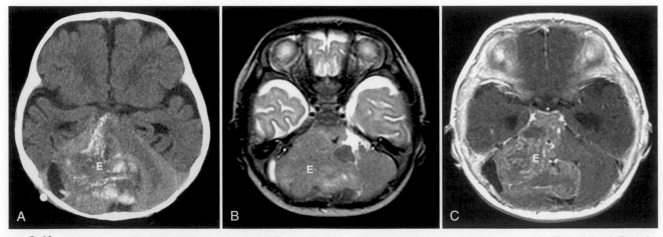

FIGURE 8-61. Ependymoma (E) with calcification on axial CT scan (**A**). Nonuniform intensity and enhancement on axial T2-weighted (**B**) and axial gadolinium-enhanced T1-weighted (**C**) MR images, respectively.

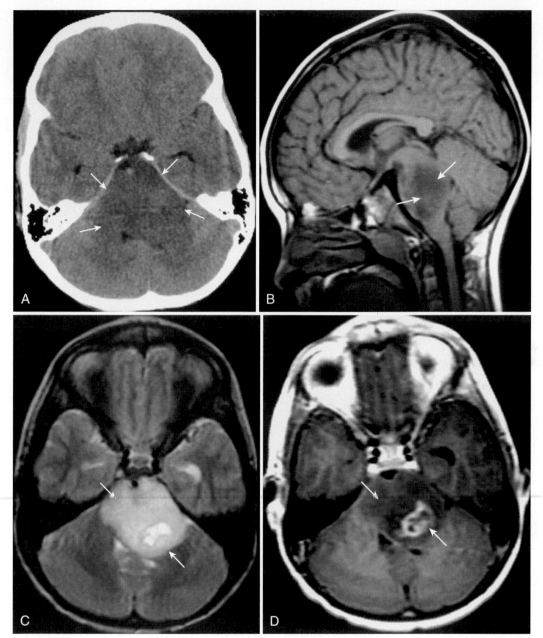

FIGURE 8-62. Pontine/diffuse brainstem glioma (*arrows*) on axial CT (**A**) as well as on sagittal T1-weighted (**B**), axial T2-weighted (**C**), and axial gadolinium-enhanced T1-weighted (**D**) MR images.

Gliomas

Gliomas constitute the largest group of neoplasms arising about the third ventricle. They may arise from the optic pathways, hypothalamus, thalamus, midbrain, foramen of Monro, or wall of the third ventricle. The optic pathway and hypothalamus are the most common sites of origin. The pilocytic astrocytoma characteristically occurs during childhood, often with slow infiltrative growth, and is more commonly solid than cystic in this region. Other astrocytic subtypes and mixed subtypes commonly occur in this region also. Ependymal, oligodendroglial, and choroid plexus tumors are somewhat unusual in this region.

Astrocytomas

Astrocytoma of the optic pathway (i.e., optic glioma) is the most common perisellar tumor of childhood and is frequently associated with NF-1. Exclusively intraorbital lesions include hamartomas, nerve sheath hypertrophy/hyperplasia, and low-grade astrocytomas. Tumors arising from the chiasm and optic tracts may range from hamartomas or low-grade astrocytomas to anaplastic astrocytomas. Multilevel visual pathway involvement also occurs. Glial neoplasms arising primarily within the hypothalamus also range from low-grade to anaplastic astrocytomas. When only a large suprasellar astrocytoma is demonstrated, it may be impossible to distinguish chiasmatic from hypothalamic origin. Diencephalic syndrome is classically associated with large astrocytomas in this region. Imaging of an optic glioma may show optic nerve, chiasm, or tract expansion with anterior or posterior extension (including lateral geniculate bodies and optic radiations). Hypothalamic gliomas are centered behind the chiasm. Astrocytomas are isodense or hypodense on CT, isointense to hypointense on T1-weighted MRI, and isointense to hyperintense on T2-weighted MRI (Fig. 8-65). Enhancement is common and may be homogeneous or irregular. Calcification, cyst, hemorrhage, or tumor hyperdensity is unusual in contrast

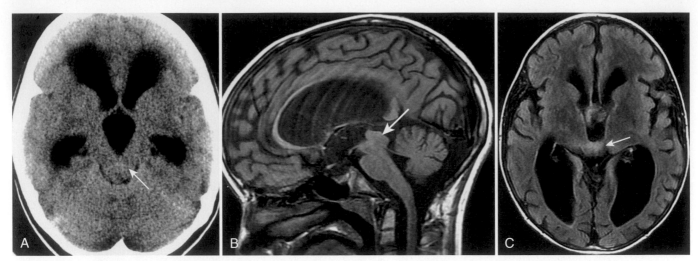

FIGURE 8-63. Tectal glioma (*arrow*) with hydrocephalus on axial CT scan (**A**) and on sagittal T1-weighted (**B**) and axial FLAIR (**C**) MR images.

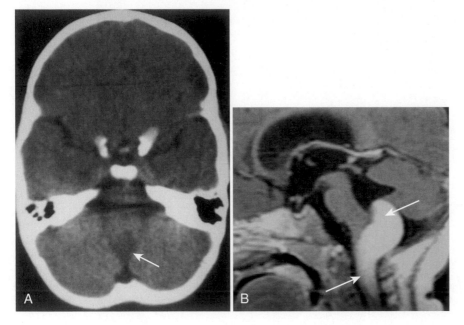

FIGURE 8-64. Cervicomedullary astrocytoma (*arrows*) on axial CT scan (**A**) and gadolinium-enhanced sagittal T1-weighted MR image (**B**).

to craniopharyngioma (calcification, cyst) or germinoma (tumor hyperdensity, hemorrhage). A nonenhancing mass along the tuber cinereum, when associated with precocious puberty, suggests a hamartoma. Differentiation from glioma is necessary especially if there are gelastic seizures. Circumscribed tumors about the third ventricle include the tectal glioma and the giant cell tumor of tuberous sclerosis. The former often manifests as hydrocephalus due to aqueductal stenosis (see "Posterior Fossa Tumors"). The subependymal giant cell tumor of tuberous sclerosis is usually situated near the foramen of Monro and produces asymmetric obstructive hydrocephalus (see "Neurocutaneous Syndromes"). In other cases, the glioma may be infiltrative and poorly marginated with anatomic distortion and extension across the midline (e.g., thalamic astrocytoma). On imaging, the density, intensity, and enhancement characteristics are variable and similar to those of glial tumors arising at other sites (as described earlier). Neuronal and mixed neuronal-glial tumors may also occur about the third ventricle (see "Cerebral Tumors").

Germ Cell Tumors

Germ cell tumors are composed of elements derived from the primitive germ layers. They most commonly arise along the midline in the hypothalamic region, pineal region, or both. Off-midline tumors occasionally occur, especially in Asian populations. This classification includes germinoma, embryonal carcinoma, endodermal sinus tumor, choriocarcinoma, and teratoma. Mixed germ cell tumors also occur. These are considered malignant tumors, except for mature teratomas, and have a tendency for CSF seeding. The "pure" germinoma is highly responsive to combined chemotherapy and radiotherapy, unlike the other "nongerminomatous" tumors. Elevated CSF and serum markers (e.g., alpha-fetoprotein, human chorionic gonadotrophin) are more often associated with the latter group. Imaging of "pure" germinomas demonstrates a midline or paramedian mass that typically is CT-isodense to hyperdense, is T1- and T2-isointense to hypointense with surrounding hyperintensity, and markedly enhances (Figs. 8-66 and 8-67). It is often associated with abnormal pineal calcification, occasionally

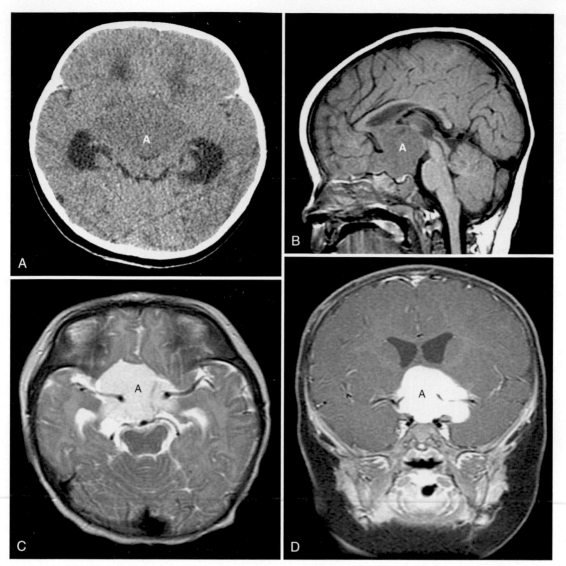

FIGURE 8-65. Optic-hypothalamic astrocytoma (A) on axial CT scan (**A**) and on sagittal T1-weighted (**B**), axial T2-weighted (**C**), and coronal gadolinium-enhanced T1-weighted (**D**) MR images.

hemorrhagic, but rarely cystic. Hypothalamic germinomas often manifest as central diabetes insipidus as indicated by absence of the normal posterior pituitary bright spot (see Figs. 8-1G and 8-66). Langerhans cell histiocytosis may have a similar presentation and imaging findings. Embryonal carcinoma, yolk sac tumor, choriocarcinoma, and teratoma often exhibit more heterogenous density, intensity, and enhancement characteristics. Teratomas are usually composed of a mixture of differentiated tissues representing derivatives of the three embryonic germ layers. They are often circumscribed and cystic masses that may contain calcification, bone, cartilage, teeth, or adipose tissue. Teratomas are divided into mature (e.g., adult tissue elements) and immature (e.g., embryonic elements) types. Mature teratomas are slow growing and benign. Immature teratomas are predominantly neuroepithelial and may be benign or malignant in behavior. Teratomas containing other germ cell tumor, carcinoma, or sarcoma elements (i.e., teratocarcinomas) are malignant. Imaging of a teratoma usually demonstrates a lobulated or cystic mass with heterogenous CT densities and MRI intensities containing fat, calcium, ossification, or cartilage (Fig. 8-68). Contrast enhancement may be more prominent in the malignant forms.

Pineal Parenchymal Tumors

Pineal parenchymal tumors include pineoblastoma, pineocytoma, and mixed/transitional pineal tumors. Pineoblastomas occur primarily in childhood. They are embryonal tumors similar to PNETs, and are considered highly malignant neoplasms with a propensity to disseminate in the CSF pathways. Imaging often shows a large lobulated pineal region mass with extensive calcification. The tumor is often CT-isodense to hyperdense, T1-isointense to hypointense, and T2-isointense to hypointense. Marked enhancement and hydrocephalus are common. Pineocytomas are generally circumscribed and may be calcified.

Malformative Tumors

The common malformative tumors occurring about the third ventricle include craniopharyngioma, Rathke cyst, colloid cyst, pineal cyst, arachnoid cyst, lipoma, hamartoma, and dermoid/epidermoid.

The *craniopharyngioma* (CPG) is a benign but aggressive squamous epithelial neoplasm arising in the suprasellar or intrasellar region. It is probably of Rathke pouch origin and most commonly occurs in childhood. CPGs are usually cystic and calcified but often have a solid component. They tend to deform, encase, or adhere

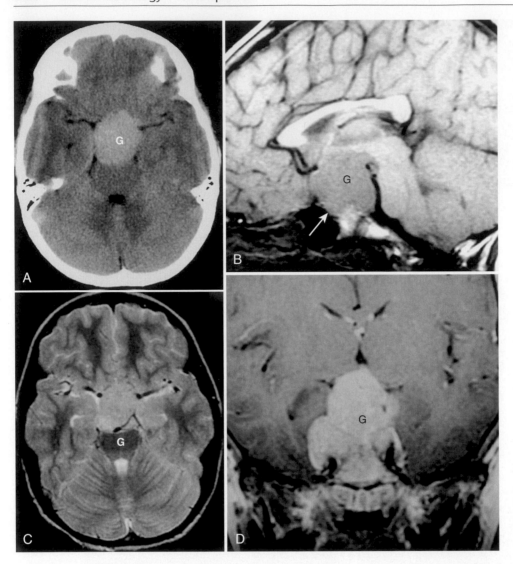

FIGURE 8-66. Hypothalamic germinoma (G) with absence of the posterior pituitary bright spot (*arrow* in **B**) on axial CT scan (**A**) as well as sagittal T1-weighted (**B**), axial T2-weighted (**C**), and coronal gadolinium-enhanced T1-weighted (**D**) MR images.

to adjacent structures and are associated with a gliotic reaction. The solid component of a CPG is CT-isodense or hypodense, T1-isointense to hypointense, and T2-isointense to hyperintense. Enhancement of the solid tumor or cyst wall is common. The calcified, ossified, or keratinized components of CPG are CT-hyperdense and of variable intensity on MRI. On CT, the cyst may be primarily hypodense (e.g., cholesterol or serous), or isodense to hyperdense (e.g., protein, hemorrhage, keratin, or calcium). On MRI, the cyst is characteristically of high intensity on all sequences, particularly on T1-weighted images (Fig. 8-69). Hypointensity may indicate keratin, calcium, or iron. The differential diagnosis may include the rare cystic or calcified glioma or teratoma. *Rathke cyst*, an epithelial cyst also of Rathke pouch origin, may be similar in appearance to CPG; however, calcification and nodular enhancement are unusual.

The *colloid cyst* is probably of neuroepithelial origin and occurs more often in adulthood. It has a fibrous wall and proteinaceous content. It arises in the wall or roof of the third ventricle at the foramina of Monro and often produces hydrocephalus. Occasionally there is hemorrhage. The colloid cyst is usually hyperdense and nonenhancing (rarely isodense or hypodense) on CT. It may be of low or high intensity on T1- and T2-weighted images.

Other neuroepithelial cysts (e.g., glioependymal) may arise in a variety of locations, including the choroid plexus and the pineal gland. They may be detected only with MRI and usually appear T1-hypointense, FLAIR-hyperintense, and T2-hyperintense. Enhancement of the cyst wall is common, although there may

be delayed enhancement within the cyst. The *pineal cyst* may be associated with deformity of the adjacent tectum and aqueduct, but hydrocephalus is rare. *Arachnoid cysts* are arachnoid-lined cysts that contain CSF, usually arise in the subarachnoid spaces, and commonly occur in the suprasellar region or about the quadrigeminal plate region (see Figs. 8-11, 8-16, and 8-17). They are CT-hypodense, conform to CSF intensities on MRI sequences (T1-hypointense, FLAIR-hypointense, T2-hyperintense, DWI-hypointense, ADC-hyperintense), do not enhance, and may have no perceptible wall. These features distinguish arachnoid cysts from neuroepithelial cysts (see earlier) and tumor cysts. Associated hemorrhage or infection, however, may change their appearance.

Lipomas are benign mesenchymal hamartomas consisting of adipose tissue (neutral fat). There may be associated muscle, fibrous, or vascular elements. They most commonly occur along the hypothalamus or stalk, quadrigeminal plate, and corpus callosum (e.g., in callosal hypogenesis). CT shows fatty hypodensity and occasional calcification. MRI demonstrates the tumor's characteristic high intensity on T1-weighted and FLAIR images, isointensity to hypointensity on T2-weighted images, chemical shift artifact, and signal loss on fat suppression sequences (Fig. 8-70A). In the suprasellar region, lipoma is to be distinguished from an ectopic posterior pituitary. Normally, the posterior pituitary is demonstrated on T1-weighted MRI as a posterior intrasellar hyperintensity (probably related to the carrier protein for antidiuretic hormone). The pituitary's presence usually indicates normal

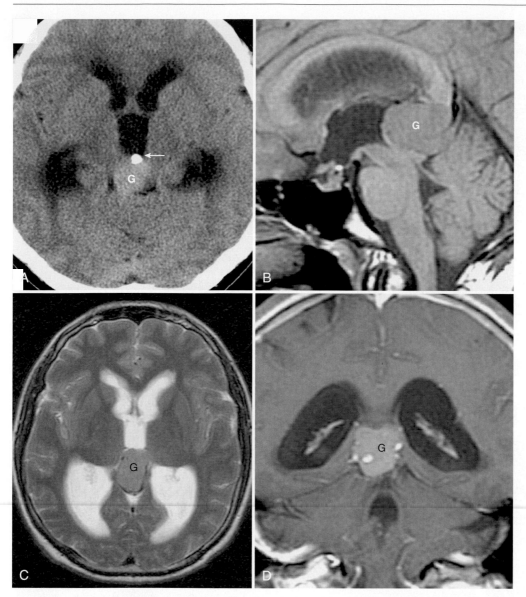

FIGURE 8-67. Pineal germinoma (G) with calcification (*arrow*) and hydrocephalus on axial CT (**A**) as well as sagittal T1-weighted (**B**), axial T2-weighted (**C**), and coronal gadolinium-enhanced T1-weighted (**D**) MR images.

antidiuretic hormone physiology (see Fig. 8-1G); its absence usually correlates with diabetes insipidus and often with hypothalamic or stalk tumor (see Fig. 8-66). Ectopic posterior pituitary is usually associated with "idiopathic" growth hormone deficiency, appears as a hypothalamic or infundibular hyperintensity on T1-weighted MRI, and is associated with absence of the normal intrasellar posterior pituitary bright spot (Fig. 8-70B). Often there is absence, interruption, or attenuation of the stalk. Lipoma and ectopic posterior pituitary are usually centered posterior to the stalk, whereas craniopharyngioma and Rathke cyst are usually more anterior.

Neuroepithelial hamartomas are composed of disorganized neuronal or glial elements. The hypothalamic location (i.e., hamartoma of the tuber cinereum) may be associated with precocious puberty, gelastic seizures, or NF-1. The hamartoma is usually CT-isodense to hypodense, T1-isointense, FLAIR-isointense to hyperintense, and T2-hyperintense (Fig. 8-71). Enhancement is unusual. Other hamartomatous lesions are ectopic masses of neural, glial, or meningeal tissue that develop in juxtacranial or extracranial locations, for example, nasal glioma. *Meningioangiomatosis* is a rare hamartomatous condition consisting of local proliferation of arachnoid cells, vessels, and Schwann cells.

Epidermoid and dermoid tumors tend to be cystic and probably result from inclusion of epithelial elements at the time of neural tube closure. Epidermoid cysts are of ectodermal origin

and are lined with keratinizing stratified squamous epithelium. They often contain desquamated cellular debris and cholesterol, the latter as a breakdown product of keratin. Dermoids are also of ectodermal origin. Additional elements are derived from skin appendages, including hair, sebaceous glands, and sweat glands. The breakdown products of these elements produce an oily lipid-like mixture. Occasionally these tumors also contain calcification, bone, cartilage, or, rarely, teeth (i.e., teratoid), thus raising the question of a link with true teratomas. Epidermoids more commonly arise off the midline and conform to CSF densities and intensities. Occasionally there is cyst wall calcification. Their hyperintense appearance on FLAIR MRI and DWI distinguish them from arachnoid cysts. Dermoid cysts arise as midline lesions, contain calcification or formed elements, have lipid densities and intensities, and are often associated with a dermal sinus or bony defect; however, it may be impossible to distinguish among these three entities. Cyst rupture may be associated with aseptic meningitis or arachnoiditis and hydrocephalus. T1-hyperintense lipid particles or lipid-CSF levels may be present.

Pituitary Tumors

The most common intrasellar neoplasms include the pituitary adenoma and the craniopharyngioma (see earlier). Pituitary adenomas are currently divided into hormonally active (about

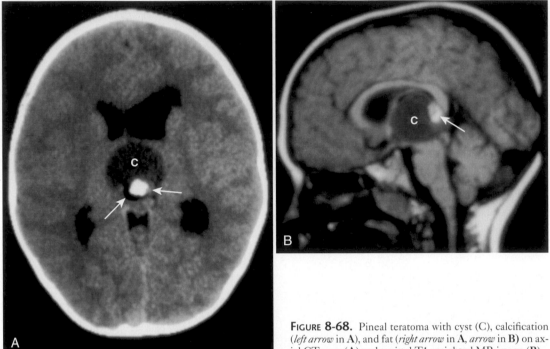

FIGURE 8-68. Pineal teratoma with cyst (C), calcification (*left arrow* in **A**), and fat (*right arrow* in **A**, *arrow* in **B**) on axial CT scan (**A**) and sagittal T1-weighted MR image (**B**).

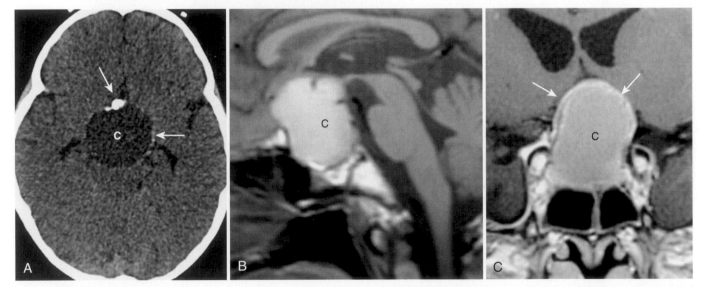

FIGURE 8-69. Craniopharyngioma with cyst (C), calcifications (*arrows* in **A**), and wall enhancement (*arrows* in **C**) on axial CT (**A**) as well as sagittal T1-weighted (**B**) and coronal gadolinium-enhanced T1-weighted (**C**) MR images.

70%) and inactive groups. They are more common in adults than in children. The most common hormonally active tumors secrete prolactin, growth hormone, or a combination. Many of the prolactin-secreting or adrenocorticotropic hormone–secreting tumors are microadenomas (<1 cm diameter). Hemorrhagic, prolactin-secreting macroadenomas characteristically occur in adolescent males. Often there is suprasellar extension of the T1-hyperintense mass, and it may be mistaken for craniopharyngioma or a Rathke cyst (Fig. 8-72).

Meningeal tumors, especially meningioma, may arise in the perisellar region or in the pineal region from the tentorium. However, these tumors are extremely rare in childhood. For meningeal tumors arising about the sella, differential diagnostic considerations include fibrous dysplasia, pituitary adenoma, and aneurysm.

Cerebral Tumors

Cerebral hemispheric tumors may manifest as seizures, hemiparesis, movement disorder, headache, other sensory phenomena, increased pressure, or cognitive disorders. Most intracranial masses or "tumors" of infancy are nonneoplastic and "cystic" (e.g., porencephaly, arachnoid cyst, Dandy-Walker cyst, galenic varix). Neoplasms, although rare in infancy, may be astrocytomas, embryonal tumors (e.g., PNET, ATRT), germ cell tumors (e.g., teratoma), choroid plexus tumors (papilloma, carcinoma), or mesenchymal tumors (e.g., sarcoma). In older children and adolescents, most intracranial tumors are of neuroepithelial origin, including gliomas, neuronal or mixed neuronal and glial tumors (e.g., ganglioglioma, neurocytoma, dysembryoplastic neuroepithelial tumor), and embryonal tumors (e.g., PNET). Nonneoplastic supratentorial masses include arachnoid cysts, abscess or empyema, hamartomas,

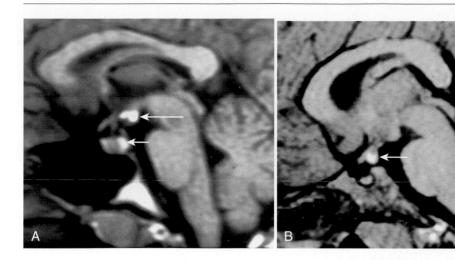

FIGURE 8-70. **A,** Hypothalamic lipoma (*long arrow*) with normal posterior pituitary bright spot (*short arrow*) on sagittal T1-weighted MR image. **B,** Ectopic posterior pituitary (*arrow*) on sagittal T1-weighted MR image.

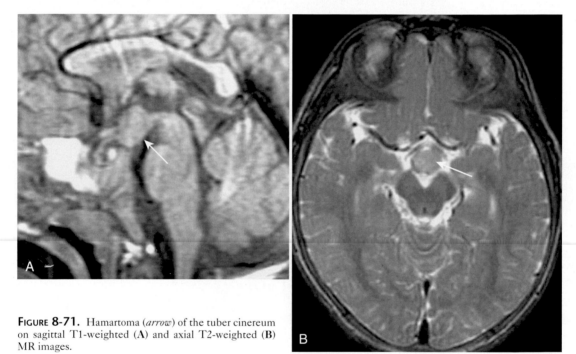

FIGURE 8-71. Hamartoma (*arrow*) of the tuber cinereum on sagittal T1-weighted (**A**) and axial T2-weighted (**B**) MR images.

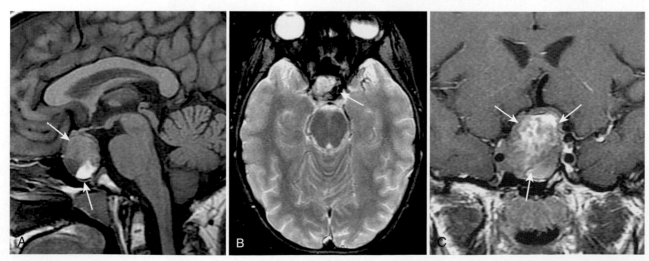

FIGURE 8-72. Hemorrhagic pituitary adenoma (*arrows*) on sagittal T1-weighted (**A**), axial GRE (**B**), and coronal gadolinium-enhanced T1-weighted (**C**) MR images.

vascular malformations (e.g., cavernous malformation), hematoma, and so forth. Extradural, calvarial, or scalp lesions (parameningeal) that may encroach upon the cerebral hemisphere include metastases (e.g., neuroblastoma), osteoma, dermoid-epidermoid, histiocytosis, hemangioma or other vascular anomaly, fibrous dysplasia, sarcomas, lymphoma, leukemia, neurofibroma, fibroma/fibromatosis, and infections.

Astrocytic Tumors

Astrocytic tumors account for the majority of gliomas and primary cerebral tumors in childhood. The tumors may be well-defined and circumscribed (e.g., pilocytic astrocytoma), ill-defined and infiltrating (e.g., fibrillary or anaplastic astrocytoma), or both (e.g., glioblastoma). These neoplasms may be cystic, solid, or calcified. Often, the tumors are CT-isodense to hypodense, T1-isointense to hypointense, and T2-isointense to hyperintense. Enhancement is variable (Fig. 8-73). A well-defined tumor in which the gadolinium enhancement matches the extent of the T2 hyperintensity may suggest a pilocytic astrocytoma. Imaging findings that may occasionally indicate the tendency for higher grades of malignancy include density or intensity heterogeneity, irregular shape and poor margination, mass effect,

edema, hemorrhage, and irregularly thick and nodular ring-like or solid enhancement (Fig. 8-74). However, density, intensity, and enhancement characteristics do not consistently correlate with grade of malignancy nor serve as accurate indicators of tumor margins (tumor vs. edema). For astrocytic tumors, as well as most other CNS neoplasia, maximum safe surgical excision or debulking is preferred to biopsy. Radiotherapy, chemotherapy, or both are important in the treatment of higher-grade tumors as well as recurrent or symptomatic lower-grade tumors. Higher-grade tumors often show faster response rates but recur earlier than lower-grade tumors. A transient increase in tumor volume, including mass effect, edema, and enhancement, may occur after radiotherapy, particularly after stereotactic radiosurgery or stereotactic (fractionated) radiotherapy.

Glioblastoma

Glioblastoma (GBM) is generally considered an anaplastic form of astrocytoma. GBM occurs primarily in the cerebrum during adolescence and is the most malignant of the neuroepithelial tumors, in terms of seeding potential and poor survival. A congenital form has also been reported. Variants include the giant cell glioblastoma and the gliosarcoma. The imaging findings are diverse and range

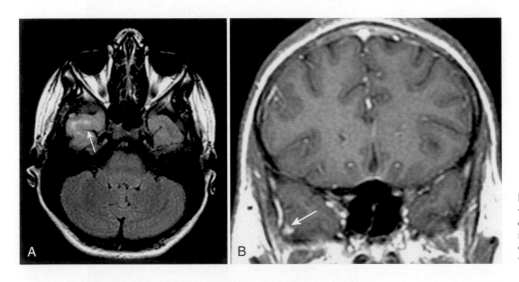

FIGURE 8-73. Temporal lobe epilepsy with astrocytoma (*arrows*) appears as focal hyperintensity on an axial FLAIR MR image (**A**) and as nodular enhancement on a coronal gadolinium-enhanced T1-weighted MR image (**B**).

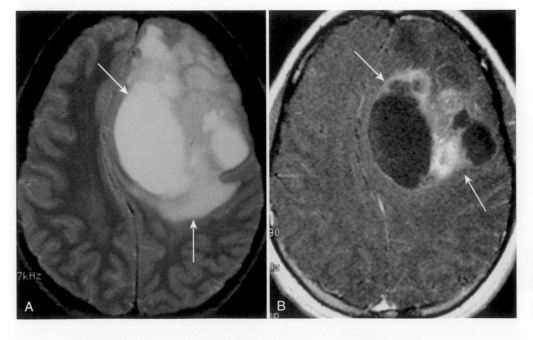

FIGURE 8-74. Frontal anaplastic astrocytoma/glioblastoma (*arrows*) on axial T2-weighted (**A**) and axial gadolinium-enhanced T1-weighted (**B**) MR images.

from a circumscribed mass to a diffuse process. Often GBMs are large, heterogenous, solid or cystic, and usually enhancing tumors with mass effect, edema, or hemorrhage (see Fig. 8-74). Calcification is occasionally present. Irregular nodular ring enhancement with a necrotic center and surrounding vasogenic edema is often characteristic. The giant cell GBM may appear as a cyst with a mural nodule. *Gliomatosis cerebri* refers to the rare entity of diffuse infiltrative glioma that involves either multiple sites or large areas of the CNS, usually the cerebral hemispheres. Pathologically, gliomatosis cerebri resembles diffuse astrocytoma, although foci of GBM may occur. It is distinguished from diffuse leptomeningeal or intraventricular spread of malignant glioma. Imaging usually underestimates the extent of tumor involvement in gliomatosis.

Other Gliomas

Ependymomas of childhood occasionally arise within the cerebrum. Oligodendrogliomas and mixed gliomas occur less often in children than in adults.

Ependymal tumors often project outward from the lateral ventricular ependyma or arise from ependymal cell rests in the cortex (i.e., cortical ependymoma). Imaging may demonstrate a heterogenous or occasionally homogeneous density or intensity mass, often with calcification and cyst formation plus irregular enhancement (Fig. 8-75). Other tumors with a similar appearance that are part of the differential diagnosis of ependymomas include PNET, ATRT, choroid plexus carcinoma, anaplastic gliomas, and GBM. Anaplastic forms may seed.

The well-differentiated or pure *oligodendroglioma* (ODG), a common tumor of adulthood, rarely occurs in childhood. It may contain other glial elements, most often astrocytic (i.e., oligoastrocytoma). Other circumscribed cerebral cortical tumors that occur more commonly in childhood and may be mistaken for ODG include dysembryoplastic neuroepithelial tumor, ganglioglioma, astrocytoma, astroblastoma (cortical ependymoma), and pleomorphic xanthoastrocytoma (PXA). These are often slow growing and circumscribed, may calcify, and may thin the cranial inner table. Rarely is there invasion or spread into the leptomeninges. The imaging appearance is often that of a circumscribed mass of uniform density or intensity that is solid, cystic, or both (Fig. 8-76). Calcification may be the major feature. The tumor itself is often CT-isodense to hypodense with calcific high density, T1-isointense to hypointense, and T2-isointense to hyperintense. Edema is often lacking, and the extent of enhancement is variable. Nonneoplastic lesions which may be revealed by CT as a solitary calcific high density are cavernous angiomas, neuroglial hamartomas (e.g., tuber), and inflammatory lesions (e.g., cysticercosis). A poorly marginated

tumor with heterogenous density/intensity characteristics, irregular enhancement, edema, or dissemination may indicate a mixed or anaplastic glioma (e.g., anaplastic ependymoma), or a mixed glioneuronal tumor (e.g., anaplastic ganglioglioma). The *subependymoma*, also rare in childhood, is a special type of mixed glioma composed of astrocytes and ependymal cells arising beneath the ventricular ependyma.

Choroid Plexus Tumors

Tumors of the choroid plexus origin are encountered primarily in early childhood and are usually associated with hydrocephalus. *Papillomas* are generally circumscribed intraventricular tumors usually involving the lateral ventricle and rarely the third or fourth ventricle (Fig. 8-77). Carcinomas are malignant and invasive, often extend beyond the ventricular margins, and are associated with mass effect and edema (Fig. 8-78). These are hypercellular and highly vascular neoplasms that often calcify or hemorrhage. These are usually CT-isodense to hyperdense, T1-isointense to hypointense, and T2-isointense to hyperintense. Marked contrast enhancement is common. ATRT may also be of choroid plexus origin.

Embryonal Tumors

The common embryonal tumors arising within the cerebral hemispheres include the *primitive neuroectodermal tumors* and, less often, the cerebral neuroblastoma or ATRT. Like other embryonal tumors (e.g., medulloblastoma), PNET is a malignant, hypercellular tumor with a tendency for seeding. Imaging commonly shows a large heterogenous mass with calcification or cyst, occasional hemorrhage, but variable edema. It is CT-isodense to hyperdense, T1-isointense to hypointense, and T2-isointense to hypointense with surrounding hyperintense edema (Fig. 8-79). Marked enhancement is common. Other tumors in the differential diagnosis with similar findings include ependymoma (see Fig. 8-75), choroid plexus carcinoma (see Fig. 8-78), and ATRT (Fig. 8-80).

Neuronal Tumors

Common neuronal, or mixed neuronal-glial, tumors of the cerebrum include ganglioglioma, dysembryoplastic neuroepithelial tumor, and neurocytoma.

Gangliogliomas are cortical tumors that are often cystic or calcified and are frequently associated with focal seizures. They are CT-isodense or hyperdense, T1-isointense to hypointense, and T2-isointense to hyperintense, and they commonly enhance (Fig. 8-81). The desmoplastic ganglioglioma characteristically occurs in infancy and is often cystic with nodular enhancement

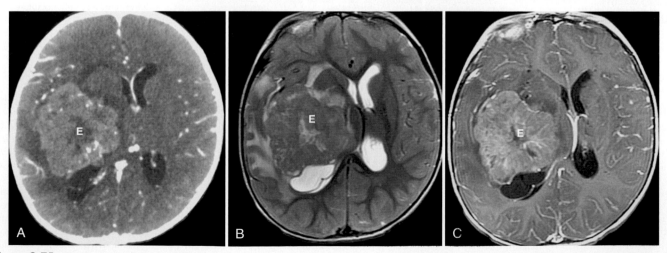

FIGURE 8-75. Cerebral ependymoma (E) on contrast axial CT scan (**A**) and on axial T2-weighted (**B**), and gadolinium-enhanced T1-weighted (**C**) MR images, which demonstrate calcifications, enhancement, and edema.

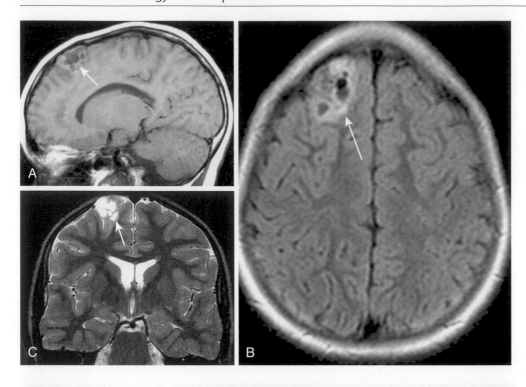

FIGURE 8-76. Frontal cortical ependymoma (*arrow*) on sagittal T1-weighted (**A**), axial FLAIR (**B**), and coronal T2-weighted (**C**) MR images; the features are similar to those of a dysembryoplastic neuroepithelial tumor.

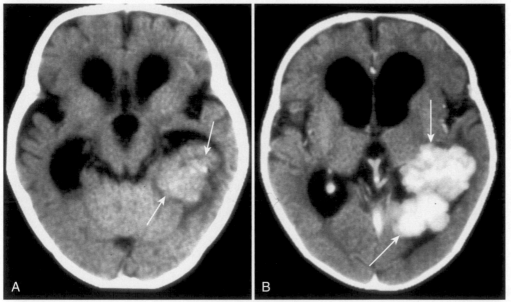

FIGURE 8-77. Choroid plexus papilloma (*arrows*) with hydrocephalus on pre-contrast (**A**) and post-contrast (**B**) CT scans, which demonstrate calcifications and enhancement.

(Fig. 8-82). It may be indistinguishable from the desmoplastic astrocytoma of infancy.

Dysembryoplastic neuroepithelial tumors are typically associated with partial seizures that may be intractable. They are well-defined cortical lesions with little or no edema. Mass effect and cortical effacement are often subtle. Nodularity, or a bubbly appearance, is characteristic, whereas focal contrast enhancement, calcification, or cystic change is less frequent (Fig. 8-83). A hyperintense rim on FLAIR MR imaging may be seen, along with thinning of the adjacent cranium.

The *central neurocytoma* typically occurs about the lateral ventricles, often in the region of the foramen of Monro. Calcification is common. The differential diagnosis may include other circumscribed periventricular tumors, such as giant cell tumor or subependymal giant cell astrocytoma (e.g., tuberous sclerosis), astrocytoma, ependymoma, and choroid plexus papilloma.

Meningeal Tumors

Meningioma occurs uncommonly in childhood. It may be sporadic, associated with NF-2, or radiation-induced. Such tumors tend to be durally based or to arise from the choroid plexus. Imaging often demonstrates a circumscribed extracerebral or intraventricular mass with calcification, marked vascularity, and lytic or blastic (hyperostosis) bony involvement. The tumor tends to be CT-isodense or hyperdense, T1-isointense to hypointense, and T2-isointense to hyperintense or hypointense, and it enhances markedly with a dural tail (Fig. 8-84). Other *nonmeningothelial mesenchymal tumors* arising from the meninges include lesions such as meningeal sarcoma and ATRT. These show a variety of findings, including density, intensity, and enhancement heterogeneity with vascular, calcific, and cystic or necrotic components. *Primary melanocytic lesions* of the meninges include melanosis (e.g., neurocutaneous melanosis),

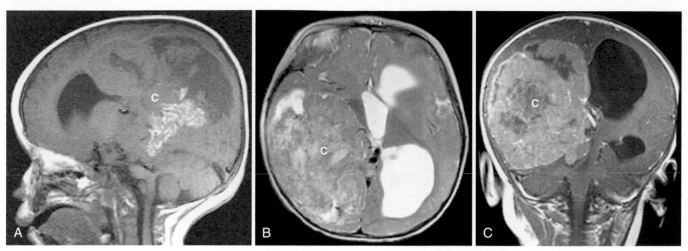

Figure 8-78. Choroid plexus carcinoma (C) on sagittal T1-weighted (**A**), axial T2-weighted (**B**), and coronal gadolinium-enhanced T1-weighted (**C**) MR images, which demonstrate calcifications, hemorrhage, and enhancement.

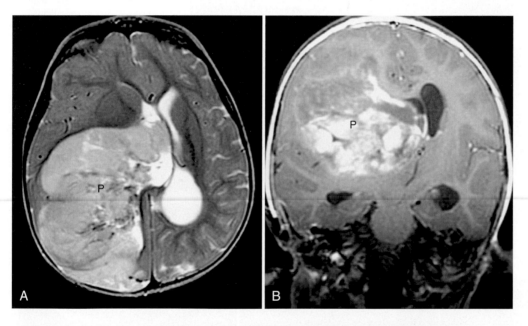

Figure 8-79. Cerebral primitive neuroepithelial tumor (P) on axial T2-weighted (**A**) and coronal gadolinium-enhanced T1-weighted (**B**) MR images.

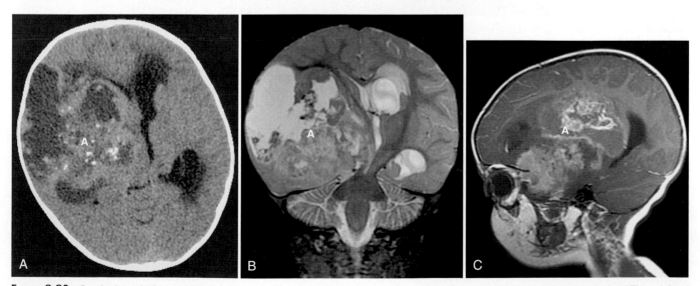

Figure 8-80. Cerebral atypical teratoid rhabdoid tumor (A) on axial CT (**A**), coronal T2-weighted (**B**), and sagittal gadolinium-enhanced T1-weighted (**C**) MR images.

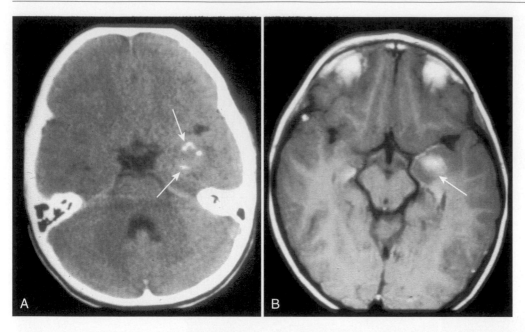

FIGURE 8-81. Temporal ganglioglioma (*arrows*) on axial CT scan (**A**) and axial gadolinium-enhanced T1-weighted MR image (**B**) showing calcification and enhancement.

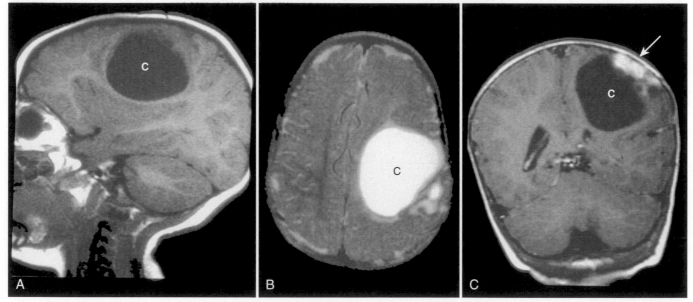

FIGURE 8-82. Desmoplastic ganglioglioma (C) on sagittal T1-weighted (**A**), axial T2-weighted (**B**) MR images. **C,** Coronal gadolinium-enhanced T1-weighted MR image demonstrates nodular enhancement (*arrow*).

melanocytoma, melanoma, and melanomatosis. Melanin-containing tumors are characteristically CT-hyperdense, T1-hyperintense, and T2-hypointense, often with hemorrhage and enhancement.

Other Tumors

Involvement of the CNS secondarily by *lymphoid and other hematologic malignancies* is uncommon in childhood. These may occur in the setting of leukemia (e.g., chloroma), lymphoma, or an underlying congenital or acquired immunodeficiency disorder (e.g., HIV-AIDS, post-transplant lymphoproliferative disorder). The lesions are often CT-isodense to hyperdense, T1-isointense to hypointense, and T2-hypointense with variable enhancement (Fig. 8-85).

Parameningeal and Metastatic Tumors

Parameningeal tumors arise outside (i.e., extradural) but are contiguous with the CNS (see Chapter 10). They may involve the intracranial or intraspinal structures without specific neurologic symptoms or signs. Parameningeal tumors of the head and neck may arise from or involve the scalp, cranial vault, cranial base, sinuses or pharynx, orbits, petrous temporal structures, or soft tissues of the face or neck. Although invasive parameningeal processes are often malignant neoplasms, benign neoplasms (e.g., epidermoid; Fig. 8-86) or nonneoplastic processes (e.g., inflammatory) may occasionally be aggressive. Dysplastic conditions may also be associated with bony defects or soft tissue masses and may mimic neoplasm (e.g., fibrous dysplasia, NF-1). The common invasive parameningeal tumors of childhood are neuroblastoma, rhabdomyosarcoma, histiocytosis (Fig. 8-87), plexiform neurofibroma, and angiofibroma.

The presence and nature of the intracranial involvement are critical to patient management. With advances in craniofacial and skull base surgery, ablation may be possible without sacrifice of function or cosmesis. In cases with intracranial involvement, surgery may serve primarily to establish the diagnosis and the extent of disease. Tumor debulking reduces the local tumor burden for chemotherapy

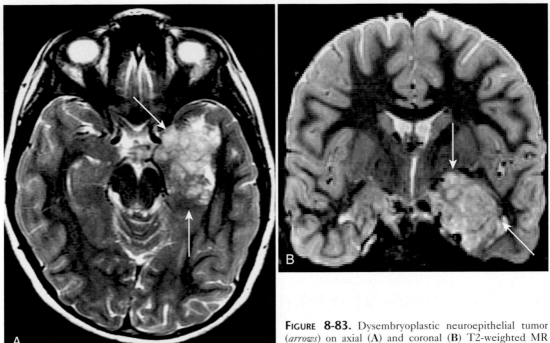

FIGURE 8-83. Dysembryoplastic neuroepithelial tumor (*arrows*) on axial (**A**) and coronal (**B**) T2-weighted MR images.

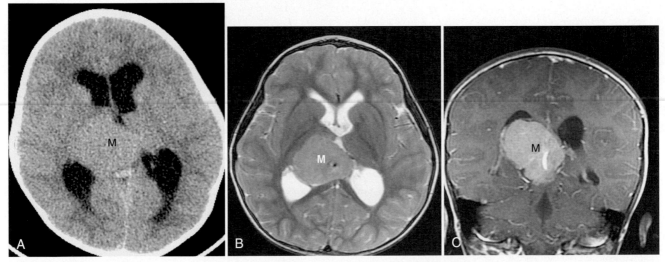

FIGURE 8-84. Meningioma (M) on axial CT scan (**A**) and on axial T2-weighted MR image (**B**). **C,** Enhancement can be seen on a coronal gadolinium-enhanced T1-weighted MR image.

and radiotherapy. Imaging often requires CT for bony involvement and calcification, and MRI for neuroanatomy and vascularity.

In addition to involvement by direct extension, the CNS may be involved by distant metastases (e.g., sarcomas; Fig. 8-88). Some primary CNS neoplasms, especially embryonal tumors, malignant gliomas, and germ cell tumors, show a propensity to disseminate in the subarachnoid space. Most metastatic neoplasms arising from non-CNS primary tumors are of hematogenous origin, although subarachnoid spread may occur, with tumors reaching the CNS originally by direct extension. CT or MRI may demonstrate single or multiple masses, which often enhance with contrast agent.

Tumor Response and Treatment Effects

Common long-term treatment effects after radiotherapy and chemotherapy include mineralization, ischemic vasculopathy (e.g., moyamoya disease), hemorrhagic vasculopathy (e.g., telangiectasia,

cavernous malformation), leukoencephalopathy, and second tumors (e.g., meningioma, sarcoma, glioma). These effects may be minimized with the use of more conformal therapies (e.g., stereotactic radiotherapy, stereotactic radiosurgery, proton beam, gamma knife). A transient increase in tumor volume, including mass effect, edema, and enhancement, may occur after radiotherapy, particularly conformal therapy. Functional imaging, including MRS, PMRI, SPECT, or PET, may be needed to distinguish treatment effects (e.g., radionecrosis) from tumor progression (Fig. 8-89).

■ NEUROCUTANEOUS SYNDROMES

The neurocutaneous syndromes, or phakomatoses, are a group of disorders primarily affecting tissues of ectodermal origin (Box 8-4). This group may also include a number of angiodysplastic syndromes of childhood (see Chapter 10). Neurologic symptoms are a prominent feature of these diseases. The common

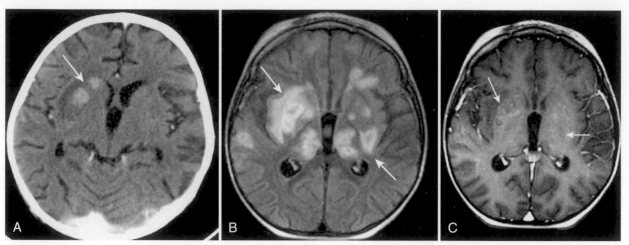

FIGURE 8-85. Post-transplant lymphoproliferative disorder with lymphoma (*arrows*) on axial CT scan (A) and on axial T2-weighted (B) and axial gadolinium-enhanced T1-weighted (C) MR images.

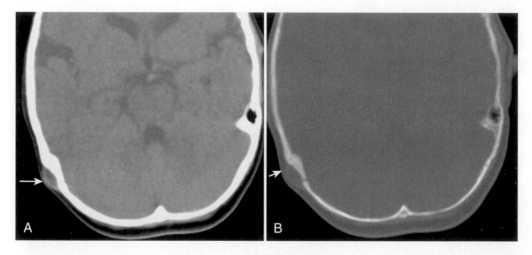

FIGURE 8-86. Cranial epidermoid (*arrows*) with bony deformity on axial CT scans using soft tissue (A) and bone (B) algorithms.

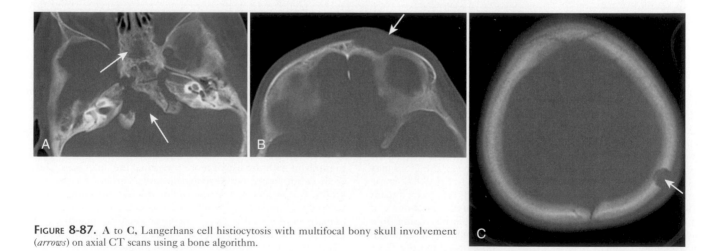

FIGURE 8-87. A to C, Langerhans cell histiocytosis with multifocal bony skull involvement (*arrows*) on axial CT scans using a bone algorithm.

neurocutaneous syndromes of childhood include neurofibromatosis 1 (NF-1), tuberous sclerosis, and Sturge-Weber syndrome. Less common are NF-2 and von Hippel–Lindau syndrome. Some of the rarer syndromes listed here are presented in greater detail in other texts.

Neurofibromatosis

Neurofibromatosis is the most common neurocutaneous disorder of childhood. To date, it has been divided into eight subgroups. NF-1 and NF-2 are the most common subtypes (NF-3 has features of both NF-1 and NF-2). NF-1 (von Recklinghausen disease) is the most common of the phakomatoses. It is inherited as an autosomal dominant disorder (chromosome 17) with variable penetrance and usually manifests in the first decade. Both dysplastic and neoplastic intracranial lesions are found in NF-1. Neurologic symptoms are often nonspecific and include developmental delay, seizures, visual disturbances, and stroke. Neuroimaging has an important role in the evaluation of optic pathway lesions and in the delineation of other neoplastic/dysplastic glial lesions and craniospinal mesodermal dysplasia that typify the disease.

The most common CNS lesions of NF-1 are the "histogenetic foci" or "NF-1 spots" (Fig. 8-90). Within the globus pallidus they are characteristically T1-hyperintense (i.e., heterotopic Schwann cells or melanin?) and do not enhance. They also appear as foci of T2/FLAIR hyperintensity (undermyelination?) in the cerebellum, brainstem, internal capsule, splenium, and thalamus. The latter are usually present before 1 year of age, increase in number and size up to puberty, and then regress (myelination?). These foci show

histologic features of hamartomas, atypical glial cells, and vacuolar myelinopathy. Increased size, mass effect, and enhancement may indicate "neoplastic transformation" (e.g., astrocytoma).

The most frequently encountered intracranial neoplasms in NF-1 are optic pathway gliomas (OPGs). These are usually low-grade and frequently pilocytic astrocytomas. The tumors may involve any part of the optic pathways. Tumors confined to the optic nerve are slow-growing and have a favorable prognosis. Lesions involving the chiasm or hypothalamus tend to be more aggressive. OPGs are usually CT-isodense to hypodense,

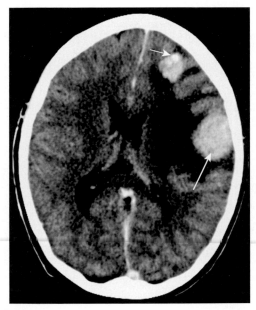

FIGURE 8-88. Metastatic cerebral osteosarcoma (*long arrow*) on axial contrast-enhanced CT scan, which demonstrates foci of bone (*short arrow*) and enhancement plus edema.

Box 8-4. Neurocutaneous Disorders and Angiodysplastic Syndromes

Neurofibromatosis 1, 2, 3 (and others)
Tuberous sclerosis
Sturge-Weber syndrome
Klippel-Trénaunay-Weber syndrome
PHACES (posterior fossa abnormalities and other structural brain abnormalities, hemangioma(s) of the cervical facial region, arterial cerebrovascular anomalies, cardiac defects, aortic coarctation and other aortic abnormalities, eye anomalies, and sternal defects and/or supraumbilical raphe)/hemangiomatosis
Wyburn-Mason syndrome
Proteus syndrome
Cowden syndrome
von Hippel–Lindau disease
Ataxia-telangiectasia
Hereditary hemorrhagic telangiectasia (Osler-Rendu-Weber syndrome)
Nevoid basal cell carcinoma syndrome (Gorlin syndrome)
Neurocutaneous melanosis
Epidermoid nevus
Linear sebaceous nevus
Hypomelanosis of Ito
Incontinentia pigmenti
Bannayan-Riley-Ruvalcaba syndrome
Encephalocraniocutaneous lipomatosis
Meningoendotheliohemangiomatosis
Facial nevi with anomalous venous return and hydrocephalus
Chédiak-Higashi syndrome
Parry-Romberg syndrome (progressive facial hemiatrophy)

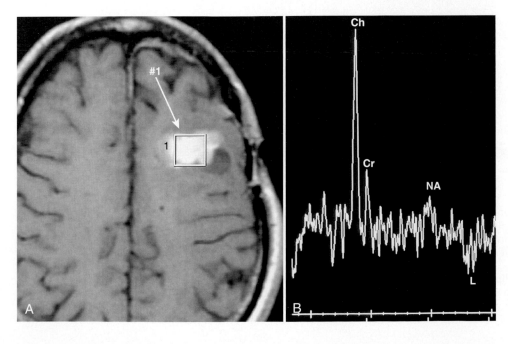

FIGURE 8-89. A, Recurrent anaplastic astrocytoma (*arrow* and *box*) on axial gadolinium-enhanced T1-weighted MR image. **B,** Spectroscopy of the tumor shows very high choline (Ch), low creatine (Cr), and low N-acetyl-aspartate (NA) concentrations as well as an inverted lactate doublet (L).

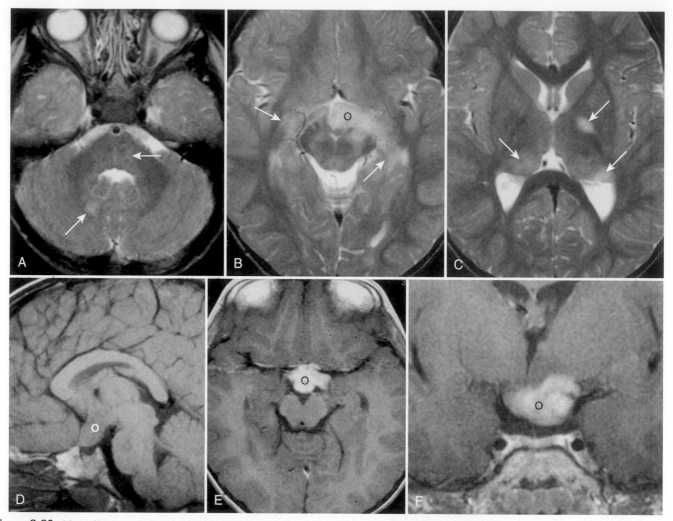

FIGURE 8-90. Neurofibromatosis 1 with "dysplastic foci" (*arrow*) and optic glioma (O) on axial T2-weighted (**A** to **C**) and sagittal T1-weighted (**D**) MR images. Axial (**E**) and coronal (**F**) gadolinium-enhanced T1-weighted MR images show tumor enhancement.

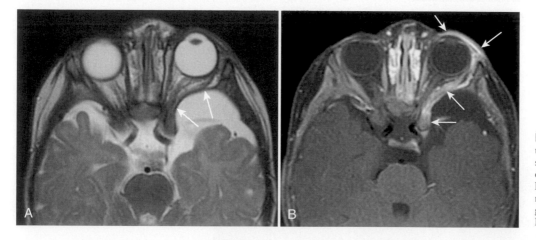

FIGURE 8-91. A, Neurofibromatosis 1 and sphenorbital dysplasia with bony deformity (*arrows*) on axial T2-weighted MR image. **B,** Enhancing orbital plexiform neurofibroma (*arrows*) on axial gadolinium-enhanced T1-weighted MR image.

T1-isointense to hypointense, and T2-isointense to hyperintense (see Fig. 8-90). Enhancement is variable but frequently intense. Cavitation or cyst formation occasionally occurs, but calcification is rare. Astrocytomas may also arise in the tectum, pons, or cerebellum. Hydrocephalus may result from tumoral or nontumoral aqueductal stenosis in NF-1.

Plexiform neurofibromas, the hallmark of NF-1, are tortuous cords of tumor composed of disorganized neurons, Schwann cells, and collagen. They commonly arise in the head and neck region, especially the scalp and orbit (Fig. 8-91). Orbital involvement is often associated with buphthalmos or glaucoma. Paraspinal involvement is also common in NF-1. The lesions are irregular, nonhomogeneous masses that are CT-hypodense, T1-hypointense, and T2-hyperintense, with variable enhancement. The "target sign" is characteristic.

Another characteristic feature of NF-1 is mesodermal dysplasia, including dural ectasia, bony defects, and vascular lesions. Optic nerve sheath ectasia may simulate OPG but is distinguished by its perioptic subarachnoid CSF intensities. Dural ectasia may produce widening of the internal auditory canal and simulate tumor; the CSF intensity character and the absence of abnormal enhancement differentiate it from tumor (e.g., acoustic neuroma). One of the most common bony defects in NF-1 is sphenoid dysplasia affecting the greater wing. The result may be an alar cephalocele producing pulsatile exophthalmos. This is often associated with intraorbital and periorbital neurofibromas (see Fig. 8-91.) A paralamboid skull defect, also characteristic of NF-1, is commonly associated with an overlying neurofibroma.

Mesodermal dysplasia also affects the spine in NF-1 (see Chapter 9). A short-segment kyphoscoliosis with vertebral deformities and scalloping is characteristic. Dural ectasia and meningoceles result in spinal canal and foraminal widening. A paraspinal meningocele is distinguished from a plexiform neurofibroma by its CSF intensities and lack of abnormal enhancement. Neurovascular complications of NF-1 include steno-occlusive disease and aneurysm formation. Cerebral infarction from arterial stenosis may occur in patients with NF-1 after radiotherapy for OPG, or as part of a systemic vascular dysplasia. When severe, the steno-occlusive disease may result in a moyamoya syndrome. Aneurysm formation is less common and occurs later in life.

NF-2 rarely occurs prior to puberty and is inherited as an autosomal dominant trait (chromosome 22). The genetic defect in NF-2 has been localized to chromosome 22. Tumors of the coverings of the brain are characteristic of NF-2 and include acoustic schwannomas and meningiomas. Schwannomas are tumors composed of abnormal Schwann cells surrounding neurons. The most commonly involved cranial nerves (CNs) are CN VIII, CN V, CN IX, and CN X. Bilateral vestibular schwannomas (aka acoustic neuromas) are diagnostic of the disorder. The tumors are typically CT-hypodense, T1-hypointense, markedly T2-hyperintense, markedly enhance, and rarely calcify (Fig. 8-92). Cystic degeneration and hemorrhage occasionally occur. Expansion of the internal auditory canal (IAC) is common with larger CN VIII lesions. Meningiomas manifest at an earlier age in patients with NF-2 than in the general population. The tumors are usually dura-based (e.g., parasagittal, convexity, or perisellar) or intraventricular. Imaging often demonstrates a circumscribed extracerebral or intraventricular mass with calcification, marked vascularity, and lytic or blastic (hyperostosis) bony involvement. The tumor tends to be CT-isodense or hyperdense, T1-isointense to hypointense, T2-isointense to hyperintense or hypointense, and to markedly enhance with a dural tail (see "Cerebral Tumors").

Tuberous Sclerosis

Tuberous sclerosis (Bourneville disease) is a multisystem, autosomal dominant disorder characterized by the clinical triad of mental retardation, seizures, and adenoma sebaceum (angiofibromas).

The brain lesions, which are neuroglial hamartomas composed of giant balloon "stem" cells (i.e., tubers), likely result from defective development of the radial glial-neuronal unit. They may arise at any point from subependymal to cortical. Subependymal, subcortical white matter, and cortical tubers are common. Calcification of the subependymal tubers is characteristic although unusual in the first year of life. In the immature brain, these lesions are typically CT-hypodense, T1-hyperintense, and T2-hypointense relative to the unmyelinated white matter (Fig. 8-93). With maturation, the lesions become isodense and isointense in relation to the myelinated white matter and appear as periventricular nodules with little or no enhancement (Fig. 8-94). Subependymal tubers near the foramen of Monro have a tendency to enlarge and develop a preponderance of giant cells (i.e., giant cell tumors or astrocytomas). Hydrocephalus may be the result. These tumors usually enhance on CT or MRI but are rarely invasive (see Fig. 8-94).

Occasionally, cysts or hemorrhage (e.g., aneurysm) may occur in tuberous sclerosis. White matter lesions consist of either hamartomatous clusters or linear bands of unmyelinated axonal fibers radiating outward from the ventricles. Calcification may occur but enhancement is not expected. Cortical tubers are a hallmark of tuberous sclerosis. They consist of giant cells, disordered myelin, and gliosis, and are associated with broad and flat gyri. Their imaging features also vary with age and generally appear T2/FLAIR-hyperintense in the mature brain (see Fig. 8-94). Enhancement of such lesions is unusual and may indicate tumor.

Sturge-Weber Syndrome

Sturge-Weber syndrome, or encephalotrigeminal angiomatosis, is a neurocutaneous disorder characterized by low-flow vascular malformations of the face, globe, and leptomeninges. A "port-wine" facial capillary nevus is almost always present, is usually unilateral, and most often follows the ophthalmic division (V1) of the trigeminal nerve. The pial capillary-venous malformation of this syndrome is likely the result of persistence of primordial sinusoids and dysgenesis or thrombosis of the cortical venous system. It typically involves the parieto-occipital or temporal region. Similar involvement of the choroid may result in buphthalmos. Seizures are common and often manifest as infantile spasms. Mental retardation, hemiparesis, and hemianopia are also frequent. Features of the Sturge-Weber syndrome may also be associated with the Klippel-Trenaunay-Weber syndrome (visceral, truncal, and extremity low-flow vascular malformations).

Enhanced MRI best demonstrates the extent of the pial malformation, which decreases with age (Fig. 8-95). Enlarged

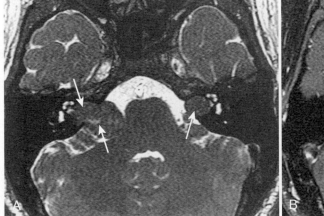
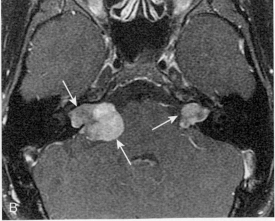

FIGURE 8-92. Neurofibromatosis 2 with bilateral acoustic neuromas (*arrows*) on axial T2-weighted (**A**) and axial gadolinium-enhanced T1-weighted (**B**) MR images.

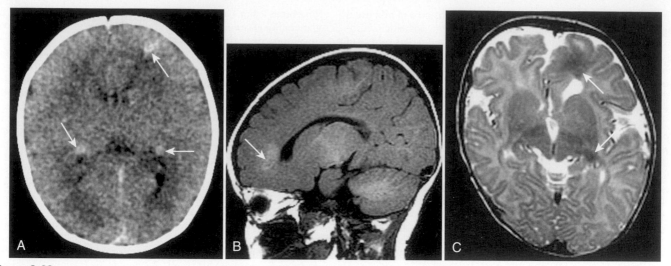

FIGURE 8-93. Infantile tuberous sclerosis with periventricular and subcortical tubers (*arrows*) on CT scan (**A**) and on sagittal T1-weighted (**B**) and axial T2-weighted (**C**) MR images.

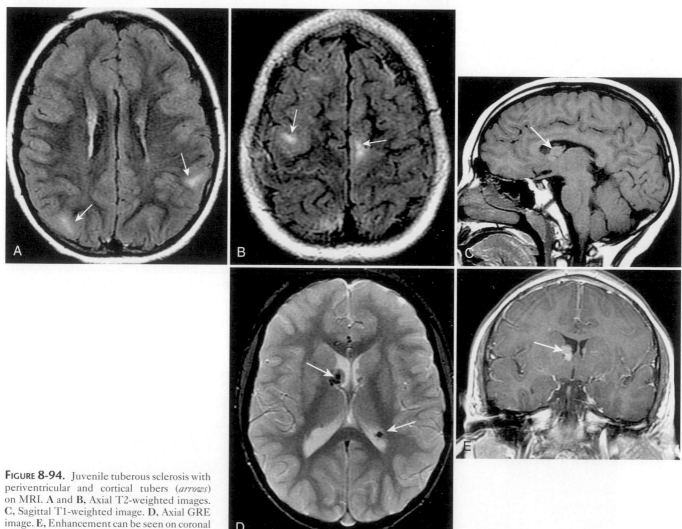

FIGURE 8-94. Juvenile tuberous sclerosis with periventricular and cortical tubers (*arrows*) on MRI. **A** and **B**, Axial T2-weighted images. **C**, Sagittal T1-weighted image. **D**, Axial GRE image. **E**, Enhancement can be seen on coronal gadolinium-enhanced T1-weighted image.

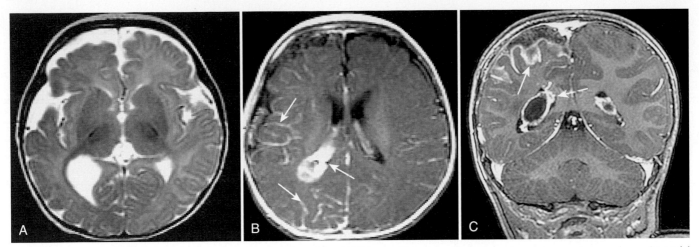

FIGURE 8-95. Sturge-Weber syndrome with atrophy on axial T2-weighted MR image. Vascular malformative enhancement can be seen (*arrows*) on axial (**B**) and coronal (**C**) gadolinium-enhanced T1-weighted MR images.

medullary and subependymal veins result from the diversion of superficial drainage. The choroid plexus is usually hypertrophied on the same side. Subjacent cortical calcification is likely related to venous ischemia, increases with age, and may not be present in infancy. It is best detected by CT. Corresponding cerebral underdevelopment, dysgenesis, hypermyelination, or atrophy is usually evident. The atrophy worsens with age. Angiography best demonstrates the malformation and associated venous abnormalities for the planning of surgery for intractable seizures. Sturge-Weber syndrome is to be distinguished from meningiangiomatosis and Wyburn-Mason syndrome.

von Hippel–Lindau Disease

Von Hippel–Lindau disease is an autosomal dominant disorder (chromosome 3) with incomplete penetrance and multisystem involvement. It is characterized by hemangioblastomas of the retina and CNS, along with renal cell carcinoma, pheochromocytoma, and cysts of the abdominal viscera. The onset of symptoms is unusual in childhood and often related to ocular complications (e.g., hemorrhage, retinal detachment, glaucoma, or cataract). CNS hemangioblastomas are highly vascular lesions that most commonly arise within the cerebellum and spinal cord. Involvement of the brainstem and cerebrum may rarely occur. CT or MRI typically shows an intensely enhancing nodule that is often associated with a cyst and prominent vessels. Occasionally there may be hemorrhage. The spinal cord lesions may be associated with hydrosyringomyelia.

Other Neurocutaneous Diseases

Ataxia-telangiectasia (Louis-Bar syndrome) is an autosomal recessive disorder characterized by capillary telangiectasias of the face and conjunctiva, progressive cerebellar atrophy, immunodeficiencies, and an increased incidence of lymphoma, leukemia, and other malignancies. The ataxia is often evident before the appearance of the telangiectasias. CT or MRI shows progressive cerebellar degeneration with atrophy involving the cerebellar hemispheres and vermis. Embolic infarction may result from associated pulmonary vascular malformations. Cerebral telangiectasias may hemorrhage.

Basal cell nevus syndrome (Gorlin syndrome) is an autosomal dominant syndrome composed of multiple basal cell carcinomas, keratocysts of the maxilla and mandible, mental retardation, seizures, hydrocephalus, dural calcification (e.g., falx), and callosal hypogenesis. There is an increased prevalence of neoplasia,

including medulloblastoma, meningioma, craniopharyngioma, ameloblastoma, and astrocytoma.

Neurocutaneous melanosis is a disorder in which large pigmented cutaneous nevi are seen in association with abnormal meningeal, perivascular, and brain melanin deposition. The anterior temporal lobe (e.g., amygdala) and the cerebellum are most often involved. The lesions tend to be CT-isodense to hyperdense, T1-hyperintense, and T2-hypointense. Enlarging and enhancing brain or leptomeningeal lesions suggest malignancy (e.g., melanoma). There may be associated hydrocephalus. Other reported findings include arachnoid cysts, Dandy-Walker spectrum, and hydrosyringomyelia.

Hypomelanosis of Ito is characterized by cutaneous hypopigmentation in association with scoliosis, skull defects, syndactyly, cleft palate, and ocular abnormalities. Seizures and mental retardation are common. Atrophy, porencephaly, white matter changes, and heterotopias have been reported.

■ METABOLIC, NEURODEGENERATIVE, AND TOXIC DISORDERS

Classification and Differential Diagnoses

The clinical hallmark of metabolic and neurodegenerative disorders is "progressive" neurologic impairment in the absence of a CNS tumor or another readily identifiable process (e.g., infection). These are rare disorders but some are specifically treatable. Many are heredofamilial, so genetic counseling and prenatal screening are important. These disorders are to be distinguished from the "nonprogressive" static encephalopathies (e.g., cerebral palsy) that may be related to maldevelopment, hypoxia-ischemia, infection, or other conditions.

Diagnosis is primarily clinical and involves metabolite testing, genetic testing, or biopsy of CNS or extra-CNS tissues. MRI is superior to CT in evaluating disease extent and anatomic distribution. In the evaluation of developmental delay (e.g., static encephalopathy versus neurodegenerative disease), MRI is the only modality that can provide an accurate assessment of brain maturation based on myelination and cortical development (including the use of MRS and DTI). Occasionally MRI may demonstrate characteristic imaging findings. Proton MRS has the potential to contribute specific metabolic characterization of these disorders. Stereotactic CT or MRI may serve as a guide for biopsy.

Metabolic, degenerative, and toxic disorders may be classified in a number of ways, including metabolic defect and anatomic predilection (Table 8-5). Clinical features are also important. For example, macrocephaly is often characteristic of maple

TABLE 8-5. Classification of Metabolic, Degenerative, and Toxic Disorders of the Central Nervous System

Metabolic and Degenerative Disorders	
Lysosomal Disorders	
Lipidoses	Fabry, Gaucher, and Niemann-Pick diseases GM$_1$ gangliosidosis GM$_2$ gangliosidosis (Tay-Sachs and Sandhoff diseases) Neuronal ceroid lipofuscinosis
Mucopolysaccharidoses (MPS)	Hurler, Scheie, Hurler-Scheie syndrome Hunter syndrome Sanfilippo types A-D Morquio syndromes A and B Maroteaux-Lamy syndrome Sly syndrome
Mucolipidoses	Mannosidosis Fucosidosis Sialidosis
Lysosomal leukodystrophies	Metachromatic leukodystrophy Globoid cell leukodystrophy (Krabbe disease)
Peroxisomal Disorders	Adrenoleukodystrophy complex Neonatal leukodystrophy Zellweger syndrome Infantile Refsum syndrome Rhizomelic chondrodysplasia punctata Hyperpipecolic acidemia Cerebrotendinous xanthomatosis
Other Leukodystrophies	Pelizaeus-Merzbacher disease Canavan disease Alexander disease Cockayne syndrome Leukodystrophy with calcifications
Mitochondrial (Respiratory Oxidative) Disorders	Leigh disease Kearns-Sayre syndrome MELAS (mitochondrial encephalomyopathy with lactic acidosis, and stroke-like episodes) syndrome MERRF (myoclonus epilepsy associated with ragged-red fibers) syndrome Alpers syndrome (poliodystrophy) Menkes disease (trichopoliodystrophy) Marinesco-Sjögren syndrome Infantile bilateral striatal necrosis Leber hereditary optic atrophy l-Carnitine deficiency
Amino Acid Disorders	Phenylketonuria Homocystinuria Nonketotic hyperglycinemia Maple syrup urine disease Glutaric aciduria, type I Glutaric aciduria, type II Methylmalonic and propionic acidurias Urea cycle defects (e.g., ornithine transcarbamylase deficiency) Oculocerebrorenal syndrome Pyridoxine dependency
Carbohydrate and Other Storage Disorders	Galactosemia Glycogen storage diseases (i.e., Pompe disease) Niemann-Pick disease Gaucher disease Farber disease Infantile sialidosis
Liver Metabolic Disorders	Wilson disease (hepatolenticular degeneration) Hallervorden-Spatz disease Hyperbilirubinemia (see "Toxic Encephalopathies") Hepatocerebral syndromes (see "Toxic Encephalopathies")
Diseases of the Cerebellum, Brainstem, and Spinal Cord	Friedreich ataxia Olivopontocerebellar atrophies Ataxia-telangiectasia Carbohydrate-deficient glycoprotein syndrome Infantile neuraxonal dystrophy
Other Metabolic and Neurodegenerative Diseases	Juvenile multiple sclerosis Molybdenum cofactor deficiency 3-Hydroxy-3-methylglutaryl–coenzyme A lyase deficiency Idiopathic leukoencephalopathy

(Continued)

TABLE 8-5. Classification of Metabolic, Degenerative, and Toxic Disorders of the Central Nervous System—cont'd

Diseases of the Basal Ganglia	Sulfur oxidase deficiency
	Parathyroid disease
	Tuberous sclerosis
	Down syndrome
	Progressive encephalopathy with basal ganglia calcifications and cerebrospinal fluid lymphocytosis
	Inflammatory, toxic, and anoxic conditions
	Radiation therapy
	Renal tubular acidosis and osteoporosis
	Huntington disease
	Fahr disease
	Hallervorden-Spatz disease
	Cockayne syndrome
	Wilson disease
Toxic Encephalopathies	
Exogenous Internal Toxicities	Hyperbilirubinemia
	Hepatocerebral syndromes
	Hypoglycemia
	Hypothermia and hyperthermia
	Paraneoplastic toxins
	Hemolytic uremic syndrome
	Uremia
	Ion imbalance disorders
	Endocrinopathies
	Porphyria
Exogenous External Toxicities	Vitamin deficiencies/depletions:
	Vitamin B_1
	Folate
	Vitamin B_{12}
	Biotin
	Vitamin K
	Vitamin C
	Vitamin D
	Toxins:
	Mercury
	Methanol
	Toluene
	Carbon monoxide
	Cyanides and sulfides
	Lead
	Alcohol
	Cocaine and heroin
	Anticonvulsants
	Drug-induced:
	Methotrexate
	Cyclosporine
	Tacrolimus
	Carmustine, cytosine arabinoside

syrup urine disease, Canavan disease, Alexander disease, and the lysosomal disorders (e.g., Tay-Sachs disease, the mucopolysaccharidoses, and metachromatic leukodystrophy). Although there is considerable overlap among the disorders, most imaging classifications use predominant anatomic involvement as follows: white matter (subcortical, periventricular), gray matter (cortical, deep), basal ganglia, brainstem, cerebellum, spinal cord, and peripheral nervous system. Specific conditions are presented in greater detail in other texts.

Disorders Primarily Affecting the Cortical Gray Matter

Disorders primarily affecting cortical gray matter include the storage diseases that result from lysosomal enzyme defects (see Table 8-5), such as the lipidoses (e.g., GM1 gangliosidosis, neuronal ceroid lipofuscinosis), the mucopolysaccharidoses, and the mucolipidosis (e.g., mannosidosis). CT and MRI show cortical atrophy (gyral thinning and sulcal/fissural widening), abnormal cortical densities and intensities, and ventriculomegaly (Fig. 8-96). Associated white matter changes reflect secondary axonal degeneration. These disorders are to be differentiated from the more common causes of cortical underdevelopment or atrophy, including the chronic static encephalopathies (e.g., maldevelopment, hypoxia-ischemia, infection, idiopathic), and atrophy related to chronic systemic disease, malnutrition, or certain types of therapy (e.g., steroids, chemotherapy, radiation, anticonvulsants, transplantation).

Disorder Primarily Affecting Deep Gray Matter

Disorders primarily affecting deep gray matter often show abnormally high or low densities and intensities of the basal ganglia or thalami, including mineralization (calcium, iron, etc.) (see Table 8-5). Third or lateral ventriculomegaly (e.g., frontal horns) may be an important finding. Disorders primarily involving the caudate and putamen include mitochondrial (e.g., Leigh syndrome; Fig. 8-97, MELAS syndrome), organic and amino acidopathies (e.g., glutaric aciduria; Fig. 8-98), juvenile Huntington disease, Wilson disease, Fahr disease (Fig. 8-99), and Cockayne syndrome (Fig. 8-100). More common causes, however, include profound hypoxia-ischemia (see Fig. 8-47), toxic exposure (e.g., methane, cyanide), osmolar myelinolysis, striatal necrosis, hypoglycemia, and meningoencephalitis. Disorders primarily involving the

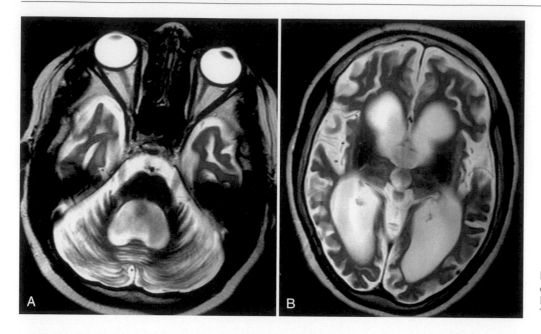

FIGURE 8-96. **A** and **B,** Neuronal ceroid lipofuscinosis with cerebellar and cerebral atrophy on axial T2-weighted MR images.

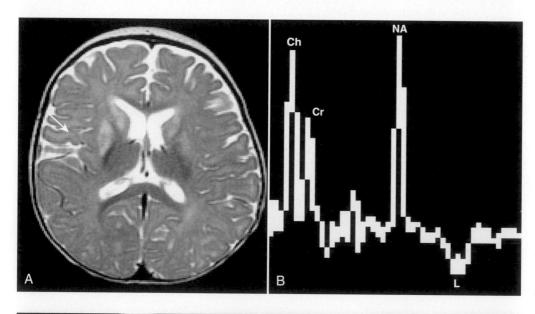

FIGURE 8-97. **A,** Leigh syndrome with bilateral caudate and putaminal high intensities on axial T2-weighted MR image. **B,** A lactate doublet (L) on MR spectroscopy.

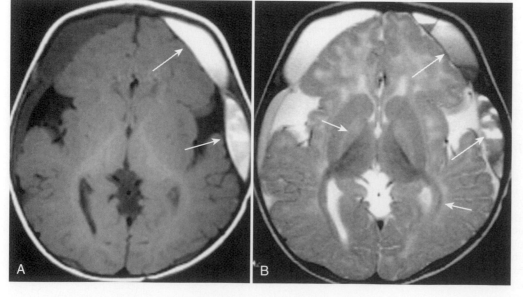

FIGURE 8-98. Glutaric acidopathy (GA1), a mimic of nonaccidental injury, with large sylvian fissures, and subdural hemorrhage (*long arrows*) as well as basal ganglia and white matter abnormalities (*short arrows* on **B**) on axial T1-weighted (**A**) and T2-weighted (**B**) MR images.

globus pallidus include pantothenate kinase–associated neurodegeneration (formerly Hallervorden-Spatz disease; Fig. 8-101) and the aminoacidopathies (e.g., methylmalonic acidopathy). More common causes include hyperbilirubinemia (bilirubin encephalopathy, kernicterus; Fig. 8-102), and toxic exposure (e.g., carbon dioxide). Isolated involvement of the thalami is unusual in metabolic disorders. However, thalamic involvement may be a feature of sulfur oxidase deficiency (Fig. 8-103), Krabbe disease, GM2 gangliosidosis, or the infantile form of Leigh disease (along with extensive brainstem, basal ganglia, and cerebral white matter involvement). Ventrolateral bithalamic lesions are often characteristic of profound perinatal hypoxia-ischemia (see Fig. 8-47).

Disorder Primarily Affecting White Matter

Disorders primarily affecting white matter, of various etiologies, are often referred to as *leukoencephalopathies*. There may be superficial involvement of the cortical/subcortical white matter (e.g., arcuate U fibers), deep involvement of the central white matter (periventricular/capsular/basal ganglia), or both (see Table 8-5). CT and MRI show abnormally low or high densities and intensities. Secondary gray matter involvement with atrophy occurs late. Traditionally, leukoencephalopathies have been divided into dysmyelinating and myelinoclastic disorders. In dysmyelinating disorders (also called leukodystrophies), there is an intrinsic (e.g., inherited, enzyme deficiency) abnormality of myelin formation, breakdown, or turnover. The cerebral involvement is often symmetric and diffuse, and spares the arcuate U fibers. Additional, symmetric cerebellar white matter involvement is common. In this category are the lysosomal disorders (e.g., metachromatic leukodystrophy, Krabbe disease), peroxisomal disorders (e.g.,

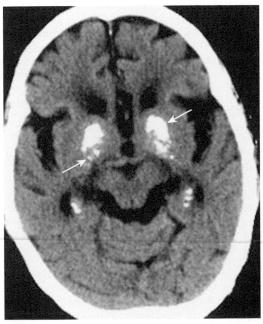

FIGURE 8-99. Fahr disease with basal ganglia calcifications (*arrows*) on CT scan.

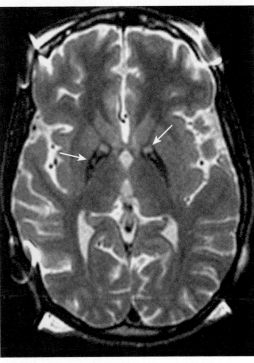

FIGURE 8-101. Pantothenate kinase-associated neurodegeneration with characteristic bilateral high- and low-intensity globus pallidus lesions (*arrows*) on axial GRE MR image.

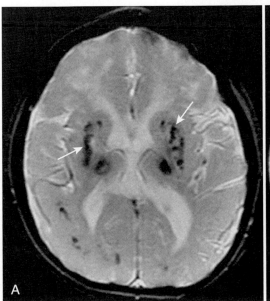
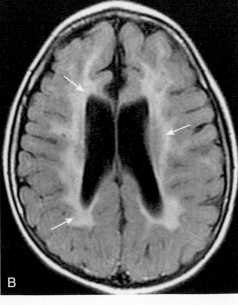

FIGURE 8-100. Cockayne syndrome with basal ganglia mineralization (*arrows*) on axial GRE MR image (**A**) and white matter disease (*arrows*) on axial FLAIR MR image (**B**).

adrenoleukodystrophies [ALDs]), and other diseases of white matter (e.g., Pelizaeus-Merzbacher disease, Canavan disease, Alexander disease, and Cockayne syndrome; see Fig. 8-100).

Certain patterns may be characteristic. Alexander disease is characterized by predominant frontal involvement, and ALD by an occipital distribution. Early subcortical white matter involvement may suggest Alexander disease (frontal U fiber involvement, macrocephaly), Canavan disease (macrocephaly and capsular involvement), galactosemia, or infantile-onset leukoencephalopathy with swelling (macrocephaly), cysts, and mild clinical course (Fig. 8-104). Early central white matter disease

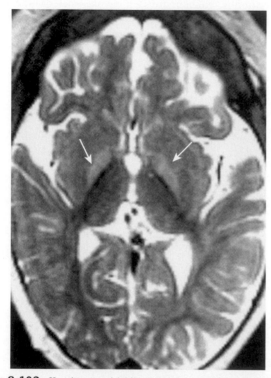

FIGURE 8-102. Kernicterus with bilateral globus pallidus lesions (*arrows*) and atrophy on axial T2-weighted MR image.

may suggest Krabbe disease (also, abnormal thalami), a peroxisomal disorder (e.g., ALD with brainstem involvement), metachromatic leukodystrophy, phenylketonuria, maple syrup urine disease (Fig. 8-105), or Lowe syndrome. The lack of myelination (hypomyelination) may suggest Pelizaeus-Merzbacher or Menkes disease.

In myelinoclastic (e.g., demyelinating) disorders, the intrinsically normal myelin sheath is damaged by exogenous or endogenous myelinotoxic factors. The cerebral pattern is often asymmetric and sharply defined, and may involve the arcuate U fibers. There may be asymmetric cerebellar, brainstem, and basal ganglia/thalamic involvement. This pattern is seen with infectious and postinfectious demyelinating diseases (e.g., HIV, CMV, ADEM [see Fig. 8-42], PML, and SSPE), chemotherapy (e.g., methotrexate, cyclosporin), radiotherapy, vasculitis (e.g., systemic lupus erythematosus), and multiple sclerosis.

Nonspecific white matter abnormalities may be seen with a variety of metabolic, neurodegenerative, infectious, postinfectious, toxic, and vascular processes. In this situation, the clinical findings must be relied upon. An important example is posterior reversible leukoencephalopathy, which may be seen in a number of conditions associated with hypertension (e.g., cyclosporine therapy in transplant recipients, renal disease [Fig. 8-106]). Also, it is important to remember that the most common causes of cerebral white matter abnormalities (particularly periventricular) and prominent Virchow-Robin spaces in children with developmental delay are static leukoencephalopathies (e.g., maldevelopmental, undermyelinated, post-inflammatory, postischemic, idiopathic).

Disorders Affecting White Matter and Cortical Gray Matter

Disorders affecting both white matter and cortical gray matter include lysosomal disorders such as the lipidoses and mucopolysaccharidoses (associated skeletal dysplasia), and mitochondrial disorders (e.g., Alpers syndrome, Menkes disease). If a diffuse cortical dysgenesis (e.g., lissencephaly, polymicrogyria) is associated with white matter abnormalities, peroxisomal disorders such as Zellweger syndrome should be considered along with congenital infections (e.g., CMV; see Fig. 8-20), and the congenital muscular dystrophies (e.g., Fukuyama syndrome, Walker-Warburg syndrome [see Fig. 8-19], and Santavuori disease).

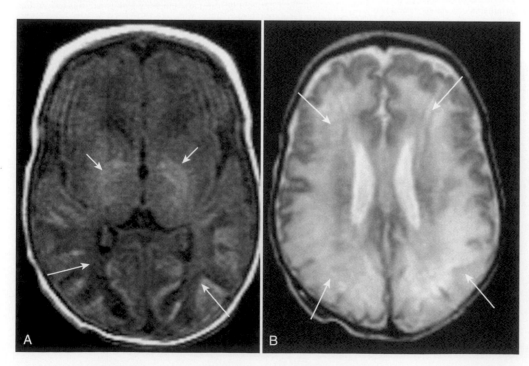

FIGURE 8-103. Sulfite oxidase deficiency with thalamic (*short arrows* on **A**) and diffuse white matter involvement (*long arrows*) on axial T1-weighted (**A**) and T2-weighted (**B**) MR images.

Disorders Affecting White Matter and Deep Gray Matter

Disorders affecting both white matter and deep gray matter include those with primarily caudate and putaminal involvement (Leigh syndrome [see Fig. 8-97], MELAS syndrome, Wilson disease, Cockayne syndrome [see Fig. 8-100]), predominant thalamic abnormalities (Krabbe disease, GM2 gangliosidosis), or primarily globus pallidus involvement (Canavan disease, maple syrup urine disease [see Fig. 8-105], methylmalonic/propionic acidopathy, Kearns-Sayre disease). More common causes are profound hypoxia-ischemia, osmolar myelinolysis, kernicterus (see Fig. 8-102), toxic exposure (e.g., carbon dioxide, methane, cyanide, radiation, chemotherapy), and infectious or postinfectious processes (e.g., TORCH diseases, HIV, ADEM).

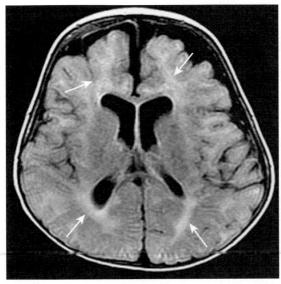

FIGURE 8-104. Infantile leukoencephalopathy (*arrows*) with macrocephaly on axial FLAIR MR image.

Magnetic Resonance Spectroscopy in Metabolic Disorders

Proton MRS is being increasingly used, including in patients with metabolic disorders. Although a number of the metabolic and neurodegenerative disorders have specific biochemical or genetic markers, some may have no differentiating features, even on MRS. Nonspecific MRS abnormalities are those that reflect brain destruction and reactive changes, including delayed maturation, neuronal loss, axonal degeneration, demyelination, and gliosis. In disorders with primary, or predominant, neuronal degeneration, there is loss of cell bodies and their projections (axons and dendrites) and myelin sheaths. Atrophy is the main pathologic result with minimal, or no, white matter changes or gliosis. The primary MRS abnormality in these disorders is a decrease in N-acetyl-aspartate (NA), which is proportional to the severity of atrophy but may be evident before atrophy is apparent. In disorders in which demyelination primarily, or predominantly, occurs there is loss of myelin sheaths with secondary axonal degeneration. Pathologically, there is loss of white matter and a reactive gliosis. Atrophy is usually not apparent unless the demyelination is severe and chronic. Active demyelination is characterized by elevated lipids and choline (Ch; increased membrane lipid turnover with increased myelin breakdown products), variable increases in lactate and glutamate/glutamine (Glx; active tissue degeneration and inflammation), and elevated inositols (gliosis). Associated neuronal damage is indicated by a decrease in NA.

More specific MRS abnormalities may be seen in a number of disorders. Abnormal MRS spectra have been reported with some of the lysosomal defects such as Niemann-Pick disease (abnormal lipid peak at 1.2 ppm), the mucopolysaccharidoses (decreased NA late), and metachromatic leukodystrophy (decreased NA, Ch, and creatine [Cr]; increased inositols and lactate). MRS abnormalities have been observed with a number of the peroxisomal disorders, including adrenoleukodystrophy (decreased NA with increased Ch, Glx, inositols, lipids, and lactate) and Zellweger syndrome (decreased NAs with increased lipids and Glx). Other leukodystrophies associated with observed MRS findings are Canavan disease (increased NA with decreased Ch and Cr plus increased inositols and lactate), Alexander disease (decreased NA with increased lactate), and Pelizaeus-Merzbacher disease (normal levels early; decreased NA and increased Ch late).

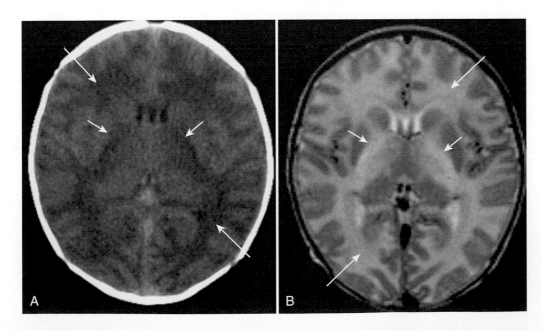

FIGURE 8-105. Maple syrup urine disease in neonate with edema of the globus pallidus (*short arrows*) and white matter (*long arrows*) on an axial CT scan (**A**) and an axial T2-weighted MR image (**B**).

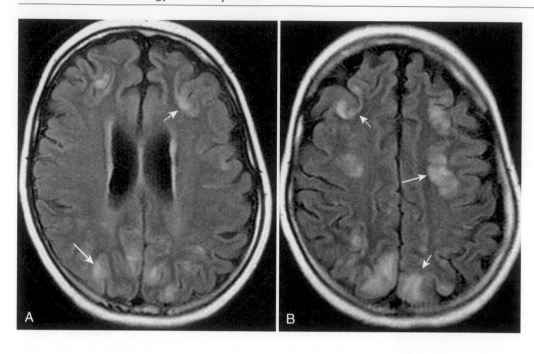

Figure 8-106. A and B, "Reversible" leukoencephaly (*long and short arrows*) on axial FLAIR MR images.

Disorders of energy metabolism have been associated with MRS findings of decreased NA and increased lactate, including mitochondrial disorders such as Leigh disease (see Fig. 8-97) and MELAS syndrome. Similar findings, however, are present with acute/subacute hypoxia-ischemia (plus elevated Glx, decreased Cr, and increased lipids). Aminoacidopathies with reportedly abnormal spectra include phenylketonuria (increased phenylalanine peak at 7.37 ppm), maple syrup urine disease (elevated leucine, isoleucine, and valine with abnormal peak at 0.9 ppm), and nonketotic hyperglycinemia (elevated glycine peak at 3.55 ppm). Other metabolic disorders associated with abnormal MRS findings include the creatine deficiencies (decrease or absence of Cr), hepatic encephalopathy (increased Glx with decreased inositols and Ch), and hyperosmolar states (increased inositols, Cr, and Ch).

▓ Suggested Readings

Ball W Jr: Pediatric Neuroradiology. Philadelphia, Lippincott-Raven, 1997.
Barkovich A: Pediatric Neuroimaging, ed 4. Philadelphia, Lippincott-Raven, 2005.
Blaser SI, Illner A, Castillo M, et al: Peds Neuro: 100 Top Diagnoses. (Pocket Radiologist.). Philadelphia, WB Saunders, 2003.
Harwood-Nash D, Fitz CR: Neuroradiology in Infants and Children. St. Louis, Mosby-Year Book, 1976.
Kirks DR: Practical Pediatric Imaging, ed 3. Philadelphia, Lippincott-Raven, 1998.

Kuhn JP, Slovis TL, Caffey J, Haller JO: Caffey's Pediatric Diagnostic Imaging, ed 10. New York, Elsevier Mosby Saunders, 2003.
Levine D: Atlas of Fetal MRI. Boca Raton, FL, Taylor and Francis Group, 2005.
Swischuk LE: Imaging of the Newborn, Infant, and Young Child. ed 5. Philadelphia, Lippincott Williams & Wilkins, 2003.
Tortori-Donati P, Rossi A: Pediatric Neuroradiology. New York, Springer, 2005.
van der Knaap MS, Valk J: Magnetic Resonance of Myelination and Myelin Disorders. ed 3. New York, Springer, 2005.
Volpe JJ: Neurology of the Newborn, ed 4. Philadelphia, WB, Saunders, 2001.
Wolpert S, Barnes P: MRI in Pediatric Neuroradiology. St. Louis, Mosby-Year Book, 1992.
Zimmerman RA, Gibby WA, Carmody RF (eds): Neuroimaging: Clinical and Physical Principles, New York, Springer, 2000.

Articles and Monographs

Barkovich AJ, Naidich TP (eds): Pediatric Neuroradiology. Neuroimaging Clin North Am 1994;4(2).
Barnes PD (ed): Imaging of the Developing Brain. Top Magn Reson Imag 2007; 18(1).
Barnes PD, Krasnokutsky M: Imaging of the central nervous system in suspected or alleged nonaccidental injury, including the mimics. Top Magn Reson Imaging 2007;18:53-74.
Edwards-Brown MK, Barnes PD (eds): Pediatric Neuroradiology. Neuroimaging Clin North Am 1999;9(1).
Mukherjee P (ed): Advanced Pediatric Imaging. Neuroimaging Clin North Am 2006;16(1).
Mukherji SK (ed): Pediatric Head and Neck Imaging. Neuroimaging Clin North Am 2000;10(1).

CHAPTER 9

Spine Imaging

Patrick D. Barnes

The central nervous system (CNS) includes the skull, brain, spine, and spinal cord. The head and neck region includes the face, eye and orbit, nasal cavity and paranasal sinuses, ear and temporal bone, oral cavity, jaw, and neck. Modalities used for the imaging of the pediatric CNS and head and neck region include plain film/computerized radiography (PF/CR), ultrasonography (US), computed tomography (CT) or multidetector CT (MDCT), magnetic resonance imaging (MRI), radionuclide imaging (RI), catheter angiography, and cerebrospinal fluid (CSF) imaging (e.g., CT myelography). Imaging modalities may be classified as structural or functional. Structural imaging modalities provide spatial resolution primarily on the basis of anatomic or morphologic data (e.g., CT). Functional imaging modalities (including molecular imaging) provide spatial resolution on the basis of physiologic, metabolic, or biologic data or markers (e.g., positron emission tomography [PET]). Some modalities may actually be regarded as providing both structural and functional information (e.g., MRI, PET-CT). The technical and procedural descriptions for angiography, myelography, and other invasive and interventional modalities are detailed in other texts. In this presentation, guidelines for their utilization are presented by region and modality.

SPINE IMAGING GUIDELINES

Plain Films/Computerized Radiography

PF/CR is commonly performed for trauma, torticollis, scoliosis, and suspected dysraphism. Occasionally, it may be the initial screening technique for evaluation of pain or any other symptoms or signs relating to the spine. Frontal and/or lateral views may be obtained initially. Oblique views are rarely needed. For scoliosis, erect posterior-anterior frontal and/or lateral views (with breast shielding) are usually obtained. Bending films may also assist in this evaluation. Flexion-extension lateral PF/CR or fluoroscopy, obtained with cooperation of the patient or supervision by a physician, may be helpful in evaluating potential instability (e.g., in craniocervical anomalies). These are x-ray–based techniques that are being increasingly displaced, or replaced, by the other modalities, especially MRI. Such techniques are best used in a limited and selective manner to minimize radiation exposure using the "as low as reasonably achievable" (ALARA) principle.

Ultrasonography

US is often helpful for evaluating the spinal contents in the fetus, newborn, and young infant. Imaging is performed, both static and real-time, with high-resolution, linear-array transducers (5- or 7-MHz) in the sagittal and axial planes. The patient is scanned in the prone position, but sometimes in the supine position, especially if cord tethering is a clinical consideration. Real-time visualization allows dynamic evaluation of the spinal cord and cauda equina nerve roots (i.e., pulsations). Scanning may be facilitated by spinal flexion to widen the interspinous acoustic window.

Computed Tomography

CT imaging of the spine has long replaced conventional tomography and is most often performed without the use of intravenous (IV) or intrathecal CSF administration of contrast material for enhancement. MDCT is replacing PF/CR and becoming the standard for the emergency evaluation of spine trauma, especially for the cervical spine. This evaluation includes high-resolution axial images with sagittal and coronal reformatting using bone and soft tissue algorithms. CT continues to be the choice for assessment of localized bony abnormalities, or a calcified component, of the spinal canal, foramina, neural arches, and articular structures, particularly when the level is precisely defined clinically or by plain film, single-photon emission CT (SPECT), or MRI (e.g., diastematomyelia, spondylolysis, spinal stenosis, spondylitis, bone tumor—i.e., osteoid osteoma, aneurysmal bone cyst). Axial sections with two-dimensional (2D) reformatting (coronal, sagittal, oblique), and/or three-dimensional (3D) reconstructions are often important in the preoperative evaluation of spine trauma, craniocervical anomalies, and congenital scoliosis as well as for the postoperative assessment of instrumentation and fusion. CT may also be obtained (with patient cooperation or physician supervision) with the spine in flexion and extension or with right and left head turning, to evaluate for translational craniocervical instability or rotatory atlantoaxial (AA) instability or fixation, respectively. CT-myelography is rarely needed except when MRI is contraindicated or spinal instrumentation does not allow adequate MRI quality. It may also assist in the more precise delineation of nerve root or other intradural lesions (e.g., cysts). A water-soluble, low-osmolar, non-ionic contrast material specifically approved for myelography is used because of its low toxicity and infrequent side effects. The technical and procedural descriptions for this and other invasive CSF imaging methods are described in detail in other texts. Again, these techniques are best used in a limited and selective manner and using ALARA guidelines to minimize radiation exposure.

Radionuclide Imaging (RI)

Bone scintigraphy, especially SPECT, is frequently helpful for evaluating children with lesions of the spinal column. Back pain, scoliosis, hip or knee pain, limp, and fever of uncertain source may be due to spondylitis, trauma, or tumor. The initial diagnosis may be suggested by bone RI findings. PET (including PET-CT) is also used in the assessment of treatment response or tumor progression in childhood neoplasia.

Magnetic Resonance Imaging

MRI using a phased-array (e.g., multichannel) surface coil system for spinal imaging, or a combined volume head coil and spine surface coil system for craniospinal imaging, has become the ideal modality for definitive evaluation of the spinal neuraxis in children with myelodysplasias (e.g., tethered cord) or myelopathy (e.g., hydrosyringomyelia). Although MRI has improved in its ability to evaluate disk and cortical bony disease, its main advantage over CT for imaging of the extradural structures is in inflammatory and neoplastic involvement of the spinal marrow and paraspinal soft tissues (e.g., osteomyelitis, neuroblastoma, plexiform neurofibroma), especially using fat suppression techniques. The addition of the contrast agent gadolinium to the fat suppression techniques further enhances the ability of MRI to evaluate inflammation and tumor, whether intramedullary, intradural, or extradural. Although MRI is the procedure of choice for initial evaluation of suspected vascular lesions (e.g., arteriovascular malformation), angiography is the definitive procedure, particularly when interventional therapy is being considered.

In general, screening spine MRI begins with sagittal T1-weighted and T2-weighted images plus axial T2-weighted images of the entire spine (as one or more series) from the posterior fossa through the coccyx. Axial T1- and T2-weighted images are obtained from the conus medullaris through the dural sac to confirm the conus level and to evaluate for filar thickening, extent of a dermal sinus, and a tethering mass (e.g., lipoma, dermoid-epidermoid). Axial images are imperative for surgical planning (e.g., lipomyelomeningocele). Coronal T2-weighted images assist in evaluating for spinal column anomalies (e.g., hemivertebra in congenital scoliosis), split-cord malformations (e.g., diastematomyelia), and renal anomalies. In cases of diastematomyelia, axial T2-weighted images through the split cord are necessary to demonstrate or rule out a tethering septum. Sagittal T2-weighted images are important for evaluating hydrosyringomyelia and Chiari I malformation along with axial T2-weighted images. Gadolinium-enhanced T1-weighted imaging is also necessary to assess for tumor as a cause of cord expansion or hydrosyringomyelia. Craniospinal imaging is often done to evaluate patients for the sequelae of repaired myelomeningocele and Chiari II malformation, including ventricular size, possible fourth ventricular isolation, and hydrosyringomyelia, as well as for sequelae at the original repair site (e.g., scarring, dermoid-epidermoid). Sagittal and axial T2-weighted MRI may also be done in flexion and extension (with patient cooperation or physician supervision) to assess craniocervical instability or fixation (e.g., craniocervical anomalies).

For evaluation of extradural traumatic, inflammatory, or neoplastic processes (e.g., ligamentous injury, disk herniation, osteomyelitis, sarcoma), sagittal T1-weighted images are performed, followed by sagittal fat-suppression T2-weighted images or short TI inversion recovery (STIR) images. Axial T2-weighted images are also important. Additional gadolinium-enhanced sagittal and axial fat-suppression T1-weighted images are necessary for evaluating neoplastic and inflammatory processes, as well as for assessing disk protrusion after surgery. These techniques allow for the complete assessment of marrow, bony, and paraspinal soft tissue involvement and extent as well as for cord, cauda equina, or nerve root compression. Diffusion-weighted MRI has been used to assist in the differentiation of traumatic vs. pathologic spinal fracture. Gadolinium enhancement is also necessary in the assessment of intramedullary tumors (e.g., astrocytoma, ependymoma, ganglioglioma), and intradural tumors (e.g., neurofibroma, schwannoma, ependymoma), and for neoplastic seeding (e.g., medulloblastoma, germ cell tumors).

Sagittal T2-weighted or STIR imaging, along with axial T2-weighted imaging, is done to evaluate for intramedullary inflammation or degeneration, including the assessment of cord atrophy. Gadolinium-enhanced imaging may also be helpful. A combination of sagittal and coronal T1- and T2-weighted imaging plus axial T2-weighted imaging is performed for screening of patients with suspected spinal vascular malformation. T2* gradient echo imaging may further detect hemorrhage. Gadolinium-enhanced imaging is occasionally needed in such patients, particularly to rule out other abnormalities. Gadolinium-enhanced MR angiography may be useful, but angiography is the "gold standard," especially for surgical planning and for interventional neuroradiologic guidance.

NORMAL DEVELOPMENT OF THE SPINAL NEURAXIS AND SPINAL COLUMN

The *spinal neuraxis* (spinal cord and nerve roots) develops through the process of *neurulation* (neural tube closure). The notochord induces the formation of the neural plate, which is neural ectoderm continuous with cutaneous ectoderm. The neural plate is the origin of both the neural tube, from which the CNS forms, and the

neural crest, from which the peripheral nervous system is derived. Closure of the neural groove forms the brain and mid- to upper spinal cord by the fourth week, including separation from the adjacent ectoderm, endoderm (i.e., neurenteric canal), and mesoderm. The dorsal root ganglia, cranial and spinal nerves, and sympathetic chain form from the neural crest. The distal conus medullaris, associated nerve roots, and filum terminale form as a result of canalization and retrogressive differentiation of the caudal neural tube (caudal cell mass origin). Rapid longitudinal growth of the spinal column occurs so that the conus is usually at or above the mid-L2 vertebral body level before 1 year postnatal age.

The *spinal column* forms as the result of membrane development (i.e., formation phase) followed by chondrification and then ossification. The notochord separates from the primitive gut and dorsal neural tube (i.e., neurenteric canal) during the fourth week of gestation. This mesenchyme subsequently forms a series of somites, or segments (i.e., segmentation phase), which become the spinal column and paraspinal tissues. Remnants of the notochord persist as the nucleus pulposus of the intervertebral disk. The components of the craniocervical junction, which arise from the primordial occipital and cervical sclerotomes, consist of the occipital bone, atlas (C1), axis (C2), and associated ligaments. More detailed descriptions of CNS embryology and development are covered in other texts. Knowledge of the normal spine and its variations of normal is important for proper image interpretation of findings of PF/CR, US, CT, and MRI. This subject is also covered in greater detail elsewhere.

DEVELOPMENTAL ABNORMALITIES
Dysraphic Myelodysplasias

The most common group of spinal neuraxis and column malformations, dysraphic myelodysplasias result from disorders of spinal neural tube closure (Box 9-1). *Dysraphism* refers to defective midline closure of neural, bony, and other mesenchymal tissues. *Spina bifida "aperta"* refers to the direct exposure of neural tissue through a dorsal bony spinal and cutaneous defect. Within this subcategory are myelocele, myelomeningocele, hydromyelia, Chiari II malformation, hemimyelocele, myeloschisis, and cranioschisis. In "occult" spinal dysraphism, the myelodysplasia lies deep to intact skin. This subcategory includes dermal sinus, lipomyelomeningocele, tight filum terminale, meningocele, myelocystocele, diastematomyelia, neurenteric cyst, the split notochord syndrome, and developmental tumors such as spinal lipomas. In both subcategories, cutaneous stigmata are common and include the exteriorized placode associated with the myelocele and myelomeningocele, as well as skin-covered lesions such as subcutaneous lipoma, hairy patch (hypertrichosis), nevus, hemangioma, and dermal sinus. Plain film findings may show formation or segmentation anomalies, congenital scoliosis or kyphosis, canal widening, or spinolaminar defects. CT is helpful for preoperative definition of the bony spinal anomalies. US is a

---

Box 9-1. Dysraphic Myelodysplasias

Myelocele and myelomeningocele
Lipomyelocele and lipomyelomeningocele
Dermal sinus
Tethered cord syndrome
Myelocystocele
Meningocele
Split notochord syndrome
Neurenteric cyst
Diastematomyelia
Caudal dysplasias
Developmental tumors

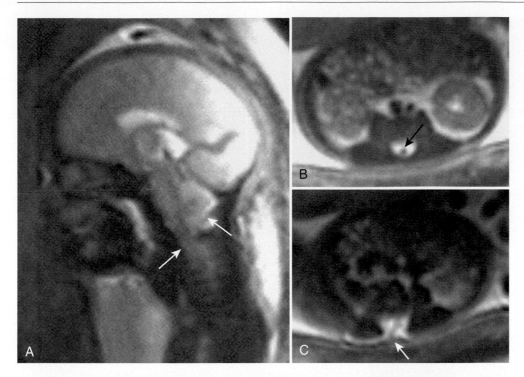

Figure 9-1. Fetal T2-weighted MR images. **A,** Chiari II malformation (*arrows*) on sagittal image. **B,** Lumbosacral myelocele with low-placed spinal cord (*arrow*) on axial image. **C,** Dysraphic defect plus placode (*arrow*) on axial image.

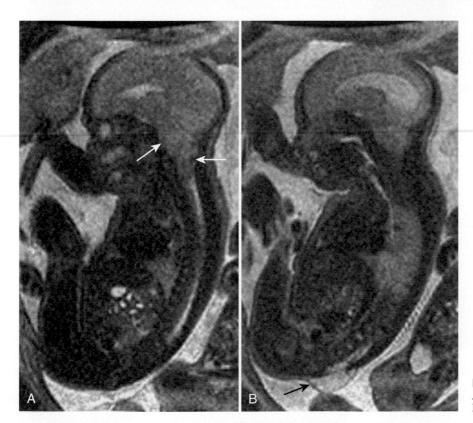

Figure 9-2. Chiari II malformation (*arrows* in A) and lumbosacral myelomeningocele (*arrow* in B) on sagittal T2-weighted fetal MR images.

useful screening modality for the fetus and young infant and is also used for intraoperative surgical guidance. MRI is the definitive modality for diagnosis, surgical planning, and follow-up.

Myelocele and Myelomeningocele

Both myelocele and myelomeningocele are the result of nondisjunction of the cutaneous ectoderm from the neural ectoderm and failure of neural tube closure. The nonneurulated cord or placode is exposed through a dural, bony, and cutaneous defect (i.e.,

myelocele; Fig. 9-1). The dorsal and ventral nerve roots exit from the ventral surface of the placode. With associated dorsal protrusion of the ventral subarachnoid space, the myelodysplasia is termed a *myelomeningocele* (Fig. 9-2). These defects commonly occur at the lumbar or sacral level. Occasionally there is an associated diastematomyelia (hemimyelomeningocele) or dermal sinus.

These defects are surgically closed shortly after birth. Hydrocephalus is often present; if so, shunting is established early. Subsequently, patients who have undergone such procedures may

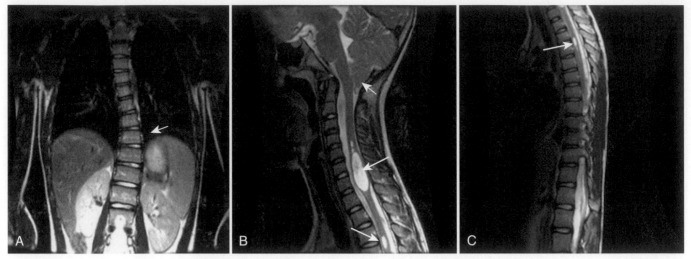

FIGURE 9-3. Chiari I malformation and cervicothoracic hydrosyringomyelia on T2-weighted MRI. **A,** Coronal image showing left thoracic curve (*arrow*). **B** and **C,** Sagittal images showing low cerebellar tonsils (*short arrow* in **B**), and cyst-like cord expansions (*long arrows* in **B** and **C**).

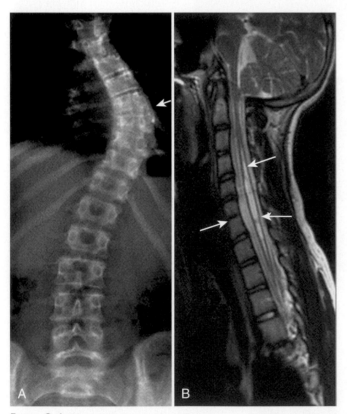

FIGURE 9-4. Klippel-Feil anomaly with hydrosyringomyelia. **A,** Frontal plain film/computerized radiograph shows left thoracic lateral curve (*arrow*). **B,** Sagittal T2-weighted MR image shows C6 to C7 bony fusion anomaly (*anterior arrow*), small C1 canal, and C3 to T2 septated cord expansion (*posterior arrows*).

undergo neuroimaging for any change in neurologic status that may be related to the Chiari II malformation (see Figs. 9-1 and 9-2), to associated anomalies, or to the sequelae of surgical closure or shunted hydrocephalus. Associated conditions or sequelae include hydrocephalus, shunt malfunction, encystment of the fourth ventricle, hydrosyringomyelia, brainstem compression or dysfunction, cervical cord compression or constriction, hemimyelocele/hemimyelomeningocele, lipoma, dermoid-epidermoid, arachnoid cyst, scarring or retethering at the operative site, dural

sac stenosis, progressive scoliosis, and cord ischemia or infarction.

Hydrosyringomyelia

Hydromyelia refers to dilatation of the central canal of the spinal cord; *syringomyelia* refers to a spinal cord cavity. Since one may be indistinguishable from the other, or the two conditions may coexist, the term *hydrosyringomyelia* is often used. This condition is most commonly associated with the Chiari malformations (e.g., Chiari I, II), spinal dysraphism, and craniocervical anomalies. MRI may demonstrate focal, segmental, or total involvement of the spinal cord (Figs. 9-3 to 9-6). Intramedullary CSF intensities are present, and the cord may be enlarged. Sacculations or septations may be present. Syrinx or cyst may also occur with trauma, infection, tumors, or arachnoiditis.

Lipomyelocele and Lipomyelomeningocele

Lipomyelocele and lipomyelomeningocele are the most common of the occult myelodysplasias. Like the myelocele and myelomeningocele, they result from faulty disjunction, but the skin is intact and there is an associated lipoma. Patients with these defects may be asymptomatic, may present with a subcutaneous mass, or may have motor or sensory loss, bladder dysfunction, or orthopedic deformities of the lower extremities. The lipoma often extends caudally, dorsally, or ventrally from the incompletely fused cord (e.g., presacral) through a dural and bony defect and is continuous with the subcutaneous fat. The spinal canal is often enlarged. Spina bifida or formation-segmentation anomalies may be present. For surgical planning, MRI demonstrates the relationships of the lipoma, which is hyperintense on T1-weighted imaging (T1-hyperintense), with the neural elements (Figs. 9-5 to 9-7). There may be an associated thickened filum or filar lipoma (Fig. 9-7).

Dermal Sinuses

Dermal sinuses are epithelial tracts, stalks, or fistulae that extend from the skin surface into the deeper tissues. They result from incomplete dysjunction of the neuroectoderm from the cutaneous ectoderm during neurulation and may occur in the lumbosacral, cervicooccipital, or thoracic region. There is often a midline dimple or ostium with an associated hairy nevus, vascular anomaly, or hyperpigmentation. The sinus often extends into the deeper tissues and enters the spinal canal. It may even extend to the dura or penetrate the dura and terminate in the subarachnoid space, the filum, or the conus medullaris. There may be an

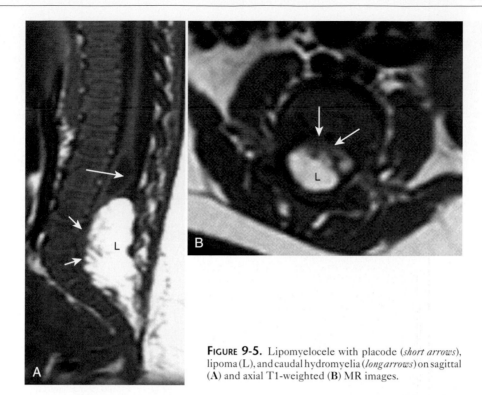

FIGURE 9-5. Lipomyelocele with placode (*short arrows*), lipoma (L), and caudal hydromyelia (*long arrows*) on sagittal (**A**) and axial T1-weighted (**B**) MR images.

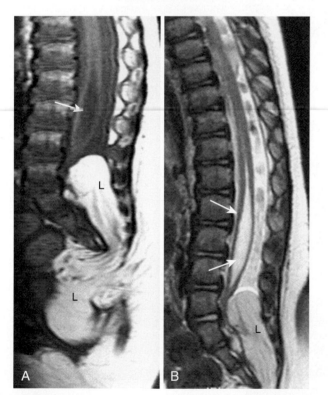

FIGURE 9-6. Lumbosacral lipomyelocele with caudal and presacral lipomas (L) and hydrosyringomyelia (*arrows*) on sagittal T1-weighted (**A**) and T2-weighted (**B**) MR images.

associated dermoid-epidermoid or lipoma (Figs. 9-8 and 9-9). Affected patients may present with abscess or meningitis. On MRI the dermal sinus usually appears as a relative hypointensity. Gadolinium may be helpful, especially when infection is present (Fig. 9-10).

The Tethered Cord Syndrome

Also known as "tight filum terminale syndrome," *tethered cord syndrome* refers to low position of the conus medullaris (below the level of mid-L2) associated with a short and thickened filum terminale. The filar thickening (usually greater than 2 mm) is usually fibrous, fatty, or cystic, and may be associated with other dysraphic myelodysplasias, including lipomyelomeningocele and diastematomyelia. The thickened filum may also terminate in a lipoma or dermoid-epidermoid. The filar abnormality is usually best demonstrated on axial T1-weighted and T2-weighted MRI (Fig. 9-11; see Fig. 9-7).

Myelocystocele

Myelocystocele is the least common of the occult myelodysplasias associated. This defect usually occurs at the lumbosacral level (rarely at the cervical level) and is often associated with other malformations of caudal cell mass origin (i.e., anorectal and urogenital anomalies—high imperforate anus, cloacal malformation, etc.). The terminal myelocystocele consists of hydromyelia and a dilated terminal ventricle of the conus-placode that is continuous with a dorsal, ependyma-lined cyst within or adjacent to a meningocele. There may be an associated lipoma (i.e., lipomyelocystocele).

Meningoceles

Meningoceles are uncommon, saccular dural protrusions that extend beyond the confines of the spinal canal and contain CSF-filled arachnoid but no cord elements. They may extend dorsally, laterally, or ventrally. Dorsal dysraphic meningoceles may occur at the occipital, cervicooccipital, or lumbosacral level. An anterior meningocele extending through a dysraphic defect may be considered a neurenteric spectrum anomaly. Presacral meningoceles associated with dysraphic defects are often associated with anorectal or urogenital anomalies in the caudal dysplasia spectrum. Meningoceles extending laterally through an intervertebral foramen, or anteriorly through a sacral foramen, may be seen with a mesodermal dysplasia such as neurofibromatosis type 1 (NF-1) or Marfan syndrome (Fig. 9-12).

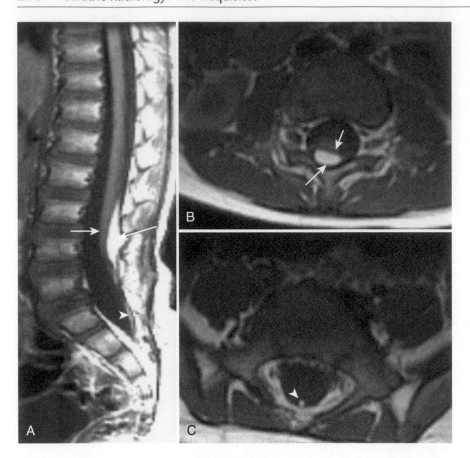

FIGURE 9-7. Sagittal (**A**) and axial (**B** and **C**) T1-weighted MR images showing tethered cord with low conus (*short arrows* in **A** and **B**), dorsal lipoma (*long arrows* in **A** and **B**), and filar lipoma (*arrowheads* in **A** and **C**).

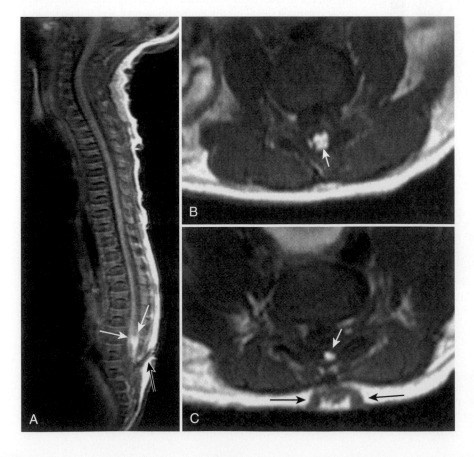

FIGURE 9-8. Sagittal (**A**) and axial (**B** and **C**) T1-weighted MR images showing lumbosacral dermal sinuses (*black arrows* on **A** and **C**) with tethered cord (*white arrows* in **A**) and lipoma (*white arrows* in **B** and **C**) in a newborn.

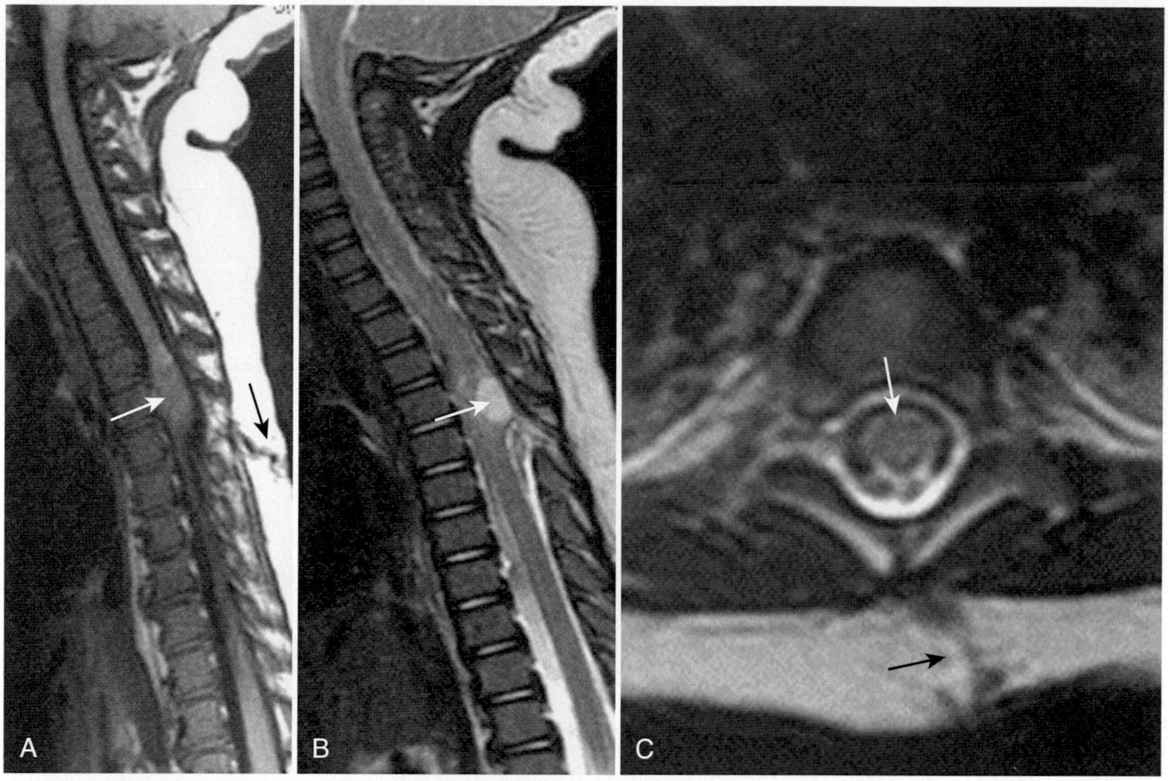

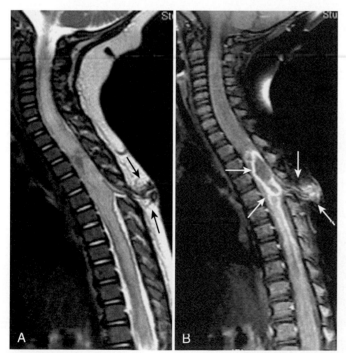

FIGURE 9-9. Thoracic dermal sinus (*black arrows*) and dermoid cyst (*white arrows*) on sagittal T1-weighted (**A**), sagittal T2-weighted (**B**), and axial T1-weighted (**C**) MR images.

FIGURE 9-10. Thoracic dermal sinus (*posterior black and white arrows* in **A** and **B**) and cyst with enhancing abscess (*anterior white arrows* in **B**) with cord edema on sagittal T2-weighted (**A**) and gadolinium-enhanced T1-weighted (**B**) MR images.

The Split Notochord Syndrome

Split notochord syndrome refers to a rare spectrum of malformations related to the incomplete separation of the endoderm and ectoderm during the formation of the notochord (i.e., complete or partial failure of obliteration of the primitive neurenteric canal). The spectrum includes dorsal enteric fistula, dorsal enteric sinus, dorsal enteric enterogenous cysts, and dorsal enteric diverticula.

Neurenteric Cyst

Neurenteric cyst is also an anomaly of the neurenteric spectrum. Such cysts usually arise in the lower cervical or thoracic region. Associated formational vertebral anomalies include butterfly vertebra, hemivertebra, and block vertebra. A classic presentation is that of a posterior mediastinal mass associated with vertebral anomalies. The intraspinal lesions are usually intradural and extramedullary in location. However, they may occur in a prevertebral or dorsal location or may involve multiple compartments. The cyst may be lined by gut or respiratory epithelium and may have serous contents similar to CSF or may contain mucoid secretions and appear T1-hyperintense.

Diastematomyelia

The most common anomaly of the neurenteric or split notochord spectrum is diastematomyelia. It consists of sagittal clefting of the cord into symmetric or asymmetric hemicords. In some cases, the split is traversed by a septum and each hemicord has its own pial, arachnoid, and dural coverings (Fig. 9-13). In other cases, the hemicords are contained within a single dural sac and there is no septum (Fig. 9-14). The septum may be bony, cartilaginous, fibrous, or may be composed of vascular elements or neuroglial tissue. The hemicords often rejoin above and below the cleft. This malformation occurs most commonly in the lumbar or thoracolumbar region and is often associated with cutaneous stigmata. PF/CR or CT may show spina bifida, intersegmental laminar fusion, anomalies of the vertebral bodies, and kyphoscoliosis. For septal definition, axial T2-weighted MRI, CT, or myelographic CT is necessary. Associated anomalies include thickened filum, developmental tumor (e.g., lipoma, dermoid-epidermoid), hydromyelia, and tethering bands (meningocele manqué).

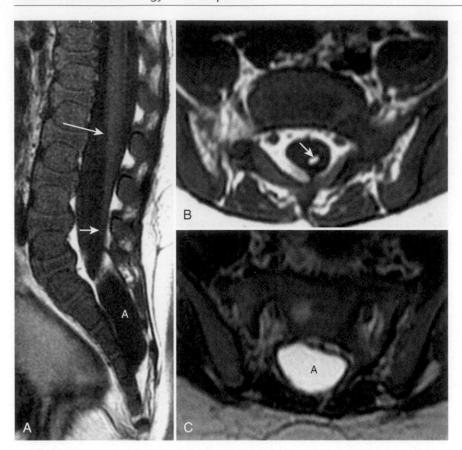

FIGURE 9-11. Tethered cord (*long arrow*), thick filum and lipoma (*short arrows*), and sacral extradural arachnoid cyst (A) on sagittal T1-weighted (**A**), axial T1-weighted (**B**), and axial T2-weighted (**C**) MR images.

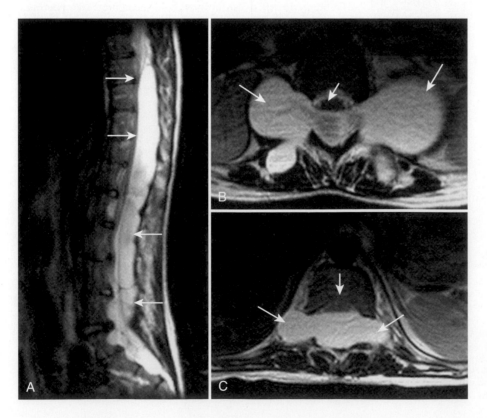

FIGURE 9-12. Sagittal (**A**) and axial (**B** and **C**) T2-weighted MR images showing dural ectasia and intradural arachnoid cysts (*arrows* in **A**) with scoliosis, cord flattening (*short arrows* in **B** and **C**), and transforaminal meningoceles (*long arrows* in **B** and **C**).

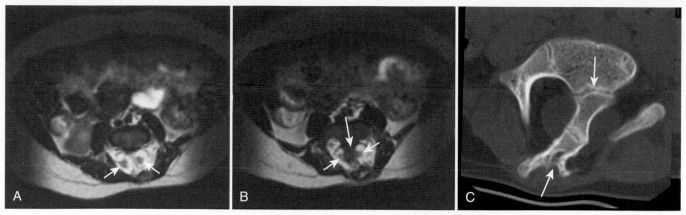

FIGURE 9-13. Lumbar diastematomyelia and split cord with two hemicords (*short arrows* in **A** and **B**), two dural sacs, and a bony septum (*long arrows* in **B** and **C**) on axial T2-weighted MR images (**A** and **B**) and an axial CT scan (**C**).

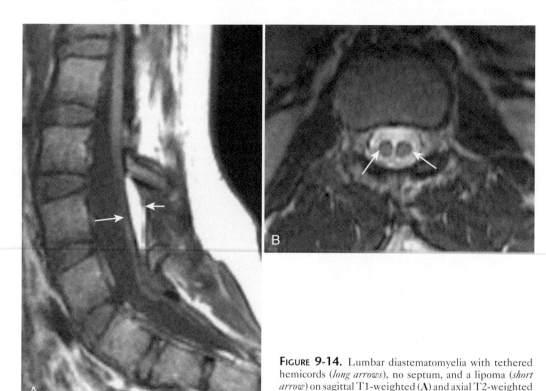

FIGURE 9-14. Lumbar diastematomyelia with tethered hemicords (*long arrows*), no septum, and a lipoma (*short arrow*) on sagittal T1-weighted (**A**) and axial T2-weighted (**B**) MR images.

The Caudal Dysplasias

The caudal dysplasias are a spectrum of malformations of caudal cell mass origin that include lumbosacral, anorectal, urogenital, and lower limb anomalies. In children with high imperforate anus, cloacal malformation, or cloacal exstrophy, there is a high prevalence of dysraphic myelodysplasia. The spinal anomalies range from dysraphism to partial to total sacral or lumbosacral agenesis. MRI may demonstrate a high-positioned and blunted or wedge-shaped conus termination (Fig. 9-15). There may be spinal canal or dural sac stenosis. Other anomalies are presacral meningocele or lipoma (see Fig. 9-6), cord tethering with filar thickening or developmental tumor, lipomyelomeningocele, and myelocystocele. The *caudal regression syndrome* is composed of lower extremity fusion (sirenomelia), lumbosacral agenesis, anal atresia, abnormal genitalia, exstrophy of the bladder, renal aplasia, and pulmonary hypoplasia. This may be associated with Potter syndrome or may be seen in infants of diabetic mothers.

Developmental Tumors

Developmental tumors of the spinal neuraxis include lipoma, dermoid-epidermoid, teratoma, arachnoid cyst, neurenteric cyst, and hamartoma.

Lipomas are the most common. They may arise as intradural lipomas, lipomyeloceles, lipomyelomeningoceles, or filar lipomas (see Figs. 9-5 to 9-8, 9-11, 9-14). Intradural lipomas usually occur as dorsal cervical or thoracic subpial masses. MRI of a lipoma demonstrates a lobulated T1-hyperintense mass adherent to or occupying a cord cleft.

Dermoids are tumors of ectodermal origin that contain elements of the dermis and epidermis (i.e., skin, hair, sweat and sebaceous glands, squamous epithelium). *Epidermoids* are composed of epidermal elements only. Both of these tumors may contain the products of squamous epithelial turnover (i.e., keratin and cholesterol). They arise most commonly from congenital rests but may also occur as implants after surgery or spinal puncture. Dermoids and epidermoids are often extramedullary but may arise within the medulla. There may be associated dermal sinus, cord tethering, abscess, or suppurative or chemical meningitis. On MRI they may be T1-isointense to hypointense and T2-hyperintense. Occasionally, there is fatlike hyperintensity or calcification (see Fig. 9-9). Enhancement may be evident because of inflammation (see Fig. 9-10).

Teratomas are neoplasms containing elements of all three germ layers. A teratoma arising in the sacrococcygeal region is common in childhood and manifests as an external perineal or gluteal mass, a pelvic mass, or a presacral mass. Two thirds are mature teratomas, and one third are immature or anaplastic teratomas. They are often lobulated and heterogeneous with solid, cystic, and calcific components. There may be associated sacral bony erosion. There is a familial form with an autosomal dominant inheritance that is associated with sacrococcygeal defects, vesicoureteral reflux, anorectal stenosis, and cutaneous stigmata (Currarino syndrome). These tumors often have heterogeneous MRI signal characteristics. Teratomas of the spinal canal are rare, are often benign, and usually occur as intramedullary or extramedullary masses at the thoracolumbar level.

Arachnoid cysts are categorized as primary or secondary (e.g., postinflammatory). Primary cysts may be intradural or extradural in location, and secondary cysts are usually intradural and associated with arachnoiditis. Although these cysts usually occur in the thoracic or lumbar region, they may be seen at any level. There may be scoliosis and spinal canal widening. MRI demonstrates a CSF-intensity cyst that displaces the cord, nerve roots, or epidural fat (see Figs. 9-11 and 9-12).

Hamartomas are masses that contain tissues of neuroectodermal or mesodermal origin—neuroglial and meningeal tissue, bone, fat, cartilage, or muscle. They are solid or cystic subcutaneous masses that occur in the mid-thoracic, thoracolumbar, or lumbar region and are often associated with cutaneous angiomas. Spina bifida and spinal canal widening are often seen with hamartomas.

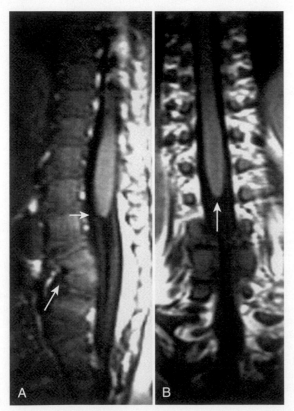

FIGURE 9-15. Caudal dysplasia with high imperforate anus, congenital lumbar kyphosis (*long arrows*), and dysplastic/hypoplastic conus medullaris (*short arrow*) on sagittal (**A**) and coronal (**B**) T1-weighted MR images.

Spondylodysplasias

Spondylodysplasia refers to any developmental abnormality of the bony spinal column (Box 9-2). This category includes idiopathic scoliosis, congenital scoliosis and kyphosis, Scheuermann disease, and the skeletal dysplasias (e.g., NF-1, mucopolysaccharidoses, spondyloepiphyseal dysplasia, achondroplasia, Down syndrome). Spinal curvature abnormalities are common in this category. As defined by clinical examination and findings on standing plain films, they include scoliosis (lateral curvature), kyphosis (posterior angulation), and lordosis (increased anterior angulation). In the skeletal dysplasias, a major concern is mechanical compromise of the spinal neuraxis due to progressive canal/foraminal stenosis, kyphoscoliosis, or craniocervical instability. Evaluation usually requires both CT and MRI.

Idiopathic Scoliosis

Idiopathic scoliosis is the most common curvature abnormality in childhood. The adolescent form, which is seen in children older than 10 years, is more common than the infantile or juvenile form. Adolescent idiopathic scoliosis is familial and most commonly seen in females. Characteristically, there is a right convex primary curve of the thoracic, thoracolumbar, or lumbar spine (Fig. 9-16). A rotatory component with pedicle asymmetry is characteristic, and a left convex secondary curve may present. Additional lordosis often occurs with curve progression. Complications of idiopathic scoliosis include curve progression, cardiopulmonary compromise, painful curves, cosmetic deformity, neurologic dysfunction, and degenerative joint disease. Curve progression usually occurs during periods of growth acceleration (e.g., infancy and prepuberty). Treatment may be required and involves bracing or surgical instrumentation and fusion (e.g., Harrington rods).

Atypical clinical or plain film findings in "presumed" idiopathic scoliosis require MRI to evaluate for an underlying abnormality such as hydrosyringomyelia (e.g., Chiari malformation), tumor, cyst, or dysraphic myelodysplasia (see Figs. 9-3, 9-4, 9-12). Atypical clinical features include early onset (prior to age 10 years), rapid curve progression, painful curves in young children, and abnormal neurologic symptoms or signs. Atypical curve patterns include a convex left primary curve, a kyphotic component, vertebral body or neural arch anomaly, pedicle thinning, and spinal canal widening.

Congenital Scoliosis and Kyphosis

Congenital scoliosis and kyphosis result from formation or segmentation anomalies (Fig. 9-17). Failure of formation may result in vertebral aplasia or hypoplasia with wedge vertebra, hemivertebra, or butterfly vertebra. Anomalies of segmentation failure include pedicle fusion bars and block vertebra. Combined anomalies are also common (e.g., block hemivertebra). Associated myelodysplasia occurs in 15% to 20% of cases of scoliosis or kyphosis (e.g., hydrosyringomyelia, diastematomyelia, neurenteric cyst,

---

Box 9-2. Spondylodysplasias

Idiopathic scoliosis
Congenital scoliosis and kyphosis
Scheuermann/Schmorl disease
Neurofibromatosis
Achondroplasia
Mucopolysaccharidoses
Down syndrome
Spondyloepiphyseal dysplasia
Craniocervical anomalies
Klippel-Feil syndrome
Spinal vascular anomalies

tethered cord) (see Figs. 9-4, 9-13, 9-17). Cardiac and genitourinary anomalies are also common. Other complications of congenital kyphosis are segmental spinal dysgenesis with congenitally dislocated spine, progressive or acute cord injury, cardiopulmonary compromise, and severe cosmetic deformity. Other causes of

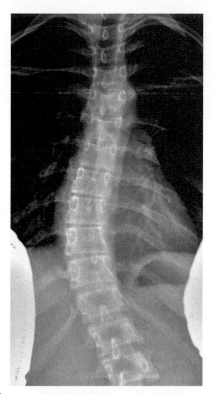

FIGURE 9-16. Idiopathic scoliosis with typical rightward thoracic lateral and rotatory curvature on a frontal plain film/computerized radiograph (obtained with breast shields in place).

kyphosis and kyphoscoliosis in childhood are posture, Scheuermann disease, neuromuscular disorder, trauma, inflammation, surgery, radiation therapy, metabolic disorders, chondrodysplasia, arthritis, and tumor. Lordotic curvature abnormalities may be congenital or acquired.

Scheuermann Disease

An osteochondrodysplasia, Scheuermann disease is a common cause of juvenile and adolescent thoracic kyphosis. An abnormality of enchondral ossification is associated with degenerative and reactive changes of the vertebral end plates. Often there is multilevel end plate irregularity, disk space narrowing, vertebral body wedging, and Schmorl nodes (Fig. 9-18). The kyphosis commonly occurs in the mid-thoracic spine. There may be progressive wedging with increasing thoracic kyphosis and lumbar lordosis. The less common lumbar form may be acute, painful, and traumatic. Limbus-like vertebral abnormalities are often seen.

Neurofibromatosis Type 1

NF-1 is a common mesodermal dysplasia of childhood (Fig. 9-19). Characteristic anomalies include a short-segment kyphoscoliosis, posterior vertebral body scalloping, vertebral body wedging, apical vertebral rotation, dural ectasia, and meningoceles (e.g., thoracic, presacral). There may also be an associated plexiform neurofibroma and other nerve sheath tumors. Other anomalies are cervical kyphosis, hypoplasia of the spinous process, transverse process, or pedicle, and twisted-ribbon ribs. Dural ectasia and meningocele formation may also be seen with Marfan or Ehlers-Danlos syndrome and in familial cases (see Fig. 9-12).

Achondroplasia

Achondroplasia is one of the osteochondrodysplasias (defective enchondral bone development) resulting in dwarfism. There is craniofacial dysmorphia with skull base constriction, including foramen magnum stenosis, short clivus, and small jugular foramina (Fig. 9-20). Macrocephaly and hydrocephalus (e.g.,

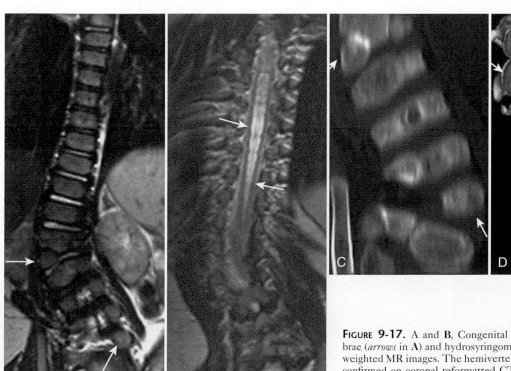

FIGURE 9-17. A and **B,** Congenital lumbar scoliosis with hemivertebrae (*arrows* in **A**) and hydrosyringomyelia (*arrows* in **B**) on coronal T2-weighted MR images. The hemivertebrae (*arrows*) and double curve are confirmed on coronal reformatted CT scan (**C**) and 3D reconstruction (**D**).

impaired venous outflow) occur, and there is enlargement of the subarachnoid spaces and ventricles. Other craniocervical abnormalities include odontoid hypoplasia, atlantoaxial (AA) instability, basilar impression, and occipitalization of the atlas. Scoliosis, kyphosis, or kyphoscoliosis may occur in about one third of patients with achondroplasia. Stenosis of the spinal canal may be cervical, thoracolumbar, lumbar, or may occur diffusely. There is platyspondyly with short pedicles, vertebral scalloping, and interpedicular narrowing. There may be associated spinal foraminal and canal compromise.

Mucopolysaccharidosis

Mucopolysaccharidosis may be associated with craniocervical abnormalities (e.g., Morquio syndrome; Fig. 9-21). They include odontoid hypoplasia, occipital hypoplasia, ligamentous laxity, AA instability, and dural sac stenosis (mucopolysaccharide deposition with fibrosis; Fig. 9-22). Foraminal and spinal canal encroachment may occur. Other vertebral anomalies are platyspondyly, beaking, wedging, gibbus deformity, and kyphoscoliosis.

Down Syndrome

Down syndrome may be complicated by craniocervical instability, such as odontoid hypoplasia, os odontoideum, atlanto-occipital (AO) subluxation, or AA subluxation (see "Craniocervical Anomalies"; Figs. 9-23 and 9-24). Scoliosis, degenerative cervical spine disease, tall vertebral bodies, vertebral fusions, and subluxations at other levels may also occur.

Spondyloepiphyseal Dysplasia

Spondyloepiphyseal dysplasia (SED) occurs as a congenita or tarda form. In the congenita form there is dwarfism, thoracolumbar kyphosis, lumbar lordosis, platyspondyly, and odontoid hypoplasia with AA instability. The tarda form of SED consists of platyspondyly, dwarfism, and early degenerative spine and hip disease. Other skeletal dysplasias associated with spinal abnormalities include diastrophic dysplasia, metatropic dysplasia, spondylometaphyseal dysplasia, Kneist dysplasia, Larsen syndrome, chondrodysplasia punctata, craniometaphyseal dysplasia, osteogenesis imperfecta, osteopetrosis, and Marfan syndrome.

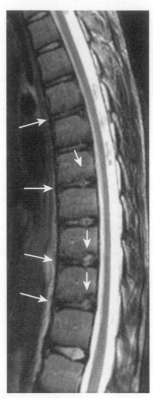

FIGURE 9-18. Scheuermann disease with multilevel, irregular thoracic disk space narrowing (*long arrows*) and Schmorl's nodes (*short arrows*).

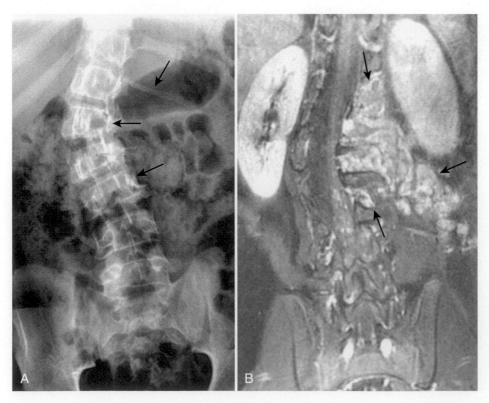

FIGURE 9-19. A, Neurofibromatosis-1 with short-segment right lumbar scoliosis plus vertebral and rib deformities (*arrows*) on frontal plain film/computerized radiograph. **B,** Enhancing paraspinal plexiform neurofibroma (*arrows*) with foraminal extension is shown on coronal gadolinium-enhanced T1-weighted MR image along with other small intradural enhancing nerve sheath tumors.

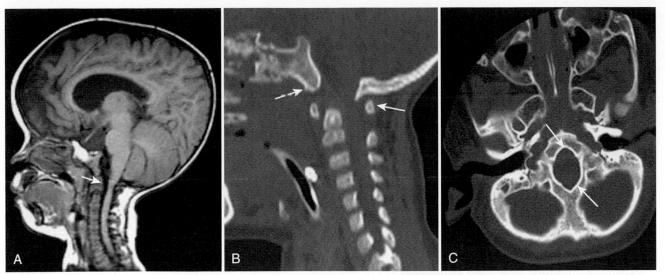

FIGURE 9-20. Achondroplasia, basilar invagination, and foramen magnum plus cervical spinal stenosis (*arrows*) on sagittal T1-weighted MR image (**A**), sagittal reformatted CT scan (**B**), and an axial CT scan (**C**). Also, there is characteristic macrocephaly and ventriculomegaly.

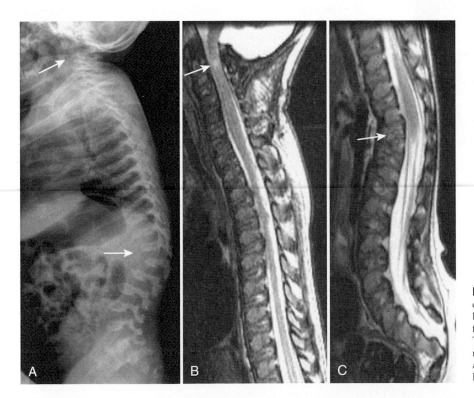

FIGURE 9-21. A, Morquio syndrome with craniocervical instability (*upper arrow*) plus thoracolumbar kyphoscoliosis (*lower arrow*) on a lateral plain film/computerized radiograph. **B** and **C,** Sagittal T2-weighted MR images show upper cervical dural sac stenosis with hyperintense cord injury (*arrow* in **B**) along with ventral cord deformity at the level of the kyphosis (*arrow* in **C**).

Craniocervical Anomalies

The craniocervical junction (CCJ) consists of the basiocciput, the atlas (C1) and axis (C2), and the ligaments of the AO and AA articulations. Imaging evaluation of this region often requires PF/CR, flexion-extension PF/CR or fluoroscopy, CT, and MRI.

A number of landmarks may be helpful in evaluating the CCJ. McRae's line defines the plane of the foramen magnum, and the dens tip should always be below it. The predental space in infants and young children (anterior atlas–dens gap) varies from 3 to a maximum of 5 mm in flexion with a 2-mm excursion from extension to flexion. The gap is normally less than 3 mm in adolescents and adults. The postdental space (dens–posterior atlas gap or dens–posterior foramen magnum gap) is at least 15 mm in children and 19 mm in adults. At the

level of C1, the spinal canal area, according to the Steel rule of thirds, should be composed of one third dens, one third cord, and one third safe zone. The dens tip should align with tip of the clivus (basion) and these two structures should not be separated by more than 1 cm.

Common anomalies of the CCJ include basilar invagination, the Klippel-Feil anomaly, occipitalization of the atlas, odontoid anomalies, and craniocervical instability. CCJ anomalies may manifest clinically as torticollis, craniofacial or craniocervical dysmorphism, limitation of motion, headache or neck pain, neck mass, or clicking. Kyphosis and scoliosis may also be seen. Patients may also be presented with symptoms or signs related to hindbrain, cervical cord, or vertebrobasilar compromise. Such abnormalities may be discovered after recent or remote trauma.

Basilar Invagination

Basilar invagination refers to an occipital dysplasia with upward displacement of the margins of the foramen magnum anteriorly, posteriorly, laterally, or combined (Fig. 9-25 and 9-26). The odontoid is superiorly displaced relative to McRae's line. In addition the posterior fossa may be of small volume with an irregularly

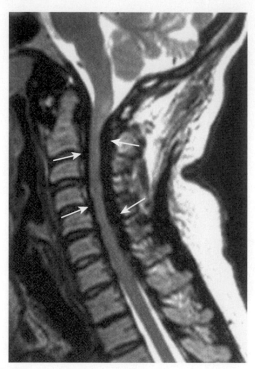

FIGURE 9-22. Scheie-type mucopolysaccharidosis with cervical dural/epidural hypointense thickening (*arrows*), dural sac stenosis, and cord thinning.

shaped foramen magnum and a short clivus. Basilar invagination may be (1) primary (i.e., developmental) and associated with other craniocervical anomalies or syndromes or (2) secondary (i.e., basilar impression) and associated with osteochondral dysplasias or metabolic disorders (e.g., rickets, fibrous dysplasia, achondroplasia, the mucopolysaccharidoses, osteogenesis imperfecta, osteomalacia, cleidocranial dysplasia). Basilar invagination may produce neural, CSF, or vascular compromise. There may be an associated Chiari I malformation, hydrocephalus, or hydrosyringomyelia.

Klippel-Feil Anomaly and Syndrome

The Klippel-Feil *anomaly*, which results from failure of segmentation, manifests as bony fusion of the cervical spine at one or more levels (see Figs. 9-4 and 9-26). The triad of low posterior hairline, short webbed neck, and limitation of neck motion represents the Klippel-Feil *syndrome*. Sprengel's deformity of the scapula and a bridging omovertebral bone may also be present in Klippel-Feil syndrome. Other associated anomalies are genitourinary, cardiac, and musculoskeletal (e.g., limbs and digits). The spinal involvement may include posterior element abnormalities, occipitalization of the atlas, basilar impression, dens anomalies, and scoliosis. Chiari I malformation, hydrosyringomyelia, neurenteric cyst, or diastematomyelia may occur. Hypermobility and instability at unfused segments and early degenerative disease may lead to foraminal or spinal canal stenosis, osteophytic spurs, subluxation, facet arthropathy, or disk herniation.

Occipitalization of the Atlas

Occipitalization of the atlas refers to complete or partial fusion of the atlas to the occiput, which may be bony or fibrous (see Fig. 9-26). Usually, the anterior arch is assimilated into the anterior rim of the foramen magnum. The involvement may also include the posterior arch or lateral masses. Associated anomalies are odontoid hypoplasia, basilar invagination, AA instability, and Klippel-Feil anomaly.

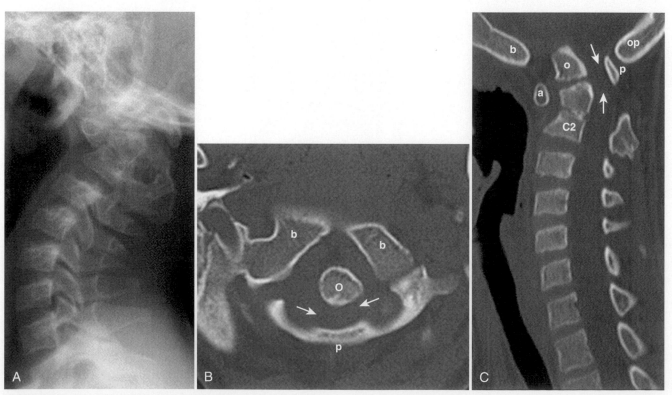

FIGURE 9-23. Lateral plain film/computerized radiograph (**A**), axial CT scan (**B**), and sagittal reformatted CT scan (**C**) showing Down syndrome with hypoplastic dens, os odontoideum (o), atlantoaxial instability, and post-dental canal stenosis (*short arrows*) with probable cord compression; C2, axis; a, anterior arch of atlas; p, posterior arch of atlas; b, basion; op, opisthion.

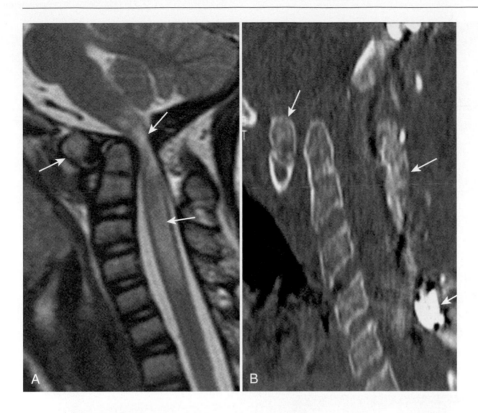

FIGURE 9-24. A, Sagittal T2-weighted MR image showing Down syndrome with hypoplastic dens, os odontoideum (*anterior arrow*), and atlantoaxial dislocation with high-intensity cervical spinal cord compressive injury (*posterior arrows*). **B,** Sagittal postoperative reformatted CT scan shows the stabilized anomaly, including the os odontoideum (*upper arrow*), decompressed canal, and metallic instrumentation plus bony fusion (*posterior arrows*).

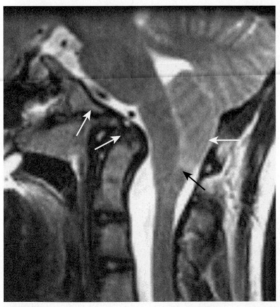

FIGURE 9-25. Basilar invagination and Chiari I malformation on sagittal T2-weighted MR image with short clivus and high dens (*anterior arrows*) plus low tonsils and low cervicomedullary junction (*posterior arrows*).

Odontoid Anomalies

Anomalies of the odontoid include aplasia, hypoplasia, and the os odontoideum (see Figs. 9-23 and 9-24). Aplasia is rare and causes severe AA dislocation. Hypoplasia leads to a short dens. Os odontoideum is a proatlas remnant or represents hypertrophy of the ossiculum terminale. Usually, there is odontoid hypoplasia, and the ossicle is located near the dens tip or the basion and lacks a normal dens fusion line. Hypertrophy of the anterior arch and hypoplasia or clefting of the posterior arch are often present. AA or occipitoaxial instability commonly occurs. Odontoid anomalies may be idiopathic or may be associated with skeletal dysplasias such as Morquio syndrome, Down syndrome, SED, and Klippel-Feil anomaly.

Craniocervical Instability

Craniocervical instability includes translational or rotary AA instability and AO instability. Craniocervical instability often results from ligamentous deficiency or insufficiency (e.g., transverse ligament in AA instabilities) and is commonly associated with odontoid anomalies (as discussed earlier). AA and AO instabilities most commonly occur with Down syndrome (see Figs. 9-23 and 9-24). Other common causes are the skeletal dysplasias (e.g., Morquio syndrome, SED), rheumatoid arthritis, and trauma. Rotary AA instability includes displacement, subluxation, or dislocation and produces torticollis. It may be spontaneous or related to trauma, infection, or CCJ anomalies (e.g., odontoid anomalies, Klippel-Feil anomaly).

Spinal Vascular Anomalies

Vascular anomalies of childhood may involve the paraspinal soft tissues, bony spinal column, spinal neuraxis, meninges, or multiple structures. The Mulliken and Glowacki biologic classification categorizes cutaneous and muscular vascular anomalies as vascular malformations (e.g., lymphatic, venous, arteriovenous), vascular tumors (i.e., hemangiomas), or angiodysplastic syndromes. These are covered in greater detail in Chapter 10. Vascular anomalies of the CNS have traditionally been classified as arteriovenous malformations (AVMs), developmental venous anomalies, cavernous malformations, telangiectasias, and aneurysms; these are covered in Chapter 8.

Intradural spinal vascular anomalies are usually AVMs or arteriovenous fistulae (AVFs) and are classified according to the anatomic site of origin or involvement. They may be classified as spinal cord AVMs (intramedullary), spinal dural AVFs, or metameric AVMs (Cobb syndrome), the last involving any or all layers of a spinal segment from the spinal cord to the skin. In spinal

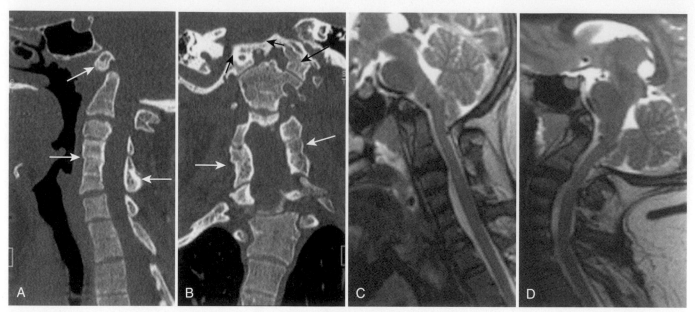

FIGURE 9-26. Sagittal (**A**) and coronal (**B**) reformatted CT scans showing Klippel-Feil anomaly, occipitalization of the atlas, and cervical spinal stenosis, including fused cervical segments (*lower arrows*), fusion of atlas to the occiput (*upper black arrows*), and a small foramen magnum and C1 canal. Flexion (**C**) and extension (**D**) T2-weighted sagittal MR images show no translational craniocervical instability.

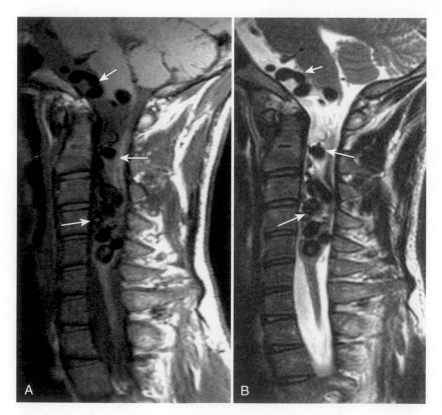

FIGURE 9-27. Cervical spinal cord arteriovenous malformation with high-flow vascular low intensities (*arrows*) on sagittal T1-weighted (**A**) and T2-weighted (**B**) MR images.

AVMs that are "high-flow" malformations, MRI may show nodular, serpiginous signal voids without tumor parenchyma, hemorrhage (subarachnoid or intramedullary), cord edema, infarct, myelomalacia, syrinx, or atrophy (Fig. 9-27). Spinal AVFs may be "high-flow" or "low-flow" malformations. Spinal angiography is necessary for full evaluation of the vascular anomaly in anticipation of surgery or interventional therapy. Cavernous angiomas of the spinal cord are rare and may manifest as hemorrhage (subarachnoid or intramedullary) or myelopathy.

■ ACQUIRED ABNORMALITIES

Trauma

Spinal Fractures

Spinal fractures occur less commonly in childhood than in adulthood and may be related to vehicular accidents, falls, diving, sports, recreation, or child abuse. In infants and young children the injuries are usually upper cervical. Owing to the relative larger head size, spinal immaturity, and higher fulcrum for

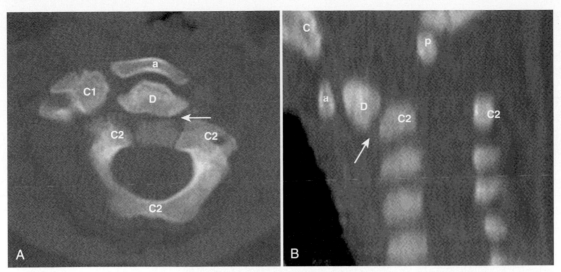

FIGURE 9-28. Infant dens fracture type 2 (*arrows*) with anterior atlantoaxial displacement/dislocation on axial (**A**) and sagittal (**B**) reformatted CT scans; a, anterior arch of C1; C, clivus; C1, atlas; C2, axis; D, dens; p, posterior arch of C1.

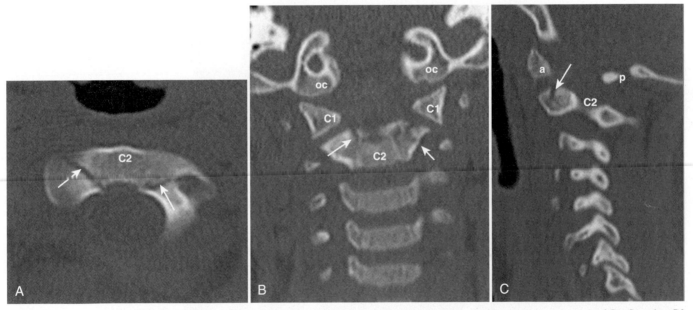

FIGURE 9-29. Hangman's C2 fracture (*arrows*) on axial (**A**), coronal (**B**), and parasagittal (**C**) reformatted CT scans; a, anterior arch of C1; C1, atlas; C2, axis; oc, occipital condyles; p, posterior arch of C1.

flexion-extension (above C2-C3), injuries in infants and young children are usually upper cervical. The spectrum includes fractures of the synchondroses of the atlas, axis, or dens and AA or occipitoatlantal (OA) dislocations (Figs. 9-28 to 9-30). After closure of the synchondroses by 8 to 10 years of age, the fulcrum shifts caudally and injuries tend to occur at the mid- to lower cervical levels (adult pattern). In the patient with spine injury, PF/CR may be performed initially with the patient properly immobilized. However, CT (e.g., MDCT) with sagittal and coronal reformatting has become the standard. MRI (with STIR) is used for further evaluation to assess for intraspinal hematoma, spinal cord injury, or ligamentous damage (Fig. 9-31).

Spinal Injury

Spinal injury results from one or a combination of basic mechanisms. *Hyperflexion* may lead to posterior ligamentous sprain, bilateral or unilateral interfacet dislocation, compression fracture,

clay shoveler fracture, flexion teardrop fracture, dens fractures (see Fig. 9-28), or lateral mass fractures of C1 or C2 (i.e., lateral flexion). *Hyperextension* may lead to anterior ligamentous sprain, avulsion fracture of the anterior arch of the atlas, C1 posterior arch fracture, extension C2 teardrop fracture, laminar fracture, hangman's fracture (i.e., traumatic C2 spondylolisthesis; see Fig. 9-29), pillar fracture, odontoid fracture, or pedicle or lamina fracture. *Axial compression* may produce Jefferson C1 fracture or burst fracture of the vertebral bodies. *Distraction forces* may result in AA or AO disassociation or chance fractures. *Translational or rotary injury* may produce AA or AO subluxation/dislocation, unilateral or bilateral facet subluxation, or fracture/dislocation (see Fig. 9-30).

Spinal injury in *neonates and young infants* may occur with birth (e.g., breech delivery), accidents, falls, or child abuse. These injuries occur primarily in the cervical spine and may result in fractures of the neurocentral synchondroses or dens

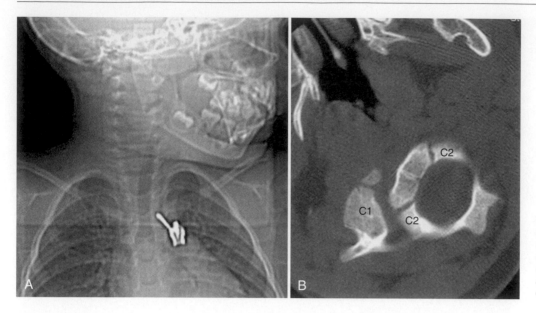

Figure 9-30. Painful torticollis on frontal plain film/computerized radiograph (**A**). Rotary C1 to C2 fixation/subluxation on axial CT scan (**B**), which also shows clockwise offset of C1 lateral mass relative to C2 lateral mass.

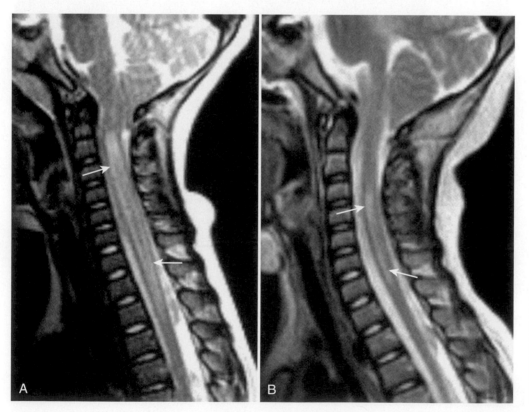

Figure 9-31. Sagittal T2-weighted MR images showing Chiari I malformation with trauma and acute hyperintense cervical cord edema (*arrows* in **A**) followed by chronic hyperintense syrinx formation (*arrows* in **B**). The differential diagnosis includes myelitis, demyelination, and ischemia, with tumor less likely.

as well as dislocations of the AO or AA articulations (see Figs. 9-28 and 9-29). Occasionally there may be an associated epidural, subdural, or subarachnoid hemorrhage. Spinal cord injury without radiographic abnormality (SCIWORA), which may occur with reversible spinal column dislocation, includes contusion, edema, avulsion, or transaction (see Fig. 9-31). Because of injury to the cervicomedullary junction, there may be respiratory arrest with otherwise unexplained hypoxic-ischemic brain injury (Fig. 9-32). PF/CR and CT findings are often negative, and MRI is needed for the diagnosis. Brachial plexus injury (e.g., shoulder dystocia) may lead to Erb palsy or Klumpke paralysis. As a result, dural tear with CSF leakage may be associated with nerve root laceration and pseudomeningocele formation.

In *older infants and children up to age 8 years*, injuries to the cervical spine also often result in fractures of the apophyses and synchondroses, including avulsions and separations of the dens, axis body, and atlas ring. The Jefferson fracture represents axial compression fractures of the anterior and posterior C1 arches, often with outward displacement of the articular masses. Less common C1 fractures include posterior arch fractures and anterior arch avulsions. Odontoid fractures occur often at the subdental synchondrosis (type 2) and less commonly at the tip (type 1) or axis body (type 3). Hangman's fracture is a bilateral hyperextension

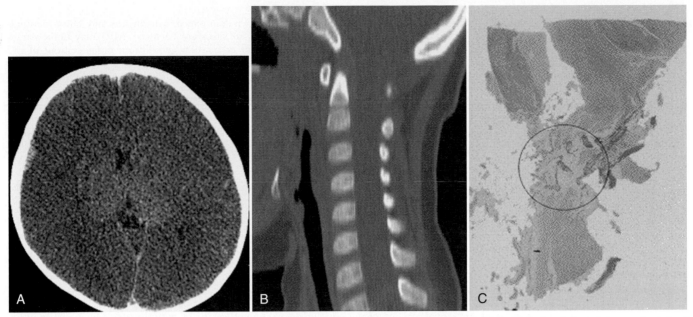

FIGURE 9-32. Spinal cord injury without radiographic abnormality (SCIWORA). **A,** axial CT scan shows hypoxic-ischemic brain injury and subdural hemorrhage. **B,** Findings on cervical spine CT scan are negative. **C,** Postmortem microsection shows partial cervicomedullary transection (*circle*).

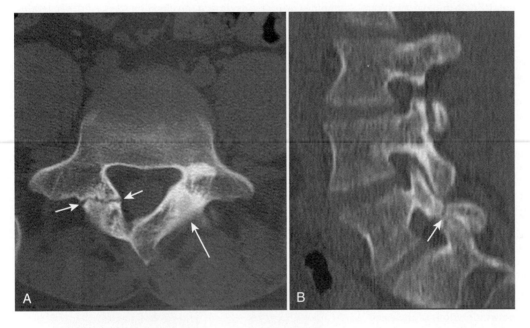

FIGURE 9-33. Spondylolysis on axial (**A**) and reformatted parasagittal (**B**) CT scans, with a hypodense pars defect on the right (*short arrows*) and more hyperdense sclerosis on the left (*long arrow*).

fracture of the C2 pars interarticularis. AA or AO instability may be associated with these fractures. AA and AO dislocations may also occur without obvious fracture and may be associated with severe spinal cord injury. In the *juvenile and adolescent*, cervical spine injuries tend to follow the adult patterns. Thoracolumbar spinal injury also occurs in childhood. The spectrum includes compression or chance fractures (horizontal body and neural arch fracture) associated with hyperflexion seat belt trauma, and axial burst fractures from falls.

Spinal Cord Injury
Spinal cord injury, including cord compression from spinal malalignment, bony fragments, disk herniation, and intraspinal hematoma, is best assessed with MRI. STIR imaging is particularly helpful in demonstrating ligamentous injury. Cord injury includes contusion, hemorrhage, edema, avulsion, and transection (see Fig. 9-31). MRI also assesses chronic sequelae, such as posttraumatic

cyst or syringomyelia, myelomalacia, arachnoiditis, arachnoid cyst, and neuroarthropathy (see Fig. 9-31).

Spondylolysis and Spondylolisthesis
Pars interarticularis defects (i.e., spondylolysis) are a common cause of back pain in childhood. Anterior slippage of the upper vertebral body upon the lower one (i.e., spondylolisthesis) is a common complication. Bilateral in most cases, spondylolysis usually occurs at L5 or L4. Although it is often associated with repetitive trauma, a developmental predisposition is likely. A dysplastic type is characterized by hypoplasia/aplasia of the L5 neural arch and S1 apophyseal joints. The extent of slippage may be assigned as Meyerding grade 1 (up to 33%), grade 2 (up to 66%), grade 3 (up to 99%), or grade 4 (100% with spondyloptosis). Although these problems are often detected by plain films or RI (e.g., SPECT), CT is preferred for complete evaluation (Fig. 9-33). MRI helps evaluate for other, or additional, causes of back pain (e.g., disk herniation, synovial cyst).

Disk Herniations and Calcifications

Herniations usually occur in adolescence from trauma (e.g., athletic activity) and are best shown by MRI. These usually arise at L4-L5 or L5-S1 and may be associated with a slipped vertebral apophysis. CT best shows the latter. Disk calcification in childhood is rare and usually of unknown etiology. It occurs mostly in boys at the cervical or thoracic level. Symptoms include pain, stiffness, and decreased motion. Anterior or posterior herniation may also occur. Although possibly detected by plain film, it is best evaluated with CT and MRI.

Infection and Inflammation

Infection may involve the disk, vertebral body, paravertebral soft tissues, epidural space, meninges, or spinal neuraxis. Infectious processes occurring during childhood include spondylitis (diskitis, vertebral osteomyelitis), sacroiliac pyarthrosis, epidural abscess or empyema, meningitis, arachnoiditis, myelitis, and spinal cord abscess. These are all best evaluated with MRI.

Infectious Spondylitis

Infectious spondylitis in childhood is most often of hematogenous origin but may also arise from contiguous spread or direct inoculation. The infecting agent is usually bacterial (e.g., *Staphylococcus aureus*) or viral. The immature and highly vascularized disk is often initially involved (i.e., diskitis). Extension with vertebral end plate involvement (i.e., osteomyelitis) is common. The lumbar level is the most common site. PF/CR findings are often negative in early infection, but results of bone scan (e.g., SPECT) may be positive. CT is more sensitive than PF/CR, but MRI is the choice for complete evaluation and as a guide for subsequent abscess aspiration or biopsy by CT. Disk space narrowing, end plate irregularities or erosions, and sclerosis may be present on CT. Additional MRI findings are T1 hypointensity, T2 hyperintensity, and gadolinium enhancement within the disk, vertebral body, and paraspinal soft tissues (Fig. 9-34). There may be an associated epidural or paraspinal abscess, or, rarely, meningitis. Sequelae include disk degeneration, vertebral destruction, osseous bridging, scoliosis, kyphosis, and Schmorl nodes.

Granulomatous spondylitis usually results from *Mycobacterium* tuberculosis, with a predilection for children from underserved or developing areas. Thoracolumbar involvement is common and may be primary or secondary (spread from other organs). Insidious onset and gradual progression are characteristic. Imaging shows anterior vertebral erosion or extensive vertebral destruction, with or without disk loss, paraspinal masses (granuloma, abscess), and calcification (Fig. 9-35). Progression to kyphosis with gibbus deformity may also be present.

Sacroiliac Pyarthrosis

Pyogenic arthritis (e.g., due to *S. aureus* infection) of the sacroiliac joint may rarely occur during late childhood and may progress to ankylosis if treatment is delayed. It may be primary or an extension from contiguous osteomyelitis of the sacrum or ileum. The presentation is often nonspecific, consisting only of back, hip, or limb pain. PF/CR findings are often negative early, but bone scan results are usually positive. MRI provides definitive evaluation.

Epidural Abscess

Epidural abscess is uncommon in childhood. It may be hematogenous in origin or may arise as a direct extension from suppurative spondylitis (e.g., due to *S. aureus*). MRI demonstrates an extradural soft tissue mass that may extend over several segments. The collection is often T1-isointense to hypointense, and T2-hyperintense. Diffuse homogeneous enhancement corresponds with phlegmon. Rim enhancement represents a necrotic abscess. Associated findings of spondylitis (described earlier) may be present.

Meningitis

Bacterial, fungal, viral, or parasitic organisms may cause meningitis. The majority of cases are bacterial. MRI may demonstrate nonspecific, linear or nodular gadolinium enhancement of the meninges, spinal cord, or nerve roots (Fig. 9-36). Similar findings may be seen with neoplastic seeding (e.g., medulloblastoma).

Arachnoiditis

Arachnoiditis may occur after infection, subarachnoid hemorrhage, intraspinal injection (e.g., for anesthesia, chemotherapy), surgery, or trauma. MRI shows nerve root thickening and clumping, often with enhancement, and occasionally a mass (see Fig. 9-36). There may be associated hydrosyringomyelia or arachnoid cysts.

Myelitis

Myelitis, which refers to spinal cord inflammation, is often viral. Viruses associated with myelitis include herpesvirus, coxsackievirus, poliovirus, and human immunodeficiency virus. Myelitis may also be post-viral or post-vaccinial, as with acute disseminated encephalomyelitis (ADEM). Other rare causes of inflammatory myelopathy in childhood include autoimmune demyelination (e.g., multiple sclerosis) and vasculitis (e.g., systemic lupus erythematosus); it may also arise as a complication of systemic malignancy, chemotherapy, or radiotherapy. Devic syndrome is the association of myelitis with optic neuritis (see Chapter 8). MRI findings include intramedullary T2 hyperintensity, cord expansion, and enhancement. The differential diagnosis for such findings includes myelitis, demyelination (e.g., ADEM), trauma, ischemia, and tumor (see Fig. 9-31).

Spinal Cord Abscess

Although rare, spinal cord abscess may occur by direct spread (e.g., dermal sinus; see Fig. 9-10), remotely by hematogenous or lymphatic spread, or in the immune-compromised child.

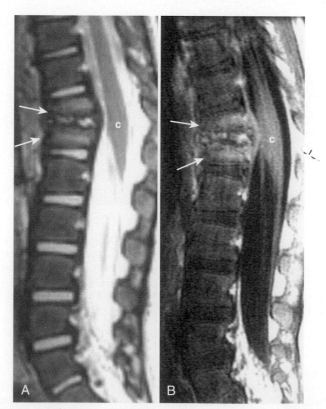

FIGURE 9-34. Sagittal T2-weighted (**A**) and gadolinium-enhanced T1-weighted (**B**) MR images show suppurative thoracolumbar diskitis/osteomyelitis (*arrows*) with disk space and end plate involvement plus T2-weighted hyperintensity and enhancement; c, conus medullaris.

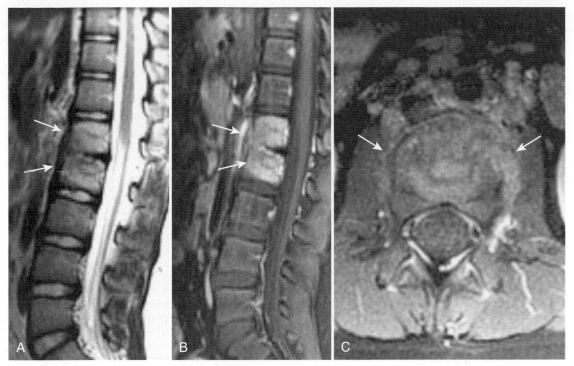

FIGURE 9-35. Lumbar tuberculous spondylitis. Sagittal T2-weighted (**A**) and gadolinium-enhanced sagittal (**B**) and axial (**C**) T1-weighted MR images show disk space narrowing, end plate irregularity, and vertebral T2-weighted hyperintensity plus enhancement (*arrows*).

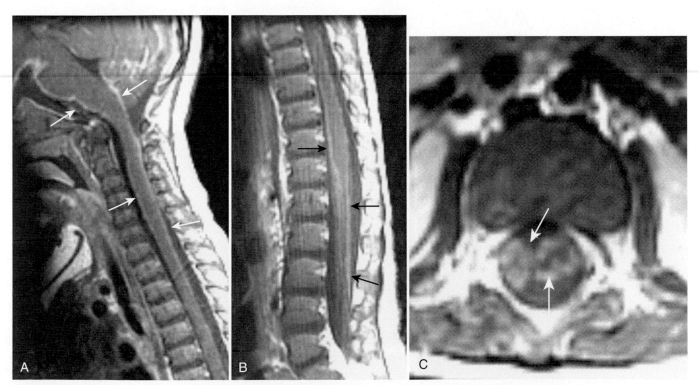

FIGURE 9-36. Tuberculous meningitis with intracranial and intraspinal involvement on sagittal (**A** and **B**) and axial (**C**) gadolinium-enhanced T1-weighted MR images, which show enhancement (*arrows*) along the brainstem, spinal cord, and nerve roots.

Neoplastic Conditions

Spinal tumors may be classified compartmentally (Table 9-1) as extradural (e.g., paraspinal, parameningeal), intradural (i.e., intrathecal, extramedullary), or intramedullary (i.e., spinal cord).

Extradural Tumors

Extradural, or parameningeal, tumors arise from the spinal column or paraspinal soft tissues. These tumors may spread to the spinal canal directly, by epidural venous extension, or by

TABLE 9-1. Neoplastic Spinal Lesions

Extradural tumors	Osteoid osteoma
	Osteoblastoma
	Osteochondroma
	Aneurysmal bone cyst
	Giant cell tumor
	Langerhans cell histiocytosis
	Leukemia and lymphoma
	Rhabdomyosarcoma
	Ewing sarcoma
	Fibromatosis
	Osteosarcoma
	Chondrosarcoma
	Chordoma
	Neuroblastoma
	Ganglioneuroblastoma
	Ganglioneuroma
	Primitive neuroectodermal tumor (PNET)
	Plexiform neurofibroma
	Metastases
Intradural (extramedullary) tumors	Schwannoma and neurofibroma
	Neoplastic seeding
	Developmental tumors
	Meningeal tumors (rare)
Intramedullary tumors	Astrocytoma
	Ganglioglioma
	Ependymoma
	Mixed glioma
	Glioblastoma
	PNET
	Hemangioblastoma
	Metastases

hematogenous, lymphatic, or CSF dissemination. This category includes benign and malignant bone and soft tissue tumors or tumor-like conditions of mesenchymal, neural crest, primitive neuroepithelial, and metastatic origins. In addition to CT and MRI, PET (e.g., PET-CT) and other nuclear imaging techniques are very helpful in the initial and follow-up evaluations of many of these tumors.

Benign Tumors of Mesenchymal Origin

Osteoid osteoma is a benign tumor with osteoid matrix and a fibrovascular nidus. A small percentage arise in the spine—most often lumbar, less often thoracic, and least often cervical—and manifest as pain, tenderness, and scoliosis. Neural arch involvement is typical. Plain films or CT may show a radiolucent nidus with calcification and surrounding sclerosis (Fig. 9-37). Increased radionuclide uptake is seen on bone scan. MRI may show extensive bone edema (T1-hypointense, T2-hyperintense), sclerosis or calcification (T1- and T2-hypointense), and the nidus (T1-isointense to hypointense, T2-hypointense or hyperintense, gadolinium-enhancing). The lesion may be treated by surgical excision or interventional ablation.

Osteoblastoma, also known as giant osteoid osteoma (> 2 cm), has a fibrovascular matrix with sclerotic osteoid mesenchyme and giant cells. It commonly occurs in the spine (e.g., cervical), is usually solitary, and typically involves the posterior elements. PF/CR or CT may show an expansile lytic lesion with bone matrix or calcific flecks. MRI shows T1 isointensity or hypointensity, T2 heterogeneity, and occasional hemorrhage. Treatment may be interventional therapy (e.g., embolization), surgical excision, or radiotherapy (e.g., for recurrence).

Osteochondroma is a benign osteocartilaginous exostosis that rarely occurs in the spine (e.g., cervical or thoracic posterior elements). It may be multiple (e.g., hereditary multiple osteochondromas). PF/CR or CT may show a bony projection with cartilaginous cap. MRI shows associated T1 isointensity or hyperintensity and T2 hyperintensity. Treatment is primarily surgical. Malignant degeneration (e.g., osteosarcoma or chondrosarcoma)

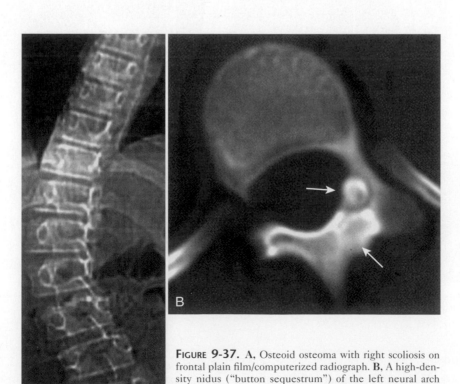

FIGURE 9-37. A, Osteoid osteoma with right scoliosis on frontal plain film/computerized radiograph. **B,** A high-density nidus ("button sequestrum") of the left neural arch with low-density collar and surrounding sclerosis (*arrows*) on axial CT scan.

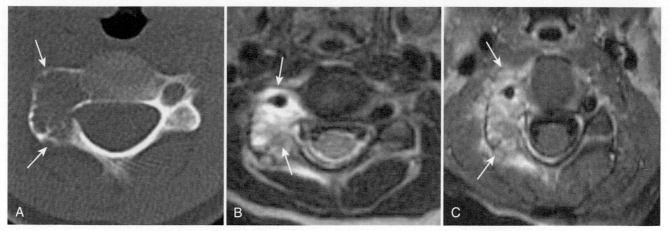

FIGURE 9-38. Aneurysmal bone cyst (*arrows*) of C3 neural arch on axial CT scan (**A**) and T2-weighted (**B**) and gadolinium-enhanced T1-weighted (**C**) MR images, which show lytic expansion, fluid levels, extensive enhancement, and vertebral artery involvement.

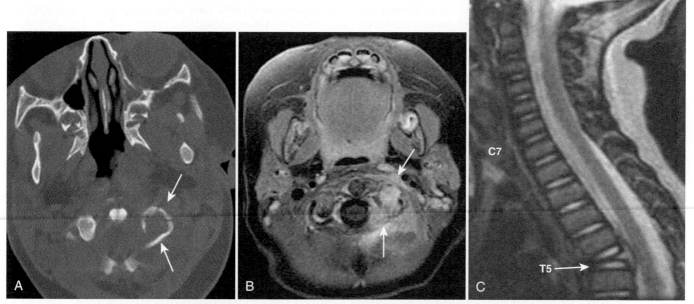

FIGURE 9-39. A, Axial CT scan shows a left C1 lateral mass lytic lesion in a patient with Langerhans cell histiocytosis with torticollis. **B,** Axial gadolinium-enhanced T1-weighted MR image shows lesion enhancement. **C,** Sagittal T2-weighted MR image shows T5 "vertebra planum" deformity (*arrow*).

is indicated by additional soft tissue mass, marrow involvement, a disorganized cap, or increased enhancement.

Aneurysmal bone cyst is a nonneoplastic bone lesion of non–endothelium-lined cavities filled with blood elements. It occasionally arises within the spine and tends to involve the posterior elements and adjacent vertebral body (Fig. 9-38). The cyst often expands into the paraspinal soft tissues or spinal canal. Aneurysmal bone cyst may occur with other lesions (e.g., giant cell tumor, osteoblastoma, chondroblastoma, nonossifying fibroma, fibrous dysplasia). PF/CR or CT may show an expansile lytic lesion with peripheral shell-like calcification and fluid-fluid levels. MRI additionally demonstrates variable intensities with varying stages of hemorrhage. Treatment is often a combination of intervention (i.e., embolization) and surgery (excision).

Giant cell tumor is an osteoclastoma composed of multinucleated giant cells, a fibroblastic stroma, and prominent vascularity. It rarely occurs in the spine (e.g., the sacrum). PF/CR or CT may show a lytic, expansile bone lesion breaking through the cortex. MRI additionally shows T1 isointensity or hypointensity, T2 isointensity or hyperintensity, associated hemorrhage or cysts, and gadolinium enhancement. Treatment is similar to that for other lesions mentioned here (e.g., osteoblastoma).

Malignant Tumors of Mesenchymal Origin

The subcategory malignant tumors or mesenchymal origin broadly includes the malignant "round cell tumors" of childhood that primarily or secondarily involve the reticuloendothelial system (e.g., Langerhans cell histiocytosis, leukemia, lymphoma, rhabdomyosarcoma, Ewing sarcoma, primitive neuroectodermal tumor [PNET], neuroblastoma). The round cell tumors have similar imaging patterns, including focal, multifocal, or diffuse involvement (e.g., marrow infiltration). Treatment for tumors in this category usually requires some combination of chemotherapy, radiotherapy, and surgery.

Langerhans cell histiocytosis describes a series of diseases characterized by abnormal histiocytes. One of the more classic forms of the disease is formerly known as "eosinophilic granuloma," which is seen in young children and often involves the lumbar and thoracic spine. PF/CR or CT may show circumscribed lytic lesions within the vertebral bodies or vertebral body collapse (i.e., vertebra plana), often without much of a soft tissue component (Fig. 9-39). Occasionally, a soft tissue mass extends into the spinal canal. MRI shows additional T1 isointensity or hypointensity, T2 hyperintensity, and gadolinium enhancement, especially with use of fat suppression (see Fig. 9-39).

Leukemia is the most common malignancy of childhood (e.g., acute lymphoblastic and acute monoblastic forms). There may be complications related to bone marrow infiltration, leukemic meningitis, or leukemic masses (chloromas). As with other round cell tumors, PF/CR may demonstrate diffuse bone marrow infiltration as osteopenia, permeative lytic destruction, or lucent bands. MRI of round cell tumors may additionally show hypercellular marrow infiltration as T1-hypointense and T2-isointense to hyperintense with gadolinium enhancement. In younger patients, it may be difficult to distinguish tumor infiltration of marrow from the hematopoietically active red marrow (also T1-hypointense, T2-isointense to hyperintense, and enhancing). Conversion to yellow marrow (increased fat content, therefore T1-hyperintense) occurs with increasing age as well as with the myelosuppressive effects of radiotherapy and chemotherapy. Marrow infiltration may then be more readily detected until there is red marrow rebound after therapeutic response (including after bone marrow transplantation). A mottled marrow pattern may represent combined tumor and treatment effects. Fat-suppression T2-weighted techniques (e.g., STIR) and fat suppression combined with gadolinium-enhanced T1-weighted sequences increase sensitivity and specificity for tumor (i.e., marked enhancement). CT may show chloromas as isodense to hyperdense, markedly enhancing masses that may be associated with bone destruction. MRI often demonstrates chloromas as T1-isointense to hypointense, T2-isointense to hypointense (or hyperintense), and markedly enhancing.

Lymphoma (Hodgkin and non-Hodgkin forms) may be focal, multifocal, or diffuse and may have imaging patterns similar to those of other round cell tumors (see Chapter 10). PET-CT is especially helpful for the initial and follow-up evaluations of lymphomas.

Rhabdomyosarcoma, one of the most common solid tumors of childhood, frequently occurs in the first decade (see Chapter 10). This tumor may involve the paraspinal soft tissues or spinal column as a mass, or may represent lymphatic or hematogenous metastasis to the bone marrow. PF/CR, CT, and MRI findings are similar to those for other round cell tumors.

Ewing sarcoma arises from the primitive reticulum stem cell (bone marrow origin) and is a common tumor of childhood. It most often occurs in the second decade as either a primary bone lesion or an extraosseous soft tissue mass with round cell infiltration. PF/CR or CT may show permeative lytic bone destruction. MRI demonstrates additional T1 hypointensity, T2 hypointensity or hyperintensity, and enhancement, especially on fat-suppression images.

Juvenile fibromatosis, an infiltrating process characterized by fibroelastic proliferation, may be focal or diffuse. A congenital form is diffuse with visceral and bone lesions. The juvenile form usually involves the musculoskeletal system. MRI shows a soft tissue mass or masses (T1-isointense to hypointense, T2-isointense to hypointense or hyperintense, with gadolinium enhancement, with use of fat-suppression techniques), that extends along tissue planes and may have bony involvement.

Other "Malignant" Tumors of Mesenchymal Origin

Osteosarcoma is an osteoid-forming neoplasm and the most common primary bone neoplasm of childhood. Subtypes include osteoblastic, chondroblastic, telangiectatic, and fibroblastic. Spinal involvement is infrequent and may be metastatic. In some cases it may be radiation-induced or may arise from an existing lesion (e.g., osteochondroma). PF/CR or CT may show a lytic, sclerotic, or mixed lesion. On MRI, intensity characteristics and enhancement vary according to the extent of tumor ossification. Treatment includes surgery, chemotherapy, and radiotherapy.

Chondrosarcoma is a bone neoplasm of cartilage origin that may originate from an existing lesion (e.g., osteochondroma). PF/CR or CT may show lytic involvement with calcific rings or nodules. MRI may additionally show a heterogenous pattern of T1 and T2 intensities and enhancement.

Chordomas arise from notochordal remnants and are most commonly found in the clivus and sacrum. They are uncommon in childhood. PF/CR or CT shows a lytic lesion with calcification and soft tissue mass. MRI demonstrates additional T1 isointensity or hypointensity, T2 hyperintensity, and enhancement, particularly with use of fat suppression techniques. Treatment includes surgery and radiotherapy.

Tumors of Neural Crest Origin

The spinal tumors of neural crest origin include neuroblastoma, ganglioneuroblastoma, ganglioneuroma, nerve sheath tumors, meningeal tumors, and PNETs. The first three tumors in the

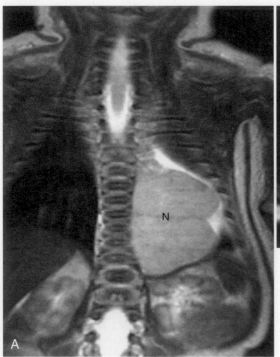

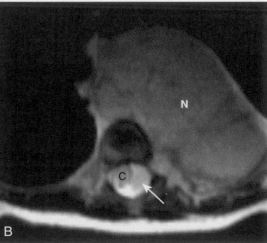

FIGURE 9-40. Infant neuroblastoma (N) on coronal (**A**) and axial (**B**) T2-weighted MR image with large left posterior mediastinal mass, thoracic intraspinal extension (*arrow*), and displacement of the spinal cord (**C**).

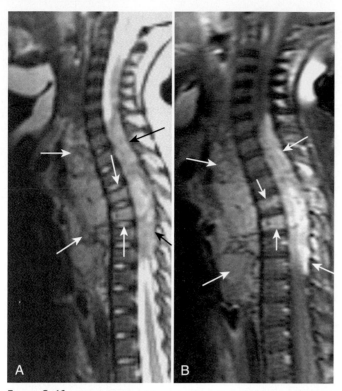

FIGURE 9-41. Thoracic neuroblastoma on sagittal T2-weighted MR image (**A**) and gadolinium-enhanced T1-weighted MR image with fat suppression (**B**). Images show a T2-weighted hyperintense and enhancing posterior mediastinal and paraspinal mass (*anterior long arrows*), intraspinal extension (*posterior long arrows*), and marrow involvement (*vertical arrows*).

previous sentence are listed, and discussed here, in order from "malignant to benign."

Neuroblastoma is the most common solid, non-CNS tumor of childhood (Figs. 9-40 and 9-41). It is composed of neuroblasts and arises within the sympathetic nervous system (e.g., paraspinal sympathetic chain, adrenal medulla, carotid body, aortic bodies, organ of Zuckerkandl). Hematogenous or lymphatic metastases to the spinal marrow often occur. Epidural and transforaminal extension may lead to cord compression. PF/CR or CT may show paraspinal masses with calcification and bony destruction. MRI may show additional T1 isointensity or hypointensity, T2 isointensity, hypointensity, or hyperintensity, and gadolinium enhancement, especially with use of fat suppression. Non-uniform intensities may be related to calcification, hemorrhage, edema, and necrosis. RI is also important because neuroblastoma tends to be avid in uptake of MIBG (iodine-131-meta-iodobenzylguanidine). Neuroblastoma may mature to one of the more benign forms.

Ganglioneuroblastoma is intermediate in malignancy. It contains both mature ganglion cells and immature neuroblast cells. Its behavior may be similar to that of neuroblastoma, including metastases and spinal canal extension.

Ganglioneuroma is a benign tumor consisting of mature ganglion cells. It commonly originates in the posterior mediastinum as a paraspinal mass. PF/CR, CT, or MRI may show a paraspinal mass that is often calcified and enhances. There may be foraminal and intraspinal extension with widening.

Nerve sheath tumors include plexiform neurofibroma (i.e., NF-1; Fig 9-42; see Fig. 9-19), neurofibroma, schwannoma, and malignant nerve sheath tumors. PNETs are rare, extra-CNS neoplasms of primitive neuroepithelial origin. Imaging findings are similar to those for other round cell tumors, including soft tissue mass, bone destruction, and calcification (as discussed earlier).

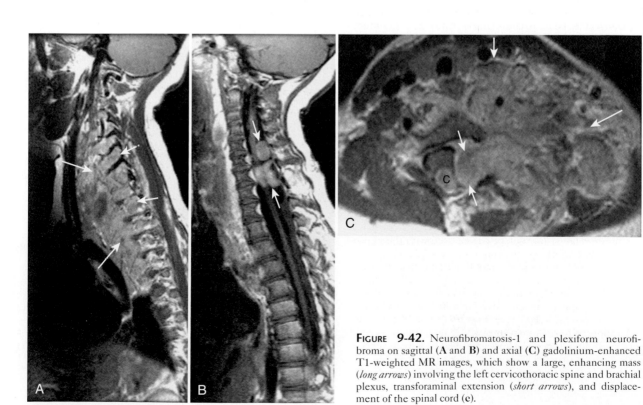

FIGURE 9-42. Neurofibromatosis-1 and plexiform neurofibroma on sagittal (**A** and **B**) and axial (**C**) gadolinium-enhanced T1-weighted MR images, which show a large, enhancing mass (*long arrows*) involving the left cervicothoracic spine and brachial plexus, transforaminal extension (*short arrows*), and displacement of the spinal cord (**c**).

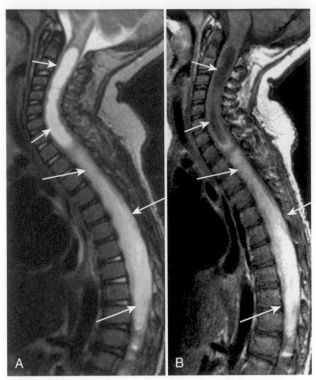

FIGURE 9-43. Cervicothoracic spinal cord astrocytoma on sagittal T2-weighted (**A**) and gadolinium-enhanced T1-weighted (**B**) MR images, which show a T2-hyperintense, enhancing tumor (*long arrows*) with a nonenhancing cystic component (*short arrows*).

Spinal Column Metastases

Metastases to the spinal column are rare in childhood but may occur with rhabdomyosarcoma, neuroblastoma, leukemia, lymphoma, histiocytosis, osteosarcoma, Ewing sarcoma, Wilms tumor, PNET, medulloblastoma, or retinoblastoma. PF/CR or CT may show focal lytic or sclerotic bone destruction (e.g., pathologic fracture), which may be associated with a paraspinal or epidural mass. There may be diffuse homogenous or inhomogeneous marrow involvement. Bone scan (e.g., SPECT) may also detect lesions, but MIBG scanning, PET-CT, or MRI may be more sensitive and specific, depending on the tumor type. MRI intensity and enhancement characteristics of spinal column metastases are similar to those described for round cell tumors.

Intradural (Extramedullary) Tumors

Intradural tumors arise within the dural sac and outside the spinal cord. This category includes tumors of nerve roots and nerve root sheaths (e.g., schwannomas, neurofibromas), neoplastic seeding, developmental tumors (discussed earlier), and meningeal tumors (rare in childhood). Schwannomas often occur sporadically in childhood. MRI shows a mass that is T1-isointense to hypointense and T2-hyperintense, with marked enhancement. Schwannomas and neurofibromas are also frequently associated with the neurofibromatoses (NF-1 or NF-2). Neurofibromas and plexiform neurofibromas consist of Schwann cells and fibroblasts and commonly occur in NF-1. Neurofibrosarcoma or malignant nerve sheath tumor may rarely occur. Extradural paraspinal and spinal involvement is common, including epidural foraminal and intraspinal extension or intradural origin (see Figs. 9-19 and 9-42). MRI shows T1 isointensity or hypointensity, T2 hyperintensity, and enhancement. A heterogenous appearance (e.g., target sign) is characteristic of plexiform neurofibroma. Spinal cord neoplasms are rare in NF-1 (e.g., astrocytoma). NF-2, which occurs more often in adolescence and adulthood, is associated with multiple spinal schwannomas, spinal cord ependymomas, and meningiomas.

Neoplastic seeding of the CSF in childhood occurs most commonly with medulloblastoma (see Chapter 8). Additional sources include other embryonal tumors (e.g., PNET, atypical teratoid rhabdoid tumor, pineoblastoma), germ cell tumors, ependymoma, and malignant glioma. Seeding may rarely occur with astrocytoma, choroid plexus tumors, lymphoma, leukemia, retinoblastoma, or rhabdomyosarcoma. MRI with gadolinium, the imaging modality of choice, may show single or multiple nodules, diffuse or patchy laminar deposits, irregular nerve root thickening or clumping, or subarachnoid space enhancement (see Chapter 8). Hemorrhagic or enhancing postoperative subdural or subarachnoid collections, and inflammatory or infectious processes may mimic neoplastic seeding.

Intramedullary Tumors

Intramedullary tumors arise within the spinal cord. The majority of the intramedullary tumors in childhood are astrocytomas and gangliogliomas, and fewer are ependymomas. Common presenting symptoms include pain, weakness, and scoliosis. MRI shows spinal cord expansion with T1 hypointensity and T2 isointensity and hyperintensity (Fig. 9-43). There may be associated edema, cysts, necrotic cavitation, or hydrosyringomyelia. The tumor often shows nodular or laminar gadolinium enhancement. Astrocytomas are often of low grade and may be circumscribed or infiltrating. Gangliogliomas and ependymomas are often more circumscribed. In childhood, ependymoma more commonly arises along the filum. It may be circumscribed or may infiltrate the conus medullaris and cauda equina nerve roots. Hemorrhage, hemosiderosis, or tumor seeding also occurs with ependymoma. Rarer intramedullary lesions of childhood include mixed gliomas, glioblastoma, PNET, hemangioblastoma (von Hippel–Lindau disease), and metastases (e.g., medulloblastoma via central canal).

▬ SUGGESTED READINGS

Ball W Jr: Pediatric Neuroradiology. Philadelphia, Lippincott-Raven, 1997.
Barkovich A: Pediatric Neuroimaging, ed 4. Philadelphia, Lippincott-Raven, 2005.
Blaser SI, Illner A, Castillo M, et al: Peds Neuro: 100 Top Diagnoses. (Pocket Radiologist.) Philadelphia, WB Saunders, 2003.
Harwood-Nash D, Fitz CR: Neuroradiology in Infants and Children. St. Louis, Mosby-Year Book, 1976.
Kirks DR: Practical Pediatric Imaging, ed 3. Philadelphia, Lippincott-Raven, 1998.
Kuhn JP, Slovis TL, Caffey J, Haller JO: Caffey's Pediatric Diagnostic Imaging. ed 10. New York, Elsevier Mosby Saunders, 2003.
Swischuk ME: Imaging of the Newborn, Infant, & Young Child, ed 5. Philadelphia, Lippincott Williams & Wilkins, 2003.
Tortori-Donati P, Rossi A: Pediatric Neuroradiology. New York, Springer, 2005.
van der Knaap MS, Valk J: Magnetic Resonance of Myelination and Myelin Disorders, ed 3. New York, Springer, 2005.
Volpe JJ: Neurology of the Newborn, ed 4. Philadelphia, WB Saunders, 2001.
Wolpert S, Barnes P: MRI in Pediatric Neuroradiology. St. Louis, Mosby-Year Book, 1992.
Zimmerman RA, Gibby WA, Carmody RF (eds): Neuroimaging: Clinical and Physical Principles, New York, Springer, 2000.

Articles and Monographs

Barkovich AJ, Naidich TP (eds): Pediatric Neuroradiology. Neuroimaging Clin North Am 1994;4(2).
Barnes PD (ed): Imaging of the Developing Brain. Top Magn Reson Imag 2007;18(1).
Edwards-Brown MK, Barnes PD (eds): Pediatric Neuroradiology. Neuroimaging Clin North Am 1999;9(1).
Mukherjee P (ed): Advanced Pediatric Imaging. Neuroimaging Clin North Am 2006;16(1).
Mukherji SK (ed): Pediatric Head and Neck Imaging. Neuroimaging Clin North Am 2000;10(1).

CHAPTER 10

Head and Neck Imaging

Patrick D. Barnes

The central nervous system (CNS) includes the skull, brain, spine, and spinal cord. The head and neck region includes the face, eye and orbit, nasal cavity and paranasal sinuses, ear and temporal bone, oral cavity, jaw, and neck. Modalities used for the imaging of the pediatric CNS and head and neck region include plain film/computerized radiography (PF/CR), ultrasonography (US), computed tomography (CT), multidetector CT (MDCT), magnetic resonance imaging (MRI), radionuclide imaging (RI), catheter angiography, and cerebrospinal fluid (CSF) imaging (e.g., CT myelography). Imaging modalities may be classified as structural or functional. Structural imaging modalities provide spatial resolution primarily on the basis of anatomic or morphologic data (e.g., CT). Functional imaging modalities (including molecular imaging) provide spatial resolution on the basis of physiologic, metabolic, or biologic data or markers (e.g., positron emission tomography [PET]). Some modalities may actually be considered to provide both structural and functional information (e.g., MRI, PET-CT). The technical and procedural descriptions for angiography, myelography, and other invasive and interventional modalities are detailed in other texts. In this chapter, guidelines for utilization are presented by region and modality.

▀ HEAD AND NECK IMAGING GUIDELINES

Plain Films and Computerized Radiography

PF/CR is only occasionally used for the initial assessment of facial, orbit, sinus, or jaw trauma (e.g., panoramic [Panorex] tomography), radiopaque foreign body, or sinus infection. For the face, orbits, and sinuses, the series usually includes straight and angled frontal views (e.g., Caldwell and Waters views, respectively) in the upright position (i.e., for air-fluid levels), and occasionally lateral views. PF/CR of the petrous temporal bone or mastoid is rarely needed (e.g., cochlear implant evaluation). This may include frontal, Towne, or angled lateral (Laws or Owens) views. Lateral neck PF/CR may be performed initially to assess upper airway abnormalities (e.g., infection) or, along with frontal neck and chest PF/CR, for foreign body ingestion or aspiration. Head and spine PF/CR is also part of the skeletal survey that may be used to assess for nonaccidental injury, skeletal dysplasia, or multiple congenital anomalies/deformities.

Ultrasonography

Real-time US is often very useful in evaluating head and neck masses with regard to size, location, and tissue characteristics. High-frequency (7.5- or 10-MHz) transducers permit the differentiation of solid from cystic elements and the detection of calcification. Oscillations may indicate the fluid nature of an apparently solid lesion (e.g., abscess). Doppler US imaging provides information about the extent of vascularity, flow direction, and pulsatility, and enables the differentiation of arterial from venous flow. This is particularly important in the assessment of vascular anomalies (e.g., hemangioma). US assessment of the thyroid gland is useful for detection and characterization of cysts and masses. Ocular US is primarily used in ophthalmology.

Computed Tomography

CT has for the most part replaced PF/CR as the primary modality for imaging of the pediatric head and neck region. In general, for imaging of the sinuses, orbits, facial bones, jaw, and temporal bones, axial and coronal (and occasionally sagittal) images using high-resolution, thin-section bone and soft tissue algorithms are necessary. This is best done using MDCT with reformatting as guided by initial frontal or lateral scout projection images.

For the most part, only nonenhanced CT is needed to delineate bony, air space, and soft tissue abnormalities. Furthermore, it is the definitive procedure for detecting and confirming calcification. Enhancement with intravenously administered contrast agents may be added or substituted to demonstrate normal vascular structures (e.g., CT angiography [CTA]), abnormal vascularity, or abnormal vascular permeability (e.g., inflammatory or neoplastic neovascularity), especially if intracranial extension is suspected. CT is preferred for evaluation of the facial bones (including the mandible and temporomandibular joint) and orbits, especially in facial trauma and craniofacial malformations, because it precisely demonstrates both bony and soft tissue structures, including the intraorbital and intracranial contents. Such an approach is particularly critical in the timely evaluation of the newborn in respiratory distress in whom nasochoanal stenosis/atresia is suspected. CT is also preferred for assessment of traumatic, neoplastic, and inflammatory involvement of the paranasal sinuses, particularly for its precise delineation of anatomy (e.g., ostiomeatal complex), bone destruction, and soft tissue changes (e.g., mucosal thickening, cyst, polyp, mucocele).

Ophthalmologic assessment and US often suffice for the evaluation of intraocular disease. However, CT and/or MRI is usually indicated for the assessment of an intraocular mass for diagnosis, extent, and treatment planning (e.g., retinoblastoma). Extraocular orbital lesions are often best evaluated first with high-resolution CT. This modality often provides definitive evaluation, especially for trauma, infection, and pseudotumor. CT may also suffice for detecting associated intracranial trauma, intracranial inflammation, and hydrocephalus. Orbital involvement in craniofacial syndromes is often best delineated by three-dimensional CT (3DCT), especially for planning of reconstructive craniofacial surgery.

CT has also replaced PF/CR and polytomography for the evaluation of the petrous and mastoid portions of the temporal bone (e.g., hearing loss, facial palsy), including developmental malformations and acquired diseases—especially inflammatory, traumatic, and neoplastic processes of the inner ear, middle ear, mastoid, and external auditory canal. CT determines the extent of bony destruction associated with cholesteatoma, mastoiditis, and tumors, including skull base and intracranial extension.

CT scanning of the neck (e.g., neck mass, infection, vascular anomaly) is usually performed after bolus intravenous administration of a contrast agent, and axial sections from the clavicles to the skull base are obtained. It is the standard for the emergency evaluation of suppurative head and neck lesions (e.g., retropharyngeal abscess). The bolus technique provides a "blood pool" effect to visualize normal neck vessels and abnormal vascularity.

Delayed post-injection imaging may demonstrate abnormal tissue enhancement (e.g., abscess). Occasionally, axial sections may be obtained prior to the enhanced study to evaluate for calcification or hemorrhage.

Radionuclide Imaging

One of the most important uses of RI in the evaluation of the neck in childhood is the imaging of the thyroid. Iodine 123 (^{123}I) and technetium Tc 99m (^{99m}Tc) pertechnetate are the agents currently used. ^{123}I is trapped and organified by the thyroid, whereas ^{99m}Tc pertechnetate is not organified. Because its biochemical behavior is identical to that of stable iodide and because it affords a higher thyroid-to-background ratio, ^{123}I is probably preferred. Common indications for thyroid RI include the identification of ectopic thyroid tissue in an extrathyroidal neck mass, the assessment of congenital hypothyroidism (in which detection of ectopic thyroid tissue is also essential), and the evaluation of a solitary thyroid nodule. PET-CT has also emerged as a primary modality in the evaluation of neoplastic processes involving the neck in childhood and adolescence (e.g., lymphoma, post-transplant lymphoproliferative disorder [PTLD]).

Magnetic Resonance Imaging

MRI is often adjunctive to CT in the assessment of head and neck lesions. However, in a number of situations MRI may be the technique of choice (e.g., vascular anomalies). In general, MRI should be considered for specific delineation of soft tissue elements, vascular components, and intracranial involvement. Disease processes and abnormalities involving the skull base are probably best evaluated with a combination of CT for bony involvement and MRI for neurovascular involvement. MR angiography (MRA) or venography (MRV) may be added to confirm vascular occlusion (e.g., dural sinus thrombosis) or to show high-flow vascular lesions such as arteriovenous malformations (AVMs) and hemangiomas. Doppler US imaging is often preferred in young infants, however, and CTA or CT venography may be better for vascular assessment in older children, especially in the diagnosis of venous thrombosis. In petrous temporal bone abnormalities, MRI is generally reserved for the detection and delineation of tumors or complicated inflammatory conditions. Clinical indications for MRI may include retrocochlear sensorineural hearing loss, facial nerve paralysis, and vertigo.

Desirable MRI techniques include fast spin echo (FSE), inversion recovery, fat suppression, and gadolinium enhancement sequences. The volume head coil, or semivolume head and neck coil, is used to obtain sagittal T1-weighted images, axial proton density images, and axial T2-weighted images. Short T1 inversion recovery (STIR) images may be preferred, however, for the additive T1 and T2 effect and the superb fat suppression provided. Gadolinium-enhanced T1-weighted images with fat suppression are often used in one or more planes, particularly for the evaluation of tumors and inflammation. High-resolution thin-section axial and coronal T1-weighted acquisitions are often used with fat suppression and gadolinium enhancement, particularly to evaluate the orbits and internal auditory canals. Gradient echo (GE) techniques are used to enhance vascular flow, CSF flow, and magnetic susceptibility effects (mineralization or hemorrhage). Non-MRA vascular flow–enhanced studies may be done using multiple single-slice or GE techniques. A number of two-dimensional (2D) and 3D time-of-flight (TOF) and phase-contrast MRA techniques are available.

▄ CONGENITAL AND DEVELOPMENTAL ABNORMALITIES

See Box 10-1.

Box 10-1. Pediatric Head and Neck Developmental Anomalies

Primary ocular abnormalities
Ocular/orbital abnormalities associated with CNS malformations
Malformative orbit lesions
Congenital nasal stenosis/atresia
Congenital nasal masses
Craniofacial anomalies
External/middle ear anomalies
Inner ear anomalies
Facial nerve anomalies
Vascular anomalies
Branchial anomalies
Thyroidal anomalies
Laryngeal anomalies
Oral cavity, tongue, salivary gland anomalies

Orbit and Globe

Normal Development

The eye and orbit develop from the neuroectoderm, the cutaneous ectoderm, and the neural crest cells. The optic primordium gives rise to the optic vesicle and stalk, which become the eye (including the retina) and the optic nerve. A transitory vascular system, the hyaloid artery and its branches, forms the primary vitreous and then involutes by the 35th gestational week. The globe lies within the fat of the orbit. The outer layer of the globe is the sclera and cornea, the middle layer is the choroid, ciliary body, and iris, and the inner layer is the retina. The retina, which is the neurovisual membrane, is continuous posteriorly with the optic nerve. The refracting media include the aqueous humor, lens, and vitreous humor. The lacrimal gland lies in the superolateral orbit and secretes tears. The tears are drained from the eye by the lacrimal canals into the lacrimal sac medially and then into the nasolacrimal duct, which empties into the inferior meatus of the nasal cavity.

The orbit contains the orbital fascia, ocular muscles, globe and its appendages, and associated arteries, veins, and nerves. The optic foramen lies at the orbital apex and transmits the optic nerve and ophthalmic artery. The superior orbital fissure lies inferolaterally to the optic foramen and transmits the third and fourth cranial nerves, the ophthalmic division of the fifth cranial nerve, the sixth cranial nerve, sympathetic nerves, and the ophthalmic vein. The extraocular muscles originate at the orbital apex and insert on the globe, forming a cone about the globe and optic nerve. The orbital fascia forms the periosteum of the orbit, and its anterior reflection about the globe is the orbital septum. This septum separates the preseptal space from the postseptal space. The postseptal space is further subdivided by the muscular cone (i.e., intraconal and extraconal space). The orbital cavity grows passively in response to the growth of the globe. The globe is 75% of adult size at birth, and its growth is complete by age 7 years.

Primary Ocular Abnormalities

It may be difficult to distinguish *anophthalmia* (congenital absence of the eye) from severe *microphthalmia* (hypoplastic eye) or orbital hypoplasia. They result from incomplete formation or degeneration of the optic vesicle. They may coexist with congenital cystic eye. Ocular structures (lens and globe) are absent in primary anophthalmia but present in microphthalmia (Fig. 10-1). Anophthalmia may be sporadic or may occur with chromosomal syndromes and complex craniofacial anomalies. Imaging shows a poorly formed and shallow orbit containing rudimentary tissue.

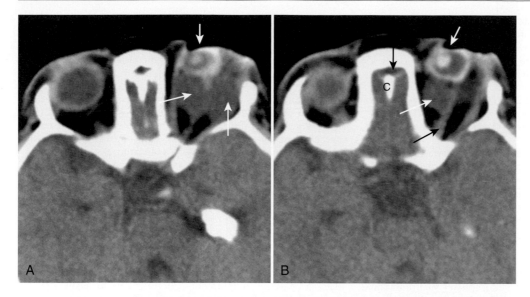

FIGURE 10-1. A and B, Axial CT scans showing microphthalmia (*short white arrows*) with coloboma (*long white arrows*) encircling the hypoplastic optic nerve (*lower black arrow* in **B**); normal foramen cecum (*upper black arrow* in **B**) and crista galli (C).

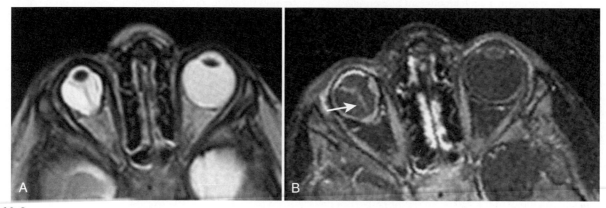

FIGURE 10-2. Right persistent hyperplastic primary vitreous with microphthalmia and vitreous band (*arrow* in **B** compared with normal left globe on axial T2-weighted (**A**) and gadolinium-enhanced T1-weighted (**B**) MR images.

Microphthalmia may be isolated or may be associated with other abnormalities (e.g., coloboma, duplication cyst, glaucoma, cataracts, septo-optic dysplasia, genetic syndromes [trisomy 1]), and the TORCH (*t*oxoplasmosis, *o*ther agents, *r*ubella, *c*ytomegalovirus, and *h*erpes simplex) infections (i.e., chorioretinitis).

Coloboma refers to any congenital or acquired ocular structural defect. Typical colobomas result from failure of embryonic choroidal fissure closure and are usually bilateral (e.g., autosomal dominant). They may also be sporadic and unilateral. On imaging, a small cyst is found behind the globe at the head of the optic nerve (see Fig. 10-1).

Optic nerve hypoplasia, defined as a subnormal number of axons, is a common and isolated anomaly. Particularly when bilateral, it may be associated with ocular, facial, endocrine, or CNS anomalies (e.g., septo-optic dysplasia or encephalocele). Imaging demonstrates small optic nerves and a small chiasm (see Fig. 10-1).

Persistent hyperplastic primary vitreous (PHPV) represents persistence and hyperplasia of the embryonic hyaloid vascular system. PHPV is usually unilateral and associated with microphthalmia. Typical clinical findings include leukocoria (white pupil), microphthalmia, and cataract. Microphthalmia and the absence of calcification are important in differentiating PHPV from retinoblastoma (calcifications in a normal-sized or enlarged globe). Complications of PHPV include glaucoma (i.e., buphthalmia), recurrent hemorrhage, retinal detachment, and phthisis bulbi. Imaging demonstrates a small globe with a bandlike hyperdensity on CT or a hyperintensity on T1-weighted MR imaging (T1 hyperintensity) that extends from the lens to the posterior globe (Fig. 10-2).

Glaucoma is abnormally elevated intraocular pressure due to disordered aqueous humor flow. Primary congenital glaucoma is usually bilateral and may occur with other disorders (e.g., phakomatoses). The increase in intraocular pressure causes ocular enlargement (i.e., buphthalmos). Secondary congenital glaucoma results from intrauterine eye inflammation (e.g., rubella), trauma, or an ocular tumor (e.g., retinoblastoma).

Coats disease is a primary retinal vascular anomaly (telangiectasia with retinal and subretinal lipoproteinaceous exudates) with peak occurrence at the end of the first decade. Retinal detachment with leukocoria makes it difficult to differentiate from retinoblastoma. Characteristic imaging findings include vitreous CT hyperdensity or T1 hyperintensity but no focal mass. Calcification sometimes occurs.

Retrolental fibroplasia, or retinopathy of prematurity, is usually bilateral and asymmetric. There may be retinal detachment or leukocoria, in which case the abnormality can mimic retinoblastoma.

Ocular and Orbital Abnormalities Associated with Central Nervous System Malformations

Orbital abnormalities are commonly associated with neural tube disorders (see Chapter 8). Cephaloceles, which commonly involve the orbit or optic pathways, can be classified as sphenoidal or frontoethmoidal. Dermal sinuses and dermoid-epidermoids (discussed later) may be associated with widening of the nasal bridge, hypertelorism, or midline anomalies (e.g., callosal hypogenesis with a lipoma). Midface hypoplasia and hypotelorism are commonly associated with the holoprosencephalies (HPE). The alobar form of HPE may also have cyclopia, ethmocephaly, cebocephaly, or median cleft lip with hypertelorism. Septo-optic dysplasia (de Morsier syndrome) involves partial or complete absence of the septum pellucidum and optic hypoplasia. Orbital deformity is commonly associated with the craniosynostoses (e.g., metopic, coronal, multiple).

Orbital abnormalities are also part of the craniofacial malformations and craniosynostosis associated with disorders such as Crouzon disease and Apert, Carpenter, and Pfeiffer syndromes. Reconstructive surgery is often required to improve function and preserve vision. Treacher Collins syndrome is another example of a craniofacial syndrome with orbital/ocular abnormalities (i.e., microphthalmia, coloboma). Neurophthalmologic involvement often occurs in the neurocutaneous syndromes and includes neurofibromatosis type 1 (NF-1) (spheno-orbital dysplasia, optic glioma), tuberous sclerosis (retinal neuroglial hamartoma), Sturge-Weber syndrome (choroidal venocapillary malformation with buphthalmos), and von Hippel–Lindau disease (retinal hemangioblastoma with retinal detachment and hemorrhage).

Migrational disorders are often associated with ocular, orbital, or optic pathway abnormalities (callosal hypogenesis, lissencephaly syndromes). Callosal hypogenesis is seen in a wide array of anomalies, including cephaloceles, dermal sinus, septo-optic dysplasia, cleft lip and palate, Apert syndrome, hypertelorism, coloboma, and Aicardi syndrome. Midface and orbital dysmorphia, as well as ocular anomalies, are frequently seen in the lissencephaly syndromes (e.g., Walker-Warburg syndrome).

Malformative Lesions

Malformative tumors, nonneoplastic and neoplastic, are aberrations of development. They are usually of neuroectodermal origin (e.g., dermoid-epidermoid) or mesodermal origin (e.g., lipoma). Some germ cell neoplasms (e.g., teratoma) and vascular anomalies are also included in this category. Malformative tumors may be cystic, solid, or mixed. In the pediatric orbit, these tumors include colobomas (see Fig. 10-1), duplication cysts, nasolacrimal duct cysts, lacrimal ectopia, dermoids-epidermoids, teratomas, and (rarely) arachnoid cysts and lipomas. It may be difficult to differentiate a coloboma from a retrobulbar duplication cyst. Hydrops and arachnoid cyst of the optic nerve sheath are exceedingly rare in the absence of suprasellar tumors or cysts.

Congenital nasolacrimal duct cyst or mucocele probably results from incomplete canalization of the duct on one or both sides. Proximal obstruction results in a lacrimal sac mucocele and manifests as a medial orbital canthal mass (dacryocystocele).

Distal obstruction produces a nasolacrimal duct mucocele that extends beneath the inferior turbinate into the nasal cavity. The two types may coexist. Bilateral involvement may clinically mimic choanal atresia. The resultant cystic dilatation often resolves in early infancy. Persistence may cause nasal airway obstruction, infection, and dacryocystitis. Imaging demonstrates a medial canthus cystic mass in continuity with an enlarged nasolacrimal duct (and canal) and an intranasal submucosal cystic mass (Fig. 10-3). The latter differentiates the mucocele from other medial canthal cystic masses (e.g., dacryocystitis, choristoma, dermoid-epidermoid, or cephalocele). With associated abscess there may be restricted diffusion on diffusion-weighted MRI (DWI), which can make it difficult to distinguish from dermoid-epidermoid.

Ectopic lacrimal gland tissue may appear as solid or cystic lesions of the orbit and may produce proptosis. Neoplastic transformation is rare (e.g., pleomorphic adenoma and adenocarcinoma).

Dermoid-epidermoid, the most common congenital lesion of the orbit, arises as a developmental sequestration of ectoderm along the sutures (Fig. 10-4). It most frequently occurs in the superolateral or medial orbit. Relatively slow growth of the cyst erodes adjacent bone (i.e., notching or scalloping) and displaces adjacent structures. CT hypodensity or fat-like T1 hyperintensity may be present along with calcification or a fat-fluid level. Restricted diffusion on DWI is also a characteristic finding that may mimic abscess (see Figs. 10-3 and 10-4).

Orbital teratoma is often benign and produces proptosis in infancy. It may be cystic, multicystic, solid, or mixed. There may be orbital expansion with ocular displacement or compression. CT or MRI may demonstrate fatty features with calcification or ossification. Mesodermal dysplasias affecting the orbit include NF-1 (spheno-orbital dysplasia; see Chapter 8) and the skeletal dysplasias (e.g., fibrous dysplasia, craniometaphyseal dysplasia, and osteopetrosis). Fibrous dysplasia produces a characteristic "ground-glass" or sclerotic appearance of the orbit, facial bones, or skull base (Fig. 10-5).

Nasal Cavity, Paranasal Sinuses, and Face

Normal Development

The mesenchymal primordia of the face form about the stomodeum (primitive mouth) and include the frontonasal prominence, maxillary prominences, and the mandibular prominences. These structures, respectively, give rise to the forehead, nose and nasal septum; turbinates, upper lip, premaxilla, maxilla, hard palate, soft palate, uvula; mandible, lower lip, chin, and lower cheek. The nasal cavities develop and ultimately communicate with the nasopharynx and oral cavity after rupture of the oronasal membrane at the level of the choanae. The paired turbinates form from the lateral wall of each nasal cavity. Specialized olfactory

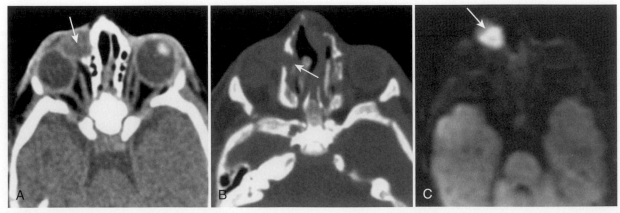

FIGURE 10-3. Right dacryocystocele (*arrows* in **A** and **C**) with large right nasolacrimal canal (*arrow* in **B**) and abscess on axial CT scans (**A** and **B**) and a diffusion-weighted MR image (**C**).

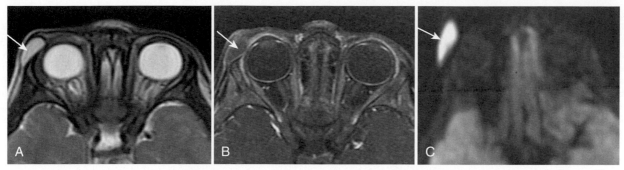

FIGURE 10-4. Right lateral orbital dermoid (*arrows*) on axial T2-weighted (**A**), gadolinium-enhanced T1-weighted (**B**), and diffusion-weighted (**C**) MR images.

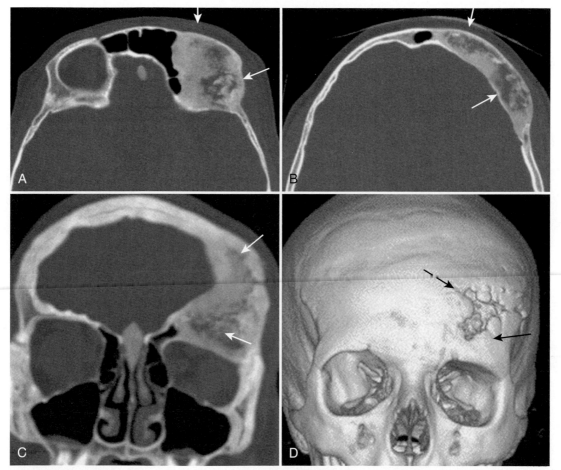

FIGURE 10-5. Left orbitofrontal fibrous dysplasia (*arrows*) with mixed sclerotic and lytic features and orbital deformity on axial (**A**) and (**B**) and coronal (**C**) CT scans and a frontal 3DCT reconstruction (**D**).

epithelium develops in the roof of each nasal cavity and connects with the olfactory bulbs of the prosencephalon. The paranasal sinuses form as diverticula of the walls of the nasal cavities and later become pneumatized.

The small size of the face relative to the head at birth results from the more rapid development of the brain. The nose is the major portal of air exchange, especially in the newborn. The nasal cavity and paranasal sinuses are covered with respiratory epithelium. The maxillary sinuses and ethmoid air cells are present at birth but may not be visible until 3 to 6 months of age (adult size by 10 to 12 years). The frontal and sphenoid sinuses may not be visualized until 6 years of age. The frontal sinuses, anterior and middle ethmoidal air cells, and maxillary sinuses drain into the middle meatus via the ostiomeatal complex. The posterior

ethmoidal air cells and sphenoidal sinuses drain into the spheno-ethmoidal recess and superior nasal meatus. During early infancy, there may be physiologic underaeration of the paranasal sinuses owing to redundant normal mucosa. Paranasal sinus disease is characterized by decreased aeration, mucosal thickening, soft tissue masses (e.g., mucus retention cyst, polyp, mucocele, tumor), air-fluid levels, and demineralization or bone destruction.

Congenital Nasal Stenosis and Atresia

Nasal airway obstruction may be the cause of respiratory distress in the newborn and infant. An obstructive abnormality is further indicated by inability to pass nasal catheters. The differential diagnosis usually includes nasal cavity and choanal stenosis or atresia, basal cephalocele, and bilateral nasolacrimal duct cysts.

Choanal stenosis and atresia, respectively, are narrowing of the posterior nasal cavity and obstruction by an atresia plate (bony, membranous, or both). The bilateral form manifests as neonatal respiratory distress (Fig. 10-6A); the unilateral form may not manifest until later (Fig. 10-6B). There may be co-existing nasal cavity stenosis or atresia and other anomalies or syndromes, such as cleft palate, cardiovascular and abdominal abnormalities, Treacher Collins syndrome, CHARGE (**c**olobomata, **h**eart defect, **a**tresia, choanal **r**etarded growth and development, **g**enital hypoplasia, and **e**ar abnormalities and/or deafness) association, fetal alcohol and Apert syndrome, and Crouzon disease.

Stenosis of the entire nasal airway is usually bony and may be associated with prematurity or maxillary hypoplasia (e.g., Apert syndrome). Atresia is extremely rare. Symptoms may not arise until there is a complicating rhinitis.

Segmental atresia, or stenosis, may occur anteriorly (i.e., piriform aperture stenosis; Fig. 10-7). This may be associated with single midline maxillary incisor (mega-incisor) and midline intracranial anomalies (e.g., holoprosencephaly). Segmental stenosis may also result from maxillary hypoplasia, turbinate hyperplasia, or nasal septal deviation.

Congenital Nasal Masses

Congenital nasal masses resulting from defective neural tube closure include cephalocele, neuroepithelial heterotopia (nasal glioma), and dermoid-epidermoid (see Chapter 8). They may manifest as bilateral nasal obstruction and respiratory distress in the newborn and are to be distinguished from nasochoanal stenosis/atresia and nasolacrimal duct cysts (discussed earlier). Later in life they may be the cause of a nasal mass or obstruction.

The fonticulus frontalis and prenasal space are transient nasofrontal structures that involute in early gestation. The fibrous tissue filled foramen cecum remains as the only remnant (see Fig. 10-1). Persistence of these primitive structures may be associated with a dural diverticulum and protrusion of intracranial contents as a nasofrontal cephalocele or a nasoethmoidal cephalocele.

With partial or complete obliteration of the intracranial connection, the cephalocele becomes a sequestered neuroepithelial heterotopia (nasal glioma; Fig. 10-8). As the dural diverticulum regresses, incorporation of surface ectoderm may form a dermal sinus. This commonly manifests as a skin dimple or mass in the nasal region. The sinus may extend to any point from the columella to the glabella. Other associated findings include nasal

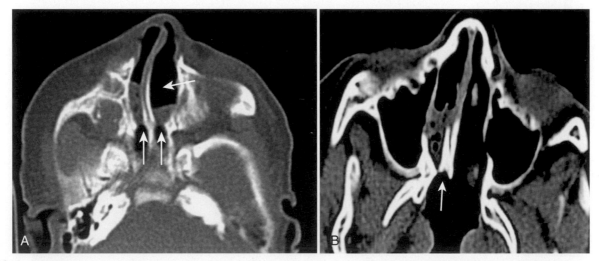

FIGURE 10-6. Axial CT scans showing choanal atresia. **A,** Bilateral choanal atresia (*lower arrows*) with retained secretions plus right nasal septal deviation (*upper arrow*). **B,** Right unilateral choanal atresia (*arrow*) with retained secretions; compare with the normal left choanal aperture.

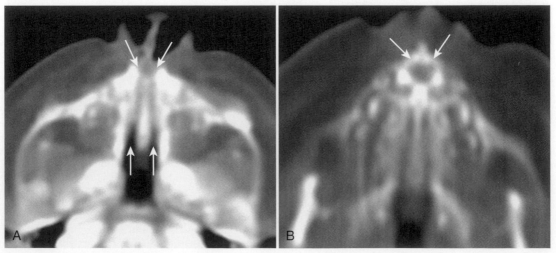

FIGURE 10-7. **A** and **B,** Axial CT scans showing neonatal piriform aperture stenosis (*upper arrows* in **A**) with bilateral open choanae (*lower arrows* in **A**) and a single midline mega-incisor (*arrows* in **B**).

or frontal bony defect, enlarged foramen cecum, dermoid, epidermoid, or lipoma (Figs. 10-9 and 10-10). The mass is often CT hypodense and calcified and has fatty T1 hyperintensity on MRI. An intracranial communication may result in recurrent meningitis, abscess, or empyema. Other rare congenital nasal masses are nasoalveolar (incisive canal) cysts, dentigerous cysts, mucous cysts, vascular anomalies, branchial cysts, hamartomas, teratoid tumors (embryoma, epignathus), and Tornwaldt cyst.

Facial Anomalies
Cleft Lip and Palate
Clefts involving the lip, alveolus, or palate are common anomalies and may be partial, complete, unilateral, or bilateral. Maxillary hypoplasia with prognathism often accompanies bilateral clefts. A complete cleft disrupts facial growth, dentition, speech, and eustachian tube function.

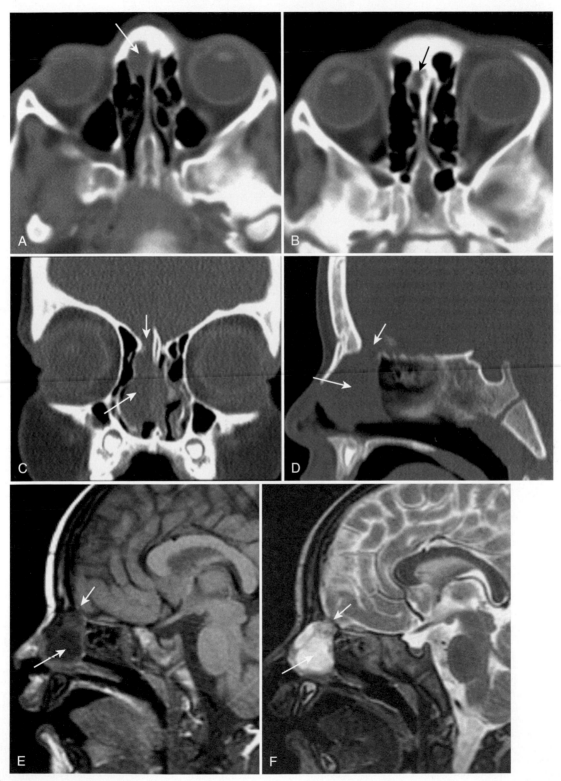

FIGURE 10-8. Right sequestered nasoethmoidal cephalocele ("nasal glioma," indicated by *long white arrows*) with extension via foramen cecum (*short black and white arrows*) on axial (**A** and **B**), coronal (**C**), and sagittal (**D**) CT scans as well as sagittal T1-weighted (**E**) and T2-weighted (**F**) MR images.

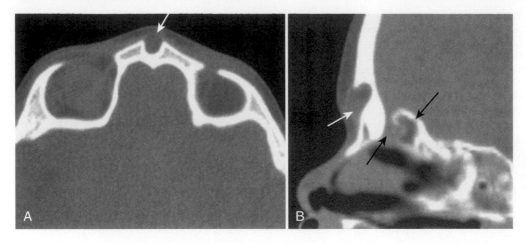

FIGURE 10-9. Glabellar dermoid (*white arrows*) with bony deformity on axial (**A**) and sagittal (**B**) CT scans. **B** also shows normal foramen cecum (*lower black arrow*) and crista galli (*upper black arrow*).

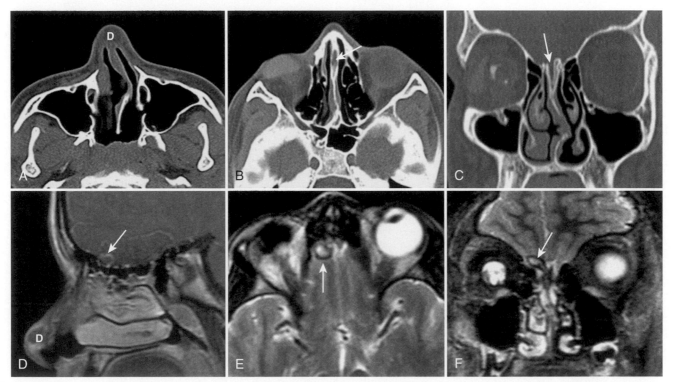

FIGURE 10-10. Nasal dermoid (D) with sinus tract (*arrows* in **B** and **C**) and intracranial extension (*arrows* in **D, E,** and **F**) on axial (**A** to **B**) and coronal (**C**) CT scans as well as sagittal gadolinium-enhanced T1-weighted (**D**) and axial (**E**) and coronal (**F**) T2-weighted MR images.

Craniofacial clefts (facial, cranial, or combined) extend along continuous axes through the eyebrow or eyelid, maxilla, nose, and lip. Facial clefts extend caudally from the lower eyelid, whereas cranial clefts extend cephalad from the upper eyelid. Associated anomalies include orbital dystopia, microphthalmos, coloboma, cephalocele, and orbital hypertelorism. Associated syndromes include median cleft syndrome, Treacher Collins syndrome, hemifacial microsomia, amniotic band syndrome, otomandibular syndrome, and Goldenhar syndrome. The *median cleft syndrome* (high and low groups) with hypertelorism may be associated with cephalocele, corpus callosum hypogenesis, intracranial lipoma, optic nerve dysplasia (coloboma), cranium bifidum, frontonasal dysplasia, microphthalmia, anophthalmia, or holoprosencephaly. *Posterior palatal defects* characteristically occur with microretrognathia (e.g., Pierre Robin sequence; Fig. 10-11).

Craniofacial Syndromes

Bilateral coronal craniosynostosis may be associated with craniofacial dysostosis (e.g., Crouzon disease) or acrocephalosyndactyly (e.g., Apert, Pfeiffer, Carpenter, Saethre-Chotzen syndromes). The associated dysmorphia includes abnormalities of the forehead, orbits (hypertelorism, exorbitism), midface, and anterior cranial base. *Cloverleaf craniofacial anomaly* results from multiple craniosynostoses and is also associated with extensive craniofacial deformities (Fig. 10-12). *Amniotic band syndrome* (congenital constrictions or amputations) manifests as facial clefts, calvarial defects, hydrocephalus, cephaloceles, or anencephaly. *Hemifacial microsomia* has facial asymmetry with maxillary and malar hypoplasia, macrostomia, mandibular hypoplasia (ramus and condyle), microtia (external ear atresia/stenosis and middle ear hypoplasia), microphthalmia, congenital cystic eye, and

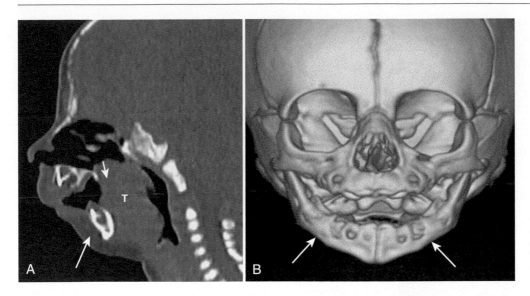

FIGURE **10-11.** Pierre-Robin sequence with microretrognathia (*long arrows*), posterior palate defect (*short arrow*), and high-riding tongue (T) with narrow airway on sagittal CT scan (**A**) and frontal 3DCT reconstruction (**B**).

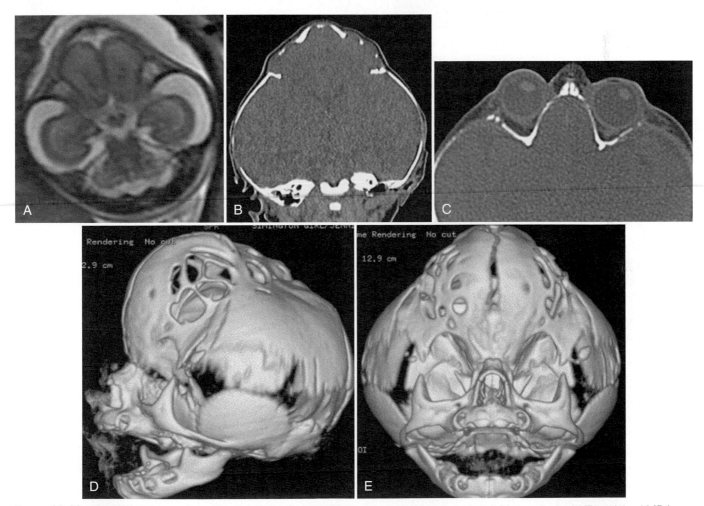

FIGURE **10-12.** Multiple craniosynostosis (bicoronal, metopic, sagittal) with cloverleaf deformity and exorbitism on fetal axial T2-weighted MR image (**A**) as well as neonatal coronal (**B**) and axial (**C**) CT scans with lateral (**D**) and frontal (**E**) 3DCT reconstructions.

coloboma. *Treacher Collins syndrome* is a mandibulofacial dysostosis (autosomal dominant) characterized by bilateral zygomatic, malar, and mandibular hypoplasia (Fig. 10-13). Also common are microtia (external and middle ear hypoplasia), colobomata,

and microphthalmia. *Goldenhar syndrome* (oculoauriculovertebral syndrome) is a mandibulofacial dysostosis with hemifacial microsomia, epibulbar dermoids or lipodermoids, and vertebral anomalies.

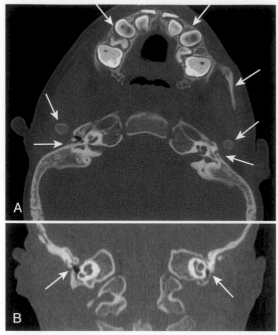

Figure 10-13. Treacher-Collins syndrome on axial (**A**) and coronal (**B**) CT scans with mandibular, maxillary, and zygomatic hypoplasia (*arrows* in **A**) and bilateral external auditory canal atresia and middle ear hypoplasia (*lower arrows* in **A**, *arrows* in **B**).

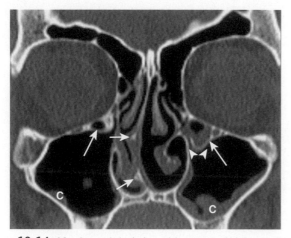

Figure 10-14. Nasal septal deviation with spurs and right nasal cavity narrowing (*short arrows*) on coronal CT scan, showing bilateral Haller cells (*long arrows*), bilateral maxillary sinus mucosal thickening, small cysts (c), and occlusion of the left ostiomeatal complex (*arrowheads*).

Developmental Variants and Anomalies of the Nose and Paranasal Sinuses

Developmental variants and anomalies may predispose to ostiomeatal complex obstruction with inflammation (Fig. 10-14). Endoscopic or open surgical procedures may be necessary for correction. Nasal septal deviation is common and is often associated with asymmetry or deformity of adjacent structures (e.g., abnormally large middle turbinate [concha bullosa], septal spur, secondary turbinate anomalies, extramural sinus pneumatization, uncinate process deviation). Extramural extension of the ethmoid cells includes pneumatization of the supraorbital ridge, superior or middle turbinate (e.g., concha bullosa), uncinate process, orbital plate of the maxilla, the sphenoid bone, agger nasi cells (anterior to the upper nasolacrimal duct), Haller cells (infraorbital; may obstruct the maxillary sinus infundibulum), and Onodi cells (sphenoid body near the optic nerve canal, internal carotid artery [ICA], cavernous sinus). Other common

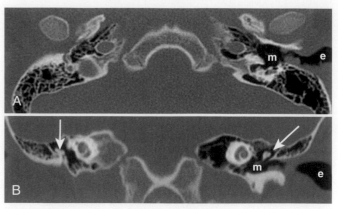

Figure 10-15. Axial (**A**) and coronal (**B**) CT scans showing right congenital aural dysplasia with external auditory canal (EAC) atresia, middle ear canal (MEC) hypoplasia, and fused ossicles (*right arrow* in **B**). Compare with normal left EAC (e), MEC (m), and ossicles (*arrow* in **B**).

anomalies are maxillary sinus hypoplasia, extramural sphenoid or maxillary sinus extension, maxillary sinus septation, and accessory ostia.

Ear and Temporal Bone

Normal Development

The external and middle ear (mastoid portion of the temporal bone) are derived from the branchial apparatus, and the internal ear is derived from the neuroectoderm. The auricle and external ear (membranous and bony portions) begin development along with the mandible. The middle ear cavity expands and incorporates the tympanic membrane, eustachian tube, auditory ossicles (malleus, incus, stapes), muscles (tensor tympani and stapedius), their tendons and ligaments, the round and oval windows, and the chorda tympani nerve, and then gives rise to the attic and mastoid antrum.

The inner ear forms from the otic vesicle, which gives rise to the membranous labyrinth. The membranous labyrinth contains endolymph, is surrounded by perilymph, and is enclosed within the bony labyrinth (otic capsule). The membranous structures (corresponding bony structures shown in parentheses) include the utricle and saccule (vestibule), semicircular ducts (semicircular canals), endolymphatic duct and sac (vestibular aqueduct), and cochlear duct–organ of Corti (cochlea, modiolus).

The petrous portion of the temporal bone contains the inner ear and transmits the cochlear aqueduct and perilymph, ICA, internal jugular vein, and cranial nerves VII (facial) and VIII (vestibulocochlear). The facial nerve extends from the internal auditory canal into the facial nerve canal, which has a labyrinthine segment (anterior genu and geniculate ganglion within the otic capsule), a tympanic segment (horizontal course within the middle ear extending to the posterior genu and facial nerve recess), and a mastoid segment (vertical course to the stylomastoid foramen). Pneumatization of the mastoid occurs rapidly and is visible by 4 to 6 months of age. Mastoid disease is characterized by decreased aeration, mucosal thickening, edema, accumulation of fluid, bony demineralization, and bone destruction.

External Auditory Canal and Middle Ear Cavity Anomalies

External auditory canal (EAC) stenosis/atresia is commonly associated with a malformed auricle (i.e., microtia), hypoplasia of the middle ear and mastoid, and, occasionally, mandibular hypoplasia (Fig. 10-15). The complex may be unilateral, bilateral, isolated, or associated with syndromes (e.g., hemifacial microsomia, Treacher Collins syndrome (see Fig. 10-13), Crouzon disease, and Goldenhar syndrome). EAC atresia may be partial or complete, and membranous or bony. Complete (osseous) atresia consists of a bony atresia plate at the tympanic membrane and fusion of the malleus to the plate. Partial (membranous) atresia consists of a soft tissue plug at the tympanic membrane (with or without fusion of the malleus).

EAC atresia may be associated with a congenital cholesteatoma (primary epidermoid) of the EAC or middle ear cavity (MEC) (Fig. 10-16). MEC hypoplasia may be mild or severe. Ossicular anomalies include absence, rotation, fusion, and dysplasia. The facial nerve is often thickened, has an aberrant course, and may be exposed (dehiscence, protrusion). First branchial arch dysplasia results in unilateral (e.g., hemifacial microsomia) or bilateral (e.g., Treacher Collins syndrome; see Fig. 10-13) mandibulofacial dysostosis with consequent anomalies of the mandible, EAC, MEC, malleus, and incus. Second branchial arch dysplasia results in anomalies of the hyoid, styloid, stylohyoid ligament, and stapes.

Inner Ear Anomalies
Congenital sensorineural hearing loss is commonly associated with inner ear anomalies. A common anomaly is vestibular aqueduct dysplasia (ranging from obliteration to dilatation; Fig. 10-17).

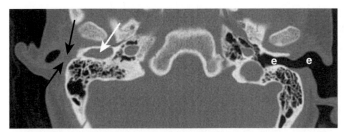

FIGURE 10-16. Right microtia with membranous external auditory canal (EAC) atresia (*black arrows*) and cholesteatoma (*white arrow*) on axial CT. Compare with normal left membranous and bony EAC (e).

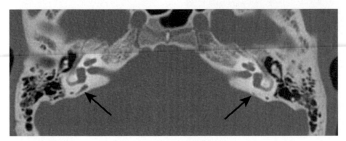

FIGURE 10-17. Dilated vestibular aqueduct (*arrow* at *right*) compared with normal aqueduct (*arrow* at *left*) on axial CT.

Dilated vestibular aqueduct (diameter > 1.5 mm, or greater than posterior semicircular canal [SCC] diameter) may be associated with malformations of the cochlea (e.g., Mondini syndrome [see later]), modiolus (hypoplasia), vestibule, SCCs, or cochlear nerve (e.g., hypoplasia). Another common anomaly is malformation of the lateral SCC. In other cases, the SCCs may be absent or may be malformed and incorporated into a dilated vestibule (Fig. 10-18).

Cochlear anomalies may be classified according to the stage of developmental arrest. Complete labyrinthine aplasia (Michel deformity) results in a single small cystic cavity. Other anomalies include a large common cavity (common chamber anomaly), cochlear aplasia or hypoplasia, and incomplete partition (Mondini syndrome—small cochlea with incomplete septation, i.e., less than two and one-half turns; Fig. 10-19). Malformations of the internal auditory canal consist of stenosis and atresia.

Facial Nerve Anomalies
Aberrant course of the facial nerve is usually associated with an anomaly of the external, middle, or inner ear. Lateral and anterior displacement of the mastoid segment is common in EAC and MEC anomalies (see Fig. 10-15). Anomalous facial nerve may be directly involved in ossicular malformations. Dehiscence of the facial nerve canal most often occurs in its tympanic portion at the level of the stapes and results in a conductive hearing loss (Fig. 10-20). Facial nerve hypoplasia has been described in syndromes, such as Goldenhar syndrome, VATER (abnormalities of **v**ertebrae, **a**nus, **t**rachea, **e**sophagus, and **r**adial and **r**enal dysplasia) association, and some trisomies. Absence of the facial nerve has been described in a few cases, including the Möbius sequence.

Neck, Oral Cavity, and Jaw
Normal Development
The branchial apparatus, which contributes to formation of the head and neck, consists of paired branchial arches, pharyngeal pouches, branchial grooves, and branchial membranes. The branchial arches form along the lateral primitive pharynx. Each arch consists of a mesenchymal core (containing neural crest cells and arterial, nerve, cartilage, and muscular elements). Each arch is separated by branchial membranes and covered externally by surface ectoderm (branchial grooves) and internally by endoderm (pharyngeal pouches). The primitive mouth (stomodeum) arises from the surface ectoderm in contact with the amniotic cavity externally and the primitive gut internally via the esophagus (after rupture of the primitive buccopharyngeal membrane). The tongue buds are mesenchymal proliferations derived from the

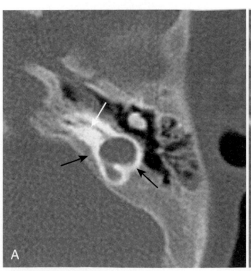

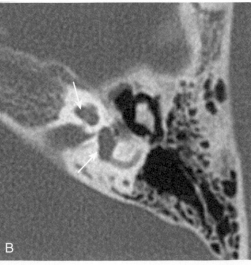

FIGURE 10-18. A, Axial CT scan showing left cochlear aplasia (*white arrow*) with common chamber anomaly (*black arrows*) and dysplastic semicircular canals (SCCs). **B,** Axial CT scan showing a normal left cochlea, vestibule, and lateral SCC (*white arrows*).

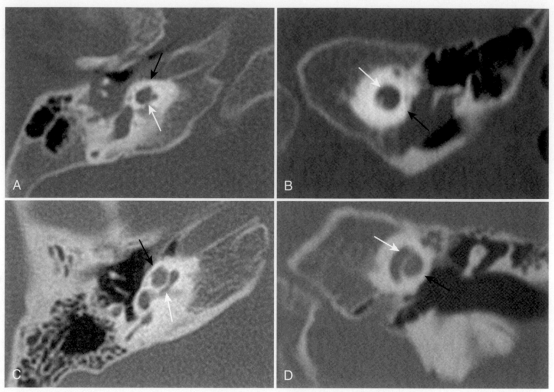

FIGURE 10-19. Right cochlear partition defect (*arrows*) on axial (**A**) and coronal (**B**) CT scans. Normal right cochlea (*arrows*) on axial (**C**) and coronal (**D**) CT scans.

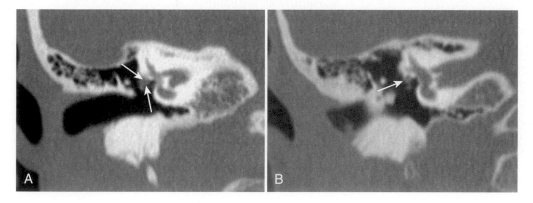

FIGURE 10-20. Coronal CT scans. **A,** Right facial nerve dehiscence/protrusion (*arrows*) onto the stapes below. **B,** Normal right facial nerve and canal (*arrow*) above the stapes.

first pair of branchial arches. The salivary glands begin as solid proliferations from epithelial buds. The developing thyroid gland is a diverticulum connected by the thyroglossal duct ventral to the hyoid to the tongue base at the foramen cecum. The thyroglossal duct normally involutes. The thymus and inferior parathyroid originate from the third pharyngeal pouch. The superior parathyroid glands arise from the fourth pharyngeal pouch. The laryngotracheal groove and tracheoesophageal folds form to become the ventral laryngotracheal tube and dorsal esophagus.

The neck is divided by the hyoid bone into the suprahyoid and infrahyoid regions. Three layers of deep cervical fascia divide the suprahyoid neck into eight compartments (parapharyngeal space, pharyngeal mucosal space, masticator space, parotid space, retropharyngeal space, perivertebral space, and posterior cervical space). The sternocleidomastoid muscle divides the infrahyoid neck into anterior and posterior triangles. The layers of the deep cervical fascia permit further subdivision of the infrahyoid neck into five major spaces that are continuous with corresponding spaces in the suprahyoid neck (carotid, visceral, posterior cervical, retropharyngeal, and perivertebral spaces).

The adenoids become conspicuous within the nasopharynx by 2 to 3 years of age and regress during adolescence. If no adenoidal tissue is seen in a young child, and in the absence of prior adenoidectomy, the possibility of immunodeficiency should be considered. The lymph nodes of the neck occur in contiguous groups and may be classified according to various systems. Normal nodes are usually homogeneous, similar in density to muscle, and oval or flat on CT. Contrast enhancement of lymph nodes is abnormal and may be seen in a variety of inflammatory and neoplastic processes. The major vessels of the head and neck include the common carotid arteries, which bifurcate into internal and external carotid arteries, the external jugular veins, the anterior jugular veins, and the internal jugular veins. The major nerves traversing the neck include cranial nerves IX through XII, the sympathetic chain, and the facial nerve.

The oral cavity contains the tongue and is bound inferiorly by the mylohyoid muscle. Within the oral cavity are the submandibular and sublingual spaces (separated by the mylohyoid muscle). The major salivary glands consist of the paired parotid, submandibular, and sublingual glands. Minor salivary glands also exist at several levels. Most muscles of the suprahyoid neck attach to the mandible. The maxilla contains the maxillary sinuses.

Branchial Anomalies

Branchial anomalies arise from incomplete development of the branchial apparatus. These anomalies are therefore classified according to the level (arch, cleft, or pouch) of origin. Defects include branchial cysts, aberrant tissue, branchial sinus (incomplete tract usually opening externally that may communicate with a cyst), and branchial fistula (epithelial tract with both external and internal openings). Fistulae and sinuses are usually identified at birth because of drainage. They are best imaged by a contrast-enhanced fistulogram (e.g., CT).

Cysts are more common in older children and adults. They usually manifest as a soft tissue mass that may enlarge with infection. US reveals a cystic or complex mass. CT and MRI show an oval or round cystic mass. Wall thickness, enhancement, content, and surrounding edema often increase with inflammation. A *first branchial cyst* usually arises as an enlarging mass about the parotid gland but may occur about the pinna, in the EAC, MEC, or nasopharynx, or submandibularly above the hyoid bone. The differential diagnosis includes an inflammatory cyst, lymphatic malformation, and necrotic adenopathy. The *second branchial cyst* is the most common of these anomalies. It usually manifests as a mass at the mandibular angle but may occur at any site along a line from the tonsillar fossa to the anterior margin of the sternocleidomastoid muscle to the supraclavicular region (Figs. 10-21 and 10-22). The differential diagnosis includes vascular anomaly, suppurative adenopathy, paramedian thyroglossal duct cyst, laryngocele, and necrotic metastatic adenopathy. The *third branchial sinus/fistula* arises from the inferior pyriform sinus and extends between the common carotid artery and vagus nerve to the lower lateral neck. The *fourth branchial sinus/fistula* usually arises from the left inferior pyriform sinus, looping beneath the aortic arch (or subclavian artery if on the right) and then upward via the carotid bifurcation to the lateral neck.

Recurrent neck abscess or suppurative thyroiditis, particularly if it contains air, should raise the possibility of a pyriform sinus/fistula (Fig. 10-23). After treatment of the infection, a swallowing study using the appropriate contrast medium is performed to demonstrate the sinus/fistula. Other branchial anomalies are exceedingly rare but include anomalies of the thymus, thyroid (see later), and parathyroid glands. These include aberrant cervical thymus (e.g., within the neck), thymic cysts, parathyroid cysts, and aberrant parathyroid tissue.

Thyroid Anomalies

Thyroglossal duct cyst arises from thyroglossal duct remnants and often occurs in childhood. They are usually midline, or paramedian, and occur at any site from the tongue base to the suprasternal region. Off-midline cysts often occur near along the outer thyroid cartilage and deep to the neck muscles. The lesion is often circumscribed and anechoic or hypoechoic on US, low density on CT, and either T1-isointense to hypointense or T1-isointense to hyperintense, with T2 hyperintensity on MRI (Fig. 10-24). Complex lesions with heterogeneity on imaging also occur (e.g., with infection), and a sinus tract may be present. The differential diagnosis includes dermoid, teratoma, vallecular cyst, mucous retention cyst, laryngocele (see Fig. 10-24), lymphatic malformation, and branchial

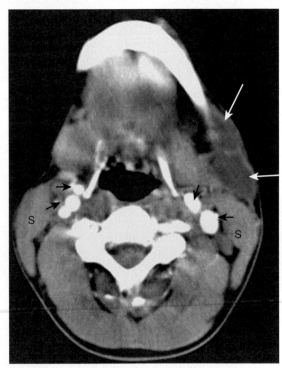

FIGURE 10-21. Left second branchial cyst (*white arrows*) on axial vascular contrast–enhanced CT scan, showing enhancement of carotid and jugular vessels (*black arrows*). S, sternocleidomastoid muscle.

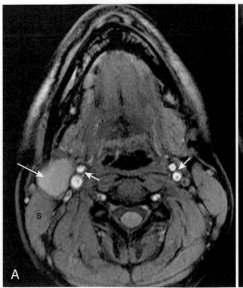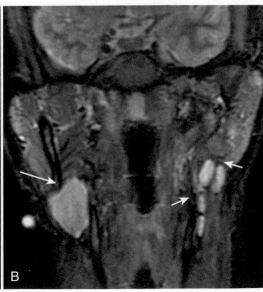

FIGURE 10-22. Axial T1-weighted (**A**) and T2-weighted coronal (**B**) MR images with fat suppression showing right second branchial cyst (*long arrows*), normal carotid and jugular vessels (*short arrows* in **A**) and normal left lymph nodes (*short arrows* in **B**). S, sternocleidomastoid muscle.

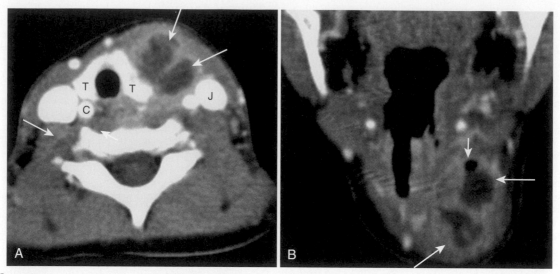

Figure 10-23. Axial (**A**) and coronal (**B**) vascular contrast–enhanced CT scans showing pyriform sinus fistula with perithyroidal abscess (*long arrows*) and air bubble (*short arrow* in **B**). C, common carotid artery; J, internal jugular vein; T, thyroid.

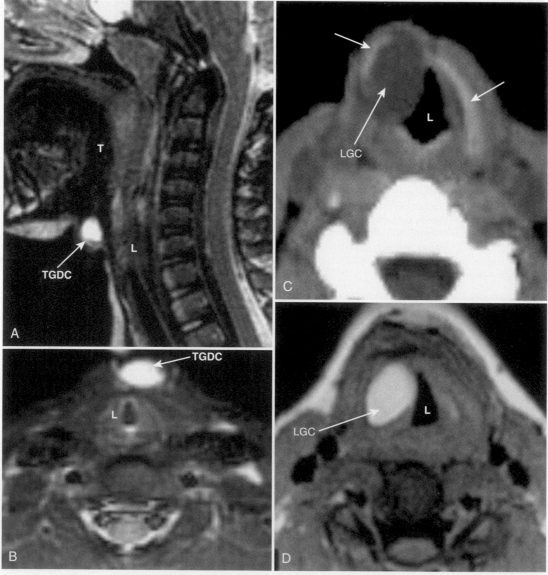

Figure 10-24. Thyroglossal duct cyst (TGDC) appears as an infrahyoid, extralaryngeal high intensity on sagittal (**A**) and axial (**B**) T2-weighted MR images. Laryngeal cyst (LGC) appears as a low-density, hyperintense laryngeal mass on axial CT scan (**C**) and T1-weighted MR image (**D**), also showing thyroid cartilage involvement (*arrows*) and extralaryngeal extension. L, larynx; T, tongue base.

anomalies. Other thyroid anomalies include hypogenesis (partial or complete) and ectopic thyroid tissue (usually near the foramen cecum at the tongue base; Fig. 10-25). In congenital hypothyroidism with absence of a normal thyroid gland, US should search for ectopic tissue. Such tissue may be shown by thyroid scintigraphy to be nonfunctional or the only functioning thyroid tissue.

Laryngocele

A laryngocele results from obstructive dilatation of the laryngeal ventricle and may be aerated or fluid-filled. The lesion may be internal, external, or translaryngeal. Complications include infection and airway compromise. The CT attenuation and MR intensity of the content vary with air and fluid content. There may be slight enhancement of the cyst wall. The differential diagnosis includes thyroglossal duct cyst and laryngeal mucosal cyst (see Fig. 10-24).

Anomalies of the Oral Cavity, Tongue, and Salivary Glands

Congenital and developmental abnormalities of the oral cavity previously described include lingual thyroid (see Fig. 10-25), thyroglossal duct cyst, and second branchial cleft cysts. Dermoid-epidermoid and vascular anomalies are also discussed elsewhere.

Agenesis of the major salivary glands is rare, causes xerostomia, and may be associated with absence of the lacrimal glands. The diagnosis can be confirmed by RI or MRI. Developmental cystic lesions of the salivary glands are uncommon. They usually involve the parotid gland and include branchial cysts and dermoid cysts. There may be painless swelling or signs of infection. These cysts are to be differentiated from lymphoepithelial cysts (e.g., acquired immunodeficiency syndrome [AIDS]). Nonobstructive sialectasis is a common anomaly of the salivary glands. Saccular ductal dilatation often involves the parotid gland. Infection exacerbates the ectasia and manifests as parotitis.

Jaw Anomalies

Mandibular and maxillary hypoplasia may be seen with a number of craniofacial syndromes (see earlier discussions). This includes mandibular hypoplasia with micrognathia and retrognathia (e.g., Pierre Robin sequence) associated with posterior palatal defects and aerodigestive compromise. 3DCT is often needed for preoperative planning (see Fig. 10-11).

Fibrous dysplasia occurs more often in the maxilla than the mandible. It appears as a unilocular or multilocular, ill-defined, expansile CT hypodensity when fibrous tissue predominates (see Fig. 10-5). Admixture of bony matrix increases the lesion's density. It may appear homogeneously hyperdense with bony expansion.

Cherubism is a benign hereditary condition misnamed "congenital fibrous dysplasia." It often appears between 2 and 5 years of age, progresses until puberty, and then regresses. The mandible and maxilla are often both involved by multiple expansile fibro-osseous lesions (Fig. 10-26).

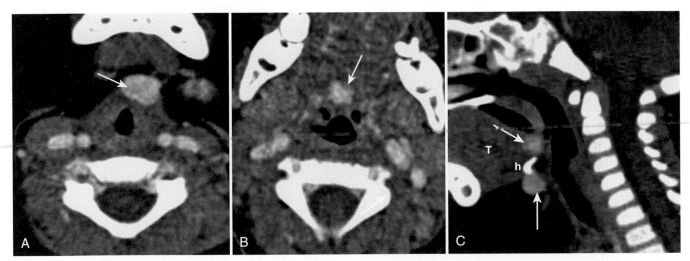

FIGURE 10-25. Ectopic thyroid as high-density suprahyoid and infrahyoid nodules (*arrows*) on axial (**A** and **B**) and sagittal (**C**) vascular contrast–enhanced CT scans. h, hyoid; T, tongue.

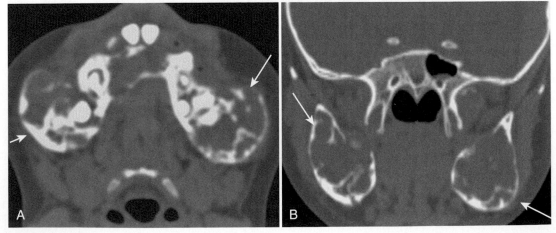

FIGURE 10-26. Cherubism (*arrows*) on axial (**A**) and coronal (**B**) CT scans.

Trauma

Orbit and Globe

Blunt and penetrating impact injuries are common in childhood.

Orbit fracture may be isolated or occur with other face or cranial fractures. *Orbit floor and inferior rim fractures* rarely occur prior to maxillary pneumatization. Frontal impact may result in a blow-out fracture of the orbital floor near the infraorbital canal (Fig. 10-27). CT may also show herniation of orbital fat or displacement of the inferior rectus or inferior oblique muscle into the fracture and maxillary sinus (upward gaze impairment). Rarely is there upward displacement of the orbital floor fragments (blow-in fracture) with impingement on the muscles or globe.

Orbit roof and superior rim fractures may be associated with CSF leak or herniation of brain tissue or meninges into the orbit. Fracture depression may rarely impinge upon the globe (upward gaze impairment).

Medial orbital wall fracture into the ethmoid may be isolated or may be associated with an orbital floor fracture (see Fig. 10-27). Orbital emphysema most commonly occurs with this fracture type. Although orbital fat herniation can occur, muscle entrapment is rare. Orbital emphysema associated with frontal or sphenoid fractures usually indicates severe or complex injury.

Orbit and ocular complications of trauma (including surgery) include hematoma, emphysema, CSF leak, traumatic cephalocele, infection, growing fracture, retinal tear, intraocular hemorrhage, ocular rupture, enophthalmos, optic nerve avulsion, vascular occlusion, pseudoaneurysm, and carotid-cavernous fistula. Penetrating orbit injury may result in retained foreign body and secondary infection.

Nasal Cavity, Paranasal Sinuses, and Face

Foreign Body

Insertion of foreign material into the nose, including that of extrinsic origin (beans, seeds, toys, beads, plastic or metal objects, etc.) and intrinsic origin (emesis or expectoration of ingested or aspirated material, inspissated mucosal secretions, bony sequestra, and mineralized concretions [rhinoliths]), is common in young children. Secondary purulent rhinitis, sinusitis, adenoiditis, or otitis media (OM) is common. CT may be needed to identify a radiopaque object or to delineate the associated infection.

Fractures

Facial fractures may be related to vehicular accident, fall, recreation, or assault. They are infrequent in young children (< 5-6 years) and tend to be greenstick in type. The high craniofacial ratio predisposes to frontal, cranial, and intracranial injuries. With maturation and increased sinus pneumatization, the adult pattern becomes more common, including midface and mandibular fractures, plus fragmentation and displacement. Frequently involved structures include the nasal bones, mandible, orbit

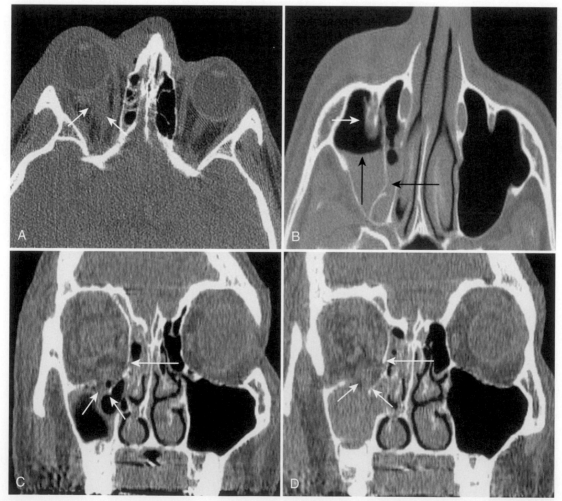

FIGURE 10-27. Right orbit and sinus trauma on axial (**A** and **B**) and coronal (**C** and **D**) CT scans. Findings include periorbital and malar swelling, perioptic edema, and hemorrhage (*arrows* on **A**); orbitoethmoid fracture (*horizontal long arrows* in **B** to **D**) and orbital floor fracture with herniation of orbital fat and inferior rectus muscle (*short arrows* in **B** to **D**); and maxillary sinus air-fluid level (*vertical black arrow* in **B**). Compare with normal left orbit and sinus structures.

and zygomaticomaxillary structures (see Figs. 10-27 and 10-28). Other system injuries are common, and midface fractures usually indicate severe trauma. Axial CT with coronal and sagittal reformatting is indicated and is performed in proper sequence according to injury priority.

Nasal fracture from minor frontal impact includes the greenstick type in younger children with splaying of the nasal bones. In older patients, such an impact usually produces bilateral distal nasal bone fractures, and the septum may be fractured and displaced. With severe impact, more extensive fractures may involve the nasal pyramid, maxilla, lacrimal and ethmoid bones, nasal septum, cribriform plate, and orbital roof (e.g., hemorrhage or CSF leak). Subchondral nasal septal hematoma may produce thickening or a mass. Surgical drainage can prevent necrosis, abscess, and perforation.

Mandibular condyle fracture, the most common *mandible fracture*, often results from a fall with impact to the chin. It is frequently bilateral and may be associated with a parasymphyseal fracture. Condylar head injury may result in underdevelopment or ankylosis. Condylar neck fractures typically occur in older children. Associated temporomandibular joint injury may rarely occur. The latter may require additional MRI. Asymmetric mandibular body fractures are commonly seen with side impact (e.g., assault) in adolescence (Fig. 10-28).

Other *midface fractures* (e.g., maxillary and zygomatic) are rare in young children but may extend bilaterally or superiorly to involve the frontal region. Associated CNS injury or CSF leak is common. In older children, the adult pattern predominates and includes isolated maxillary alveolar fractures, partial fractures of the maxilla, palatal fractures, the LeFort fractures, and lateral midface or trimalar fractures.

Frontal bone fractures occur most commonly in younger children, are of the greenstick type (nonpneumatized frontal sinus), and may extend into the skull or orbital roof. In older children, frontal sinus fractures may result from direct impact or from extension of a skull fracture. Intracranial injury is common. Posterior wall fracture may be associated with CSF leak, pneumocephalus, or CNS infection.

Sphenoid fractures rarely occur but indicate severe trauma, including other skull base fractures. CT may show sinus opacification, air-fluid level, or pneumocephalus. CTA may be indicated to evaluate for associated carotid arterial or cavernous sinus injury (e.g., carotid-cavernous fistula; see Chapter 8).

Ear and Temporal Bone

Petrous and mastoid trauma may result in external auditory canal hemorrhage, hemotympanum, CSF otorrhea, hearing loss, vertigo, or facial nerve palsy. CT may show opacification of the EAC,

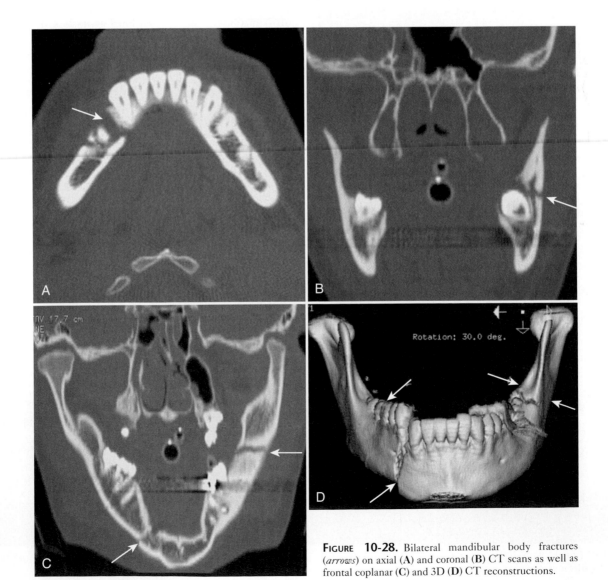

FIGURE 10-28. Bilateral mandibular body fractures (*arrows*) on axial (**A**) and coronal (**B**) CT scans as well as frontal coplanar (**C**) and 3D (**D**) CT reconstructions.

MEC, or mastoid air cells. Local pneumocephalus is common, and there may be intracranial hemorrhage or brain injury.

Fractures are classified according to their course relative to the long axis of the petrous bone. *Longitudinal fractures* often result from lateral impact and commonly involve the mastoid (Fig. 10-29). The result may be tympanic membrane rupture, ossicular disruption, and fracture of the tegmen tympani. The inner ear is often spared. Fractures may not heal except for fibrous union. Facial nerve paralysis may result from injury distal to the geniculate ganglion.

Transverse fractures usually result from an occipital or frontal impact and may involve the mastoid (Fig. 10-30) or the otic capsule and internal auditory canal. With the latter fracture, there may be sensorineural hearing loss and vertigo. Facial nerve paralysis is often due to injury proximal to the geniculate ganglion. Combined longitudinal and transverse, or oblique, fractures usually result in petrous bone fragmentation. Because of the incompletely developed mastoid, the facial nerve is also susceptible to trauma in the neonate and young infant.

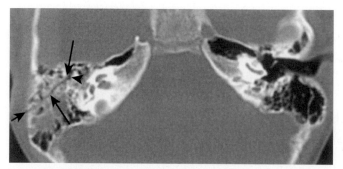

FIGURE 10-29. Right longitudinal mastoid fracture (*arrows*) on axial CT scan.

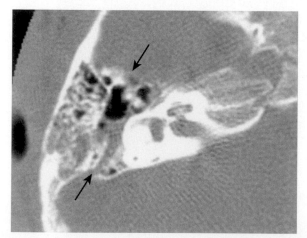

FIGURE 10-30. Right transverse mastoid fracture (*arrows*) on axial CT scan.

Oral Cavity and Neck

Trauma mechanisms in the oral cavity and neck include vehicular accidents, bites, knife or gun wounds, surgery, burns, and oral penetration by foreign objects. CT may show edema, contusion, laceration, hematoma, or air. Soft tissue emphysema may result from external penetration or injury of the airway, thorax (i.e., pneumothorax), or esophagus. There may be airway compression, airway or esophageal perforation, vascular injury, retained foreign body, or subsequent infection. Intravenous contrast agents may be used to delineate vessels or to evaluate infection. Oral or esophageal contrast enhancement may show pharyngeal or esophageal penetration. Vascular injury may include laceration, transection, contusion, dissection, false aneurysm, arteriovenous fistula, thrombosis, and embolization. CTA or CT venography using MDCT may be preferred to MRA/MRV, although angiography may be necessary. Salivary gland trauma may cause emphysema, hematoma, duct stricture or transection, fistula, sialocele, or subsequent infection.

Vascular Abnormalities

Vascular abnormalities of the head and neck may include variants, anomalies, and tumors. These are presented here according to category and region. The Mulliken and Glowacki biologic classification of vascular anomalies involving cutaneous and muscular tissues includes hemangiomas and vascular malformations. Hemangiomas are congenital endothelial tumors, whereas vascular malformations are endothelial-lined anomalies. They are distinguished both by clinical criteria and imaging features (high flow vs. low flow), especially on US with Doppler imaging and MRI. The orbit, parotid, face, scalp, oral cavity, and neck are frequent sites of origin.

Hemangioma is the most common tumor of the head and neck in childhood. It evolves from a cellular proliferative phase to a plateau phase, and then to an involuting phase. Proliferating hemangiomas are high-flow benign neoplasms that appear as vascular flow voids (hypointensity) on spin echo (SE) sequences, hyperintensity on GE vascular flow or MRA sequences, and marked tumor enhancement on gadolinium-enhanced sequences (Figs. 10-31 to 10-33). There may be arteriovenous shunting. Involuting hemangiomas demonstrate decreasing flow characteristics, decreasing tumor size, and increased fibrofatty tissue. Involution is usually complete by age 7 to 8 years and may mimic a lipoma or low-flow malformation. Hemangiomas may be further categorized as congenital hemangioma, endangering hemangioma (e.g., orbit, airway, spontaneous hemorrhage), noninvoluting congenital hemangioma, multiple hemangioma or hemangiomatosis, kaposiform hemangioendothelioma, and Kasabach-Merritt syndrome (consumptive coagulopathy).

Vascular malformations are subclassified as capillary, arterial, venous, lymphatic, and combined. Venous malformation (VM) and lymphatic malformation (LM) are low-flow anomalies (no vascular high-flow voids) consisting of septated or cystic channels, and often with a fibrofatty stroma. VMs are characterized by phleboliths and

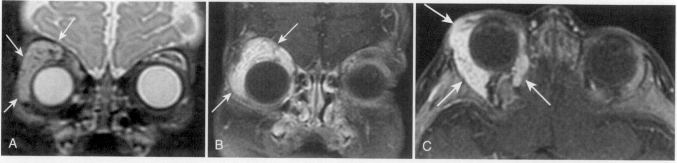

FIGURE 10-31. Orbit hemangioma (*arrows*) on coronal T2-weighted (**A**) as well as coronal (**B**) and axial (**C**) gadolinium-enhanced T1-weighted MR images, all with fat suppression, which also show intrinsic vascular high-flow voids.

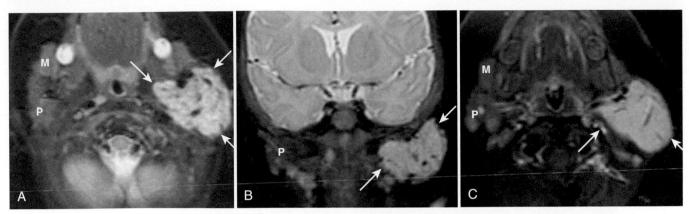

FIGURE 10-32. Left parotid hemangioma (*arrows*) on axial T2-weighted (**A**), coronal T2-weighted (**B**), and axial gadolinium-enhanced T1-weighted (**C**) MR images, all with fat suppression, which also show vascular high-flow voids. M, masseter muscle; P, parotid gland.

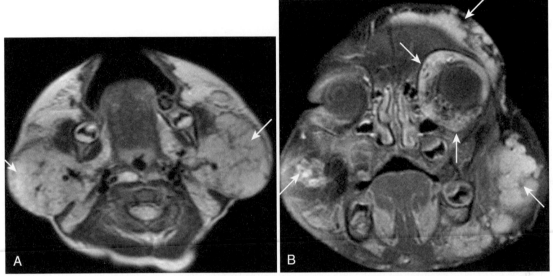

FIGURE 10-33. PHACE (posterior fossa abnormalities, facial hemangioma, arterial abnormalities, cardiovascular defects, eye abnormalities) syndrome with multiple hemangiomata (*arrows*) on axial T2-weighted MR image with fat suppression (**A**) and coronal gadolinium-enhanced T1-weighted MR image (**B**), which show facial, scalp, parotid, and orbit involvement.

gadolinium enhancement of the cavernous blood-filled spaces (Fig. 10-34). There may also be prominent draining or anomalous veins (hyperintensity on GE vascular flow or MRV sequences). LMs may be macrocystic (e.g., cystic hygroma), microcystic, or mixed (Figs. 10-35 and 10-36). Only the septa (separating the lymph-filled spaces) show enhancement. Proteinaceous or hemorrhagic fluid-fluid levels are characteristic. Rapid enlargement may be seen with hemorrhage or infection. Common combined malformations include venolymphatic malformation (VLM) and AVM. VLMs share features of both VM and LM. It may be difficult to distinguish VLM from mixed microcystic/macrocystic LM. AVM is a high-flow anomaly without a tumor component, although reactive tissue intensities may be present. It is composed of arterial feeding vessels, vascular nidus, and venous draining vessels. In some cases there are one or more direct AV connections or fistulae without a nidus.

A number of syndromes in childhood are associated with vascular anomalies. Examples are PHACE association (**p**osterior fossa abnormalities, facial **h**emangioma, **a**rterial abnormalities, **c**ardiovascular defects, **e**ye abnormalities; see Fig. 10-33), Sturge-Weber syndrome (facial cutaneous capillary or telangiectatic malformation in a trigeminal distribution), Beckwith-Wiedemann syndrome (facial capillary or telangiectatic malformation), Klippel-Trenaunay-Weber syndrome (capillary, venous, and lymphatic malformations), Maffucci syndrome (multiple venous malformations), Rendu-Osler-Weber (hereditary hemorrhagic

telangiectasia) syndrome (capillary or telangiectatic malformation), and blue rubber bleb nevus syndrome.

Orbit and Globe

Hemangioma is the most common tumor of the pediatric orbit (as previously discussed) and may be preseptal, extraconal, intraconal, or multicompartmental (see Figs. 10-31 and 10-33). VM or LM may occasionally involve the orbit. Other vascular abnormalities of the orbit include varices, AVM, aneurysm, angiodysplastic syndromes, and vascular occlusive disease. Primary varices are venous malformations that drain to the cavernous sinus, face, or scalp veins. Secondary varices are associated with AV shunting (e.g., intracranial AVM, carotid-cavernous or dural AV fistulae, hemangioma) or venous occlusion (dural sinus or jugular venous atresia [smallness or absence of jugular foramina], stenosis, or thrombosis). The varices may be associated with VM or an angiodysplastic syndrome (e.g., Klippel-Trenaunay-Weber). Varices appear as prominent, tortuous flow voids whose size may vary with respiration, Valsalva maneuver, or arterial pulsation. Blood pool enhancement on CT or MRI is characteristic, but hemorrhage is rare.

Aneurysms and pseudoaneurysms of the orbit are very rare in childhood (e.g., AVM, hemangioma, carotid dissection). Prominent ophthalmic arterial collateral vessels may be seen with moyamoya disease (see Chapter 8). Other vascular anomalies and abnormalities may occur in association with cervicofacial hemangiomas.

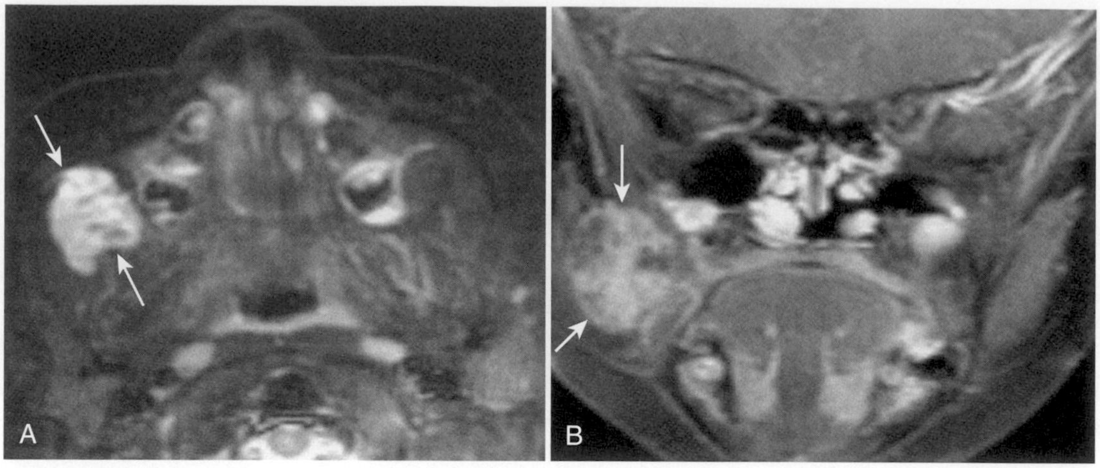

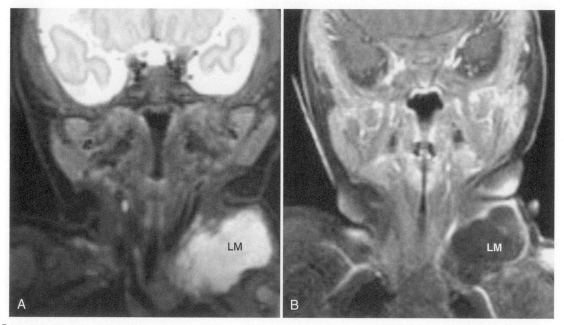

FIGURE 10-34. Venous malformation (VM) of the right masseter muscle appears as a high-intensity and enhancing area (*arrows*) on axial T2-weighted MR image with fat suppression (**A**) and coronal gadolinium-enhanced T1-weighted MR image (**B**). Low intensities within the VM represent phleboliths.

FIGURE 10-35. Left neck macrocystic lymphatic malformation (LM) (cystic hygroma) on coronal T2-weighted MR image with fat suppression (**A**) and coronal gadolinium-enhanced T1-weighted MR image (**B**), showing septal and rim enhancement.

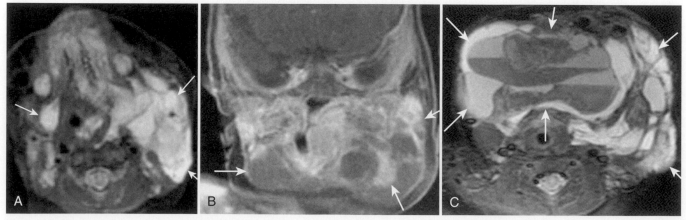

FIGURE 10-36. Macrocystic and microcystic lymphatic malformation (*arrows*) on axial T2-weighted MR image with fat suppression (**A**) and coronal gadolinium-enhanced T1-weighted MR image (**B**). Subsequent axial T2-weighted MR image (**C**) shows enhancing septations and hemorrhagic levels.

The Wyburn-Mason syndrome is an ocular vascular malformation with orbital and intracranial components (i.e., pituitary-hypothalamic and brainstem).

Nasal Cavity, Paranasal Sinuses, and Face

Vascular abnormalities may manifest as epistaxis, nasosinus obstruction, or cosmetic deformity. The nose and nasal cavity are vascularized by terminal branches of the internal and external carotid arteries. Common causes of epistaxis in childhood are infections, allergic rhinitis, and trauma (e.g., fracture, foreign body, excoriation). Severe or recurrent epistaxis may be related to coagulopathy, neoplasia (e.g., angiofibroma), or vascular anomalies (e.g., telangiectasia in hereditary hemorrhagic telangiectasia syndrome). CT and CTA may be performed initially. MRI or angiography may be necessary, particularly if intervention is needed for control of the bleeding.

Ear and Temporal Bone

A *high jugular bulb* is the most common vascular anomaly of the temporal bone. There is a thin bony covering, a poorly pneumatized mastoid, and dehiscence of the floor with protrusion of the jugular bulb into the middle ear cavity (Fig. 10-37). Symptoms may include pulsatile tinnitus, headache, or conductive hearing loss. An enhancing mass is present in the middle ear at the bony defect on CT or MRI. The anomalous vein is vulnerable to trauma or surgical procedures. Atresia or stenosis of the jugular vein may occur in isolation or in Crouzon disease, achondroplasia, and other similar conditions. The foramen is absent or small, and venous collaterals are present.

Anomalies of the ICA include aberrancy and partial or complete absence. They may be symptomatic (e.g., tinnitus, hearing loss). Aberrant ICA results from absence of the bony plate of the carotid canal. The aberrant ICA may protrude into the middle ear cavity and lie against the tympanic membrane, making it vulnerable to trauma or surgery. Partial absence of the ICA most often involves the vertical petrous segment, including atresia of that segment of the canal. Reconstitution occurs through an enlarged inferior tympanic artery. These anomalies appear as an enhancing mass in the hypotympanum. Complete agenesis of the ICA is associated with an atretic carotid canal. Angiography shows the arterial collateralization.

Persistent stapedial artery may occur with aberrant ICA or may be isolated (see Fig. 10-37). This anomaly is suspected when there is absence of the foramen spinosum and an anterior tympanic facial canal mass (i.e., aberrant middle meningeal artery). Hemangiomas

and vascular malformations (as discussed previously) may involve the auricle and EAC but are uncommon in the temporal bone.

Neck, Oral Cavity, and Jaw

LM (i.e., cystic hygroma), VM, and hemangiomas are the most common vascular anomalies arising in the neck in childhood (see Figs. 10-32 to 10-36). They may be small and localized, or large and extensive, involving many compartments, including the mediastinum.

Jugular vein and carotid artery variants, or anomalies, are also common. The internal jugular veins are almost always asymmetric, the right larger than left. Occasionally they are multiple. The external and anterior jugular veins are also asymmetric and may be multiple or absent. The term *phlebectasia* (i.e., varix or ectasia) describes a normal vein that appears dilated in the supine position and may cause soft tissue fullness. The pterygoid venous plexus may be asymmetric and appears on CT or MRI as a pseudomass in the parapharyngeal space. The ICA may be tortuous, swing medially, and cause a pulsatile submucosal retropharyngeal mass. An aberrant medial course is also found in the velocardio facial syndrome and must be documented before corrective palatal surgery.

Infections and Inflammatory Processes

See Box 10-2.

> ### Box 10-2. Pediatric Head and Neck Infections and Inflammatory Processes
>
> Periorbital/orbital cellulitis/abscess
> Inflammatory pseudotumor
> Chorioretinitis/endophthalmitis/optic neuritis
> Acute rhinitis/sinusitis
> Allergic rhinitis
> Subacute/chronic sinonasal infections
> Otitis externa
> Otitis media and mastoiditis
> Chronic otitis media and cholesteatoma
> Adenotonsillar/pharyngeal infection
> Lymphadenitis/cellulitis/abscess
> Thyroiditis
> Sialadenitis
> Osteomyelitis (e.g., mandible)

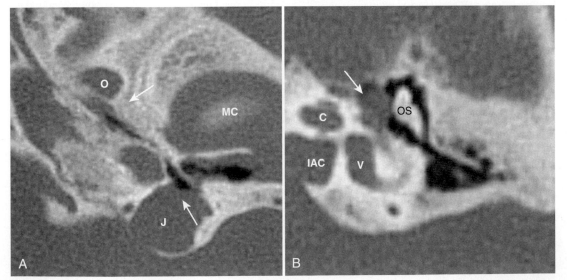

FIGURE 10-37. A and **B,** Axial CT scans of left jugular vein dehiscence and persistent stapedial artery anomaly. **A,** Absence of the jugular bony strut (*lower arrow*) and of the foramen spinosum (*upper arrow*). **B,** Mass (*arrow*) near the anterior tympanic portion of the facial nerve canal. C, cochlea; IAC, internal auditory canal; J, jugular bulb; MC, mandibular condyle; O, foramen ovale; os, ossicles; V, vestibule.

Orbit and Globe

The orbit is a common site of infection or inflammation, whether primary or secondary (especially from the paranasal sinuses). The infecting agent is usually bacterial and less often viral, mycotic, parasitic, or tuberculous. Noninfectious or postinfectious orbital inflammation may be seen as orbital pseudotumor with myositis. Infection may also be seen after penetrating trauma, especially if there is a foreign body. Unusual inflammations include endophthalmitis, dacryoadenitis, and optic neuritis.

Suppurative Infection

The most common orbital disease of childhood is bacterial infection (e.g., staphylococcal, streptococcal, pneumococcal, or from *Haemophilus*). *Preseptal (periorbital) cellulitis* involves the eyelid and adjacent face without intraorbital (postseptal) involvement. In infants, it is commonly of hematogenous origin (e.g., *Haemophilus*). *Postseptal (orbital) cellulitis* is usually extraconal and subperiosteal, but usually manifests with a preseptal component (Fig. 10-38). It is usually associated with ethmoid sinusitis (e.g., younger children) but may occur with maxillary or frontal sinusitis (e.g., older children, adolescents).

Orbital infection (extraconal or intraconal) may also result from facial infection, from sinus or facial fracture, or from penetrating trauma with a retained foreign body. Infection may also complicate an existing anomaly (e.g., cephalocele, nasolacrimal mucocele). Other complications of orbital infection may result in osteomyelitis, orbital or cavernous sinus thrombophlebitis (Fig. 10-39), epidural abscess, subdural empyema, meningitis, cerebritis, or brain abscess (see Chapter 8). Infection may also be confined to, or extend from, the lacrimal gland or duct (i.e., dacryoadenitis; see Fig. 10-3). Imaging of orbital inflammation may show edema, cellulitis, or abscess. Abscess may demonstrate central fluid or air content and rim enhancement. Preseptal infection and subperiosteal infection tend to be localized. Postseptal involvement of the extraconal or intraconal space results in increased density of the orbital fat and may obscure the optic nerve, muscle, and ocular landmarks. Follow-up imaging after antibiotic treatment and reduced inflammation may uncover an existing lesion (e.g., cephalocele, tumor, cyst, fracture, foreign body).

Inflammatory Pseudotumor

Also common in childhood, *inflammatory pseudotumor* refers to idiopathic inflammatory lymphoid infiltration of the orbit (Fig. 10-40). CT or MRI may demonstrate unilateral or bilateral enlargement of one or more extraocular muscles and tendons, uveoscleral thickening, or a retro-ocular mass. Enhancement is common, but bony involvement is rare. The disease often responds to steroid treatment. Orbital pseudotumor differs from Graves disease by its asymmetric muscular involvement, painful proptosis, and the lack of thyroid disease. Occasionally, inflammatory pseudotumor may arise within the paranasal sinuses and cause bony destruction and infiltration of the orbit. In these cases, it must be differentiated from infection, neoplasm (e.g., lymphoma, rhabdomyosarcoma), and Wegener granulomatosis. The *Tolosa-Hunt syndrome* is a painful, steroid-responsive ophthalmoplegia that may be seen in adolescence. It results from idiopathic granulomatous inflammation of the orbital apex and cavernous sinus. It may be complicated by orbital venous and cavernous sinus thrombosis (see Fig. 10-39). The differential diagnosis includes fungal infection, lymphoma, and, rarely, dermatomyositis, sarcoidosis, tuberculosis, or meningioma.

Other Inflammatory Processes

Orbital invasion may follow an aggressive fungal sinus infection (e.g., mucormycosis, aspergillosis), especially in immunocompromised individuals. Vascular and cavernous sinus involvement may cause thrombosis, infarction, or hemorrhage. Other complications of sinusitis which may rarely involve the orbit include mucoceles, retention cysts, papillomas, polyps, and granulomas (as discussed below).

Ocular and Optic Inflammatory Processes

Sclerosing endophthalmitis is a granulomatous uveitis due to *Toxocara canis* infestation. Chorioretinitis is often present, including calcification and retinal detachment. A vitreous high density or hyperintensity without a discrete mass is often present on CT or MRI. The findings are similar to those in Coats disease. Chorioretinitis may also be seen with the TORCH infections, particularly cytomegalovirus, and may have similar findings (e.g., calcifications). Optic neuritis rarely occurs in childhood (see Chapter 8). It may be viral or postviral or may be associated with inflammatory pseudotumor, vasculitis, leukemia, granulomatous disease, or juvenile multiple sclerosis. Imaging may show optic or perioptic thickening with marked enhancement.

Nasal Cavity, Paranasal Sinuses, and Face
Acute Rhinitis and Sinusitis

Upper respiratory tract inflammation is very common in childhood and usually viral or allergic. Bacterial infection is usually secondary and results from swelling, obstruction, or stasis (Fig. 10-41). The infecting agents include group A *Streptococcus*, *Pneumococcus*, *Haemophilus*, *Staphylococcus*, and *Moraxella catarrhalis*. Acute, recurrent, and chronic sinusitis may subsequently develop because of ostiomeatal obstruction from persistent swelling or from mucociliary disorders. The difficulty is differentiating viral or allergic inflammation from secondary bacterial infection, which requires antibiotics. Persistent ostial obstruction or mucociliary impairment allows the proliferation of anaerobic microbes. Persistent nasal discharge suggests sinusitis. Other causes of rhinitis/sinusitis are obstruction from foreign body, nasochoanal stenosis/atresia,

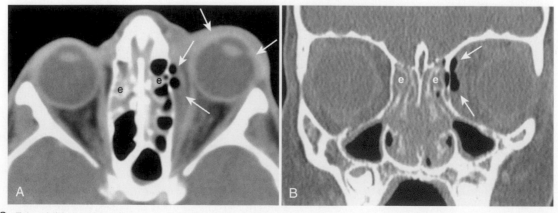

FIGURE 10-38. Ethmoiditis (e) with preseptal periorbital cellulitis (*upper arrows* on **A**) and subperiosteal orbital abscess with air (*medial arrows* in **A** and *arrows* in **B**) on axial soft tissue (**A**) and coronal bone (**B**) contrast-enhanced CT scans.

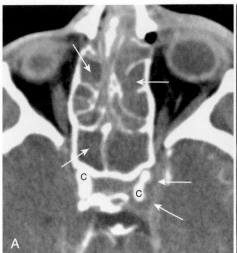
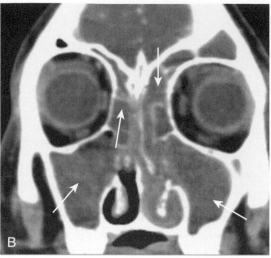

FIGURE **10-39.** Pansinusitis (*upper arrows* in **A**, *arrows* in **B**) with left cavernous sinus thrombosis (*lower left arrows* in **A**), including narrowing of the left internal carotid artery (C) and perioptic and preseptal swelling, on axial (**A**) and coronal (**B**) contrast-enhanced CT scans.

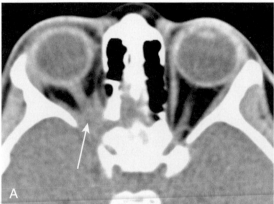
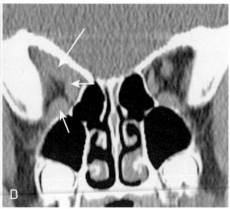

FIGURE **10-40.** Right orbital pseudotumor on axial (**A**) and coronal (**B**) CT scans showing muscle enlargement (*short arrows*) and orbit apex mass (*long arrows*). Compare with normal left musculature.

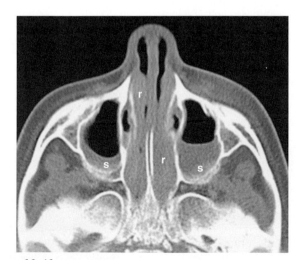

FIGURE **10-41.** Acute rhinitis (r) with turbinate congestion and bilateral acute maxillary sinusitis (s) and air-fluid levels on axial CT scan.

septal deviation, polyp, and tumor. Sinus infection may occasionally be of dental origin, including periodontitis, periapical abscess, minor trauma, and surgery (e.g., perforation with oroantral fistula). Developmental bony defects and dental cysts may also provide a direct pathway for sinusitis.

Allergic Rhinitis

Allergic rhinitis is another common cause of nasal or sinus obstruction and rhinorrhea in children (Fig. 10-42). Mucostasis with ostial obstruction is often followed by bacterial infection. Differentiating infectious from allergic sinusitis is difficult because they often coexist. The involvement is usually bilateral and diffuse in allergic sinusitis. The nasal turbinates are often edematous or thickened. Nodular thickening may be present, but air-fluid levels are unusual. Polyps often result from chronic mucosal hyperplasia and are commonly multiple. Unilateral involvement suggests ostiomeatal obstruction, and an air-fluid level suggests an infectious process. Intraluminal sinonasal fungal infections (including aspergillosis) may manifest as polypoid lesions or as fungus balls in patients with atopy (Fig. 10-43). Relative CT hyperdensity or T2 hypointensity may be seen along with marked enhancement.

Subacute and Chronic Sinonasal Infection

Fungal infection tends to be seen in chronically ill or immunocompromised children (e.g., patients with cancer and transplant recipients). Mucormycosis and aspergillosis are the most common pathogens. They are aggressive and fulminant fungal infections that invade the orbit, cavernous sinus, and neurovascular structures (Fig. 10-44; see Fig. 10-39). The result may be thrombosis, infarction, hemorrhage, or abscess. *Adenoidal and tonsillar hyperplasia* may cause obstruction; acute obstruction may lead to purulent rhinorrhea, and chronic obstruction to alveolar hypoventilation, cor pulmonale, and sleep apnea. Nasal obstruction and

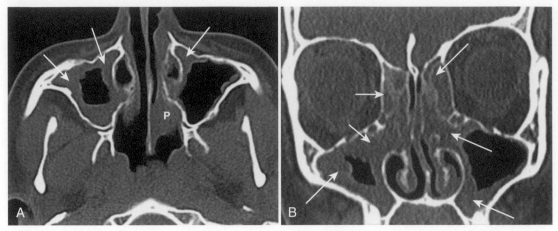

FIGURE 10-42. Asthma with allergic rhinitis and pansinusitis on axial (**A**) and coronal (**B**) CT scans showing chronic asymmetric mucosal thickening (*arrows*), polyps (**P**), and right maxillary sinus air-fluid level.

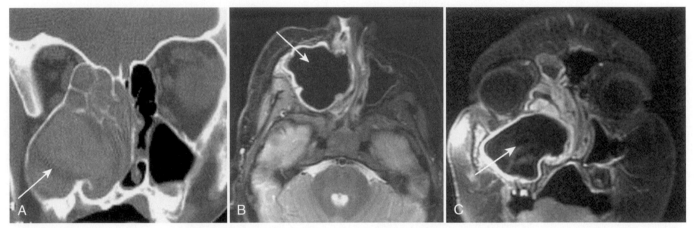

FIGURE 10-43. Right maxillary and ethmoid fungal mycetoma with polyposis (*arrows*) is isodense to hyperdense on coronal CT scans (**A**) and hypointense on axial T2-weighted (**B**) and coronal gadolinium-enhanced T1-weighted (**C**) MR images.

rhinorrhea may occur with cerebral palsy, familial dysautonomia, midface anomalies, or tumors.

Sinonasal obstruction and rhinorrhea are common manifestations of *cystic fibrosis* (Fig. 10-45). There is chronic sinusitis with mucosal thickening, mucus inspissation, and nasal polyps. Inflammatory sinonasal disease also occurs in systemic lupus erythematosus, other rheumatoid or connective tissue diseases, Wegener granulomatosis, sarcoidosis, Churg-Strauss syndrome, and atrophic rhinitis. Nasal septal or bony sinus destruction is characteristic of these conditions.

Inflammatory pseudotumor is a chronic inflammatory lesion that may result from an exaggerated immune response. These are histologically diverse masses of acute and chronic inflammation with a variable fibrous response, often a plasmacytic component, and no granulomatous elements. These pseudotumors may respond to steroid therapy. They mimic lymphoma and chloroma.

Imaging Findings
The imaging findings in sinonasal congestion or inflammation may not correlate with clinical sinusitis. Acute sinusitis may show sinus opacification (i.e., edema and secretions) or mucosal thickening with air-fluid levels (see Figs. 10-41 and 10-42). Air-fluid levels may also occur from trauma, barotrauma, lavage, intubation, hemorrhage, or CSF rhinorrhea. Chronic sinusitis may appear on imaging as mucosal thickening, retention cysts, polyps, sinus opacification, loss of the mucoperiosteal margin, and osteopenia or sclerosis (see Figs. 10-14, 10-42 to 10-45). Mucosal thickening, edema, and mucous secretions are CT-isointense to hypodense,

T1-hypointense, and T2-hyperintense. With inspissation, the secretions may become concretions and are CT-hyperdense, T2-hypointense, and T1-hypointense or hyperintense. Tumor is often isointense, whereas fibrosis is usually hypointense on all MR sequences. Acute or subacute inflammatory mucosal thickening usually demonstrates contrast enhancement, whereas chronic, fibrotic thickening often does not. Secretions and edema usually do not enhance. Single, or unilateral, turbinate enlargement may reflect the normal nasal cycle rather than inflammation.

Complications of Sinusitis
Mucous and serous *retention cysts* result from obstruction of submucosal mucinous glands or from a serous effusion (see Fig. 10-14). *Polyps* result from mucosal hyperplasia (see Figs. 10-42, 10-43, 10-45). They may be solitary or multiple and usually are allergic or occur with cystic fibrosis. *Antrochoanal polyps* are usually solitary and arise from the maxillary antra. They often extend through the ostium into the middle meatus, enlarge the sinonasal cavity, and may also extend into the posterior choana and nasopharynx. On imaging, cysts and polyps are homogeneous soft tissue masses with an air interface. They have CT and MRI characteristics similar to those of mucosal inflammation. Polyps often appear as rounded masses associated with ostial enlargement, sinonasal expansion, and bony attenuation. Polyps are often T2-hyperintense and may show diffuse or surface enhancement. Occasionally, they are fibrous with high CT density and T2 hypointensity. There may be trapped secretions intermixed with mucoceles.

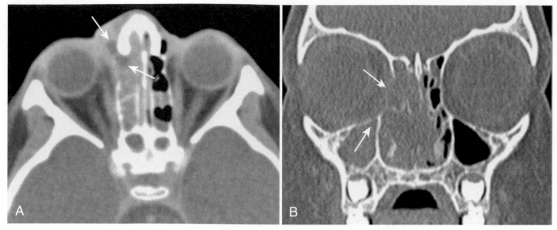

FIGURE 10-44. Right maxillary and ethmoid sinus aspergillosis with bony destruction (*arrows*) on axial (**A**) and coronal (**B**) CT scans.

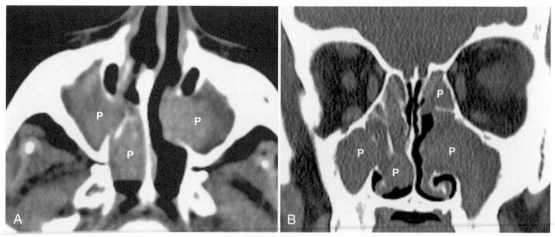

FIGURE 10-45. Cystic fibrosis with sinonasal polyposis (P) on axial (**A**) and coronal (**B**) CT, which show relative high densities and nasosinus expansion.

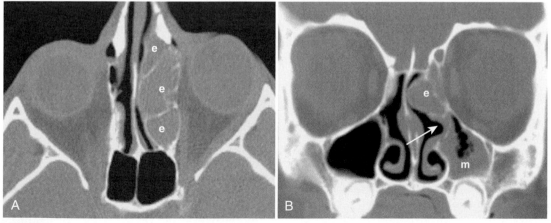

FIGURE 10-46. Left ethmoidal mucocele (e) and left ostiomeatal obstruction (*arrow*) as well as chronic left maxillary sinusitis (m) on axial (**A**) and coronal (**B**) CT scans.

A *mucocele* develops from sinus ostial obstruction and results in opacification and expansion of the sinus (Fig. 10-46). An air-fluid level may suggest a mucopyocele. On CT and MRI, the peripheral enhancement of a mucocele distinguishes it from neoplasm. CT hyperdensity, T2 hypointensity, or T1 hyperintensity may represent chronic inspissated secretions, mycetoma (e.g., aspergillosis), hemorrhage, a sinolith, or an intrasinus tooth.

Orbital complications of sinusitis include preseptal periorbital cellulitis, postseptal or orbital cellulitis, and orbital abscess (see Fig. 10-38). Intracranial complications include meningitis, empyema, abscess, thrombophlebitis, and cavernous sinus thrombosis (see Chapter 8). Osteomyelitis rarely complicates sinonasal infection but may occur with trauma, surgery, or hematogenous spread. Osteopenia progresses to bone destruction. With chronic osteomyelitis, there is irregular thickening and sclerosis with

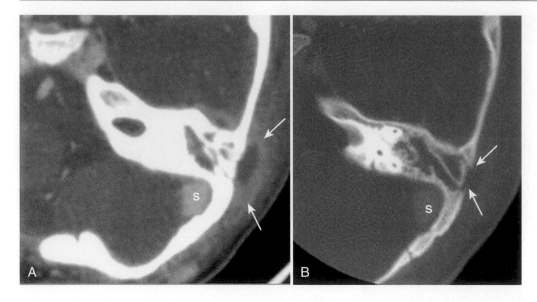

FIGURE 10-47. A and B, Axial contrast-enhanced CT scans showing coalescent mastoiditis with lateral bony erosion (*arrows* in **B**) and subperiosteal abscess (*arrows* in **A**). s, normal sigmoid sinus.

sequestra formation. Imaging may show an irregular, mottled pattern (similar to that in radiation osteitis).

Ear and Temporal Bone
Otitis Media and Mastoiditis
Acute and chronic forms of otitis media characteristically produce a conductive hearing loss. In the acute form there is mucosal edema, effusion, and stasis. Tympanic membrane rupture, otorrhea, and middle ear atelectasis may also occur. Initially the infection may be viral or allergic. Secondary bacterial infection is common (e.g., with *Haemophilus influenzae, Streptococcus, Moraxella catarrhalis*). Middle ear cavity and mastoid air cell opacification (CT isodensity, T2 hyperintensity) usually results from eustachian tube dysfunction or obstruction, especially in infants and young children. The opacification may represent either serous or purulent acute otitis media.

Mastoiditis results from occlusion of the aditus ad antrum and may be a complication of acute OM or the result of chronic OM (e.g., cholesteatoma). CT or MRI shows patchy mastoid opacification (i.e., mucosal edema, mucus, or purulent exudates). *Coalescent mastoiditis* refers to bony trabecular osteopenia or destruction (Fig. 10-47). Complications include suppurative labyrinthitis (MRI enhancement), facial nerve palsy (MRI enhancement), subperiosteal abscess, and neck abscess (Bezold abscess).

Gradenigo syndrome is the triad of petrous apex mastoiditis, eighth cranial nerve palsy, and deep trigeminal pain (Fig. 10-48). Intracranial complications result from bony erosion or septic thrombophlebitis and include epidural abscess, subdural empyema, meningitis, cerebritis, cerebellitis, brain abscess (usually in the temporal lobe or cerebellum), and dural venous sinus thrombosis.

Chronic Otitis Media and Cholesteatoma
Chronic OM results from persistent atelectasis or tympanic perforation, recurrent infection, and chronic effusion. Granulation tissue may be soft or fibrous, contain cholesterol or hemorrhage, and may coexist with cholesteatoma (Fig. 10-49). Enhancement may be seen only on MRI.

Cholesteatomas are stratified squamous epithelial masses with exfoliated keratin (CT-isodense, T2-isointense to hyperintense, nonenhancing). They may be congenital (see also under "Neoplastic Processes") or acquired. Primary acquired cholesteatomas result from eustachian or attic obstruction with tympanic membrane (superior pars flaccida) retraction. They begin in Prussak's space and extend to the mastoid antrum and air cells, often with extension to the posterior tympanic recesses. Secondary acquired

cholesteatomas arise from chronic OM with tympanic membrane perforation (pars tensa). They tend to involve the posterior recesses. Cholesteatomas may also involve the petrous apex. Complications are related to bony erosion or deformity that may involve the scutum, ossicles, mastoid, tegmen tympani, sigmoid sinus plate, facial nerve canal, or lateral semicircular canal (e.g., labyrinthine fistula). Restricted diffusion (DWI-hyperintense, ADC-hypointense) assists in distinguishing cholesteatoma from other inflammatory masses (e.g., granulation). Rare intracranial complications include meningitis, abscess formation, venous sinus thrombosis, and CSF rhinorrhea. Labyrinthine or facial nerve involvement may result in enhancement on MRI. Other causes of conductive hearing loss in chronic otitis media (without cholesteatoma) include ossicular erosion (e.g., incus, stapes), ossicular fixation (e.g., fibrosis, ossification), and tympanosclerosis (hyalinized collagenosis).

Cholesterol Granuloma
Cholesterol granuloma, which may also result from middle ear or mastoid obstruction, contains hemorrhage plus cholesterol crystals. It rarely occurs in childhood and may arise at any point from the middle ear cavity to the petrous apex, or within a mastoidectomy defect. It appears as a nonenhancing soft tissue mass with sharply marginated bone destruction. Hyperintensity on T1- and T2-weighted MRI, which is due to hemoglobin breakdown, is characteristic.

Otitis Externa
Otitis externa is often self-limiting. In immunocompromised patients, a severe necrotizing form may develop that extends to the middle ear and mastoid (e.g., *Pseudomonas aeruginosa*). There may be bony involvement, but rarely intracranial extension.

The Mastoidectomy Ear
A simple mastoidectomy results in removal of mastoid air cells but preservation of the external canal wall and ossicles. Modified radical mastoidectomy preserves the ossicular chain, the bulk of which is removed in a radical mastoidectomy. CT evaluates the surgical defects, residual debris, ossicular chain, the inner ear for possible fistula, and the facial nerve canal.

The Neck, Oral Cavity, and Jaw
Pharyngeal and Retropharyngeal Infection
Inflammatory processes are common in childhood and may manifest as fever, sore throat, jaw pain, dysphagia, drooling, stridor, or torticollis. Intrinsic airway inflammation (e.g., epiglottitis, croup)

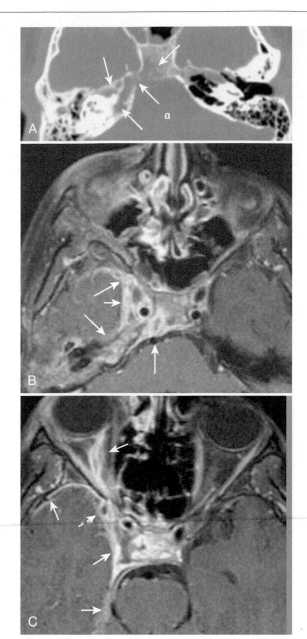

FIGURE 10-48. Gradenigo syndrome on axial CT scan (**A**) and axial gadolinium-enhanced T1-weighted MR images (**B** and **C**). Note the right petrous apex opacification, enhancement, and bony destruction (*arrows* in **A**) as well as the right dural, cavernous sinus, and orbit involvement (*arrows* in **B** and **C**).

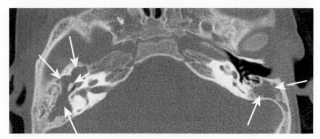

FIGURE 10-49. Bilateral chronic otitis media (*long arrows*) and cholesteatomas on axial CT scan. Because of ossicular destruction, only a portion of the right incus remains (*short arrow*).

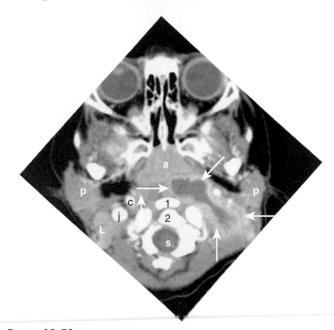

FIGURE 10-50. Retroparapharyngeal and posterior paracervical abscess (*arrows*) on vascular contrast-enhanced CT scan. a, adenoids; c, internal carotid artery; j, internal jugular vein; L, lymph nodes; p, parotid gland; s, cervical spinal cord; 1, anterior arch of atlas; 2, dens of axis.

is covered elsewhere in this book. Acute tonsillitis often occurs in older children and adolescents and may occasionally result in peritonsillar cellulitis or abscess or may extend to the parapharyngeal and retropharyngeal spaces. Parapharyngeal or retropharyngeal lymphadenitis may do the same, especially in infants and young children (Fig. 10-50). The retropharyngeal space extends from the skull base to the mediastinum and contains lymph nodes that drain the sinonasal structures and pharynx, including the eustachian tube. Unilateral or bilateral posterior pharyngeal swelling is often seen on CT. This is to be distinguished from the more midline perivertebral space edema that may follow vertebral osteomyelitis or epidural abscess. Imaging findings include thickening of the retropharyngeal soft tissues and anterior displacement of the airway. The presence of gas in the abscess, although uncommon, is diagnostic in the absence of acute trauma, foreign body ingestion, and recent surgery. There may be anteroposterior, rotary, or transverse displacement of C1 on C2,

or C2 on C3, caused by intense muscle spasm or direct inflammatory ligamentous involvement. US may be used to differentiate between adenitis and abscess (i.e., fluid content), and provides guidance for aspiration. Contrast-enhanced CT will demonstrate the location and extent of the disease and often distinguishes cellulitis from suppurative adenopathy and abscess. Complications include airway encroachment, osteomyelitis, sinus or orbital involvement, internal jugular vein thrombosis, carotid artery rupture, intracranial sepsis, and mediastinal spread. The source of infection may be apparent on CT. Examples are dental infection, penetrating foreign body, and sialolithiasis.

Lymphadenitis, Cellulitis, and Abscess
Lymphadenitis is the most common cause of lymphadenopathy in childhood. It may be primary or may follow adenotonsillar, pharyngeal, or dental infection. Acute adenitis may be bilateral (e.g., systemic infection or viral pharyngitis) or unilateral (e.g., primary streptococcal or staphylococcal infection). Persistent adenitis after antibiotic therapy may be seen with Kawasaki disease or infectious mononucleosis. Subacute or chronic lymphadenitis is more typical of mycobacterial infections, cat-scratch disease, toxoplasmosis, and AIDS. Noninflammatory adenopathy raises suspicion for malignancy (e.g., leukemia, lymphoma). US, CT, or MRI shows lymphadenopathy as one or more nodular masses along the cervical lymphatic chains that are more than 1.0 to 1.5 cm in diameter. Uniform contrast enhancement is common with viral processes. Abscess formation is characteristic of

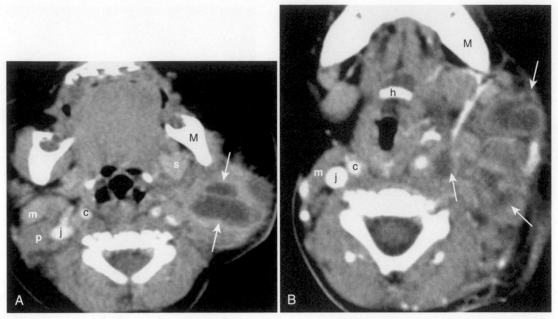

FIGURE 10-51. **A** and **B,** Left suppurative lymphadenitis with abscesses (*arrows*) on axial contrast-enhanced CT scans. c, internal carotid artery; h, hyoid; j, internal jugular vein; M, mandible; m, sternocleidomastoid muscle; p, parotid gland; s, submandibular gland.

bacterial infection (Fig. 10-51). Cat-scratch disease (i.e., due to *Rochalimaea henselae*) may mimic neoplasm, including marked nodal enlargement with necrosis and adjacent edema. Mycobacterial adenitis (tuberculous or nontuberculous) is suggested by a nodal mass with central liquefaction, thick margin enhancement, and extension to the skin (Figs. 10-52 and 10-53). Calcification is common but may also be seen in other granulomatous infections, treated lymphoma, and metastatic disease. Lymphadenopathy associated with salivary gland enlargement and multiple parotid cysts is characteristic of human immunodeficiency virus (HIV)/ AIDS. Sarcoidosis may produce lymphadenopathy and parotid enlargement.

Cellulitis refers to diffuse bacterial or viral inflammation with edema, swelling, and fat plane obliteration, but no distinct mass. Extensive soft tissue infiltration of multiple tissue planes, including muscle, suggests the more severe condition of fasciitis.

Abscess is a more discrete suppurative collection. US shows one or more complex masses with partially anechoic centers. Contrast-enhanced CT shows a discrete hypodense mass that may contain gas and has rim enhancement with adjacent edema. Differentiation from necrotic adenitis may not be possible. MRI demonstrates an encapsulated mass that is T1-hypointense and T2-hyperintense and shows gadolinium ring enhancement. In addition to antibiotic therapy, surgical drainage may be necessary to prevent or address complications such as airway obstruction, rupture with aspiration, mediastinal spread, and vascular involvement (e.g., jugular venous thrombosis).

Thyroid Inflammation

Hashimoto thyroiditis is the most common acquired thyroid disorder of childhood, including hypothyroidism. US, CT, and MRI show diffuse and homogeneous enlargement of the thyroid gland. Acute suppurative thyroiditis with abscess suggests a congenital pyriform sinus fistula (see Fig. 10-23). Multinodular goiter is of mixed echogenicity, density, and intensity on US, CT, and MRI.

Salivary Gland Inflammation

Acute sialadenitis is usually viral or bacterial. Suppurative sialadenitis most commonly affects the parotid gland and usually follows prior infection, dehydration, trauma, surgery, irradiation, certain

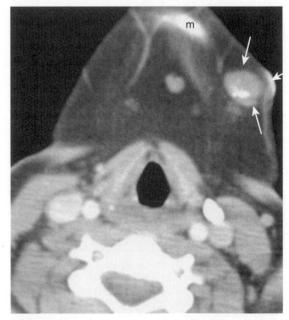

FIGURE 10-52. Nontuberculous mycobacterial infection (*arrows*) with calcification and skin involvement on axial CT scan. m, mandible.

medications, or duct obstruction from stone or tumor. It may also be seen in premature neonates. Rarely is there an abscess. Suppurative submandibular sialadenitis is usually related to sialolithiasis. In sialadenitis, CT and MRI show diffuse swelling of the gland with adjacent lymphadenopathy (Fig. 10-54). A calcified stone appears as a focal ductal CT hyperdensity. There may be contrast enhancement of the gland and duct walls with ductal dilatation. Thickened, enhancing duct walls indicate sialodochitis. Abscess appears as one or more "liquid" foci with rim enhancement. Sialography is contraindicated during acute infection.

In *sialolithiasis*, stones are usually solitary and arise within Wharton's duct. Complications include obstruction, infection, stricture, mucocele, swelling, and progression to atrophy. Calcified stones are usually visible on CT. Noncalcified stones may be diagnosed only with sialography.

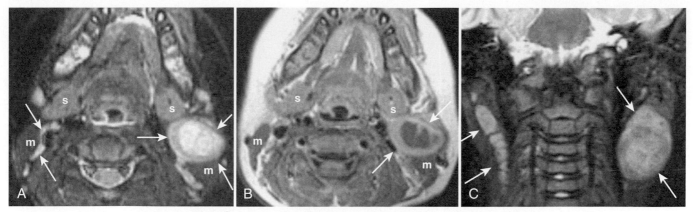

FIGURE 10-53. Left nontuberculous mycobacterial infection (*left arrows*) on axial (**A**) and coronal T2-weighted (**C**) MR images, both with fat suppression, as well as axial gadolinium-enhanced T1-weighted MR image (**B**). Note the central liquefaction and normal right lymph nodes (*right arrows*). m, sternocleidomastoid muscle; s, submandibular gland.

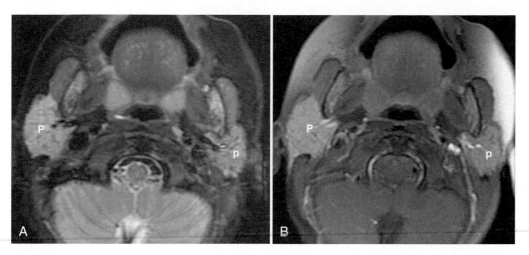

FIGURE 10-54. Right parotitis (P) as enlargement with marked hyperintensity and enhancement on axial T2-weighted (**A**) and gadolinium-enhanced T1-weighted (**B**) MR images. Compare with the normal left parotid gland (p).

Ranula results from obstruction and fluid expansion of a sublingual gland duct and manifests as a unilateral mass in the floor of the mouth (Fig. 10-55). Extension below the mylohyoid muscle anterior to the submandibular gland is called a "plunging ranula."

Chronic sialadenitis may be idiopathic or result from recurrent bacterial infection, ductal obstruction (especially submandibular gland), granulomatous disease, prior irradiation, or autoimmune disease. The diagnosis is suggested by recurrent sialadenitis with fluctuating size or progressive gland enlargement. Sjögren syndrome is an autoimmune disease that may be limited to the salivary or lacrimal glands or may also have systemic involvement. Imaging shows glandular enlargement with sialectasis. The disease may be complicated by lymphoma. HIV/AIDS, tuberculosis, or sarcoidosis may also cause salivary gland enlargement or enlargement of intraglandular lymph nodes. Glandular involvement in HIV/AIDS includes bilateral parotid enlargement with lymphocytic infiltration, lymphoepithelial cysts, and diffuse neck lymphadenopathy. Such involvement is to be distinguished from infection and lymphoma.

Sialosis is nonneoplastic, noninflammatory recurrent or chronic salivary gland enlargement. The parotid is most commonly involved including gland enlargement but normal ducts.

Osteomyelitis

Osteomyelitis of the mandible may result from direct inoculation (e.g., trauma), hematogenous origin (e.g., distant infection, vascular catheter), or contiguous spread (e.g., dental or sinus infection). Imaging may show permeative bone destruction, soft tissue edema, cellulitis, or abscess. Chronic periosteal reaction, sequestrum formation, and bony sclerosis indicate chronicity. A chronic sclerosing form may be seen and may be associated with systemic disorders.

Neoplastic Processes

See Box 10-3.

Orbit and Globe

Neoplastic processes of the orbit and globe include ocular tumors, orbital tumors, sinus or craniofacial tumors that involve the orbit, and optic pathway tumors. Pathologically, these may be neoplastic processes of mesenchymal, neural, or malformative origin. Malformative tumors are also addressed in earlier sections of this chapter. The most common benign primary orbital "tumors" of childhood are dermoid-epidermoid (Fig. 10-56), hemangioma, lymphatic malformation, plexiform neurofibroma, and teratoma. The most common primary malignant orbital tumors are retinoblastoma, optic nerve glioma, and rhabdomyosarcoma. The most common secondary orbital tumors are leukemia (e.g., chloroma), neuroblastoma, rhabdomyosarcoma, other sarcomas, Langerhans cell histiocytosis (LCH), and lymphoma. Tumors most often arising extraconally include dermoid-epidermoid, hemangioma, lymphatic malformation, plexiform neurofibroma, teratoma, neuroblastoma, rhabdomyosarcoma, histiocytosis, and lymphoma. The most common intraconal tumors are optic nerve glioma and hemangioma.

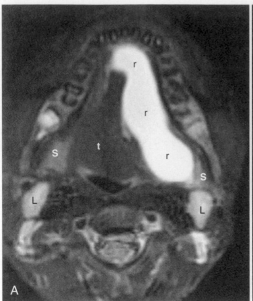
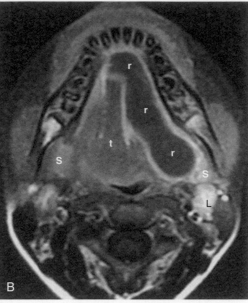

FIGURE 10-55. Left ranula (r) on axial T2-weighted MR image with fat suppression (**A**) and gadolinium-enhanced T1-weighted MR image (**B**). L, lymph nodes; S, submandibular gland; t, tongue.

Box 10-3. Pediatric Head and Neck Neoplastic Processes

Malformative/benign:
  Dermoid-epidermoid
  Lipoma
  Teratoma
  Hemangioma
  Vascular malformations
  Fibromatosis coli
  Fibrous dysplasia/fibromas
  Osteoma/osteochondroma
  Osteoblastoma/giant cell tumor/ABC
  Jaw cysts
Mesenchymal tumors:
  Angiofibroma
  Rhabdomyosarcoma
  Langerhans cell histiocytosis
  Leukemia/lymphoma
  Fibromatosis
  Sarcomas (Ewing, osteosarcoma, chondrosarcoma, fibrosarcoma)
  Chordoma
Neurogenic:
  Retinoblastoma
  Optic glioma
  Neuroblastoma
  Esthesioneuroblastoma
  Primitive neuroectodermal tumor
  Progonoma
  Schwannoma/neurofibroma (e.g., plexiform)
  Paraganglioma
Cutaneous and mucosal epithelial:
  Papilloma
  Carcinoma (e.g., sinonasal, thyroid, salivary gland)
Jaw tumors
Metastatic disease

Mesenchymal Tumors

Rhabdomyosarcoma is the most common malignant tumor of the head and neck region. Common origins are the orbit, sinuses, pharynx, temporal bone, and neck. They may also arise elsewhere and metastasize to the orbit. These aggressive, invasive neoplasms are usually of the embryonal or alveolar subtype. Like other small round cell malignancies—neuroblastoma, Ewing sarcoma, primitive neuroectodermal tumor (PNET), lymphoma, leukemia, histiocytosis—these hypercellular tumors are often large soft tissue masses that infiltrate tissue planes and cause permeative bone destruction (Fig. 10-57). There may be intracranial extension and regional or systemic metastases. Also like other small round cell tumors, rhabdomyosarcomas are often CT isodense to hyperdense and show enhancement. MRI shows T1 isointensity to hypointensity, T2 isointensity to hypointensity or occasional hyperintensity, and variable gadolinium enhancement.

Reticuloendothelial and lymphoreticular neoplasms that involve the orbit include LCH, leukemia, and lymphoma. In *Langerhans cell histiocytosis*, there may be solitary or multiple soft tissue masses with lytic bony destruction of the orbit, sinuses, cranial base, or calvaria (see Chapter 8). Intracranial involvement may also occur. CT usually shows isodense to hyperdense, or occasionally hypodense, masses that enhance. MRI often shows T1 isointensity to hypointensity, T2 isointensity to hypointensity or occasional hyperintensity, and gadolinium enhancement. There may be bone marrow replacement (e.g., T1 hypointensity, T2 hyperintensity). There may also be pituitary-hypothalamic involvement with diabetes insipidus, absence of the posterior pituitary bright spot, and hypothalamic or stalk enhancement (see Chapter 8).

Leukemic infiltration of the orbit may occur in acute lymphoblastic leukemia. *Chloromas* are leukemic masses and occur more often with the myeloblastic forms (Fig. 10-58). Orbital involvement by *non-Hodgkin lymphoma* (e.g., Burkitt lymphoma) is more common than Hodgkin lymphoma. *Juvenile angiofibroma* is an invasive fibrovascular mesenchymal tumor of adolescent males that arises in the nasal cavity and may involve the orbit along with other structures (see paranasal sinus tumors).

Fibromas are mesenchymal tumors that may be isolated and relatively benign. When aggressive and malignant, they range from fibromatosis to fibrosarcoma. Benign or malignant *osteochondral tumors* rarely involve the orbit in childhood. Examples are osteoma, osteochondroma, aneurysmal bone cyst, giant cell tumor,

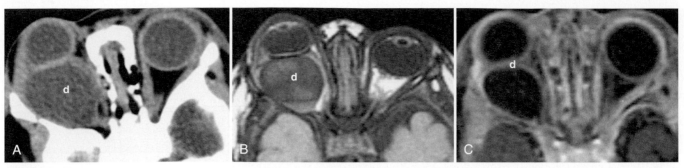

FIGURE 10-56. Large right orbital dermoid (d), including orbital expansion and proptosis, on axial CT scan (**A**) as well as FLAIR (**B**) and gadolinium-enhanced T1 weighted (**C**) MR images.

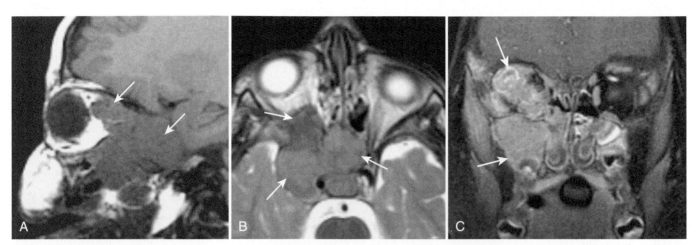

FIGURE 10-57. Sphenorbital rhabdomyosarcoma (*arrows*) on sagittal T1-weighted (**A**), axial T2-weighted (**B**), and coronal gadolinium-enhanced T1-weighted (**C**) MR images, which show orbit, sinus, and intracranial extension.

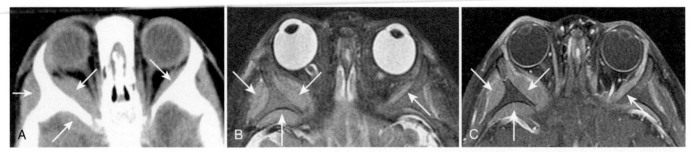

FIGURE 10-58. Bilateral orbit chloromas (*arrows*) without bone destruction on axial CT scan (**A**) as well as axial T2-weighted (**B**) and axial gadolinium-enhanced T1-weighted (**C**) MR images.

osteoblastoma, Ewing sarcoma, osteosarcoma, chondrosarcoma, and fibrosarcoma, which are discussed later.

Neural Tumors

Neural tumors of the orbit include retinoblastoma, medulloepithelioma, neuroblastoma, esthesioneuroblastoma, PNET, progonoma, schwannoma, neurofibroma, and plexiform neurofibroma.

Retinoblastoma is by far the most common primary intraocular malignancy. Retinoma (retinocytoma) is a benign variant. Retinoblastoma may be multifocal, bilateral, or familial. Bilateral retinoblastoma is usually hereditary and may be associated with a pineoblastoma (trilateral retinoblastoma), additional hypothalamic involvement (quadrilateral retinoblastoma), and radiation-induced or second nonocular malignancies (e.g., osteosarcoma, fibrosarcoma, rhabdomyosarcoma). Retinoblastoma is the most important lesion to be ruled out in the differential diagnosis of leukocoria or

strabismus (Fig. 10-59). Calcification occurs in more than 90% of cases. CT usually shows a high-density intraocular mass that often enhances. MRI commonly shows T1 isointensity to hypointensity, T2 isointensity to hypointensity, and gadolinium enhancement. Spread may occur along the optic nerve or by lymphatic or hematogenous means. Retinoblastoma is to be differentiated from other ocular lesions, such as retinoma, Coats disease, PHPV, retrolental fibroplasia, chronic retinal detachment, sclerosing endophthalmitis, congenital cataract, coloboma, retinal hemangioblastoma, choroidal or retinal hemangioma, and medulloepithelioma.

Neuroblastoma is the most common neural tumor to invade the orbit secondarily (Figs. 10-60 and 10-61). It is usually a nodular infiltrating mass causing permeative, blastic, or spiculated bone destruction. Esthesioneuroblastoma, PNETs, and progonomas are other neural tumors that have similar imaging findings (see later). *Nerve sheath tumors* rarely involve the orbit but include schwannoma, neurofibroma, and

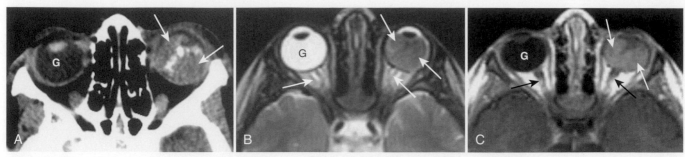

FIGURE 10-59. Left retinoblastoma (*arrows*) with calcified ocular mass on axial CT scan (**A**). The tumor (*upper right arrows*) shows as a hypointensity on an axial T2-weighted MR image (**B**) and enhances on an axial gadolinium-enhanced T1-weighted MR image (**C**). Optic nerves are normal (*lower arrows* in **B** and **C**). G, normal right globe.

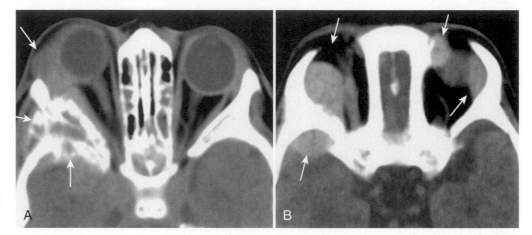

FIGURE 10-60. **A** and **B**, Axial contrast-enhanced CT scans showing bilateral orbital neuroblastoma (*arrows*) including high-density and enhancing masses and bony destruction of the right sphenoid buttress.

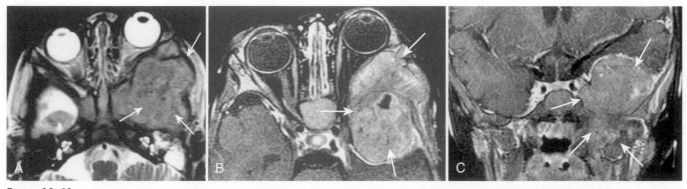

FIGURE 10-61. Left sphenorbital neuroblastoma (*arrows*) on axial T2-weighted (**A**) and gadolinium-enhanced T1-weighted axial (**B**) and coronal (**C**) MR images, which show proptosis and intracranial extension.

plexiform neurofibroma (e.g., spheno-orbital dysplasia of NF-1; Fig. 10-62).

Optic Pathway Tumors

Optic pathway tumors are common tumors of childhood and are often associated with NF-1 (Fig. 10-63). Solitary intraorbital lesions are rare and include hamartomas, arachnoidal hyperplasia, and low-grade astrocytomas. Tumors arising from the chiasm and optic tracts range from hamartomas and low-grade astrocytomas to anaplastic astrocytomas. Often there is combined intraorbital, intracanalicular, and intracranial optic pathway involvement. Optic gliomas must be distinguished from perioptic tumors such as a schwannoma, neurofibroma, and meningioma.

Nasal Cavity, Paranasal Sinuses, and Face

Tumors of childhood arising in the nasal cavity, sinuses, and face may be neoplastic or nonneoplastic (e.g., dysplastic), and circumscribed, expanding, or infiltrating. They may be of mesenchymal, neural, cutaneous or mucosal origin. The extent of regional involvement, including orbital or intracranial, is important for treatment. Combined therapies may be required (e.g., surgery, chemotherapy, and radiotherapy). Mesenchymal tumors are of vascular, soft tissue, reticuloendothelial, osteochondroid, dental, and notochordal origin. Neural tumors include those of neuroepithelial, neural crest, and nerve sheath origins. Neoplastic lesions of cutaneous or mucosal epithelial origin are rare. The most common and important tumors arising in the nasal cavity, paranasal sinuses, and nasopharynx are juvenile

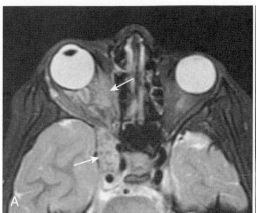

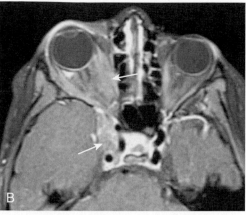

FIGURE 10-62. Neurofibromatosis type 1. Right sphenorbital dysplasia with orbital plexiform neurofibroma (*arrows*) on axial T2-weighted (**A**) and gadolinium-enhanced T1-weighted (**B**) MR images, which show palpebral and cavernous sinus involvement.

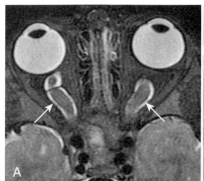

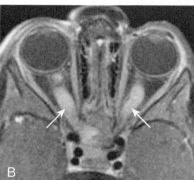

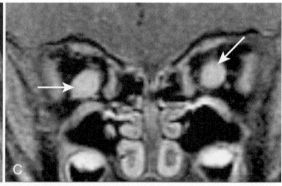

FIGURE 10-63. Neurofibromatosis type 1 with bilateral optic nerve gliomas (*arrows*) on axial T2-weighted (**A**) and axial (**B**) and coronal (**C**) gadolinium-enhanced T1-weighted MR images.

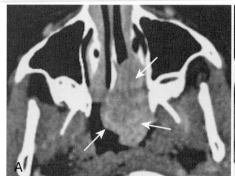

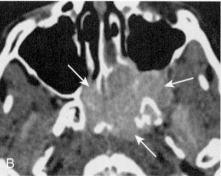

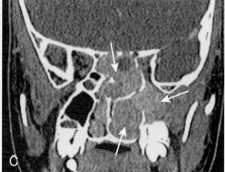

FIGURE 10-64. Left juvenile nasal angiofibroma (*arrows*) on contrast-enhanced axial (**A** and **B**) and coronal (**C**) CT scans, which show the high-density, enhancing tumor and bony destructive changes.

angiofibroma, rhabdomyosarcoma, neuroblastoma, LCH, chondrosarcoma, leukemia, lymphoma, and fibrous dysplasia. Vascular anomalies and tumors and cysts of dental origin are discussed elsewhere.

Vascular Tumors

Juvenile nasal angiofibroma (JNA) is a common benign but aggressive fibrovascular tumor that occurs primarily in adolescent boys. Arising from the posterolateral nasal cavity near the pterygopalatine fossa and sphenopalatine foramen, it manifests as nasal obstruction, epistaxis, facial swelling, proptosis, otitis media, or headache (Figs. 10-64 and 10-65). These are isodense or low-density masses that enhance markedly on CT. Bony expansion and erosion are common, including widening of the

pterygopalatine fossa and anterior bowing of the posterolateral maxillary sinus wall. Extension often occurs into the sphenoid, maxillary, and ethmoid sinuses as well as the orbit, middle cranial fossa, and cavernous sinus. Vascular, neural, and intracranial involvement are best evaluated on MRI. The MRI findings reflect varying components of increased vascularity (flow signal voids), fibrous tissue (hypointensity), tumor matrix (marked gadolinium enhancement), edema (T2 hyperintensity), cysts, cavitation, and hemorrhage. Sinus or otomastoid obstruction with mucosal edema and retained secretions is common. Preoperative catheter angiography and therapeutic embolization often facilitate surgical excision.

Angiomatous polyp and hemangiopericytoma are very rare in childhood but may be mistaken for angiofibroma.

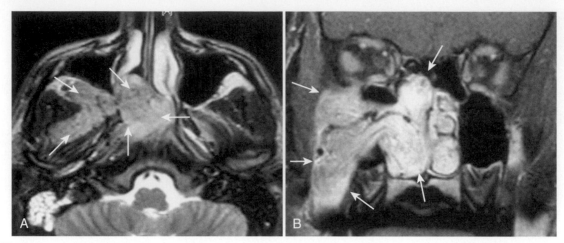

FIGURE 10-65. Right juvenile nasal angiofibroma (*arrows*) with extensive retromaxillary and infratemporal involvement and hypervascular flow voids on axial T2-weighted (**A**) and coronal gadolinium-enhanced T1-weighted (**B**) MR images.

Soft Tissue and Reticuloendothelial System Tumors

Common malignant soft tissue tumors of the head and neck region in childhood include rhabdomyosarcoma, lymphoma, Ewing sarcoma, histiocytosis, leukemia, neural origin tumors (neuroblastoma, PNET), and fibromatous tumors.

The orbit and paranasal sinuses are common sites of origin of *rhabdomyosarcoma* (see Fig. 10-57). Similar to the other small "blue" round cell tumors, these are hypercellular tumors that often manifest as infiltrating soft tissue masses with bone destruction and regional or systemic metastases. They are often isodense to hyperdense on CT with iodinated contrast enhancement, and T1-isointense to hypointense, T2-isointense to hypointense (or occasionally hyperintense), with variable gadolinium enhancement on MRI.

Langerhans cell histiocytosis is a reticuloendothelial disorder histologically characterized by tissue infiltration with reticulum cells, histiocytes, plasmocytes, and leukocytes (see Chapter 8). The involvement may be isolated (formerly eosinophilic granuloma), or there may be dissemination with cutaneous, visceral, and bony involvement.

Lymphoma is another common malignant tumor of the head and neck region in childhood. Hodgkin disease often manifests as cervical lymphadenopathy and spreads contiguously along nodal chains. Non-Hodgkin lymphoma is often widespread with noncontiguous nodal involvement. The origin may be in the nasopharynx, sinuses, adenotonsillar region (Waldeyer ring), or salivary glands. Head and neck lymphomas may be associated with childhood AIDS or PTLD (see Chapter 8).

Leukemia rarely involves the nasal cavity or paranasal sinuses. Such involvement is more often due to infection or hemorrhage. Occasionally, a chloroma (e.g., in myeloblastic leukemia) is seen as an osseous or soft tissue mass that may expand or destroy bone. It is often CT-isodense to hyperdense and T2-isointense to hypointense, and shows enhancement.

Fibromatous tumors are mesenchymal neoplasms that may be isolated and benign (solitary fibroma) or aggressive and malignant (fibromatosis, fibrosarcoma). The fibromatous tumor is a locally infiltrating pseudoneoplastic process characterized by fibroelastic proliferation. Desmoid tumor is a well-differentiated form with no tendency to metastasize. Wide tissue infiltration and recurrence after resection is common. Progression to fibrosarcoma may occur despite therapy. In other forms there may be widespread visceral and bony involvement without metastases (e.g., congenital or infantile form). The juvenile form usually involves musculoskeletal structures but not the viscera. Imaging shows an infiltrating soft tissue mass or masses that involve bone. CT and MRI may show isodensity to hypodensity and hypointensity, respectively, in the more fibrous forms. There may be minimal or no enhancement. CT hypodensity, T2 hyperintensity, and contrast enhancement may be seen in the more aggressive, malignant forms.

Osseous and Chondroid Tumors

Osseous and chondroid tumors may arise from the facial bones or from the skull base and may secondarily involve the nasal cavity, sinuses, and nasopharynx.

Osteoma, a benign osseous neoplasm, is rare in childhood, but most often arises in the frontal or ethmoid sinus. It may be asymptomatic or associated with headache, sinus obstruction, CSF rhinorrhea, or Gardner syndrome. The imaging appearance depends on the histologic subtype (cortical, cancellous, or fibrous), varying from a sclerotic lesion to a soft tissue density.

Osteochondroma is a benign osteocartilaginous exostosis that may arise from the mandible, maxilla, sphenoid bone, zygoma, or nasal septum. Multiple lesions occur in familial cases and in Ollier disease. They may arise after radiotherapy. Malignancy (e.g., osteosarcoma or chondrosarcoma) is rare except in familial cases. Imaging shows a miniature metaphysis, growth plate, and cartilaginous cap that are continuous with the bone of origin. Malignant degeneration is indicated by a disorganized appearance and involvement of the parent bone.

Fibrous dysplasia is an idiopathic and benign fibro-osseous disorder that may be monostotic, polyostotic, or part of the McCune-Albright syndrome. The maxilla and mandible are most frequently involved, unilaterally or bilaterally (Fig. 10-66). There may be encroachment upon the neurovascular foramina, orbit, nasal structures, or sinuses (see Fig. 10-5). Lesion growth may continue after skeletal maturation, but conversion to sarcoma is rare. CT and MRI findings include inhomogeneous soft tissue density or intensity, a "ground-glass" appearance, or sclerotic bony thickening. Marked enhancement may mimic neoplasm. *Ossifying fibroma* is a circumscribed fibrous neoplasm that progressively ossifies. The CT and MRI appearances may mimic those of fibrous dysplasia, although this tumor tends to be expansile, grows faster, and recurs. *Cementifying fibroma* is another fibro-osseous tumor that is aggressive and tends to recur.

Giant cell tumor, giant cell reparative granuloma, aneurysmal bone cyst, and *osteoblastoma* (Fig. 10-67) are benign osseous tumors rarely arising in this region in childhood. These often have overlapping pathologic findings, and combined lesions are well known. On CT and MRI, these lesions often are lytic and expansile and have a bony matrix or calcification, cortical erosion, soft tissue mass, and a thin calcified shell. Cavitation, cyst formation, and hemorrhage may be observed. Moderate contrast enhancement is common. A multiloculated appearance with fluid-fluid levels is

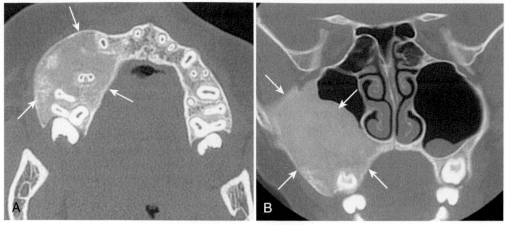

FIGURE 10-66. Right maxillary fibrous dysplasia (*arrows*) on axial (**A**) and coronal (**B**) CT scans.

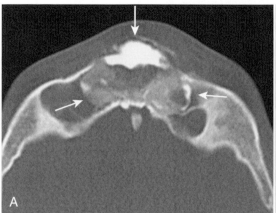

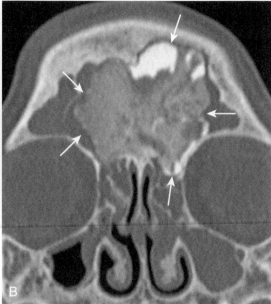

FIGURE 10-67. Frontoethmoidal osteoblastoma (*arrows*) appears as mixed isodensity and high-density masses on axial (**A**) and coronal (**B**) CT scans.

suggestive of aneurysmal bone cyst. The latter finding, however, has also been reported with lymphatic malformation, venolymphatic malformation, and telangiectatic osteosarcoma.

As previously discussed, *cherubism* is an autosomal dominant disorder with progressive giant cell tumor involvement of the mandible and maxilla in childhood (misnomer "congenital fibrous dysplasia"—see Fig. 10-26).

Chondrosarcoma is a malignant bone neoplasm of cartilage origin that may arise de novo, from an osteochondroma, or following radiotherapy. It is occasionally found in the sphenoid bone or sphenooccipital synchondrosis. On CT and MRI, this expansile mass is often of nonspecific soft tissue density, intensity, and enhancement. Chondroid matrix calcifications may not be present.

Chordoma is a rare tumor that arises from intraosseous notochordal remnants in the skull base near synchondroses. These tumors are locally invasive, destroy bone, and may metastasize. The chondroid form of chordoma may be indistinguishable from chondrosarcoma on imaging.

Osteosarcoma, *fibrosarcoma*, and *Ewing sarcoma* are other rare mesenchymal neoplasms that arise in this region as primary or secondary neoplasms (e.g., after radiation therapy for retinoblastoma). These invasive tumors spread regionally and metastasize. Osteosarcoma may appear as a soft tissue mass with bony destruction and spiculated periosteal bone reaction, or as a partially calcified or ossified osteoid matrix mass. Fibrosarcoma and Ewing sarcoma produce soft tissue masses and permeative bony destruction, but no osteoid or chondroid matrix elements.

Neural Tumors

Neuroepithelial or neural crest tumors include neuroblastoma, PNET, esthesioneuroblastoma, retinoblastoma, and progonoma. *Neuroblastoma*, the most common of these tumors, may arise in or involve the skull base, nose, sinuses, or orbit, usually as part of metastatic disease (see Figs. 10-60 and 10-61). *Esthesioneuroblastoma* (olfactory neuroblastoma) is a very rare tumor that arises from the olfactory groove and produces extensive destruction of the sinuses, orbit, and adjacent skull base and extends intracranially. *Primitive neuroectodermal tumors* are rare extra-CNS malignancies of primitive neuroepithelial origin. They are characterized by small round cell infiltrations similar to those of neuroblastoma. *Progonomas* are rare retinal anlage tumors, often contain melanin, tend to arise from the cranial base, and invade the adjacent nasosinus structures or orbit. All of these tumors tend to have similar imaging appearances, consisting of a soft tissue mass with CT-isodensity to hyperdensity, T2-isointensity to hypointensity, prominent contrast enhancement, permeative bone destruction, and calcification. Schwannomas, neurofibromas, and plexiform neurofibromas rarely arise in the nasal cavity, paranasal sinuses, or nasopharynx.

Tumors of Cutaneous and Mucosal Epithelial Origin

Nasal *papillomas* are benign mucosal tumors that often extend into the maxillary, ethmoid, sphenoid, or frontal sinuses. Malignant transformation is extremely rare. CT and MRI often demonstrate a small or large polypoid nasal cavity mass with remodeling and ostiomeatal obstruction. Cylindric cell and inverted papillomas tend to be more aggressive. Complete surgical excision may be difficult, and recurrence is common. *Squamous cell carcinoma* and *adenocarcinoma* of the nasal cavity and sinuses are extremely rare in childhood. Imaging often demonstrates a sinus mass of homogeneous density and intensity with bone destruction. Contrast enhancement is uncommon. Necrosis and hemorrhage may occur, along with regional extension, nodal spread, and distant metastases.

Ear and Temporal Bone

Congenital cholesteatoma grows from ectopic epithelial rests (Fig. 10-68). Classically, there is no prior inflammation, trauma, or surgery. The most common site is the anterior middle ear cavity, although it may also arise in the external canal, petrous apex, or mastoid, or deep to an atresia plate (see Fig. 10-16). Usually there is conductive hearing loss and a white mass behind an intact tympanic membrane. The mass tends to be circumscribed, CT-isodense, T1-hypointense, and T2-hyperintense. Occasionally, it may be more extensive and may produce bony erosion.

Temporal bone involvement is uncommon and usually monostotic in *fibrous dysplasia*. Painless fibro-osseous expansion may be associated with external canal narrowing, hearing loss, or secondary cholesteatoma. CT shows expansion with "ground-glass" appearance, sclerosis, or lytic destruction. The differential diagnosis may include other fibro-osseous lesions, benign or malignant.

Exostosis is a common, benign bony hyperplasia of the external canal. It arises from the sutures of the tympanic ring, is usually localized, and is often bilateral. There may be hearing loss, pain, infection, or tinnitus. CT often shows nodular bony thickening with canal narrowing. *Osteoma* is an uncommon benign bony tumor that is usually unilateral and more often arises in the outer bony canal.

Of the *nerve sheath tumors* in the region, neurofibromas (e.g., plexiform, NF-1) may involve the auricle and external canal. Acoustic or vestibular schwannoma is rare in childhood, suggests neurofibromatosis, and must be considered in retrocochlear hearing loss (see Chapter 8). CT may show only widening or shortening of the IAC. MRI is the study of choice, on which the tumor tends to be T2-hyperintense and gadolinium-enhancing. Schwannomas of other cranial nerves (e.g., VII, IX-XII) in this region are rare in children. Characteristically, there is an enhancing mass that expands the facial canal, jugular foramen, or hypoglossal canal.

Paragangliomas (glomus tumors) are also rare in childhood. They may be hereditary, familial, multicentric, or hormonally active. Paragangliomas are vascular, but slow-growing, tumors that may arise within the jugular bulb (glomus jugulare), middle ear cavity (glomus tympanicum), or the auricular branch of the vagus nerve (glomus vagale). Conductive hearing loss, pulsatile tinnitus, and a red retrotympanic mass are characteristic. The mass may be obscured by otitis media. Differentiation from carotid and jugular anomalies is necessary. CT may show an expanding and enhancing mass. MRI shows a T2-heterogenous mass ("salt-and-pepper" appearance), with multiple vascular flow voids and marked gadolinium enhancement. Angiography and therapeutic embolization are helpful for surgical management.

Rhabdomyosarcoma is a common malignancy in this region (Fig. 10-69). Extensive local involvement is frequent, along with intracranial invasion and metastases. CT and MRI show an enhancing soft tissue mass with bony destruction. Vascular complications include internal jugular vein invasion, compression, and thrombosis.

Langerhans cell histiocytosis occasionally involves the temporal bone and may be bilateral (Fig. 10-70). CT and MRI often show enhancing soft tissue masses with marginated bony destruction. Other skeletal lesions and intracranial involvement should be sought.

Metastasis

The most common metastatic tumors of the temporal bone are neuroblastoma and leukemia. Permeative, lytic bone destruction on CT is often seen. Differentiation from coalescent mastoiditis may be difficult. MRI better delineates intracranial involvement.

Neck, Oral Cavity, and Jaw

Benign "tumors" of the neck may be developmental, inflammatory, or neoplastic. Such lesions include cysts, ectopias, vascular anomalies, fibromatosis colli, dermoid-epidermoid, teratoma, lipoma, and nerve sheath tumors. These are to be distinguished from lymphadenopathy, cellulitis, and abscess.

Primary malignant tumors of the pediatric head and neck vary with the age of the patient. Malignant teratoma is primarily congenital. Neuroblastoma usually arises in infants and young children. Rhabdomyosarcoma typically occurs in the preschool years. Other sarcomas and non-Hodgkin lymphoma occur over a broad age range but particularly in later childhood. Hodgkin disease, thyroid carcinoma, nasopharyngeal carcinoma, and salivary gland neoplasms most often occur in adolescence. These tumors may be asymptomatic with variable size and growth. Other symptoms and signs may be related to associated lymphadenopathy, paranasal sinus or ear involvement, aerodigestive compromise, or headache.

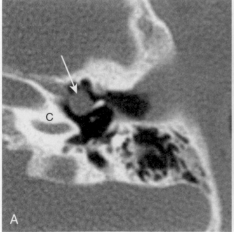
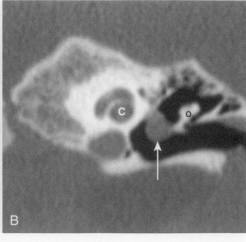

FIGURE 10-68. Left congenital cholesteatoma (*arrows*) on axial (**A**) and coronal (**B**) CT scans. C, cochlea; o, ossicles.

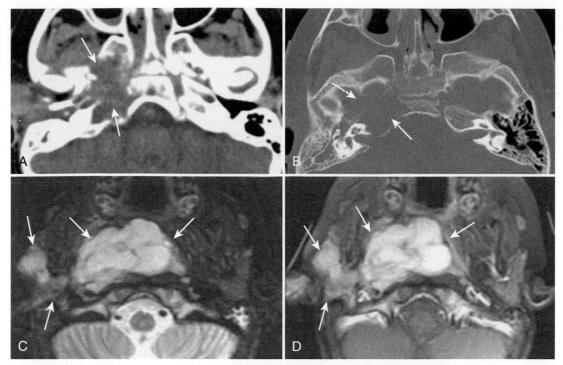

FIGURE 10-69. Right petromastoid rhabdomyosarcoma (*arrows*) with soft tissue masses and bony destruction with extension into infratemporal space and nasopharynx on axial CT scans (**A** and **B**), an axial T2-weighted MR image with fat suppression (**C**), and a gadolinium-enhanced T1-weighted MR image (**D**).

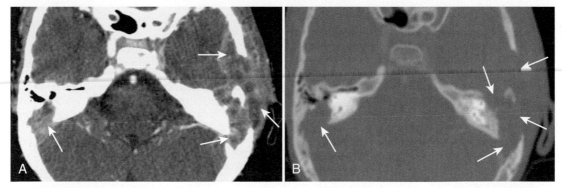

FIGURE 10-70. **A** and **B**, Bilateral mastoid Langerhans cell histiocytosis (*arrows*) on axial contrast-enhanced CT scans, which show enhancing masses and bony destruction.

Fibromatosis colli (also known as congenital muscular torticollis) is a common benign condition of the neonate and young infant (Fig. 10-71). A firm, nontender, fibrous mass is usually palpated in the sternocleidomastoid muscle (SCM). Suggested causes include in utero deformation and birth trauma. There is venous hemorrhage evolving to fibrosis. SCM enlargement often occurs early, followed by muscle contracture and atrophy with torticollis. Ipsilateral hemifacial microsomia or plagiocephaly may also be seen. US shows a mass, or enlargement, of the SCM with variable echogenicity. CT shows an isodense SCM mass, hemorrhage, or calcification. MRI may show hemorrhage or mineralization along with enhancement. Treatment usually consists of physical therapy, but surgery may be required.

Dermoid (epidermoid) cysts are of ectodermal origin, usually occur as near-midline upper neck or scalp lesions, and may be asymptomatic (Figs. 10-72 and 10-73). They may also be associated with a dimple and dermal sinus and manifest as infection. US shows a circumscribed and thin-walled echogenic mass. CT and MRI demonstrate an encapsulated mass with fatty density or intensity. Particularly when occurring in the midline scalp,

dermoid-epidermoid is to be distinguished from cephalocele (see Chapter 8) and vascular anomalies (e.g., venous malformation, hemangioma; Fig. 10-74).

Teratomas arise from pluripotential cells and usually manifest at birth as large neck masses causing respiratory or swallowing problems (Fig. 10-75). About one fifth are malignant. There is a higher incidence of polyhydramnios, stillbirth, and prematurity in infants with teratomas. Imaging shows a heterogeneous mass containing cystic areas, calcification, and variable amounts of fat.

Lipoma is a benign tumor composed of fat cells that tend to follow somatic growth (Fig. 10-76). On US, CT, and MRI, the mass has the same echogenicity, density, and intensity, respectively, as adipose tissue. The presence of other soft tissue characteristics, including enhancement, may require a differential diagnosis that includes teratoma, lipoblastoma, and liposarcoma.

Nerve sheath tumors (neurofibromas and schwannomas) arise from cranial or peripheral nerves in the neck. They may be sporadic or may occur as part of neurofibromatosis. Plexiform neurofibromas, which are pathognomonic of NF-1, consist of multiple nerve masses that incorporate adjacent soft tissues (Fig. 10-77).

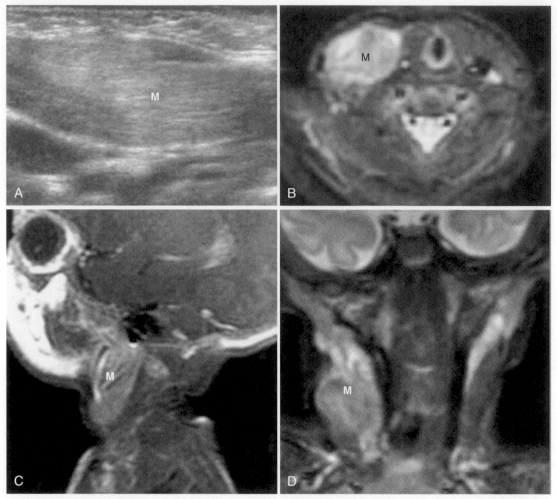

FIGURE 10-71. Fibromatosis coli of the sternocleidomastoid muscle (M) on a longitudinal US image (**A**) as well as axial T2-weighted (**B**), sagittal gadolinium-enhanced T1-weighted (**C**), and coronal T2-weighted (**D**) MR images.

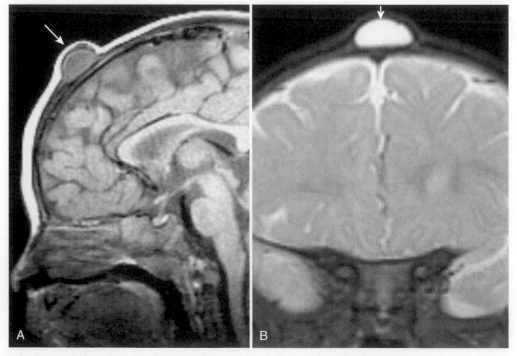

FIGURE 10-72. Anterior fontanelle dermoid (*arrows*) on sagittal T1-weighted (**A**) and coronal STIR (**B**) MR images.

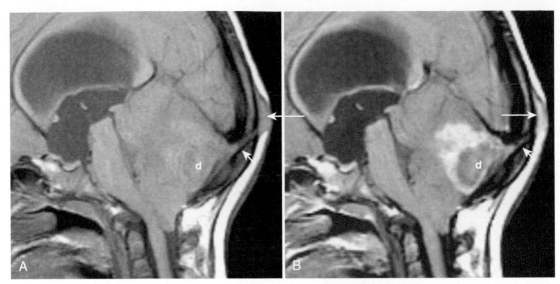

FIGURE 10-73. Occipital dermoid (*long arrows*) and sinus (*short arrows*) with cerebellar dermoid (d) and enhancing abscess on sagittal T1-weighted (**A**) and gadolinium-enhanced T1-weighted (**B**) MR images.

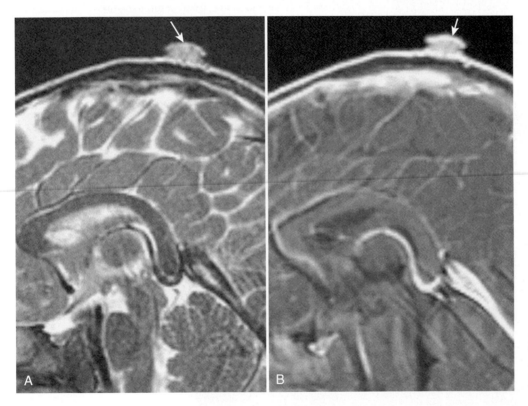

FIGURE 10-74. Vertex parietal scalp hemangioma (*arrows*) on sagittal T2-weighted (**A**), and gadolinium-enhanced T1-weighted (**B**) MR images, which show enhancement and vascular high-flow voids.

The tumors are CT isodense to hypodense, T1-isointense to hypointense, and T2-isointense to hyperintense ("target sign"), and they enhance irregularly. Malignant degeneration occurs in a small percentage. Nerve sheath tumors are to be differentiated from neuroblastoma (Fig. 10-78).

Paragangliomas are exceedingly rare in this region in childhood.

Hodgkin *lymphoma* tends to involve contiguous nodal groups (Fig. 10-79). Non-Hodgkin lymphoma tends to be extranodal (e.g., adenotonsillar, nasal cavity, paranasal sinuses). Developmental or acquired immunodeficiency (e.g., PTLD; Fig. 10-80) predisposes to non-Hodgkin lymphoma. Asymptomatic lymphadenopathy is a common mode of presentation. Imaging findings include lymphadenopathy in several locations, usually with a dominant larger node or aggregate of nodes. Adenotonsillar involvement usually is bilateral and associated with airway obstruction. Necrosis and mineralization are uncommon except after treatment. These tumors are CT-isodense (relative to muscle), T1-isointense, T2-hyperintense, and variably enhancing. Local bone destruction may occur. Hypermetabolic activity on PET-CT correlates with tumor.

Rhabdomyosarcoma, typically the embryonal subtype, often originates in the head and neck (see Figs. 10-57 and 10-69). Other, less common sarcomas of childhood include fibrosarcoma, Ewing sarcoma, chondrosarcoma, osteosarcoma, malignant schwannoma, hemangiopericytoma, and Kaposi sarcoma.

Thyroid adenoma and carcinoma are unusual in childhood. Carcinoma may be sporadic or may be associated with prior irradiation or multiple endocrine neoplasia type II. The papillary and follicular types are more common than the medullary type. A common presentation is an asymptomatic, firm, but mobile neck

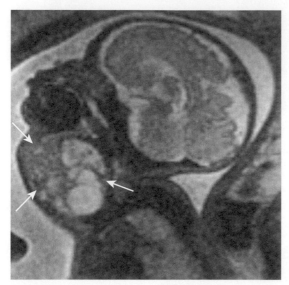

FIGURE 10-75. Fetal cystic neck teratoma (*arrows*) on sagittal T2-weighted MR image.

mass (Fig. 10-81). Rapid growth, fixation, aerodigestive symptoms, or cervical lymphadenopathy suggests malignancy. US may show an isoechoic to hypoechoic thyroid mass. Cystic masses can be aspirated. Solitary thyroid nodules are usually evaluated with ^{99m}Tc or ^{123}I scanning. Fine-needle aspiration for cytologic analysis, or open biopsy, is considered for nodules that lack, or show variable, radionuclide uptake.

Metastatic disease involving the head and neck may occur with neuroblastoma or leukemia. Primary neuroblastoma may rarely occur in the neck. Metastatic disease from a primary abdominal, thoracic, or pelvic neuroblastoma may also involve the skull, orbit, jaw, and neck nodes.

Salivary gland tumors of childhood most commonly involve the parotid gland. Hemangioma is the most common benign neoplasm (see Figs. 10-32 and 10-33), followed by the pleomorphic adenoma. Malignant tumors are more common in older children and adolescents. Mucoepidermoid carcinoma is the most common "low-grade" malignancy. Salivary gland tumors are often asymptomatic, solitary, firm, and slow-growing. Rapid growth, pain, facial nerve involvement, and cervical adenopathy suggest higher-grade malignancy. US may be used for localization and to differentiate solid from cystic masses. MRI is the best procedure for evaluating tumor character and extent. Most neoplasms (other than hemangioma) are T1-hypointense and T2-hyperintense with variable enhancement. T2 hypointensity suggests a highly cellular lesion, and local invasion often indicates malignancy.

Cysts and tumors of the jaw (maxilla and mandible) are categorized as odontogenic (dental origin) or nonodontogenic. Odontogenic cysts arise from tooth derivatives. The *radicular cyst*

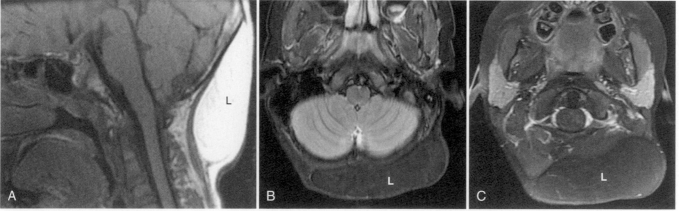

FIGURE 10-76. Posterior neck lipoma (L) appears as a high intensity on a sagittal T1-weighted MR image (**A**) and as a low intensity on an axial STIR MR image (**B**) and a gadolinium-enhanced T1-weighted MR image with fat suppression (**C**).

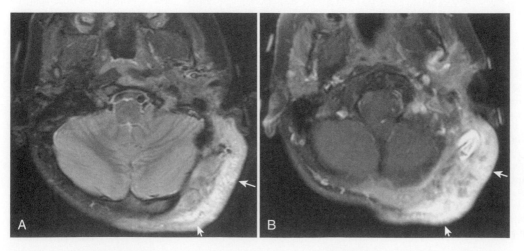

FIGURE 10-77. Left head and neck plexiform neurofibroma (*arrows*) on an axial STIR MR image (**A**) and a gadolinium-enhanced T1-weighted MR image with fat suppression (**B**), which show the characteristic dysplastic occipital bone defect.

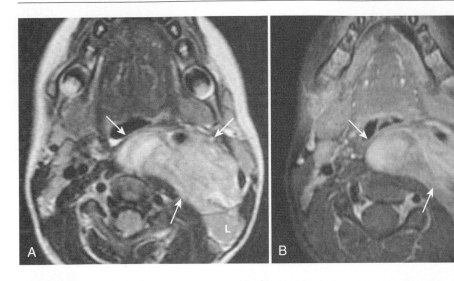

FIGURE 10-78. Left neck ganglio-neuroblastoma (*arrows*) with involvement of the carotid space and lymphadenopathy (L) on an axial T2-weighted MR image (**A**) and a gadolinium-enhanced T1-weighted MR image with fat suppression (**B**).

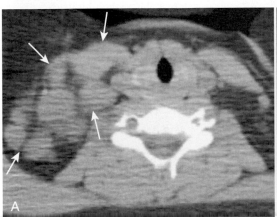

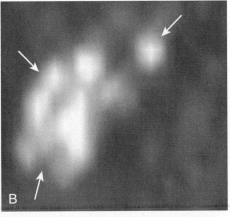

FIGURE 10-79. Hodgkin lymphoma with large right isodense and hypermetabolic lower neck nodes (*arrows*) on CT (**A**) and PET (**B**) scans.

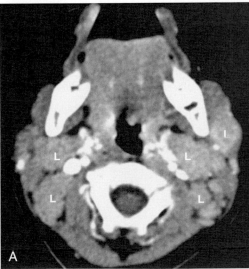

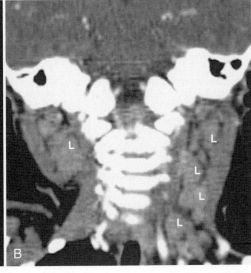

FIGURE 10-80. Post-transplant lymphoproliferative disorder with extensive lymphadenopathy (L) on contrast-enhanced axial (**A**) and coronal (**B**) CT scans.

arises from the tooth apex, is circumscribed, and is surrounded by a thin rim of cortical bone. It is CT-hypodense and similar in appearance to periapical granuloma. The *dentigerous cyst* is a sharply defined unilocular or multilocular CT-hypodense cyst of the crown of an unerupted tooth (mandibular or maxillary; Fig. 10-82). The *keratocyst* is a unilocular or multilocular, keratin-containing, CT-hypodense cyst (usually mandibular). There may be cortical thinning and expansion. Multiple keratocysts are characteristic of the basal cell nevus syndrome.

Nonodontogenic cysts include fissural, hemorrhagic, and Stafne cysts. The *fissural cyst* occurs along bony fusion lines. It is usually a small, circumscribed, and corticated CT hypodensity. *Hemorrhagic bone cysts* tend to be mandibular, unilocular, and scalloped. *Stafne cyst* represents an anatomic variant (i.e., deep fossa of the submandibular gland) and is a well-defined, round or oval CT hypodensity near the mandibular angle.

Benign odontogenic tumors may be partially cystic; they include the ameloblastoma, calcifying epithelial odontogenic

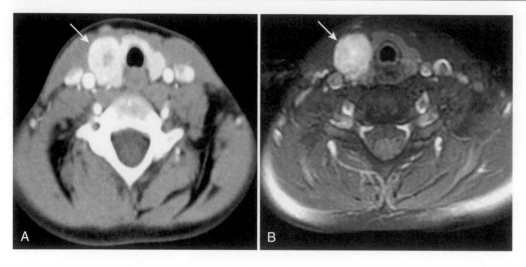

FIGURE 10-81. Cowden syndrome with right thyroid adenoma vs. carcinoma on a contrast-enhanced CT scan (**A**) and a gadolinium-enhanced T1-weighted MR image (**B**).

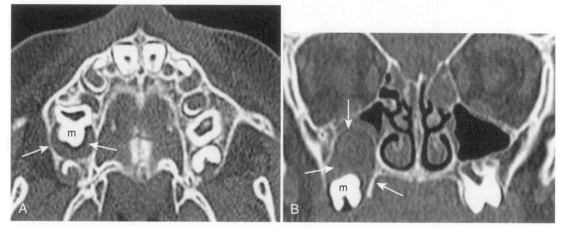

FIGURE 10-82. Right maxillary dentigerous cyst (*arrows*) on axial (**A**) and coronal (**B**) CT scans. m, molar tooth.

tumors, and mixed epithelial odontogenic tumors (e.g., odontoma and cementoma). *Ameloblastoma* is the most common. It is benign but locally aggressive. It appears as a unilocular or multilocular lesion with distinct borders. There may be marginal sclerosis, expansion, a "soap-bubble" appearance, or cortical disruption with a soft tissue mass. CT often shows hypodensities interspersed with isodensities. MRI shows heterogeneous T1 and T2 intensities. Benign nonodontogenic tumors may be solid or partially cystic. These include the exostosis, osteoma, giant cell lesions, aneurysmal bone cyst, and fibro-osseous lesions.

Malignant jaw tumors may be of primary bone origin, may represent spread from an adjacent soft tissue tumor, or may be metastatic. Examples, respectively, include sarcoma, Langerhans cell histiocytosis, neuroblastoma, leukemia, and lymphoma.

■ SUGGESTED READINGS

TEXTS

Barkovich A: Pediatric Neuroimaging, ed 4. Philadelphia, Lippincott-Raven, 2005.

Blaser SI, Illner A, Castillo M, et al: Peds Neuro: 100 Top Diagnoses. (Pocket Radiologist.) Philadelphia, WB Saunders, 2003.

Bluestone C, Stool S, Alper C, et al: Pediatric Otolaryngology, ed 4. Philadelphia, WB Saunders, 2003.

Harnsberger HR, Hudgins P, Wiggins R, Davidson C: Diagnostic Imaging: Head and Neck. Philadelphia, WB Saunders, 2004.

Harwood-Nash D, Fitz CR: Neuroradiology in Infants and Children. St. Louis, Mosby-Year Book, 1976.

Kirks DR: Practical Pediatric Imaging, ed 3. Philadelphia, Lippincott-Raven, 1998.

Kuhn JP, Slovis TL, Caffey J, Haller JO: Caffey's Pediatric Diagnostic Imaging, ed 11. New York, Elsevier Mosby Saunders, 2007.

Som PM, Curtin HD (eds): Head and Neck Imaging, ed 4. St. Louis, Mosby-Year Book, 2003 .

Swischuk ME: Imaging of the Newborn, Infant, and Young Child, ed 5. Philadelphia, Lippincott Williams & Wilkins, 2003.

Tortori-Donati P, Rossi A: Pediatric Neuroradiology. New York, Springer, 2005.

Wolpert S, Barnes P: MRI in Pediatric Neuroradiology. St. Louis, Mosby-Year Book, 1992.

Monographs

Edwards-Brown MK, Barnes PD (eds): Pediatric Neuroradiology. Neuroimaging Clin North Am 1999;9(1).

Mukherji SK (ed): Pediatric Head and Neck Imaging. Neuroimaging Clin North Am 2000;10(1).

Index

Note: Page numbers followed by *b*, *f* and *t* indicate boxes, figures and tables, respectively.